Molecular
Biotechnology

Molecular Biotechnology

MD Morris

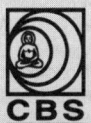

CBS Publishers & Distributors Pvt Ltd

New Delhi • Bengaluru • Chennai • Kochi • Kolkata • Mumbai • Pune
Hyderabad • Nagpur • Patna • Vijayawada

Molecular Biotechnology

ISBN: 978-81-239-2865-4 (Soft Cover)

ISBN: 978-81-239-2915-6 (Hard Cover)

Copyright © Publisher

First Edition: 2016

Published by Satish Kumar Jain and produced by Varun Jain for
CBS Publishers & Distributors Pvt Ltd
4819/XI Prahlad Street, 24 Ansari Road, Daryaganj, New Delhi 110 002, India.
Ph: 23289259, 23266861, 23266867   Website: www.cbspd.com
Fax: 011-23243014   e-mail: delhi@cbspd.com; cbspubs@airtelmail.in.
Corporate Office: 204 FIE, Industrial Area, Patparganj, Delhi 110 092
Ph: 4934 4934   Fax: 4934 4935   e-mail: publishing@cbspd.com; publicity@cbspd.com

Branches

- **Bengaluru:** Seema House 2975, 17th Cross, K.R. Road,
  Banasankari 2nd Stage, Bengaluru 560 070, Karnataka
  Ph: +91-80-26771678/79   Fax: +91-80-26771680   e-mail: bangalore@cbspd.com
- **Chennai:** 7, Subbaraya Street, Shenoy Nagar, Chennai 600 030, Tamil Nadu
  Ph: +91-44-26680620, 26681266   Fax: +91-44-42032115   e-mail: chennai@cbspd.com
- **Kochi:** Ashana House, No. 39/1904, AM Thomas Road, Valanjambalam, Eranakulam 682 018,
  Kochi Kerala
  Ph: +91-484-4059061-65   Fax: +91-484-4059065   e-mail: kochi@cbspd.com
- **Kolkata:** 6/B, Ground Floor, Rameswar Shaw Road, Kolkata-700 014, West Bengal
  Ph: +91-33-22891126, 22891127, 22891128   e-mail: kolkata@cbspd.com
- **Mumbai:** 83-C, Dr E Moses Road, Worli, Mumbai-400018, Maharashtra
  Ph: +91-22-24902340/41   Fax: +91-22-24902342   e-mail: mumbai@cbspd.com
- **Pune:** Bhuruk Prestige, Sr. No. 52/12/2+1+3/2 Narhe, Haveli
  (Near Katraj-Dehu Road Bypass), Pune 411 041, Maharashtra
  Ph: +91-20-64704058, 64704059, 32392277   Fax: +91-20-24300160 e-mail: pune@cbspd.com

Representatives

- **Hyderabad** 0-9885175004 • **Nagpur** 0-9021734563
- **Patna** 0-9334159340 • **Vijayawada** 0-9000660880

Printed at India Binding House, Noida, UP

Preface

Molecular biotechnology is an exciting revolutionary scientific discipline that is based on the ability of a researcher to transfer specific units of genetic information from one organism to another. The objective of recombinant DNA technology is often to produce a useful product or a commercial process.

Genetic engineering provides a means to create, rather than merely isolate highly productive strains. Micro-organisms and eukaryotic cells could be used as 'biological factories' for the production of insulin, interferon, growth hormone, viral antigens and a variety of other proteins. Recombinant DNA technology (molecular cloning) could also be used to facilitate the biological production of large amounts of useful lower molecular weight compounds and macromolecules that occur naturally in minute quantities. This technology facilitates the development of radically new medical therapies and diagnostic systems. Thus, the union of recombinant DNA technology with biotechnology creates a vibrant, highly competitive field of study that has been called 'Molecular Biotechnology'. Molecular biotechnology ought to contribute unprecedented benefits to humanity.

In this reference textbook each chapter covers an important aspect with an accurate and up-to-date account of each topic. Chapter 1 gives a review on molecular biotechnology. Molecular cloning (recombinant DNA technology) the basis of modern biotechnology is dealt in chapter 2. Biotechnology for most part uses micro-organisms on a large scale for the production of commercially important products. Chapter 3 focuses on research procedures in molecular biotechnology, these techniques include the chemical synthesis of DNA, DNA sequences, polymerase chain reaction, and production of monoclonal antibodies. Chapter 4 is devoted to regulation of gene expression in prokaryotes which includes the processes that cells and viruses use to turn the information in genes into gene products. Gene regulation is also essential for viruses, prokaryotes and eukaryotes as it increases the versatility and adaptability of an organism by allowing the cell to express protein when needed. Chapter 5 deals with heterologous proteins in production of eukaryotic cells and also discusses heterologous production of proteins, yeast and cultured insect cell expression systems, etc. Chapter 6 concentrates on changing genes: site-directed mutagenesis and protein engineering. Various directed and oligonucleotide mutagenesis procedures along with random mutagenesis are briefly discussed. Chapter 7 provides information on microbial synthesis of commercial and allied products. The chapter also describes number of proteins that have potential as pharmaceutical agents as the major use of recombinant DNA technology today is production of proteins. Chapter 8 is devoted to molecular diagnostics and antibodies. Molecular diagnostics has been extremely successful in the area of infectious diseases where viral and bacterial genotyping has made rapid progress. Traditionally, vaccines are either inactivated or attenuated infection agents that are injected into an antibody producing organism to produce immunity. Monoclonal antibodies combined with recombinant DNA technology also can be used to create therapeutic agents for treating animal or human diseases. Considering this chapter 9 focuses on vaccines and therapeutic agents. Chapter 10 deals with bioremediation and microbial biomass utilisation. Bioremediation is the term applied to any process that uses micro-organisms, fungi, green plants or their enzyme to return the natural environment altered by contaminants to its original conditions. On the other hand biomass is a renewable energy source, is a biological material derived from living or recently living organisms, such as wood, waste, alcohol fuels, etc. Chapter 11 provides information on plant growth-promoting bacteria and nitrogen fixation. Nitrogenase, the nitrogen-fixing enzyme, hydrogen metabolism, modulation its genetic engineering and siderophores are also discussed in detail. Chapter 12 describes microbial insecticides and pesticides which has led to the large scale production of *Bacillus thruingiensis*, a promising fungi and various other compounds. Chapter 13 provides information on production of proteins from recombinant micro-organisms. The chapter discusses microbial growth kinetics, batch and continuous fermentation, large scale fermentation systems and downstream processing. Genetic engineering can be used to introduce specific traits into plants. Genes that might make plant resistant to insect predation, infection by viruses, and herbicides have been introduced into different plants and have shown promising results. Keeping this in mind chapter 14 is devoted to genetic engineering of plants. Chapter 15 deals with transgenic animals which have been genetically transformed by splicing and inserting foreign animal or human genes into their chromosomes. Chapter 16 focuses on isolation of human genes. The main objective of this chapter is isolation and characterisation of the disease-causing gene and then devise remedial therapies. Chapter 17 concentrates on human somatic cell gene therapy. Various aspects like *ex vivo*, *in vivo* gene therapy and antisense therapy are discussed in detail. Chapter 18 provides information on regulating the use of biotechnology. Chapter 19 is devoted to biotechnology patents and intellectual property rights. For a patent to be granted, an invention must be novel and useful.

Glossary and index have been provided at the end for quick reference. This reference textbook of *Molecular Biotechnology* is essential reading for all students, teachers, professionals, researchers and industrialists involved with biochemical engineering, microbiology, biotechnology, life sciences, environmental science, and chemical engineering. The reference textbook also caters to the requirement of the syllabus prescribed by various Indian universities for undergraduate and postgraduate students pursuing these courses. Constructive suggestions are always welcome from users of this book.

MD Morris

Contents at a Glance

Contents

Chapter 1

Molecular Biotechnology: A Review

INTRODUCTION

The term biotechnology is derived from a fusion of biology and technology. True to its name, it concerns with the exploitation of biological agents or their components for generating useful products/services. By its nature, the area covered under biotechnology is very vast and techniques involved are highly divergent; this has often made a precise definition of the subject rather difficult. Some standard definitions of biotechnology are reproduced below with a view to orient the readers to the nature and scope of the discipline. Biotechnology is 'the integrated use of biochemistry, microbiology and engineering sciences in order to achieve technological application of the capabilities of micro-organisms, cultured tissues/ cells and parts thereof'.

Biotechnology may be defined as 'the use of living organisms in systems or processes for the manufacture of useful products; it may involve algae, bacteria, fungi, yeast, cells of higher plants and animals or subsystems of any of these or isolated components from living matter'.

Biotechnology operates at the molecular levels of life, where the seemingly solid boundaries between species disappear. Down among those molecules there lies little difference between a man and a bacterium. What biotechnology does is to choreograph the complex dances among the molecules that ultimately make every living thing what it is.

Biotechnology has rapidly emerged as an area of activity having a marked realised as well as potential impact on virtually all domains of human welfare, ranging from food processing, protecting the environment, to human health. As a result, it now plays a very important role in employment, production and productivity, trade, economics and economy, human health, and the quality of human life throughout the world. This is clearly reflected in the emergence of numerous biotechnology companies throughout the world, including India, and the movement of noted scientists.

MOLECULAR BIOTECHNOLOGY

Molecular biotechnology is an exciting revolutionary scientific discipline that is based on the ability of a researcher to transfer specific units of genetic information from one organism to another. The objective of recombinant DNA technology is often to produce a useful product or a commercial process. In early 1970, traditional biotechnology was not well known as a scientific discipline. Research in this area was carried out in chemical engineering departments. Biotechnology involves all works carried out with the aid of living things. More formally, biotechnology may be defined as 'the application of scientific and engineering principles to the processing of material by biological agents to provide goods and services'.

In 1961, Swedish microbiologist Carl Gordon Heden redefined biotechnology as 'the industrial production of goods and services by processing using biological organisms, and it is firmly ground on expertise in microbiology, biochemistry and chemical engineering'. However the nature of biotechnology was changed forever by the development of recombinant DNA technology. With these techniques, the optimisation of any biotechnological process was achieved more directly.

Genetic engineering provided a means to create, rather than merely isolate highly productive strains. Micro-organisms and eukaryotic cells could be used as 'biological factories' for the production of insulin, interferon, growth hormone, viral antigens and a variety of other proteins. Recombinant DNA technology could also be used to facilitate the biological production of large amounts of useful lower molecular weight compounds and macromolecules that occur naturally in minute quantities. This, technology facilitated the development of radically new medical therapies and diagnostic systems. Thus, the union of recombinant DNA technology with biotechnology created a vibrant, highly competitive field of study that has been called 'Molecular Biotechnology'. Molecular biotechnology ought to contribute unprecedented benefits to humanity.

1. It should provide opportunities to accurately diagnose and prevent or cure a wide range of infectious and genetic diseases.
2. Significant increase in crop yield may be obtained by generating disease-, pathogen- or herbicide-resistant varieties.
3. Micro-organisms that will produce chemicals, antibiotics, polymers, amino acids, enzymes, etc. can be developed.
4. Livestock and other animals that have enhanced genetically determined attributes can be developed. Molecular biotechnology with much fuss and fanfare has become a comprehensive scientific venture, both commercially and academically, in a remarkably short time.
5. A number of new scientific and business publications are devoted to molecular biotechnology. Both graduate and undergraduate programmes and courses have been created at many universities throughout the world.

Although it is exciting and important to emphasise the positive aspects of new advances, there are also social concerns and consequences that must be addressed. Because molecular biotechnology is so broadly based, its potential impact on society must be considered.

Many issues have been considered and discussed extensively by government commissions, and debated by individuals in popular and academic publications. There has been an active and extensive participation by both scientists and the general public in deciding how molecular biotechnology should proceed, although some controversies still remain.

Finally, molecular biotechnology is the third scientific revolution after the industrial and computer revolution, which is going to change the lives and future of humankind on this earth. The ability to manipulate genetic material to achieve specified outcome in living organisms promises major changes in many aspects of modern life.

Biomolecule is any organic molecule that is produced by a living organism, including large polymeric molecules such as proteins, polysaccharides, and nucleic acids as well as small molecules such as primary metabolites, secondary metabolites, and natural products. A more general name for this class of molecules is a biogenic substance. As organic molecules, biomolecules consist primarily of carbon and hydrogen, nitrogen, and oxygen, and, to a smaller extent, phosphorus and sulphur. Other elements sometimes are incorporated but are much less common.

Monoclonal Antibodies

Monoclonal antibodies (mAb or moAb) are monospecific antibodies that are the same because they are made by identical immune cells that are all clones of a unique parent cell. Given almost any substance, it is possible to create monoclonal antibodies that specifically bind to that substance; they can then serve to detect or purify that substance. This has become an important tool in biochemistry, molecular biology and medicine. When used as medications, the nonproprietary drug name ends in -*mab*. The idea of a 'magic bullet' was first proposed by Paul Ehrlich, who, at the beginning of the 20th century, postulated that, if a compound could be made that selectively targeted a disease-causing organism, then a toxin for that organism could be delivered along with the agent of selectivity.

In the 1970s, the B-cell cancer multiple myeloma was known, and it was understood that these cancerous B-cells all produce a single type of antibody (a paraprotein). This was used to study the structure of antibodies, but it was not yet possible to produce identical antibodies specific to a given antigen. Production of monoclonal antibodies involving human–mouse hybrid cells was described by Jerrold Schwaber and remains widely cited among those using human-derived hybridomas, but claims to priority have been controversial.

Bioprocess Technology

Like other applications of biotechnology, modern bioprocess technology is an extension of ancient techniques for developing useful products by taking advantage of natural biological activities. When our early ancestors made alcoholic beverages, they used a bioprocess: the combination of yeast cells and nutrients (cereal grains) formed a fermentation system in which the organisms consumed the nutrients for their own growth and produced by-products (alcohol and carbon dioxide gas) that helped to make the beverage. Although more sophisticated, today's bioprocess technology is based on the same principle: combining living matter (whole organisms or enzymes) with nutrients under the conditions necessary to make the desired end product.

Bioprocesses have become widely used in several fields of commercial biotechnology, such as production of enzymes (used, for example, in food processing and waste management) and antibiotics. As techniques and instrumentation are refined, bioprocesses may have applications in other areas where chemical processes are now used.

Because bioprocesses use living material, they offer several advantages over conventional chemical methods of production: they usually require lower temperature, pressure, and pH (the measure of acidity); they can use renewable resources as raw materials; and greater quantities can be produced with less energy consumption.

In most bioprocesses, enzymes are used to catalyse the biochemical reactions of whole micro-organisms or their cellular components. The biological catalyst causes the reactions to occur, but is not itself changed. After a series of such reactions (which take place in large vessels called fermenters or fermentation tanks), the initial raw materials are chemically changed to form the desired end product. Although it sounds quite simple, this procedure presents two major challenges.

Fermentation and mammalian cell culture

Companies commercially manufacture a wide variety of biotechnology products through large-scale fermentation and mammalian cell culture, two types of bioprocessing technologies that reply on the cellular enzymes that synthesise chemical substances. Because of the scale of the production systems, these technologies represent triumphs of both chemical engineering and molecular biology.

The oldest and most familiar bioprocessing technology is microbial fermentation. Originally, the microbial fermentation products people used were derived from the series of enzyme-catalysed reactions that microbes use to break down glucose. In the process of metabolising glucose to acquire energy, microbes synthesise useful by-products: carbon dioxide for leavening bread, ethanol for brewing wine and beer, lactic acid for making yogurt, and acetic acid (vinegar) for pickling foods (Fig. 1.1).

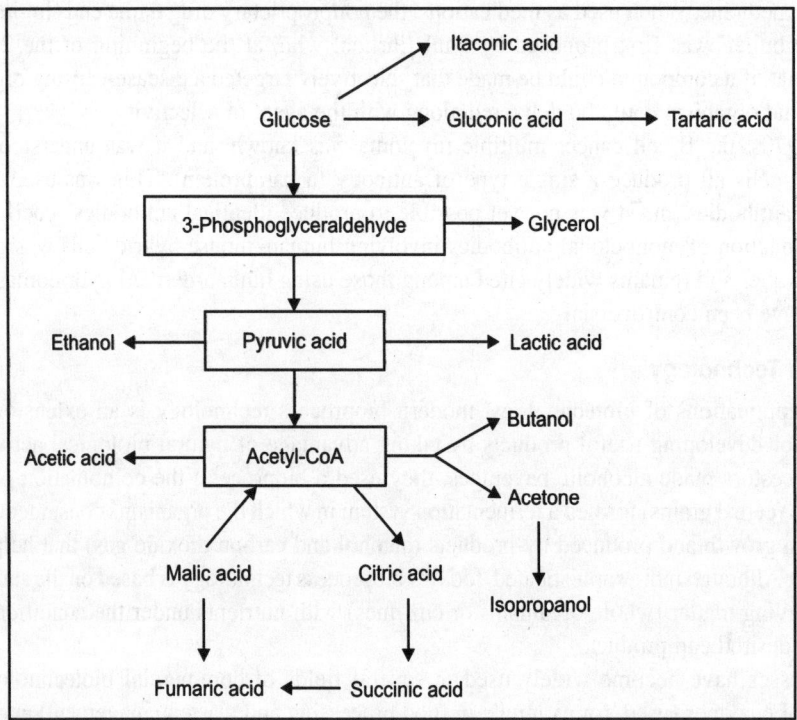

Fig. 1.1. Useful metabolic products (in boldface type) of glucose breakdown provided by various micro-organisms.

Microbial biodegradation

Interest in the microbial biodegradation of pollutants has intensified in recent years as humanity strives to find sustainable ways to cleanup contaminated environments. These bioremediation and biotransformation methods endeavour to harness the astonishing, naturally occurring, ability of microbial xenobiotic metabolism to degrade, transform or accumulate a huge range of compounds including hydrocarbons (e.g. oil), polychlorinated biphenyls (PCBs), polyaromatic hydrocarbons (PAHs), heterocyclic compounds (such as pyridine or quinoline), pharmaceutical substances, radionuclides and metals.

Major methodological breakthroughs in recent years have enabled detailed genomic, metagenomic, proteomic, bioinformatic and other high-throughput analyses of environmentally relevant micro-organisms providing unprecedented insights into key biodegradative pathways and the ability of organisms to adapt to changing environmental conditions.

Biological processes play a major role in the removal of contaminants and they take advantage of the astonishing catabolic versatility of micro-organisms to degrade/convert such compounds.

Cell Culture

Cell culture is the complex process by which cells are grown under controlled conditions. In practice, the term 'cell culture' has come to refer to the culturing of cells derived from multicellular eukaryotes, especially animal cells. The historical development and methods of cell culture are closely interrelated to those of tissue culture and organ culture.

Culture of non-mammalian cells

Plant cell culture methods

Plant cell cultures are typically grown as cell suspension cultures in liquid medium or as callus cultures on solid medium. The culturing of undifferentiated plant cells and calli requires the proper balance of the plant growth hormones auxin and cytokinin.

Animal cell culture

Plant cell culture is not the only type of cell culture being applied to agriculture. Using insect cell culture to grow viruses that infect insects may enable agricultural scientists to broaden the application of species-specific viruses in insect pest control. Mammalian cell culture is also being used in livestock breeding. Large number of brovine zygotes from genetically superior bulls and cows can be produced and cultured before being implanted into surrogate cows.

Bacterial/Yeast culture methods

For bacteria and yeast, small quantities of cells are usually grown on a solid support that contains nutrients embedded in it, usually a gel such as agar, while large-scale cultures are grown with the cells suspended in a nutrient broth.

Viral culture methods

The culture of viruses requires the culture of cells of mammalian, plant, fungal or bacterial origin as hosts for the growth and replication of the virus. Whole wild type viruses, recombinant viruses or viral products may be generated in cell types other than their natural hosts under the right conditions. Depending on the species of the virus, infection and viral replication may result in host cell lysis and formation of a viral plaque.

Biosensor

A biosensor is a device for the detection of an enalyte that combines a biological component with a physicochemical detector component. A common example of a commercial biosensor is the blood glucose biosensor, which uses the enzyme glucose oxidase to break blood glucose down. In doing so it first oxidises glucose and uses two electrons to reduce the FAD (a component of the enzyme) to $FADH_2$. This in turn is oxidised by the electrode (accepting two electrons from the electrode) in a number of steps. The resulting current is a measure of the concentration of glucose. In this case, the electrode is the transducer and the enzyme is the biologically active component.

Protein Engineering

Protein engineering is the process of developing useful or valuable proteins. It is a young discipline, with much research taking place into the understanding of protein folding and recognition for protein design principles.

There are two general strategies for protein engineering, rational design and directed evolution. These techniques are not mutually exclusive; researchers will often apply both. In the future, more detailed knowledge of protein structure and function, as well as advancements in high-throughput technology, may greatly expand the capabilities of protein engineering. Eventually, even unnatural amino acids may be incorporated thanks to a new method that allows the inclusion of novel amino acids in the genetic code.

Enzyme engineering

Enzyme engineering (or enzyme technology) is the application of modifying an enzyme's structure (and thus its function) or modifying the catalytic activity of isolated enzymes to produce new metabolites, to allow new (catalysed) pathways for reactions to occur, or to convert from some certain compounds into others (biotransformation). These products will be useful as chemicals, pharmaceuticals, fuel, food or agricultural additives. An enzyme reactor consists of a vessel containing a reactional medium that is used to perform a desired conversion by enzymatic means. Enzymes used in this process are free in the solution.

Abzyme engineering

Although most of the protein engineering work has been directed at changing the catalytic properties of existing enzymes, scientists have also invented a way to synthesise novel catalysts. Some researchers are synthesising enzymes essentially from scratch, while others are creating antibodies with catalytic abilities, or abzymes. Antibodies resemble enzymes because both are proteins that bind to specific molecules. However, the similarity ends there. Antibodies bind for the sake of binding; enzymes bind to make reactions happen.

Cloning and Technology

Cloning is creating an exact copy of a living organism from a single cell, using a genderless organism where the organism inherits the genetical characteristics from the parent who donated the cell. Scientist have been studying and experimenting the concept of cloning for the last fifty years. Cloning in regards to technology has its advantages and disadvantages.

Some of these advantages of cloning with the help of technology help to increase of population, farm better livestock for human, child cloned for unfertile parents, cloning lost family members, and decrease in developing a serious disease. The disadvantages of cloning is decrease in genetic diversity, technology is new and very unstable, and maybe in human.

Antisense Technology

Antisense refers to short DNA or RNA sequences, termed oligonucleotides, which are designed to be complementary to a specific gene sequence. The goal is to alter specific gene expression resulting from the binding of the antisense oligonucleotide to a unique gene sequence.

In principle, antisense technology is supposed to prevent protein production from a targeted gene. The exact mechanism by which this occurs remains uncertain. Proposed mechanisms include triplex formation, blocking RNA splicing, preventing transport of the mRNA antisense complex into the cytoplasm, increasing RNA degradation, or blocking the initiation of translation. Initially, cellular nucleases dramatically reduce the effectiveness of antisense oligonucleotides by rapidly degrading these molecules after administration.

Metabolic engineering

Metabolic engineering is the practice of optimising genetic and regulatory processes within cells to increase the cells' production of a certain substance. Metabolic engineers commonly work to reduce cellular energy use (i.e. the energetic cost of cell reproduction or proliferation) and to reduce waste production. Producing beer, wine, cheese, pharmaceuticals, and other biotechnology products often involves metabolic engineering.

Microarray Technology

Microarray technology is transforming laboratory research because it allows scientists to analyse tens of thousands of samples simultaneously. For example, thousands of different DNA, RNA, or protein molecules are placed on glass slides in a grid-like array to create DNA chips, RNA chips, and protein chips. Recent developments in microarray technology utilise customised beads in place of glass slides, but the principle remains the same.

DNA microarray

A DNA microarray is a multiplex technology used in molecular biology and in medicine. It consists of an arrayed series of thousands of microscopic spots of DNA oligonucleotides, called features, each containing picomoles (10^{-12} moles) of a specific DNA sequence, known as probes (or reporters). This can be a short section of a gene or other DNA element that are used to hybridise a cDNA or cRNA sample (called target) under high-stringency conditions.

Protein microarray

A protein microarray, sometimes referred to as a protein binding microarray, provides a multiplex approach to identify protein–protein interactions, to identify the substrates of protein kinases, to identify transcription factor protein-activation, or to identify the targets of biologically active small molecules. The array is a piece of glass on which different molecules of protein or specific DNA binding sequences (as capture probes for the proteins) have been affixed at separate locations in an ordered manner thus forming a microscopic array. The most common protein microarray is the antibody microarray, where antibodies are spotted onto the protein chip and are used as capture molecules to detect proteins from cell lysate solutions.

Other microarrays

Microarray technology was developed originally for genetic analysis, but the fundamental principle underlying this technology has inspired researchers to create many types of microarrays to answer scientific questions and discover new products.

Tissue microarrays, which allow the analysis of thousands of tissue samples on a single glass slide, are being used to detect protein profiles in healthy and diseased tissues and to validate potential drug targets. Brain tissue samples arrayed on slides with electrodes allow researchers to measure the electrical activity of nerve cells exposed to certain drugs.

Bioinformatics

Bioinformatics is the application of statistics and computer science to the field of molecular biology. Bioinformatics now entails the creation and advancement of databases, algorithms, computational and statistical techniques and theory to solve formal and practical problems arising from the management and analysis of biological data. Common activities in bioinformatics include mapping and analysing DNA and protein sequences, aligning different DNA and protein sequences to compare them and creating and viewing 3-D models of protein structures. The primary goal of bioinformatics is to increase the understanding of biological processes. What sets it apart from other approaches, however, is its focus on developing and applying computationally intensive techniques (e.g. pattern recognition, data mining, machine learning algorithms, and visualisation) to achieve this goal.

Nanobiotechnology

Nanobiotechnology is the branch of nanotechnology with biological and biochemical applications or uses. Nanobiotechnology often studies existing elements of nature in order to fabricate new devices. The term bionanotechnology is often used interchangeably with nanobiotechnology, though a distinction is sometimes drawn between the two. If the two are distinguished, nanobiotechnology usually refers to the use of nanotechnology to further the goals of biotechnology, while bionanotechnology might refer to any overlap between biology and nanotechnology, including the use of biomolecules as part of or as an inspiration for nanotechnological devices. Nanobiotechnology is that branch of one, which deals with the study and application of biological and biochemical activities from elements of nature to fabricate new devices like biosensors.

APPLICATIONS OF BIOTECHNOLOGY

Most of the commercial applications of biotechnology arein human health, agriculture and environmental management are shown in Fig. 1.2.

Medical Biotechnology

Biotechnology has already provided us with quicker and more accurate diagnostic tests, therapeutic compounds with fewer side effects, and safer vaccines.

Diagnostics

A physician's success in managing or curing a disease depends on diagnosing it accurately and early. Physicians can now detect many diseases and medical conditions more quickly and with greater accuracy because of the sensitivity of new diagnostic tools and techniques developed through biotechnology, such as MAbs, biosensors, DNA probes, DNA microarrays, restriction fragment length polymorphisms, and the polymerase chain reaction (PCR).

Certain cancers are now diagnosed by simply taking a blood sample, thus eliminating the need for invasive and costly surgery. In some cases, the molecule that is uses as the basis for diagnosis is secreted by precancerous cells, permitting intervention before cells turn cancerous and metastasize. Molecular footprints that are secreted by cells as the disease progresses from one stage to the next are known as biomarkers.

In certain cases, biotechnology has also decreased the cost of disease diagnosis. A new blood test, developed through biotechnology, measures the amount of low-density lipoprotein, or 'bad' cholesterol, in blood. Conventional methods require separate and expensive tests for total cholesterol, triglycerides, and high density lipoprotein cholesterol. Also, a patient must fast for 12 hours before the test. The new biotechnological test measures low-density lipoprotein in one test, and fasting is not necessary. We now use biotechnology-based tests to diagnose certain cancers, such as prostate and ovarian cancers, by taking a blood sample, eliminating the need for invasive and costly surgery.

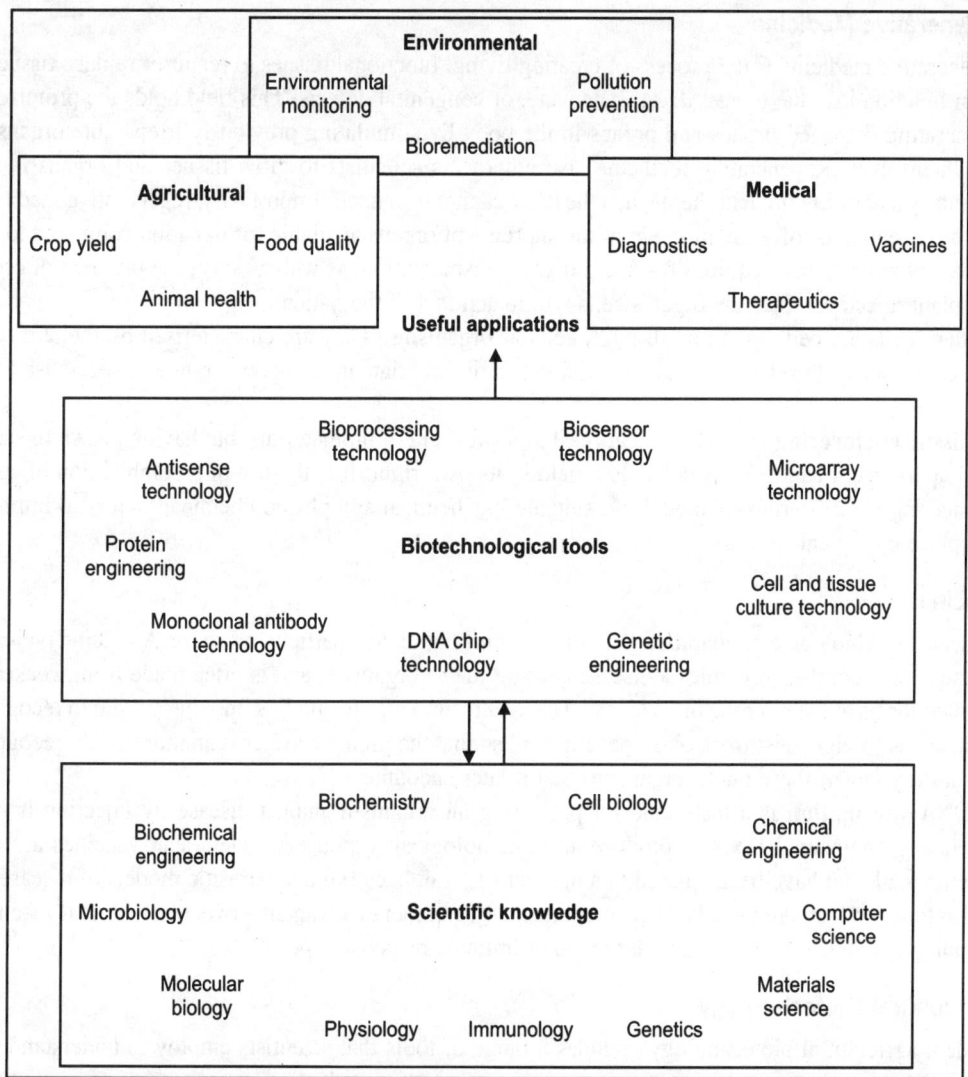

Fig. 1.2. Synthesis of scientific and technical knowledge from many academic disciplines has produced a set of enabling technologies—the biotechnologies. Any one technology will be applied to a number of industries to produce an even broader array of products.

Biotechnology-based diagnostics are also altering health care provision. Many of the new tests are portable, so physicians carry out tests and interpret results right at the patient's bedside. These point-of-care tests allow doctors to make decisions immediately rather than waiting hours or days for test results to come from a centralised hospital laboratory.

Therapeutics

Biotechnology will provide improved versions of today's therapeutic regimens, as well as treatments that would not be possible without these new techniques.

Regenerative Medicine

Regenerative medicine is the process of creating living, functional tissues to repair or replace tissue or organ function lost due to age, disease, damage, or congenital defects. This field holds the promise of regenerating damaged tissues and organs in the body by stimulating previously irreparable organs to heal themselves. Regenerative medicine also empowers scientists to grow tissues and organs in the laboratory and safely implant them when the body cannot heal itself. Importantly, regenerative medicine has the potential to solve the problem of the shortage of organs available for donation compared to the number of patients that require life-saving organ transplantation, as well as solve the problem of organ transplant rejection, since the organ's cells will match that of the patient.

Stem cells are cells found in all multi cellular organisms. They are characterised by the ability to renew themselves through mitotic cell division and differentiate into a diverse range of specialised cell types.

Tissue engineering was once categorised as a sub-field of biomaterials, but having grown in scope and importance it can be considered as a field in its own right. It is the use of a combination of cells, engineering and materials methods, and suitable biochemical and physio-chemical factors to improve or replace biological functions.

Vaccine

A vaccine is a biological preparation that improves immunity to a particular disease. A vaccine typically contains an agent that resembles a disease-causing micro-organism, and is often made from weakened or killed forms of the microbe or its toxins. The agent stimulates the body's immune system to recognise the agent as foreign, destroy it, and 'recognise' it, so that the immune system can more easily recognise and destroy any of these micro-organisms that it later encounters.

DNA vaccination is a technique for protecting an organism against disease by injecting it with genetically engineered DNA to produce an immunological response. Nucleic acid vaccines are still experimental, and have been applied to a number of viral, bacterial and parasitic models of disease, as well as to several tumour models. DNA vaccines have a number of advantages over conventional vaccines, including the ability to induce a wider range of immune response types.

Agricultural Biotechnology

Modern agricultural biotechnology includes a range of tools that scientists employ to understand and manipulate the genetic make-up of organisms for use in the production or processing of agricultural products. Some applications of biotechnology, such as fermentation and brewing, have been used for millennia. Other applications are newer but also well established. For example, micro-organisms have been used for decades as living factories for the production of life-saving antibiotics including penicillin, from the fungus Penicillium, and streptomycin from the bacterium Streptomyces. Modern detergents rely on enzymes produced via biotechnology, hard cheese production largely relies on rennet produced by biotech yeast and human insulin for diabetics is now produced using biotechnology.

Animal agriculture

Animal agriculture is an integral part of food-producing systems, with foods of animal origin representing about one-sixth of human food energy and one-third of the human food protein on a global basis. Animals convert forages, crop residues, and food and fibre processing by-products to high quality human food; provide draught power for about half the world's crop production; and provide manure to help maintain soil fertility. Animal production makes important contributions to agricultural economies throughout the world and to food security in developing countries.

Food processing

Food processing is the set of methods and techniques used to transform raw ingredients into food or to transform food into other forms for consumption by humans or animals either in the home or by the food processing industry. Food processing typically takes clean, harvested crops or butchered animal products and uses these to produce attractive, marketable and often long shelf-life food products. Similar processes are used to produce animal feed.

Environmental Biotechnology

Environmental biotechnology is when biotechnology is applied to and used to study the natural environment. Environmental biotechnology could also imply that one try to harness biological process for commercial uses and exploitation.

The International Society for Environmental Biotechnology defines environmental biotechnology as 'the development, use and regulation of biological systems for remediation of contaminated environments (land, air, water), and for environment-friendly processes (green manufacturing technologies and sustainable development)'.

Bioremediation

Today, the health of the environment seems to be forefront all over the globe. Everywhere people are talking about critical environmental conditions, and how something needs to be done so future generations can have a part in the world as it was before it was polluted. This has led governments, groups, and organisations to step up to try to at least slow down the increasingly degraded conditions of the planet. There are many possible solutions to this problem, but one particular idea stands out. That concept is bioremediation.

Bioremediation can be defined as the use of organisms to break-down harmful environmental contaminants, to restore the environment to a healthier state. Bioremediation can utilise fungi, which is called mycoremediation, plants, which is called phytoremediation, or bacteria, which is called bacterial bioremediation.

Mycoremediation is the one of the more modern methods of bioremediation. It is used to remove chemicals, such as diesel, from soil. This process uses fungi to decompose these substances. This is done by certain enzymes and acids that the fungi secrete. These enzymes and acids break down lignin and cellulose, the main components of plant fibres.

Biodegradable and ecofriendly products

Physical and chemical methods of pollution control were always in the forefront because they were easy to understand, easy to control and were reproducible. Biodegradation, the real mechanism of nature of balancing the material, was always found to be incompletely understood, unpredictable and uncontrollable if we have to adapt it in the form of biological treatment methods. A better option then is to modify our materials, processes and products in such a way that we can rely upon the biodegradation in nature and recalcitrance, bioaccumulation problems are overcome.

Biodegradation mechanisms which occur in the soil, aquatic environment though slow are important for us as they do not involve any cost of treatment when it occurs naturally, and are safer and bring about complete degradation and not mere conversion. Hence incorporating biodegradability or aiming for biodegradability is an obvious approach while carrying out production of different items. The agricultural products, food products, commodities hereafter will carry a label of ecofriendly in most of the countries.

Environmental monitoring

Environmental monitoring describes the processes and activities that need to take place to characterise and monitor the quality of the environment. Environmental monitoring is used in the preparation of environmental impact assessments, as well as in many circumstances in which human activities carry a risk of harmful effects on the natural environment.

Chapter 2

Recombinant DNA Technology

INTRODUCTION

Deoxyribonucleic acid (DNA) is a nucleic acid that contains the genetic instructions used in the development and functioning of all known living organisms and some viruses. The main role of DNA molecules is the long-term storage of information. DNA is often compared to a set of blueprints, like a recipe or a code, since it contains the instructions needed to construct other components of cells, such as proteins and RNA molecules. The DNA segments that carry this genetic information are called genes, but other DNA sequences have structural purposes, or are involved in regulating the use of this genetic information. Chemically, DNA consists of two long polymers of simple units called nucleotides, with backbones made of sugars and phosphate groups joined by ester bonds. These two strands run in opposite directions to each other and are therefore anti-parallel. Attached to each sugar is one of four types of molecules called bases. It is the sequence of these four bases along the backbone that encodes information. This information is read using the genetic code, which specifies the sequence of the amino acids within proteins. The code is read by copying stretches of DNA into the related nucleic acid RNA, in a process called transcription.

Within cells, DNA is organised into long structures called chromosomes. These chromosomes are duplicated before cells divide, in a process called DNA replication. Eukaryotic organisms (animals, plants, fungi, and protists) store most of their DNA inside the cell nucleus and some of their DNA in organelles, such as mitochondria or chloroplasts. In contrast, prokaryotes (bacteria and archaea) store their DNA only in the cytoplasm. Within the chromosomes, chromatin proteins such as histones compact and organise DNA. These compact structures guide the interactions between DNA and other proteins, helping control which parts of the DNA are transcribed.

A few DNA sequences in prokaryotes and eukaryotes, and more in plasmids and viruses, blur the distinction between sense and antisense strands by having overlapping genes. In these cases, some DNA sequences do double duty, encoding one protein when read along one strand, and a second protein when read in the opposite direction along the other strand. In bacteria, this overlap may be involved in the regulation of gene transcription, while in viruses, overlapping genes increase the amount of information that can be encoded within the small viral genome.

DNA can be twisted like a rope in a process called DNA supercoiling. With DNA in its 'relaxed' state, a strand usually circles the axis of the double helix once every 10.4 base pairs, but if the DNA is twisted the strands become more tightly or more loosely wound. If the DNA is twisted in the direction of the helix, this is positive supercoiling, and the bases are held more tightly together. If they are twisted in the opposite direction, this is negative supercoiling, and the bases come apart more easily. In nature, most DNA has slight negative supercoiling that is introduced by enzymes called topoisomerases. These enzymes are also needed to relieve the twisting stresses introduced into DNA strands during processes such as transcription and DNA replication.

RECOMBINANT DNA TECHNOLOGY

A recombinant DNA molecule is produced by joining together two or more DNA segments usually originating from different organisms. More specifically, a recombinant DNA molecule is a vector (e.g. a plasmid, phage or virus) into which the desired DNA fragment has been inserted to enable its cloning in an appropriate host. This is achieved by using specific enzymes for cutting the DNA (restriction enzymes) into suitable fragments and then for joining together the appropriate fragments (ligation). In this manner, a recombinant DNA molecule may be produced which contains a gene from one organism joined to regulatory sequences from another organism; such a gene is called chimaeric gene. Clearly, the capability to produce recombinant DNA molecules has given man the power and opportunity to create novel gene combinations to suit specific needs.

Recombinant DNA molecules are produced with one of the following three objectives: (i) to obtain a large number of copies of specific DNA fragments, (ii) to recover large quantities of the protein produced by the concerned gene, and (iii) to integrate the gene in question into the chromosome of a target organism where it expresses itself. Even for the later two objectives, it is essential to first obtain a large number of copies of the concerned genes. To achieve this, the DNA segments are integrated into a self-replicating DNA molecule called vector; most commonly used vectors are either bacterial plasmids or DNA viruses. All these steps concerned with piecing together DNA segments of diverse origin and placing them into a suitable vector together constitute recombinant DNA technology.

The vectors containing DNA segments to be cloned, called DNA inserts (chimaeric vectors) are then introduced into a suitable organism, usually a bacterium; this organism is called host, while the process is called transformation. The transformed host cells are selected and cloned. The vector present in such clones would replicate either in synchrony with or independent of the host cell; the gene present in the vector may or may not express itself by directing the synthesis of concerned polypeptide. The step concerned with transformation of a suitable host with a chimaeric vector, and cloning of the transformant cells is called DNA cloning or gene cloning. However, often DNA or gene cloning is taken to include both the development of chimaeric vectors as well as their cloning in a suitable host.

A clone consists of asexual progeny of a single individual or cell, while the process/technique of producing a clone is called cloning. As a result, all the individuals of a clone have the same genotype which is also identical with that of the individual from which the clone was derived. Therefore, the genomes present in members of a single clone are also identical; this applies to the recombinant DNA as well. Therefore, gene or DNA cloning produces large number of copies of the gene/DNA being cloned.

Similarly, often the term recombinant DNA technology is used as a synonym for DNA or gene cloning used in the broader sense. A rather popular term for these activities is genetic engineering.

STRUCTURE AND FUNCTION OF DNA

DNA, the information molecule of all living cells, is made up of nucleotide chains wound in a helix. It's structure and function are intertwined, and understanding these aspects of DNA helps biology students understand the basics of genetics. The structure of DNA – nucleotides, sugars and phosphates: DNA, along with RNA, is a nucleic acid, a macromolecule made up of a strand of nucleotides. Nucleotide molecules are made of a nucleotide base, a five-carbon sugar and phosphate groups. DNA, deoxyribonucleic acid, is made of two long strands of nucleotide bases with a sugar and phosphate backbone. The sugar-phosphate backbones are on the outside and the nucleotide bases are attached in the middle by hydrogen bonds and the strands are coiled around each other to create a helical ladder-like form. This double helix is then coiled and folded many times to fit inside a chromosome, which resides in the nucleus of the cell.

Nucleotide bases adenine, thymine, guanine and cytosine form base pairs: There are four nucleotide bases in DNA. Adenine, thymine, guanine, and cytosine. They are often referred to by their first letters, A, T, G and C. These nucleotides pair up in the middle of DNA, but they can only match up with specific other bases, because they are two different types of nucleotide bases. Adenine and Guanine are both purines, while thymine and cytosine are pyrimidines. When joining together, adenine and thymine always pair up together and guanine and cytosine always make a pair. The specific order of the nucleotide bases, read from the 5′ end to the 3′ end, makes up the genetic code, which directs the production of all of the components of a cell.

Adenine is a nucleobase (a purine derivative) with a variety of roles in biochemistry including cellular respiration, in the form of both the energy-rich adenosine triphosphate (ATP) and the cofactors nicotinamide adenine dinucleotide (NAD) and flavin adenine dinucleotide (FAD), and protein synthesis, as a chemical component of DNA and RNA. The shape of adenine is complementary to either thymine in DNA or uracil in RNA. Adenine forms several tautomers, compounds that can be rapidly interconverted and are often considered equivalent.

Adenine

Purine metabolism involves the formation of adenine and guanine. Both adenine and guanine are derived from the nucleotide inosine monophosphate (IMP), which is synthesised on a pre-existing ribosome through a complex pathway using atoms from the amino acids glycine, glutamine, and aspartic acid, as well as fused with the enzyme tetrahydrofolate. In *Saccharomyces cerevisiae* (yeast), the adenine pathway converts P-ribosyl-PP into adenine through a seven-step process.

Adenine is one of the two purine nucleobases (the other being guanine) used in forming nucleotides of the nucleic acids. In DNA, adenine binds to thymine via two hydrogen bonds to assist in stabilising the nucleic acid structures. In RNA, which is used for protein synthesis, adenine binds to uracil.

Adenine forms adenosine, a nucleoside, when attached to ribose, and deoxyadenosine when attached to deoxyribose. It forms adenosine triphosphate (ATP), a nucleotide, when three phosphate groups are added to adenosine. Adenosine triphosphate is used in cellular metabolism as one of the basic methods of transferring chemical energy between chemical reactions.

Guanine is one of the four main nucleobases found in the nucleic acids DNA and RNA, the others being adenine, cytosine, and thymine. In DNA, guanine is paired with cytosine. With the formula $C_5H_5N_5O$, guanine is a derivative of purine, consisting of a fused pyrimidine-imidazole ring system with conjugated double bonds. Being unsaturated, the bicyclic molecule is planar. The guanine nucleoside is called guanosine.

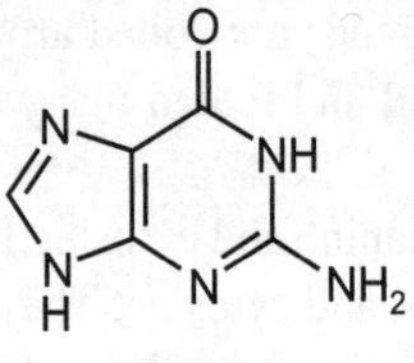

Guanine

Guanine, along with adenine and cytosine, is present in both DNA and RNA, whereas thymine is usually seen only in DNA, and uracil only in RNA. Guanine has two tautomeric forms, the major keto form and rare enol form. It binds to cytosine through three hydrogen bonds. In cytosine, the amino group acts as the hydrogen donor and the C-2 carbonyl and the N-3 amine as the hydrogen-bond acceptors. Guanine has a group at C-6 that acts as the hydrogen acceptor, while the group at N-1 and the amino group at C-2 act as the hydrogen donors.

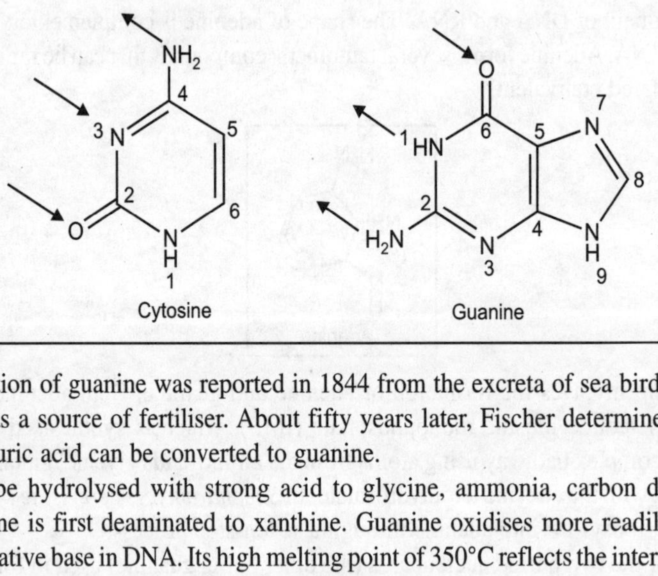

Cytosine   Guanine

The first isolation of guanine was reported in 1844 from the excreta of sea birds, known as guano, which was used as a source of fertiliser. About fifty years later, Fischer determined the structure and also showed that uric acid can be converted to guanine.

Guanine can be hydrolysed with strong acid to glycine, ammonia, carbon dioxide, and carbon monoxide. Guanine is first deaminated to xanthine. Guanine oxidises more readily than adenine, the other purine-derivative base in DNA. Its high melting point of 350°C reflects the intermolecular hydrogen bonding between the *oxo* and amino groups in the molecules in the crystal. Because of this intermolecular bonding, guanine is relatively insoluble in water, but it is soluble in dilute acids and bases. Trace amounts of guanine are formed by the polymerisation of ammonium cyanide (NH_4CN).

Two experiments conducted by Levy showed that heating 10 mol·L^{-1} NH_4CN at 80°C for 24 hours gave a yield of 0.0007 per cent, while using 0.1 mol·L^{-1} NH_4CN frozen at –20°C for 25 years gave a 0.0035 per cent yield. These results indicate guanine could arise in frozen regions of the primitive earth. Yuasa reported a 0.00017 per cent yield of guanine after the electrical discharge of NH_3, CH_4, C_2H_6, and 50 ml of water, followed by a subsequent acid hydrolysis. However, it is unknown whether the presence of guanine was not simply a resultant contaminant of the reaction.

$$5NH_3 + CH_4 + 2C_2H_6 + H_2O \rightarrow C_5H_8N_5O \text{ (guanine)} + (25/2)H_2$$

A Fischer-Tropsch synthesis can also be used to form guanine, along with adenine, uracil, and thymine. Heating an equimolar gas mixture of CO, H_2, and NH_3 to 700°C for 15 to 24 minutes, followed by quick cooling and then sustainted reheating to 100° to 200°C for 16 to 44 hours with an alumina catalyst, yielded guanine and uracil.

$$5CO + (1/2)H_2 + 5NH_3 \rightarrow C_5H_8N_5O \text{ (guanine)} + 4H_2O$$

Another possible abiotic route was explored by quenching a 90 per cent N_2–10 per cent CO–H_2O gas mixture high-temperature plasma. Traube's synthesis involves heating 2,4,5-triamino-1,6-dihydro-6-oxypyrimidine (as the sulphate) with formic acid for several hours.

In 1656 in Paris, François Jaquin (a rosary maker) extracted from scales of some fishes the so-called pearl essence, crystalline guanine forming G-quadruplexes. In the cosmetics industry, crystalline guanine is used as an additive to various products (e.g. shampoos), where it provides a pearly iridescent effect. It is also used in metallic paints and simulated pearls and plastics. It provides shimmering luster to eye shadow and nail polish. Guanine crystals are rhombic platelets composed of multiple transparent layers, but they have a high index of refraction that partially reflects and transmits light from layer to layer, thus producing a pearly luster. It can be applied by spray, painting, or dipping. It may irritate the eyes. Its alternatives are mica, faux pearl (from ground shells), and aluminium and bronze particles.

Spiders and scorpions convert ammonia, as a product of protein metabolism in the cells, to guanine as it can be excreted with minimal water loss. Guanine is found in integumentary system of many fish such as sturgeon. It is also present in the reflective deposits of the eyes of deep-sea fish and some reptiles such as Crocodiles.

Thymine is one of the four nucleobases in the nucleic acid of DNA that are represented by the letters G–C–A–T. The others are adenine, guanine, and cytosine. Thymine is also known as 5-methyluracil, a pyrimidine nucleobase. As the name suggests, thymine may be derived by methylation of uracil at the 5th carbon. In RNA, thymine is replaced with uracil in most cases. In DNA, thymine(T) binds to adenine (A) via two hydrogen bonds to assist in stabilising the nucleic acid structures.

Thymine

Thymine combined with deoxyribose creates the nucleoside deoxythymidine, which is synonymous with the term thymidine. Thymidine can be phosphorylated with one, two, or three phosphoric acid groups, creating, respectively, TMP, TDP, or TTP (thymidine mono-, di-, or triphosphate). One of the common mutations of DNA involves two adjacent thymines or cytosine, which, in presence of ultraviolet light, may form thymine dimers, causing 'kinks' in the DNA molecule that inhibit normal function. Thymine could also be a target for actions of 5-fluorouracil (5-FU) in cancer treatment. 5-FU can be a metabolic analog of thymine (in DNA synthesis) or uracil (in RNA synthesis). Substitution of this analog inhibits DNA synthesis in actively-dividing cells. Thymine bases are frequently oxidised to hydantoins over time after the death of an organism.

Recombinant DNA (rDNA) has various definitions, ranging from very simple to strangely complex. The following are three examples of how recombinant DNA is defined:

1. A DNA molecule containing DNA originating from two or more sources.
2. DNA that has been artificially created. It is DNA from two or more sources that is incorporated into a single recombinant molecule.
3. According to the NIH guidelines, recombinant DNA are molecules constructed outside of living cells by joining natural or synthetic DNA segments to DNA molecules that can replicate in a living cell, or molecules that result from their replication.

Recombinant DNA, also known as *in vitro* recombination, is a technique involved in creating and purifying desired genes. Molecular cloning (i.e. gene cloning) involves creating recombinant DNA and introducing it into a host cell to be replicated. One of the basic strategies of molecular cloning is to move desired genes from a large, complex genome to a small, simple one. The process of *in vitro* recombination makes it possible to cut different strands of DNA, *in vitro* (outside the cell), with a restriction enzyme and join the DNA molecules together via complementary base pairing.

Techniques of DNA

Some of the molecular biology techniques utilised during recombinant DNA include:

1. The study and/or modification of gene expression patterns: Gene expression is the process by which a gene's coded information is converted into the structures present and operating in the cell. Expressed genes include those that are transcribed into mRNA (messenger RNA) and then translated into protein, and those that are transcribed into tRNA (transfer RNA) and rRNA (ribosomal RNA). Gene expression can be studied using microarray analysis, which is a method of visualising the patterns of gene expression of thousands of genes using fluorescence or radioactive hybridisation.
2. Gene cloning: Gene cloning utilising recombinant DNA technology is the process of manipulating DNA to produce multiple copies of a single gene or segment of DNA.
3. DNA sequencing: DNA sequencing is a lab technique used to determine the sequence of nucleotide bases in a molecule of DNA.
4. Creation of transgenic plants and animals: A transgenic plant or animal is one who has been genetically engineered, and usually contains genetic material from at least one unrelated organism, such as from a virus, other plant, or other animal.

Processes

The following is a summary of the process of making recombinant DNA (Fig. 2.1):

1. Treat the DNA taken from both sources with the same restriction endonuclease.
2. The restriction enzyme cuts both molecules at the same site.
3. The ends of the cut have an overhanging piece of single-stranded DNA called 'sticky ends'.

4. These sticky ends are able to base pair with any DNA molecule that contains the complementary sticky end.
5. Complementary sticky ends can pair with each other when mixed.
6. DNA ligase is used to covalently link the two strands into a molecule of recombinant DNA.
7. In order to be useful, the recombinant DNA needs to be replicated many times (i.e. cloned). Cloning can be done *in vitro*, via the Polymerase Chain Reaction (PCR), or *in vivo* (inside the cell) using unicellular prokaryotes (e.g. *E. coli*), unicellular eukaryotes (e.g. yeast), or mammalian tissue culture cells.

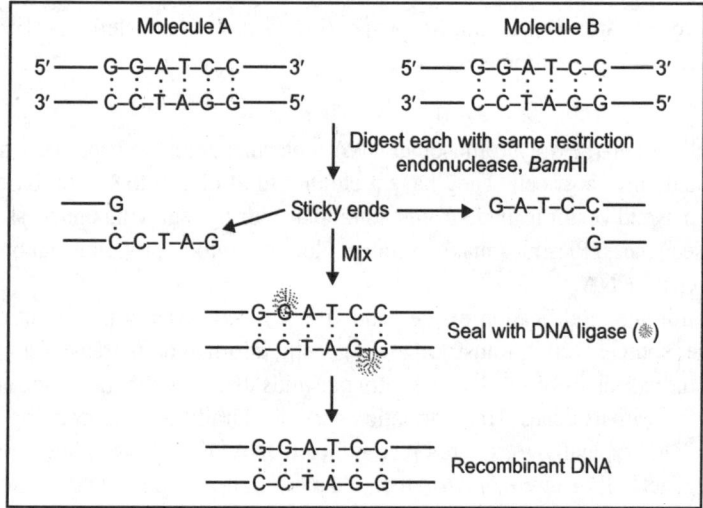

Fig. 2.1. A pictorial representation of the recombinant DNA process.

Examples

Some examples of the therapeutic products made by recombinant DNA techniques include:

1. Blood proteins: Erythropoietin; factors VII, VIII, IX; tissue plasminogen activator; urokinase.
2. Human hormones: Epidermal growth factor; follicle stimulating hormone; insulin; nerve growth factor; relaxin; somatotropin.
3. Immune modulators: α-interferon; β-interferon; colony stimulating factor; lysozyme; tumour necrosis factor.
4. Vaccines: Cytomegalovirus; hepatitis B; measles; rabies.

Cloning vectors

A cloning vector is a DNA molecule that carries foreign DNA into a host cell (usually bacterial or yeast), where it replicates, producing many copies of itself along with the foreign DNA. There are three features required for all cloning vectors:

1. Sequences that will permit the propagation of itself in bacteria or in yeast.
2. A cloning site to insert the foreign DNA; the most versatile vectors contain a site that can be cut by many restriction enzymes.
3. A method of selecting for bacteria or yeast containing a vector with foreign DNA; this is usually accomplished by selectable markers for drug resistance.

General steps of cloning with vectors

1. Prepare the vector and the DNA to be cloned by digestion with restriction enzymes to generate complementary ends.
2. Ligate (join) the foreign DNA into the vector with the enzyme DNA ligase.
3. Introduce the DNA into bacterial cells or yeast cells by transformation.
4. Select cells containing foreign DNA by screening for selectable markers (commonly drug resistance).

Types of cloning vectors

Types of cloning vectors are: (i) plasmid, (ii) phage, (iii) cosmid, (iv) bacterial artificial chromosomes (BAC), and (v) yeast artificial chromosomes (YAC).

Plasmids

Plasmids are small, circular, extrachromosomal DNA molecules found in bacteria, which can replicate on their own, outside of a host cell. They have a cloning limit of 100 to 10,000 base pairs or 0.1–10 kilobases (kb). A plasmid vector is made from natural plasmids by removing unnecessary segments and adding essential sequences. Plasmids make excellent cloning vectors for various laboratory techniques, including recombinant DNA.

Transformation is the modification of the genotype of a cell (usually prokaryotic) by introducing DNA from another source. During transformation, genetic information is transferred via the uptake of free DNA. Often these sources of DNA come from plasmids that are deliberately introduced into a cell, transforming the cell with its genes. Transformation occurs naturally, and the resulting uptake of foreign DNA by the cell is not typically considered recombinant DNA. If the plasmid being introduced to the cell has not been genetically altered, *in vitro*, then the plasmid is not considered to contain recombinant DNA. Plasmids that have been genetically altered, such as by the insertion of an antibiotic resistance gene, do contain recombinant DNA because the original genetic composition of the plasmid has been artificially altered. These plasmids can be used to incorporate bacterial cells with the antibiotic resistance gene via transformation.

Phages

Phages are derivatives of bacteriophage lambda (λ phage), a virus which infects *E. coli*. They are linear DNA molecules, whose region can be replaced with foreign DNA without disrupting its life cycle. The major advantage of the λ phage vector is its high transformation efficiency, which is about 1000 times greater than that of the plasmid vector. They also have a larger cloning limit than plasmids, consisting of 8–25 kb.

Cosmids

Cosmids are extrachromosomal circular DNA molecules that combine features of plasmids and phages. They also have a high transformation efficiency, and their cloning limit of 35–50 kb is larger than that of plasmids or phages.

Bacterial artificial chromosomes (BAC)

BACs are based on bacterial mini-F plasmids, which are small pieces of episomal bacterial DNA that give the bacteria the ability to initiate conjugation with adjacent bacteria. They have a cloning limit of 75–300 kb.

Yeast artificial chromosomes (YAC)

YACs are artificial chromosomes that replicate in yeast cells. They consist of:

1. Telomeres, which are ends of chromosomes involved in the replication and stability of linear DNA.
2. Origin of replication sequences necessary for the replication in yeast cells.
3. A yeast centromere, which is a specialised chromosomal region where spindle fibres attach during mitosis.
4. A selectable marker for identification in yeast cells.
5. Ampicillin resistance gene for selective amplification.
6. Recognition sites for restriction enzymes.

The procedure for making YAC vectors is as follows:

1. The target DNA is partially digested by a restriction endonuclease, and the YAC vector is cleaved by restriction enzymes.
2. The cleaved vector segments are ligated with a digested DNA fragment to form an artificial chromosome.
3. Yeast cells are transformed to make a large number of copies.
4. They are the largest of the cloning vectors, with a cloning limit of 100–1000 kb, however they have very low efficiency.

Yeast

Yeasts, eukaryotic unicellular fungi, contribute a great deal to the study of molecular genetics. They are popular organisms to clone and express DNA in because they are eukaryotes, and can therefore splice out introns, the noncoding sequences in the middle of many eukaryotic genes. For the past two decades *Saccharomyces cerevisiae*, a species of yeast, has been an important model system for biological research because its entire genome has been base sequenced, and is used as a reference to human and other higher eukaryotic genes. This is because the basic cellular mechanics of replication, recombination, cell division and metabolism are generally conserved between yeast and larger eukaryotes, including mammals. Also, yeast is easily genetically manipulated, which allows for convenient analysis and the functional dissecting of gene products from other eukaryotes.

Gene therapy

Gene therapy can be defined as the transfer of genetic material into the cells of an individual resulting in a therapeutic benefit to the individual. It involves the intentional modification of genetic material with the aim of preventing, diagnosing, or curing a disease. These modifications include the correction of a genetic defect resulting from the absence or alteration of a protein, or the addition of genetic information to modify cellular characteristics. Gene therapy allows the modification of specific genes without having to alter the disease phenotype using agents that either interact with the gene products (proteins), or are gene products themselves. The genetic modifications can be done *in vitro* or directly *in vivo* by using vectors that are capable of genetic transfer. Products used in gene therapy include viral vectors, genetically modified cells, and free or complex nucleic acids. Currently the most efficient method for gene transfer is viral vectors. They cause infection of the target cell and transfer the therapeutic gene using their natural biological mechanisms. Viral vectors used in gene therapy must be unable to replicate and have no lytic (ability to rupture a cell) activity. The result of gene therapy is the permanent treatment of disease, hopefully with few or no side effects in the process.

Viral vectors

A viral vector is a virus that carries a modified or foreign gene. They are commonly used in gene therapy where the viral vector delivers the desired gene to a target cell. Some of the viruses used as vectors in gene therapy include: (i) retroviruses, (ii) adenoviruses, (iii) parvoviruses, (iv) herpesviruses, and (v) poxviruses.

Retrovirus

Retroviruses are viruses belonging to the family *Retroviridae*. They are composed of a single RNA strand and use the enzyme reverse transcriptase to copy their genome into the DNA of the host cell's chromosomes. They are relatively genetically simple, and have the ability to infect a wide variety of cell types with high efficiency. Retroviruses are the cause of many infections and cancers in vertebrates, including human T-cell leukemia and HIV. They also cause a variety of haematopoetic and neurological conditions, including paralysis, wasting, ataxia, arthritis, dementia, and neuropathy. Although vertebrate infection is mainly focused on, retroviruses have also been identified in virtually all organisms including invertebrates. The genome of all retroviruses consists of two molecules of RNA, which are single stranded, (+) sense, and have 5′ cap and 3′ poly-(A) (which is equivalent to mRNA). They vary in size from approximately 8 to 11 kb. Retrovirus genomes have four unique features:

1. They are the only viruses that are truly diploid (i.e. contain a full set of genetic material which consists of paired chromosomes).
2. They are the only RNA viruses whose genome is produced by cellular transcriptional machinery, *i.e.* they do not require participation by a virus-encoded polymerase.
3. They are the only viruses whose genome requires tRNA for replication.
4. They are the only (+) sense RNA viruses whose genome does not serve directly as mRNA immediately after infection.

Avian and murine retroviruses are commonly used as cloning vectors in gene therapy. Lentiviruses are a sub-group of retroviruses that are able to infect nondividing cells or terminally differentiated cells, such as neurons. The main lentivirus vectors are derived from immunodeficiency viruses, including HIV.

Adenovirus

Adenovirus can be defined as a group of DNA containing viruses, which most commonly cause respiratory disease (ranging from one form of the common cold to pneumonia, croup, and bronchitis), and can also cause gastrointestinal illness, eye infections, cystitis, and rash in humans. Adenoviruses can also be genetically modified and used in gene therapy to treat cystic fibrosis, cancer, and potentially other diseases. Some of the characteristic features of adenoviruses include:

1. They are widespread in nature, infecting birds, and many mammals including humans. There are two genera: Aviadenovirus (avian) and Mastadenovirus (mammalian).
2. They can undergo latent infection in lymphoid tissues, and become reactivated at a later time.
3. Several types have oncogenic (cancer-causing) potential.

Adenoviral vectors can be used to express a wide variety of viral and cellular genes in mammalian cells. They can also be used to transfect cells for protein expression and *in vivo* characterisation studies. Transfection is the uptake, incorporation, and expression of recombinant DNA by eukaryotic cells.

Adenoviral vectors are great to use for transfection because the adenovirus efficiently infects many different cell lines. The virus enters the cell but it does not replicate because the essential E1 (viral genes which are expressed early in the viral life cycle) are absent. This is termed abortive infection, and it can be used as a transfection system for introducing a functional gene into cells. Adenoviral vectors are used in gene therapy when a high level of expression of the transferred gene is required for brief periods of time. The advantages of using adenovirus for the introduction of genes into cells include:

1. The process is quick, simple, and does not require any special equipment.
2. It is well tolerated, contrary to other methods. Post-infection viability is near 100 per cent which means adenovirus can transfer genetic material into cells without toxic effects.
3. Adenovirus can infect most cell types.
4. Gene expression can be analysed as early as a few hours after infection.
5. More than one protein can be expressed simultaneously.

Adenoviruses are medium-sized, nonenveloped, regular icosahedrons of 65–100 nanometers in diameter. The genome of adenoviruses is a linear double-stranded DNA molecule containing 30,000–42,000 nucleotides.

Example

The following is an example of how adenovirus can be used in gene therapy to treat cystic fibrosis: Adenoviruses are good vectors for use in human gene therapy because it can infect cells *in vivo*, rather than manipulating the cells *in vitro*, and returning the cells to the body. In order to become a vector, the genome of the adenovirus must first be altered by removing all the viral DNA, except for the minimum necessary for the virus to live and infect the cells. Genetically engineered viral vectors like these are harmless and typically cannot live outside of the laboratory. A copy of the Cystic Fibrosis gene is then inserted into the viral genome via *in vitro* recombination. The viral genome is now considered recombinant. Then purified proteins and enzymes are used to build a new virus, or 'package' the DNA. To do this, the recombinant DNA is mixed with all of the protein components of the virus along with some viral enzymes that assemble the virus, and in the test tube a whole, intact virus is created with the new DNA inside. After infecting some cells in the laboratory, the new virus makes millions of copies of itself (carrying the Cystic Fibrosis gene), which can be purified and used for gene therapy.

Parvovirus

Parvoviruses are small DNA viruses that cause several diseases in mammals, such as canine parvovirus in dogs. Parvovirus B-19, which causes Fifth disease (erythema infectiosum) in humans, is the only form that is pathogenic to humans. In fact, many parvoviruses exhibit oncosuppressive properties (suppression of cancer-causing genes). Parvovirus-based vectors can be used to target the expression of therapeutic genes in tumours.

Herpesviruses

Herpesviruses include infectious human viruses including herpes simplex virus type-1 (HSV-1), which is common in the general population, but in rare cases can cause encephalitis. It is one of the most commonly used vector systems because it has a broad host cell range, the ability to transduce neurons, and a capacity to receive large inserts.

Poxviruses

Poxviruses are the largest and most complex viruses known. There are at least nine different poxviruses that are pathogenic to humans, the most common being vaccinia and variola virus (smallpox), which has since been erradicated. Poxviral vectors are successful in immunogenetic therapy protocols, due to their strong immnuogenicity (ability to induce a high immune response). They cause the activation of immune responses against tumour antigens transported in dendritic cells.

RESTRICTION ENZYME/ENDONUCLEASES

A restriction enzyme (or restriction endonuclease) is an enzyme that cuts double-stranded or single stranded DNA at specific recognition nucleotide sequences known as restriction sites. Such enzymes, found in bacteria and archaea, are thought to have evolved to provide a defense mechanism against invading viruses. Inside a bacterial host, the restriction enzymes selectively cut up foreign DNA in a process called restriction; host DNA is methylated by a modification enzyme (a methylase) to protect it from the restriction enzyme's activity. Collectively, these two processes form the restriction modification system. To cut the DNA, a restriction enzyme makes two incisions, once through each sugar-phosphate backbone (i.e. each strand) of the DNA double helix. After isolating the first restriction enzyme, *Hind*II, in 1970, and the subsequent discovery and characterisation of numerous restriction endonucleases, the 1978 Nobel Prize for Physiology or Medicine was awarded to Daniel Nathans, Werner Arber, and Hamilton O. Smith. Their discovery led to the development of recombinant DNA technology that allowed, for example, the large scale production of human insulin for diabetics using *E. coli* bacteria. Over 3000 restriction enzymes have been studied in detail, and more than 600 of these are available commercially and are routinely used for DNA modification and manipulation in laboratories.

Recognition Site

Restriction enzymes recognise a specific sequence of nucleotides and produce a double-stranded cut in the DNA. While recognition sequences vary between 4 and 8 nucleotides, many of them are palindromic, which correspond to nitrogenous base sequences that read the same backwards and forwards. In theory, there are two types of palindromic sequences that can be possible in DNA. The mirror-like palindrome is similar to those found in ordinary text, in which a sequence reads the same forward and backwards on the same DNA strand (i.e. single stranded) as in GTAATG. The inverted repeat palindrome is also a sequence that reads the same forward and backwards, but the forward and backward sequences are found in complementary DNA strands (i.e. double stranded) as in GTATAC (Notice that GTATAC is complementary to CATATG). The inverted repeat is more common and has greater biological importance than the mirror-like (Fig. 2.2).

5′-GTATAC-3′

: : : : : :

3′-CATATG-5′

Fig. 2.2. A palindromic recognition site reads the same on the reverse strand as it does on the forward strand.

EcoRI digestion produces 'sticky' ends,

G|AATTC
CTTAA|G

whereas *Sma*I restriction enzyme cleavage produces 'blunt' ends

CCC|GGG
GGG|CCC

Recognition sequences in DNA differ for each restriction enzyme, producing differences in the length, sequence and strand orientation (5′ end or the 3′ end) of a sticky-end 'overhang' of an enzyme restriction. Different restriction enzymes that recognise the same sequence are known as neoschizomers. These often cleave in a different locales of the sequence; however, different enzymes that recognise and cleave in the same location are known as an isoschizomer. Bacteria prevent their own DNA from being cut by modifying their nucleotides via DNA methylation.

Types

Restriction endonucleases are categorised into three general groups (Types I, II and III) based on their composition and enzyme cofactor requirements, the nature of their target sequence, and the position of their DNA cleavage site relative to the target sequence.

Type I

Type I restriction enzymes were the first to be identified and are characteristic of two different strains (K-12 and B) of *E. coli*. These enzymes cut at a site that differs, and is some distance (at least 1000 bp) away, from their recognition site. The recognition site is asymmetrical and is composed of two portions—one containing 3–4 nucleotides, and another containing 4–5 nucleotides—separated by a spacer of about 6–8 nucleotides. Several enzyme cofactors, including S-Adenosyl methionine (AdoMet), hydrolysed adenosine triphosphate (ATP), and magnesium (Mg^{2+}) ions, are required for their activity. Type I restriction enzymes possess three subunits called HsdR, HsdM, and HsdS; HsdR is required for restriction; HsdM is necessary for adding methyl groups to host DNA (methyltransferase activity) and HsdS is important for specificity of cut site recognition in addition to its methyltransferase activity.

Type II

Typical type II restriction enzymes differ from type I restriction enzymes in several ways. They are composed of homodimeric two subunit; their recognition sites are usually undivided and palindromic and 4–8 nucleotides in length, they recognise and cleave DNA at the same site, and they do not use ATP or AdoMet for their activity—they usually require only Mg^{2+} as a cofactor. These are the most commonly available and used restriction enzymes. In the 1990s and early 2000s, new enzymes from this family were discovered that did not follow all the classical criteria of this enzyme class, and new subfamily nomenclature was developed to divide this large family into subcategories based on deviations from typical characteristics of Type II enzymes. These subgroups are defined using a letter suffix.

Type IIB restriction enzymes (e.g. *Bcg*I and *Bpl*I) are multimers, containing more than one subunit. They cleave DNA on both sides of their recognition to cut out the recognition site. They require both AdoMet and Mg^{2+} cofactors. Type IIE restriction endonucleases (e.g. *Nae*I) cleave DNA following interaction with two copies of their recognition sequence. One recognition site acts as the target for cleavage, while the other acts as an allosteric effector that speeds up or improves the efficiency of enzyme cleavage. Similar to type IIE enzymes, type IIF restriction endonucleases (e.g. NgoMIV) interact with two copies of their recognition sequence but cleave both sequences at the same time. Type IIG restriction endonucleases (Eco57I) do have a single subunit, like classical Type II restriction enzymes, but require the cofactor AdoMet to be active.

Type IIM restriction endonucleases, such as *Dpn*I, are able to recognise and cut methylated DNA. Type IIS restriction endonucleases (e.g. FokI) cleave DNA at a defined distance from their non-palindromic asymmetric recognition sites. These enzymes may function as dimers. Similarly, Type IIT restriction enzymes (e.g. *Bpu*10I and *Bsl*I) are composed of two different subunits. Some recognise palindromic sequences while others have asymmetric recognition sites.

Type III

Type III restriction enzymes (e.g. EcoP15) recognise two separate non-palindromic sequences that are inversely oriented. They cut DNA about 20-30 base pairs after the recognition site. These enzymes contain more than one subunit and require AdoMet and ATP cofactors for their roles in DNA methylation and restriction, respectively.

Nomenclature

Since their discovery in the 1970s, more than 100 different restriction enzymes have been identified in different bacteria. Each enzyme is named after the bacterium from which it was isolated using a naming system based on bacterial genus, species and strain. For example, the name of the EcoRI restriction enzyme was derived as shown in the Table 2.1.

Table 2.1. Derivation of the EcoRI name.

Abbreviation	Meaning	Description
E	*Escherichia*	Genus
co	*coli*	Species
R	RY13	Strain
I	First identified	Order of identification in the bacterium

Applications

Isolated restriction enzymes are used to manipulate DNA for different scientific applications. They are used to assist insertion of genes into plasmid vectors during gene cloning and protein expression experiments. For optimal use, plasmids that are commonly used for gene cloning are modified to include a short polylinker sequence (called the multiple cloning site, or MCS) rich in restriction enzyme recognition sequences. This allows flexibility when inserting gene fragments into the plasmid vector; restriction sites contained naturally within genes influence the choice of endonuclease for digesting the DNA since it is necessary to avoid restriction of wanted DNA while intentionally cutting the ends of the DNA. To clone a gene fragment into a vector, both plasmid DNA and gene insert are typically cut with the same restriction enzymes, and then glued together with the assistance of an enzyme known as a DNA ligase.

Restriction enzymes can also be used to distinguish gene alleles by specifically recognising single base changes in DNA known as single nucleotide polymorphisms (SNPs). This is only possible if a SNP alters the restriction site present in the allele. In this method, the restriction enzyme can be used to genotype a DNA sample without the need for expensive gene sequencing. The sample is first digested with the restriction enzyme to generate DNA fragments, and then the different sized fragments separated by gel electrophoresis.

In general, alleles with correct restriction sites will generate two visible bands of DNA on the gel, and those with altered restriction sites will not be cut and will generate only a single band. The number of bands reveals the sample subject's genotype, an example of restriction mapping.

In a similar manner, restriction enzymes are used to digest genomic DNA for gene analysis by Southern blot. This technique allows researchers to identify how many copies (or paralogues) of a gene are present in the genome of one individual, or how many gene mutations (polymorphisms) have occurred within a population. The latter example is called restriction fragment length polymorphism (RFLP).

Cloning Vector

A cloning vector is a small piece of DNA into which a foreign DNA fragment can be inserted. The insertion of the fragment into the cloning vector is carried out by treating the vehicle and the foreign DNA with the same restriction enzyme, then ligating the fragments together. There are many types of cloning vectors. Genetically engineered plasmids and bacteriophages (such as phage λ) are perhaps most commonly used for this purpose. Other types of cloning vectors include bacterial artificial chromosomes (BACs) and yeast artificial chromosomes (YACs).

Common features

Most commercial cloning vectors have key features that have made their use in molecular biology so widespread. In the case of expression vectors, the main purpose of these vehicles is the controlled expression of a particular gene inside a convenient host organism (e.g. *E. coli*). Control of expression can be very important; it is usually desirable to insert the target DNA into a site that is under the control of a particular promoter. Some commonly used promoters are T7 promoters, *lac* promoters (*bla* promoter) and cauliflower mosaic virus's 35s promoter (for plant vectors).

To allow for convenient and favourable insertions, most cloning vectors have had nearly all their restriction sites engineered out of them and a synthetic multiple cloning site (MCS) inserted that contains many restriction sites.

MCSs allow for insertions of DNA into the vector to be targeted and possibly directed in a chosen orientation. A selectable marker, such as an antibiotic resistance [e.g. beta-lactamase (Fig. 2.3)] is often carried by the vector to allow the selection of positively transformed cells. All plasmids must carry a functional origin of replication.

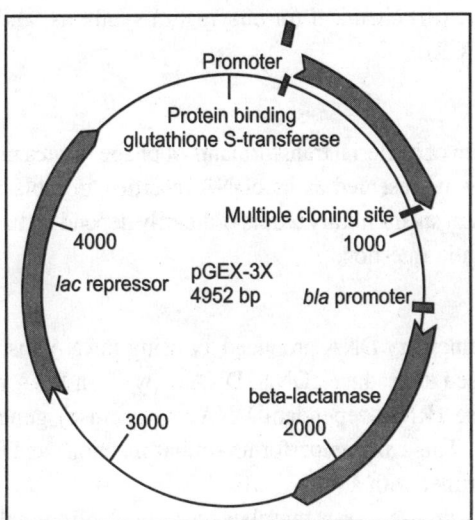

Fig. 2.3. The pGEX-3x plasmid is a popular cloning vector.

Some other possible features present in cloning vectors are: *vir* genes for plant transformation, integrase sites for chromosomal insertion, *lac*Za fragment for a complementation and blue-white selection, and/or reporter genes in frame with and flanking the MCS to facilitate the production of recombinant proteins [e.g. fused to the Green fluorescent protein (GFP) or to the glutathione S-transferase (Fig. 2.3)].

Many general purpose vectors such as *p*UC19 usually include a system for detecting the presence of a cloned DNA fragment, based on the loss of an easily scored phenotype. The most widely used is the gene coding for *E. coli* β-galactosidase, whose integrity can easily be detected by the ability of the enzyme it encodes to hydrolyse the soluble, colourless substrate X-gal (5-bromo-4-chloro-3-indolyl-beta-D-galactoside) into an insoluble, blue product (5,5′-dibromo-4,4′-dichloro indigo). Cloning a fragment of DNA within the vector-based gene encoding the β-galactosidase prevents the production of an active enzyme. If X-gal is included in the selective agar plates, transformant colonies are generally blue in the case of a vector with no inserted DNA and white in the case of a vector containing a fragment of cloned DNA.

STEPS IN GENE CLONING

The entire procedure of cloning or recombinant DNA technology may be classified into the following five steps for the convenience in description and on the basis of the chief activity performed.

1. Identification and isolation of the desired gene or DNA fragment to be cloned.
2. Insertion of the isolated gene in a suitable vector.
3. Introduction of this vector into a suitable organism/cell called host (transformation).
4. Selection of the transformed host cells.
5. Multiplication/expression/integration followed by expression of the introduced gene in the host.

Isolation of the Desired Gene

The identification and isolation of the desired gene or DNA fragment, called DNA insert, to be cloned is a critical step in gene cloning. The desired DNA inserts can be obtained from the following: (i) cDNA libraries, (ii) genomic library, (iii) chemical (or enzymatic) synthesis, and (iv) amplification through polymerase chain reaction (PCR).

cDNA library

A cDNA library is a population of bacterial transformants or phage lysates in which each mRNA isolated from an organism or tissue is represented as its cDNA insertion in a plasmid or a phage vector. The frequency of a specific cDNA in such a library would ordinarily depend on the frequency of the concerned mRNA in the tissue/organism in question.

Preparation of cDNA

cDNA is the copy or complementary DNA produced by using mRNA (usually) as a template. In fact, any RNA molecule can be used to produce cDNA. DNA copy of an RNA molecule is produced by the enzyme reverse transcriptase (RNA-dependent DNA polymerase) generally obtained from avian myeloblastosis virus (AMV). This enzyme performs similar reactions as DNA polymerase, and has an absolute requirement for a primer with a free 3′-OH.

When eukaryotic mRNA is used as a template, a poly-T oligonucleotide (more specifically, oligodeoxynucleotide) is conveniently used as the primer since these mRNAs have a poly-A tail at their 3′ ends. But special tricks are required to utilise primers for other RNAs, e.g. prokaryotic mRNA, rRNA, RNA virus genomes, etc. In such cases, a poly-A tail may be added to 3′ end of the RNA to make it analogous to eukaryotic mRNA (oligo-T is now used as primer); this reaction is catalysed by the enzyme poly-A polymerase. Alternatively, a oligonucleotide complementary to a region, preferably at the 3′ end, of the RNA molecule may be used as a primer; for this approach, the sequence of a segment of the RNA must be known.

The appropriate oligonucleotide primer (oligo-T for eukaryotic mRNA) is annealed with the mRNA; this primer will base-pair to the 3′ end of mRNA (Fig. 2.4). Reverse transcriptase extends the 3′ end of the primer using mRNA molecule as a template. This produces a RNA . DNA hybrid molecule; the DNA strand of this hybrid is obviously the DNA copy (cDNA) of the mRNA strand. The RNA strand is digested either by RNAase H or alkaline hydrolysis; this frees the single stranded cDNA. Curiously, the end of this cDNA serves as its own primer and provides the free 3′-OH required for the synthesis of its complementary strand; therefore, a primer is not required for this step (Fig. 2.4). The complementary strand of cDNA single strand is synthesised by either the reverse transcriptase itself or by DNA polymerase I. Since the 3′ end of cDNA single strand is used as the primer for this reaction, a short hairpin loop is generated at this end. The hairpin loop is cleaved by a single strand-specific nuclease to yield a regular DNA duplex (Fig. 2.4).

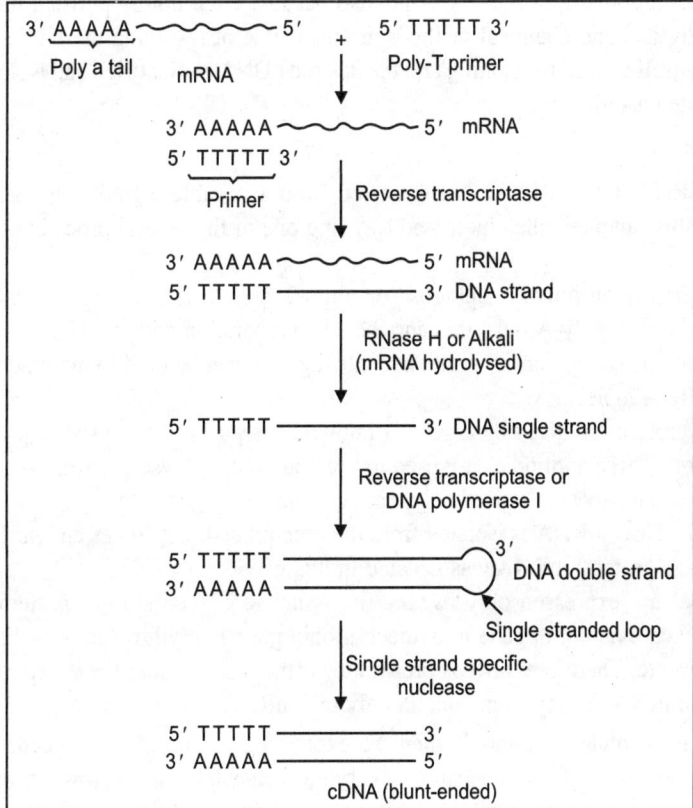

Fig. 2.4. Production of cDNA (complementary or copy DNA) from an mRNA molecule used as template by the enzyme reverse transcriptase.

Problems in cDNA preparation

The ideal situation of Fig. 2.4 is rare. In fact, starting with even a pure mRNA preparation, the end product consists of a mixture of cDNAs most of which are somewhat shorter than the complete RNA molecule. This is because of the following problems: (i) incomplete copying of the: mRNA by reverse transcriptase (5′ end of mRNA missing from cDNA), (ii) incomplete copying of the cDNA single strand so that the 3′ end of mRNA will be missing from cDNA, and (iii) the nuclease used for cleaving the hairpin loop- may also nibble away the ends of the duplex.

Elaborate strategies have been developed to overcome these problems. For example, incomplete copying of the RNA can be ameliorated by using a specially designed *E. coli* vector to which the RNA is attached before copying; all subsequent steps are performed in association with this vector. Similarly, the use of single-strand specific nuclease can be avoided by adding a poly-A, poly-Tor poly-C tail to the 3′ end of the cDNA single strand produced by copying of the mRNA; the complementary oligonucleotide (Poly-T, Poly-A, poly-G, respectively) is now used as a primer for the synthesis of complementary strand to yield double-stranded cDNA without a hairpin loop. This can be combined with PCR to obtain a large number of copies of the cDNA.

The double strand cDNA preparations are always a mixture of different kinds of molecules due to the above problems in copying of the RNA and also because even highly purified mRNAs are never absolutely pure. Physical and chemical methods are incapable of resolving these mixtures. Therefore, the cDNA mixture itself is used for cloning and the desired cDNA is identified and isolated in pure form from the appropriate bacterial clone.

Isolation of mRNA

For isolation of mRNA, total RNA is first extracted from a suitable organism/tissue. The amount of desired mRNA in this sample is then increased by using one of the several procedures, some of which are listed below.

1. Chromatography on poly-U sepharose or oligo-T cellulose which retains mRNA molecules since they have 3′ poly-A tails; this enriches the preparation with mRNAs of all kinds.

2. In some specific cases, density gradient centrifugation can be used to increase the frequency of desired mRNA molecules.

3. When the protein produced by a gene is known, it is purified and used to produce antibodies specific to it. These antibodies are used to precipitate the polysomes (mRNAs associated with ribosomes and newly synthesised polypeptide chains) engaged in the synthesis of the concerned polypeptide. Now mRNA is isolated from the precipitated polysomes and purified. Maize zein (seed storage protein) mRNA was isolated in this way.

4. Some genes are expressed only in specific tissues, e.g. seed storage proteins in developing seeds, chicken ovalbumin gene in oviduct, globin gene in erythrocytes, insulin gene in β cells of pancreas, etc. Therefore, mRNA preparations from such tissues are exceptionally rich in the concerned mRNA or may even contain only this mRNA.

Use of cDNA is absolutely essential when the expression of an eukaryotic gene is required in a prokaryote, e.g. a bacterium. This is because eukaryotic genes have introns which must be removed from their transcripts to yield mature mRNA. Bacteria do not possess the enzymes necessary for removal of introns; therefore, they do not have the ability to produce mature ready-to-translate mRNA molecules from the transcripts of complete native eukaryotic genes. In contrast, functional mRNA molecules do not have introns; hence their cDNA is also free from introns and can be cloned and expressed in bacteria. For example, cDNA for interferon, blood clotting factor VIII C (both human) and several other mRNAs have been expressed in bacteria.

Genomic Library

A genomic library is a collection of plasmid clones or phage lysates containing recombinant DNA molecules so that the sum total of DNA inserts in this collection, ideally, represents the entire genome of the concerned organism. However, inspite of all the care taken in the production of genomic libraries, certain DNA fragments should be expected to be under- or over-represented or even missing. The possible reasons for this may be that certain fragments code for a toxic product, or might replicate slowly or might have been altered by recombinational events during cloning. In addition, endonuclease cleavage sites are often not recognised equally well. Certain DNA fragments may therefore never appear in partial digests by a restriction endonuclease used for the construction of genomic libraries.

Construction of a genomic library

For preparation of a genomic library, the total genomic DNA of an organism is extracted. The DNA is broken into fragments of appropriate size either by mechanical shearing (this generates blunt-ended fragments), or sonication, or by using a suitable restriction endonuclease for partial digestion of the DNA; complete digestion is avoided since it generates fragments that are too heterogeneous in size. For partial digestion, restriction enzymes having 4-base (tetrameric) recognition sequences are employed in preference to those having 6-base (hexameric) target sites. This is because a given 4-base recognition site is expected to occur every 4^4 (= 256) base pairs in a DNA molecule, while a 6 base target site would occur only after every 4^6 (= 4096) base pairs. (It is assumed here that the arrangement of the 4 bases in DNA molecules is random).

Therefore, the fragments produced in partial digests with enzymes having 4 base recognition sites are more likely to be of appropriate size for cloning than those generated by enzymes having 6 base recognition sites. Single or mixed digestions with the enzymes AluI (AG/CT), HaeIII (GG/CC) or Sau3A (/GATC) have been used for constructing genomic libraries. The use of restriction enzymes has the advantage that the same set of fragments are obtained from a DNA each time a specific enzyme is used, and many of the enzymes produce cohesive ends.

The partial digests of genomic DNA are subjected to agarose gel electrophoresis or sucrose gradient centrifugation for separation from the mixture of fragment of appropriate size. These fragments are then inserted into a suitable vector for cloning. This constitutes the shotgun approach to gene cloning. In principle, any vector can be used, but λ vectors and cosmids have been the most commonly used since DNA inserts of up to 23–25 kb (kilobase pairs) can be cloned in these vectors, particularly in replacement vectors. The vectors containing the inserts are cloned in a suitable bacterial host.

The minimum size (number of clones or bacterial colonies) of a genomic library depends on the following two factors: (i) the complexity of the genome (the more complex the genome the larger the size), and (ii) the insert or fragment length used for cloning (the smaller the fragment size, the larger the number of clones for the same genome). The minimum number of colonies in a genomic library constructed with 20 kb inserts for a 99 per cent probability of all the genomic sequences being represented would be 1157 for or E. coli (genome of 3.75×10^3 kb), 3462 for yeast (genome, 1.5×10^4 kb), 38,000 for Drosophila (genome, 1.65×10^5 kb), and 6,90,819 for man (genome, 3×10 kb).

Identification of the desired clone

Identification of the bacterial colony containing the desired DNA fragments from among those making up the library generally employs a suitable hybridisation probe in colony hybridisation. The probe may be mRNA of the gene, cDNA of its mRNA, homologous gene from another organism, or a synthetic oligonucleotide representing the sequence of a part of the desired gene/DNA fragment. In order to detect hybridisation, the probe must be labelled, usually with a radioactive isotope.

VECTOR

A vector is a DNA molecule that has the ability to replicate in an appropriate host cell, and into which the DNA fragment to be cloned (called DNA insert) is integrated for cloning. Therefore, a vector must have an origin of DNA replication (denoted as on) that functions in the host cell. Any extra-chromosomal small genome, e.g. plasmid, phage and virus, may be used as a vector.

Properties of a Good Vector

A good vector must have the following properties:

1. It should be able to replicate autonomously. When the objective of cloning is to obtain a large number of copies of the DNA insert, the vector replicon must be under relaxed control so that it can generate multiple copies of itself in a single host cell.
2. It should be easy to isolate and purify.
3. It should be easily introduced into the host cells, i.e. transformation of the host with the vector should be easy.
4. The vector should have suitable marker genes that allow easy detection and/or selection of the transformed host cells.
5. When the objective is gene transfer, it should have the ability to integrate either itself or the DNA insert it carries into the genome of the host cell.
6. The cells transformed with the vector molecules containing the DNA insert (recombinant or chimaeric vector) should be identifiable or selectable from those transformed by the vector molecules only.
7. A vector should contain unique target sites for as many restriction enzymes as possible into which the DNA insert can be integrated without disrupting an essential function.
8. When expression of the DNA insert is desired, the vector should contain atleast suitable control elements, e.g. promoter, operator and ribosome binding sites; several other features may also be important.

It should be kept in and that (i) the DNA molecules used as vectors have coevolved with their specific natural host species, and hence are adapted to function well in them and in their closely related species. Therefore, the choice of vector depends largely on the host species into which the DNA insert or gene is to be cloned. In addition, (ii) most naturally occurring vectors do not have all the required functions; therefore, useful vectors have been created by joining together segments performing specific functions (called modules) from two or more natural entities. A brief description of some of the important vectors used in different hosts is given below.

Cloning and Expression Vectors

All vectors used for propagation of DNA inserts in a suitable host are called cloning vectors. But when a vector is designed for the expression of, i.e. production of the protein specified by, the DNA insert, it is termed as expression vector. As a rule, such vectors contain at least the regulatory sequences, i.e. promoters, operators, ribosomal binding sites, etc. having optimum function in the chosen host. It is desirable that all cloning vectors have relaxed replication control so that they can produce multiple copies per host cell.

When an eukaryotic gene to be expressed in a prokaryote, the eukaryotic coding sequence has to be placed after prokaryotic promoter and ribosome building site since the regulatory sequences of eukaryotic are not recognised in prokaryotes. In addition, eukaryotic genes, as a rule, contain introns (noncoding regions) present within their coding regions. These introns must be removed to enable the proper expression of eukaryotic genes since prokaryotes lack the machinery needed for their removal from the RNA transcripts. When eukaryotic genes are isolated as cDNA they are intron-free and, hence, suitable for expression in prokaryotes.

Several strategies have been attempted for the construction of expression vectors using regulatory sequences of the appropriate hosts. These approaches may be grouped into the following two broad, categories.

1. Construction of vectors allowing the synthesis of fusion proteins comprising amino acids coded by a sequence in the vector and those encoded by the DNA insert (translational fusion).
2. Development of vectors permitting the synthesis of pure proteins encoded exclusively by the DNA inserts (transcriptional fusion).

Examples of the first strategy producing fusion proteins are: the expression of rat insulin, rat growth hormone, structural protein VP1 of foot and mouth disease, virus, human growth hormone, etc. Some examples of the second approach producing unique proteins are: rabbit β-globin; small *t*-antigen of SV 40, human fibroblast interferon, human IGF-I protein. It may be pointed out that the undesired amino acids encoded by the vector sequence in cases of translational fusion must be removed from the fusion proteins by a suitable chemical cleavage.

Several other problems are faced when eukaryotic genes are expressed in a prokaryotic system, e.g. removal of signal sequences from precursor proteins to obtain active mature protein molecules. Various strategies are being rapidly devised to effectively overcome these problems.

E. Coli VECTORS

Bacteria are the hosts of choice for DNA cloning. Among them, *E. coli* occupies a prominent position since cloning and isolating DNA inserts for structural analysis is the easiest in this host. Therefore, the initial cloning experiments are generally carried out in *E. coli*. The *E. coli* strain K12 is the most commonly used; it has several substrains, e.g. C 600, RRI, HB 101, etc. each of which has some specific features important in cloning. For example, the substrain RRI has, in addition to certain other features, the mutation *hsdR* which inactivates the restriction enzyme endogenous to *E. coli* K12; this minimises the degradation of recombinant DNA introduced into it.

Properties of a Good Host

A good host should have the following features: (i) is easy to transform, (ii) supports the replication of recombinant DNA, (iii) is free from elements that interfere with replication of recombinant DNA, (iv) lacks active restriction enzymes, e.g. *E. coli* K12 substrain HB 101, (v) does not have methylases since these enzymes would methylate the replicated recombinant DNA which, as a result, would become resistant to useful restriction enzymes, and (vi) is deficient in normal recombination function so that the DNA insert is not altered by recombination events.

E. coli supports several types of vectors, some natural, some constructed, which can be grouped as follows: (i) plasmids, (ii) bacteriophages (both natural), (iii) cosmids, (iv) plasmids, and (v) shuttle vectors (the last three constructed by man). A brief description of these vectors follows.

Plasmids

A plasmid is a DNA molecule, other than the bacterial chromosome, that is capable of independent replication and transmission. Plasmids are circular and may exist either independent of or may become integrated into the bacterial chromosome; generally they are not essential for the host cell except under specific environments.

There are several types of bacterial plasmids, but the three widely studied types are: (i) F plasmids (responsible for conjugation), (ii) R plasmids (carry genes for resistance to antibiotics), and (iii) Col plasmids (code for colicins, the proteins that kill sensitive *E. coli* cells; they also carry genes that provide immunity to the particular colicin).

The plasmids may either be conjugative or transmissible (mediate DNA transfer through conjugation, and as a result spread rapidly among the bacterial cells of a population), e.g. F plasmids, many R plasmids and some Col plasmids, or nonconjugative (do not mediate DNA transfer through conjugation), e.g. many R plasmids and most Col plasmids.

Stringent and relaxed replication

Each plasmid is maintained in the bacterial cell at a characteristic copy number mainly due to its replication control system. In this respect the plasmids are of two types: (i) single copy, and (ii) multicopy plasmids. The replication control of single copy plasmids is the same as that of their bacterial host cells so that they replicate and segregate with the bacterial chromosome; this is called stringent replication. In contrast, the replication control of multicopy plasmids is different from that of their bacterial host genome so that they undergo more than one replication for each replication of their host genome; this is referred to as relaxed replication.

Modular organisation

Plasmids may be visualised as constructed from modular DNA segments. A module may be regarded as a DNA segment or sequence performing a specific function; each module may contain one or more genes. The various modules present in the different plasmids are: (i) replication module (essential for all plasmids; it functions only in the natural host or closely related species); (ii) sex factors (found in conjugative plasmids; represented by *tra* genes in F factor and RTF, resistance transfer factor, in R plasmids); (iii) R-determinant module (specific to R plasmids; genes contained in it produce proteins that inactivate antibiotics); (iv) Col module (contains genes for colicins, antibacterial agents produced by bacteria); (v) modules specifying restriction modification systems, e.g. *Eco* RI system; and (vi) *IS* (insertion sequences) elements which enable transposition (movement from one DNA molecule into another) of the modules flanked by them, e.g. R-determinant modules of many R plasmids. Each plasmid must have the replication module; in addition it may or may not contain one or more of the other modules.

PLASMID VECTORS

Many different *E. coli* plasmids are used as vectors. The natural plasmids have been modified, shortened, reconstructed and recombined both *in vitro* and *in vivo* to create plasmids of enhanced utility and also with specific functions; the best ones include genes (Table 2.2) that allow easy selection of the recombinant or chimaeric vectors (vectors containing DNA inserts). Some *E. coli* plasmid vectors are briefly described below.

Table 2.2. Antibiotic resistance genes found in R plasmids, their proteins and mechanism of antibiotic resistance.

Antibiotic (gene conferring resistance)	Protein produced by the gene	Mechanism of resistance
Ampicillin (amp)	Penicillinase or β-lactamase	Hydrolysis of C-N bond in β-lactam ring
Kanamycin (kan)	Kanamycin acetyltransferase*	N-acetylation of the antibiotic
Neomycin (neo)	Aminogycoside phosphotransferase*	O-phosphorylation of the antibiotic
Streptomycin (str)	Streptomycin phosphotransferase	Phosphorylation of OH on the antibiotic
	Streptomycin adenylate synthetase	Adenylation of the OH on the antibiotic.

*The antibiotics kanamycin and neomycin are related; hence neo product also inactivates kanamycin, and *kan* product inactivates neomycin as well.

Selection of Recombinant Vectors

It may be pointed out that when an experiment is performed to insert a DNA fragment into a vector, two types of vector molecules are obtained: (i) many vector molecules will contain the DNA insert (recombinant or chimaeric vector), but (ii) many others will contain only the vector sequences (unaltered vector or simply vector). This mixture of vector molecules is used for transformation of host cells: (i) some host cells will receive the recombinant vector, (ii) some others will contain the normal unaltered vector, while (iii) the majority of them will contain no vector, i.e. will not be transformed. In a cloning experiment it is critical to effectively select for the low frequency of cells transformed by the recombinant vector from among the cells containing the unaltered vector and the nontransformed cells.

Selection of host cells transformed by the recombinant vector is easily achieved by placing two selectable makers, e.g. antibiotic resistance genes, such as, ampicillin resistance (amp^r) and tetracycline resistance (tet^r), in the vector. The DNA insert is integrated within one of the two selectable markers. If the DNA insert is integrated within the ampicillin resistance gene, the cells containing the recombinant vector will be resistant to tetracycline but sensitive to ampicillin. In contrast, nontransformed cells will be sensitive to both the antibiotics, while those containing the unaltered vector will be resistant to both. Therefore, following transformation with the above recombinant vector, cells are plated on a tetracycline supplemented medium; this eliminates the nontransformed cells.

The remaining colonies are now replica-plated on ampicillin containing medium to identify sensitive colonies; these colonies contain the recombinant vector, and are isolated from the master plate. Further, transformed cells tend to lose the recombinant vector, since cells lacking such vectors divide much faster. The use of a vector having two selectable markers allows the maintenance of cells containing the recombinant vector on antibiotic medium (tetracycline in the above case) which eliminates the vector-free cells produced during culture.

pSC101

This earliest plasmid vector contains the replication module (*ori*) for replication in *E. coli*, tet^r gene for resistance to tetracycline and single recognition sites for restriction endonucleases *Eco*RI (outside tet^r gene), *Hind*III, *Bam*HI and *Sal*I (within the tet^r gene; Fig. 2.5). Insertion of DNA insert into the *Eco*RI site leaves the tet^r gene intact and functional; as a result, *E. coli* cells transformed by pSC101 become tetracycline resistant but such cells may either have a nonrecombinant pSC101 (without the DNA insert) or a recombinant one (having the DNA insert). On the other hand, insertion of the DNA fragment into the *Hind*III, *Bam*HI or *Sal*I sites disrupts the tet^r gene and makes it nonfunctional. Therefore, cells transformed by such a recombinant pSC101 are sensitive to tetracycline and hence can be easily distinguished from those containing the nonrecombinant plasmid which are resistant to the antibiotic. But nontransformed cells too are tetracycline sensitive hence they can not be separated from those having the recombinant pSC101.

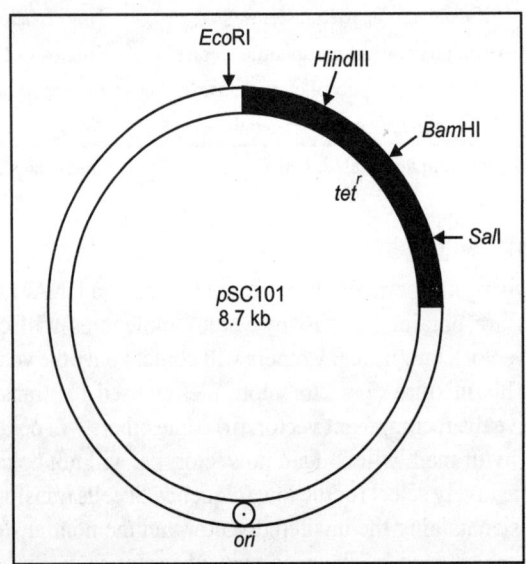

Fig. 2.5. Structural features of pSC101. The open circle denotes the replication module, tet^r specifies tetracycline resistance, while EcoRI, $Hind$III , BamHI and SalI represent the recognition sites for these restriction enzymes.

Clearly pSC101 does not permit a direct selection of cells containing the recombinant vector. In addition, it contains unnecessary DNA, and has stringent regulation of replication. Subsequently, several novel plasmid vectors were designed to overcome these deficiencies.

pBR322

An ideal plasmid vector must have the following functions: (i) minimum amount of DNA, (ii) relaxed replication control, (iii) atleast two selectable markers, (iv) only one (unique) recognition site for atleast one restriction endonuclease, and (v) for easy selection of the recombinant vector, this unique restriction site must be located within one of the two selectable markers. Almost all such vectors have been constructed from naturally occurring DNA sequences using both classical genetic (recombination) and recombinant DNA techniques.

The name pBR denotes the following: p signifies plasmid, B is from Boliver, and R is from Rodriguez, the two scientists who developed pBR322. Some other plasmid names derive from the names of the places they were developed at, e.g. pUC gets its name from University of California. pBR322 is the most popular and most widely used plasmid of 4362 bp. Its entire base sequence is known. It has the replication module of $E. coli$ plasmid Col E1. This module has been incorporated in many other plasmid vectors since it permits plasmid replication even when chromosome replication and cell division are inhibited by amino acid starvation or chloramphemicol; as a result under such conditions, each cell accumulates several thousand copies of the plasmid so that one litre of bacterial culture easily yields a milligram of plasmid DNA. It has two selectable markers (tetracycline, tet^r, and ampicillin, amp^r, resistance genes), and only single or unique recognition sites for 12 different restriction enzymes (two, *Pst*I and *Pvu*I, located within the *amp^r* gene, and 4, e.g. *Bam*HI, *Sal*I, etc. within *tet^r* gene) (Fig. 2.6).

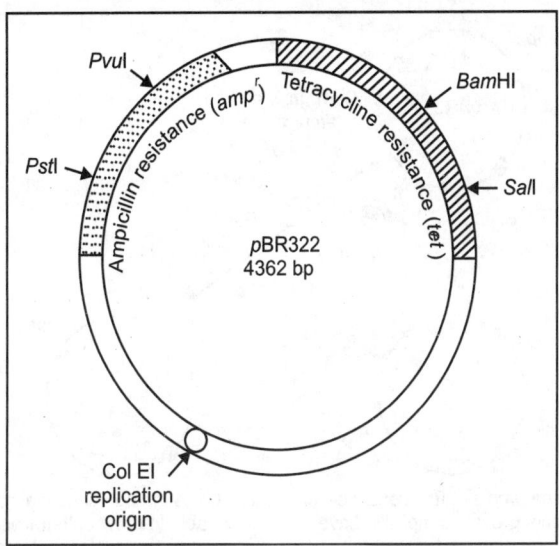

Fig. 2.6. Structural features of *p*BR322. Col E1 origin of replication allows production of multiple copies per cell, and the two resistance markers (*tet^r* and *amp^r*) allow easy selection of the recombinant vectors.

The presence of restriction sites within the markers *tet^r* and amp permits an 'easy selection for cells transformed with the recombinant *p*BR322. Insertion of the DNA fragment into the plasmid using restriction enzyme *Pst*I or *Pvu*I, places the DNA insert within the gene *amp^r* and thus makes it nonfunctional. Bacterial cells containing such a recombinant *p*BR322 will be unable to grow in the presence of ampicillin, but will grow on tetracycline. Similarly, when restriction enzyme. *Bam*HI or *Sal*I is used, the DNA insert is placed within the gene *tet^r* making it nonfunctional. Bacterial cells possessing such a recombinant pBR322 will, therefore, grow on ampicillin but not on tetracycline (Fig. 2.7). This feature allows an easy selection of a single bacterial cell having recombinant *p*BR322 from among 10^8 other types of cells.

Transformed *E. coli* cells are first plated on an agar medium containing the antibiotic within the resistance gene for which the DNA fragment is not inserted, i.e. for which the bacterial cells having the recombinant plasmid are expected to be resistant. This eliminates nontransformed bacterial cells; the resulting bacterial colonies will posses either recombinant or unaltered *p*BR322. The colonies so obtained are then replica-plated on agar plates containing the other antibiotic (within the gene for which the DNA insert is placed); all the colonies that develop on this plate will contain the unaltered *p*BR322. Therefore, the antibiotic sensitive colonies are identified and recovered from the master plate; these colonies will have the recombinant *p*BR322. This entire process may take 1–2 days.

*p*BR322 has a *nic-bom* (*bom* = basis of mobility) region which is responsible for its mobilisation. Mobilisation refers to the cell to cell transfer of an otherwise nonconjugative plasmid in the presence of a conjugative plasmid inside the same cell as the former. The *nic-bom* region also interferes with replication efficiency of extrachromosomal DNA in monkey cells; such prokaryotic sequences are called poison sequences. The poison sequence of *p*BR322 has been deleted to yield *p*BR327 (deletion between bases 1442 and 2502 of *p*BR322) and *p*ATl53 (deletion between bases 1644 and 2345). These modified plasmids are used to construct shuttle vectors for *E. coli* and monkey cells; they also produce three times as many copies per *E. coli* cell as the parent *p*BR322.

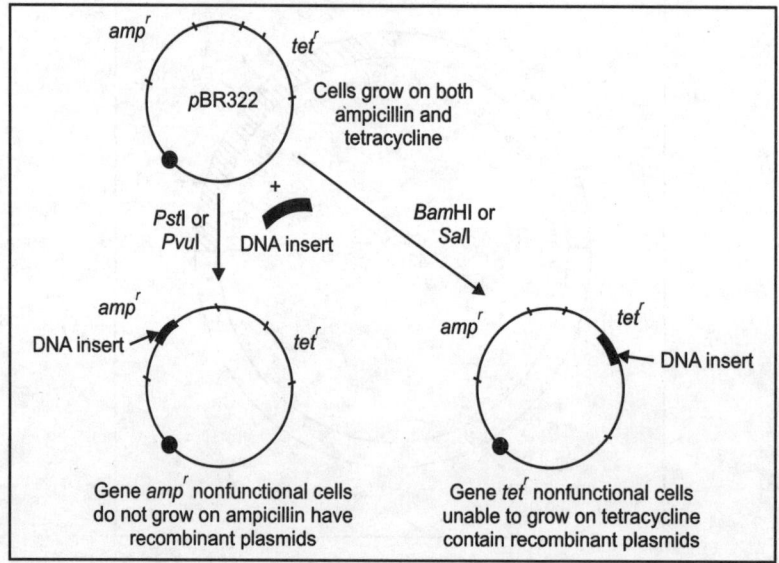

Fig. 2.7. The consequences of insertion of a DNA fragment within *amp*[r] or *tet*[r] gene or *p*BR322. Cells containing the recombinant vector are resistant to only one antibiotic, they are not resistant to the antibiotic within the marker gene for which the DNA insert is integrated. In contrast, nontransformed cells are sensitive to both the antibiotics, while those transformed by the unaltered *p*BR322 are resistant to both ampicillin and tetracycline.

*p*UC7

It is a derivative of *p*BR322 and is much smaller (2.7 kb); it has all the essential parts of *p*BR322, e.g. (i) ampicillin resistance gene, and (ii) Col E1 origin. The second scrobale marker is due to *E. coli* gene *lacZ*α encoding the α fragment of β-galactosidase, the enzyme that hydrolyses galactose. The *E. coli* strains, e.g. JM103, JM109, used as hosts for the *p*UC series vectors have the *lacZ*α deleted from their lac operons. When *p*UC enters such an *E. coli* cell, the host genome and the plasmid encode for different parts of the β-galactosidase enzyme which interact with each other to produce the active enzyme enabling these cells to hydrolyse galactose. β-galactosidase also hydrolyses X-gal (5-Bromo-4-chloro-3-indolyl-β-D-galactoside) to yield a blue dye. Therefore appropriate *lacZ*⁻ *E. coli* cells transformed by the *p*UC vectors behave as *lacZ*⁺ and produce blue coloured colonies on a X-gal containing medium. A polylinker sequence located within the *lacZ*α provides several unique restriction sites for DNA insertion. The polylinker sequence by itself does not interfere with *lacZ*α expression, but when a DNA insert is placed within it *lacZ*α expression is prevented.

The unique restriction sites used for integration of DNA inserts into *p*UC vectors interrupt the *lacZ*α fragment so that appropriate *E. coli* cells possessing recombinant *p*UC vectors are β-galactosidase deficient and, as a result, produce white colonies on X-gal medium. Therefore, appropriate *E. coli* cells transformed with *p*UC vectors are first grown on ampicillin containing medium to eliminate nontransformed cells. The colonies so obtained are replica-plated on X-gal containing medium; the white colonies are selected as they contain the recombinant vector (in contrast, blue colonies will contain the unaltered vector). The other vectors in *p*UC series are *p*UC 8, *p*UC 9, *p*UC 12, *p*UC 13, etc.

Cosmid

A cosmid, is a type of hybrid plasmid (often used as a cloning vector) that contains *cos* sequences, DNA sequences originally from the Lambda phage. Cosmids can be used to build genomic libraries. Cosmids are able to contain 37 to 52 kb of DNA, while normal plasmids are able to carry only 1–20 kb. They can replicate as plasmids if they have a suitable origin of replication: for example SV40 ori in mammalian cells, *Col*E1 ori for double-stranded DNA replication or f1 ori for single-stranded DNA replication in prokaryotes. They frequently also contain a gene for selection such as antibiotic resistance, so that the transfected cells can be identified by plating on a medium containing the antibiotic. Those cells which did not take up the cosmid would be unable to grow. Unlike plasmids, they can also be packaged in phage capsids, which allows the foreign genes to be transferred into or between cells by transduction. Plasmids become unstable after a certain amount of DNA has been inserted into them, because their increased size is more conducive to recombination. To circumvent this, phage transduction is used instead. This is made possible by the cohesive ends, also known as *cos* sites. In this way, they are similar to using the lambda phage as a vector, but only that all the lambda genes have been deleted with the exception of the *cos* sequence.

Cos sequences are ~200 base pairs long and essential for packaging. They contain a *cosN* site where DNA is nicked at each strand, 12bp apart, by terminase. This causes linearisation of the circular cosmid with two 'cohesive' or 'sticky ends' of 12bp. (The DNA must be linear to fit into a phage head.) The *cosB* site holds the terminase while it is nicking and separating the strands. The *cosQ* site of next cosmid (as rolling circle replication often results in linear concatemers) is held by the terminase after the previous cosmid has been packaged, to prevent degradation by cellular DNases.

Cosmid features and uses

Cosmids are predominantly plasmids with a bacterial *oriV*, an antibiotic selection marker and a cloning site, but they carry one, or more recently two *cos* sites derived from bacteriophage lambda. Depending on the particular aim of the experiment broad host range cosmids, shuttle cosmids or 'mammalian' cosmids (linked to SV40 oriV and mammalian selection markers) are available. The loading capacity of cosmids varies depending on the size of the vector itself but usually lies around 40–45 kb. The cloning procedure involves the generation of two vector arms which are then joined to the foreign DNA. Selection against wildtype cosmid DNA is simply done via size exclusion. Cosmids, however, always form colonies and not plaques. Also the clone density is much lower with around 105–106 CFU per µg of ligated DNA.

After the construction of recombinant lambda or cosmid libraries the total DNA is transferred into an appropriate *E. coli* host via a technique called *in vitro* packaging. The necessary packaging extracts are derived from *E. coli* cI857 lysogens (red- gam- Sam and Dam (head assembly) and Eam (tail assembly) respectively). These extracts will recognise and package the recombinant molecules *in vitro*, generating either mature phage particles (lambda-based vectors) or recombinant plasmids contained in phage shells (cosmids). These differences are reflected in the different infection frequencies seen in favour of lambda-replacement vectors. This compensates for their slightly lower loading capacity. Phage library are also stored and screened easier than cosmid (colonies) libraries.

Target DNA: the genomic DNA to be cloned has to be cut into the appropriate size range of restriction fragments. This is usually done by partial restriction followed by either size fractionation or dephosphorylation (using calf-intestine phosphatase) in order to avoid chromosome scrambling, i.e. the ligation of physically unlinked fragments.

Molecular Tool: Electroporation

Electroporation is a mechanical method used to introduce polar molecules into a host cell through the cell membrane. In this procedure, a large electric pulse temporarily disturbs the phospholipid bilayer, allowing molecules like DNA to pass into the cell.

Many research techniques in molecular biology require a foreign gene or protein material to be inserted into a host cell. Since the phospholipid bilayer of the plasma membrane has a hydrophobic exterior and a hydrophobic interior (Fig. 2.8), any polar molecules, including DNA and protein, are unable to freely pass through the membrane.

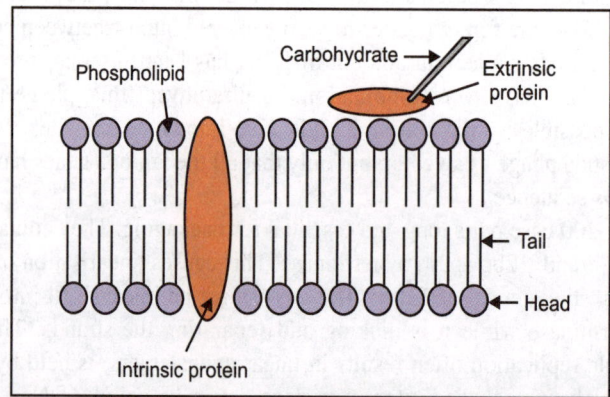

Fig. 2.8. Diagram of the Phospholipid Bilayer. This image shows the chemical components of the plasma membrane. The polar head groups face outward while the hydrophobic tail groups face inward and interact with one another to hold the membrane together. Polar molecules cannot pass through this membrane without external aid.

Many methods have been developed to surpass this barrier and allow the insertion of DNA and other molecules into the cells to be studied. One such method is electroporation. The concept of electroporation capitalises on the relatively weak nature of the phospholipid bilayer's hydrophobic/hydrophilic interactions and its ability to spontaneously reassemble after disturbance. Thus, a quick voltage shock may disrupt areas of the membrane temporarily, allowing polar molecules to pass, but then the membrane may reseal quickly and leave the cell intact.

Procedure

The host cells and the molecules to be inserted into these cells are suspended in solution. The electroporation apparatus is typically commercially produced and purchased, but the basic process inside such an apparatus may be represented in a schematic diagram (Fig. 2.9). When the first switch is closed, the capacitor charges up and stores a high voltage. When the second switch is closed, this voltage discharges through the liquid of the cell suspension. Typically, 10,000–100,000 V/cm (varying with cell size) in a pulse lasting a few microseconds to a millisecond is necessary for electroporation. This electric pulse disturbs the phospholipid bilayer of the membrane and causes the formation of temporary aqueous pores.

The electric potential across the membrane of the cell simultaneously rises by about 0.5–1.0 V so that charged molecules (such as DNA) are driven across the membrane through the pores in a manner similar to electrophoresis. As charged ions and molecules flow through the pores, the cell membrane discharges and the pores quickly close, and the phospholipid bilayer reassembles. The intended molecules should now be inside the cell for further use or study.

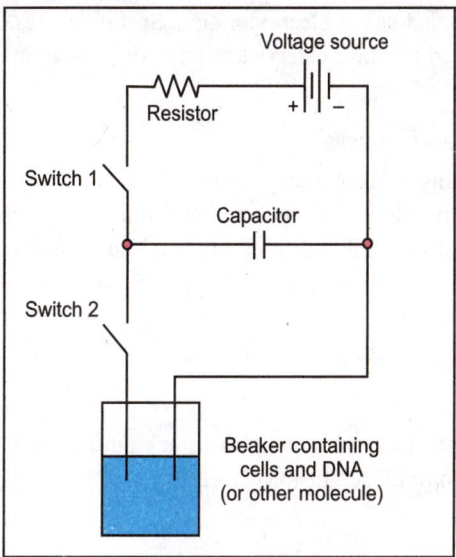

Fig. 2.9. Diagram of the basic circuit setup of the electroporation apparatus. This diagram shows the basic electric circuit that provides the voltage for electroporation.

Advantages and disadvantages of electroporation

Several methods other than electroporation are used to transfer polar molecules like DNA into host cells. These other methods include microprecipitates, microinjection, liposomes, and biological vectors. Electroporation has both advantages and disadvantages compared to these methods.

Advantages

1. Versatility: Electroporation is effective with nearly all cell and species types.
2. Efficiency: A large majority of cells take in the target DNA or molecule. In a study on electrotransformation of *E. coli*, for example, 80 per cent of the cells received the foreign DNA.
3. Small Scale: The amount of DNA required is smaller than for other methods.
4. *In vivo*: The procedure may be performed with intact tissue.

Disadvantages

1. Cell damage: If the pulses are of the wrong length or intensity, some pores may become too large or fail to close after membrane discharge causing cell damage or rupture.
2. Nonspecific transport: The transport of material into and out of the cell during the time of electropermeability is relatively nonspecific. This may result in an ion imbalance that could later lead to improper cell function and cell death.

Applications

As previously mentioned, electroporation is widely used in many areas of molecular biology research and in the medical field.

Some applications of electroporation include:

DNA transfection or transformation

This is likely the most widespread use of electroporation. Specific genes can be cloned into a plasmid and then this plasmid introduced into host cells (bacterial or otherwise) in order to investigate gene and protein structure and function.

Direct transfer of plasmids between cells

Bacterial cells already containing a plasmid may be incubated with another strain that does not contain plasmids but that has some other desireable feature. The voltage of electroporation will create pores, allowing some plasmids to exit one cell and enter another. The desired cells may then be selected by antibiotic resistance or another similar method. This type of transfer may also be performed between species. Thus, large numbers of plasmids may be grown in rapidly multiplying bacterial colonies and then transferred to yeast cells by electroporation for study.

Induced cell fusion

The disruption of the membrane that occurs with the quick pulse of electricity in the electroporation procedure has also been shown to induce fusion of cells.

Trans-dermal drug delivery

Just as electroporation causes temporary pores to form in plasma membranes, studies suggest that similar pores form in lipid bilayers of the stratum corneum the outermost dead layer of skin. These pores could allow drugs to pass through to the skin to a target tissue. This method of drug delivery would be more pleasant than injection for the patient (not requiring a needle) and could avoid the problems of improper absorption or degradation of oral medication in the digestive system.

Cancer tumour electrochemotherapy

Scientists are investigating the potential of electroporation to increase the effectiveness of chemotherapy. As in electroporation for DNA transfection, the applied electrical pulse would disrupt the membrane of the tumour cell and increase the amount of drug delivered to the site. Some studies have suggested that increased tumour reduction is seen when this method is applied to cancerous cells in animal model systems.

Gene therapy

Much like drug delivery, electroporation techniques can allow vectors containing important genes to be transported across the skin and into the target tissue. Once incorporated into the cells of the body, the protein produced from this gene could replace a defective one and thus treat a genetic disorder (Fig. 2.10).

Bacterial Conjugation

Bacterial conjugation is the transfer of genetic material between bacterial cells by direct cell-to-cell contact or through a bridge-like connection between two cells. Discovered in 1946 by Joshua Lederberg and Edward Tatum, conjugation is a mechanism of horizontal gene transfer as are transformation and transduction although these mechanisms do not involve cell-to-cell contact.

Bacterial conjugation is often incorrectly regarded as the bacterial equivalent of sexual reproduction or mating since it involves the exchange of genetic material. During conjugation the donor cell provides a conjugative or mobilisable genetic element that is most often a plasmid or transposon. Most conjugative plasmids have systems ensuring that the recipient cell does not already contain a similar element.

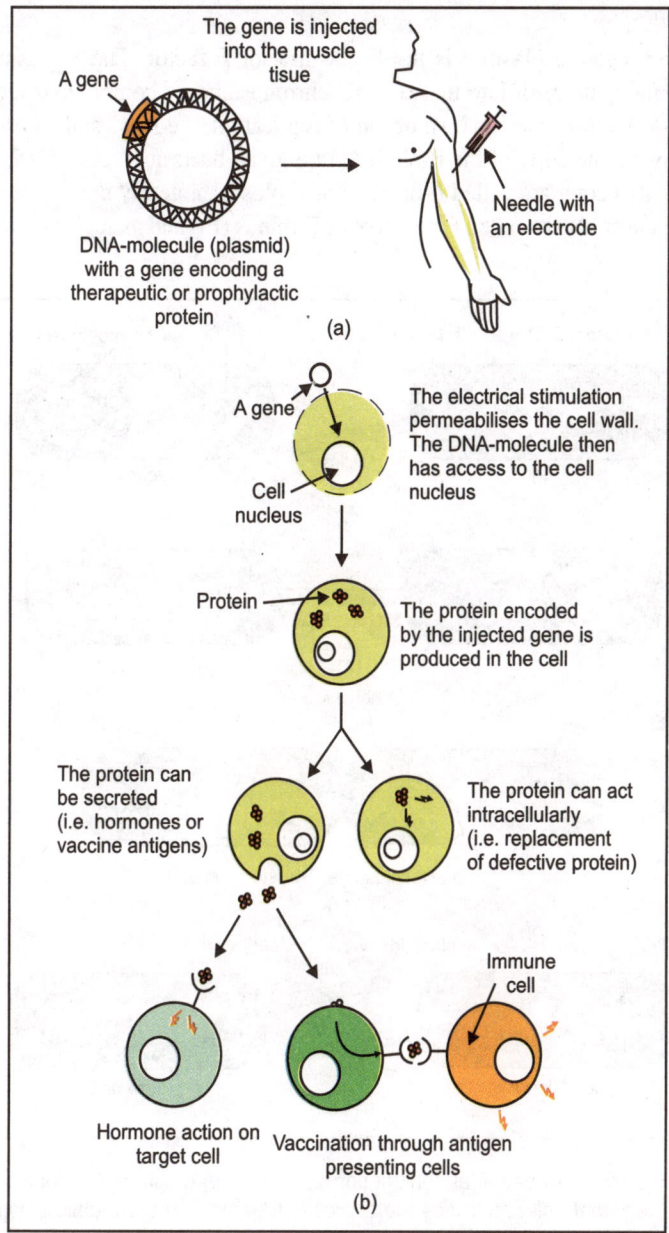

Fig. 2.10. Diagram of the method of gene therapy using electroporation.

The genetic information transferred is often beneficial to the recipient cell. Benefits may include antibiotic resistance, xenobiotic tolerance or the ability to use new metabolites. Such beneficial plasmids may be considered bacterial endosymbionts.

Other elements, however, may be viewed as bacterial parasites and conjugation as a mechanism evolved by them to allow for their spread.

Mechanism

The prototypical conjugative plasmid is the F-plasmid, or F-factor. The F-plasmid is an episome (a plasmid that can integrate itself into the bacterial chromosome by homologous recombination) with a length of about 100 kb. It carries its own origin of replication, the *oriV*, and an origin of transfer, or *oriT*. There can only be one copy of the F-plasmid in a given bacterium, either free or integrated, and bacterium that possess a copy are called F-positive or F-plus (denoted F$^+$).

Cells that lack F plasmids are called F-negative or F-minus (F$^-$) and as such can function as recipient cells (Fig. 2.11).

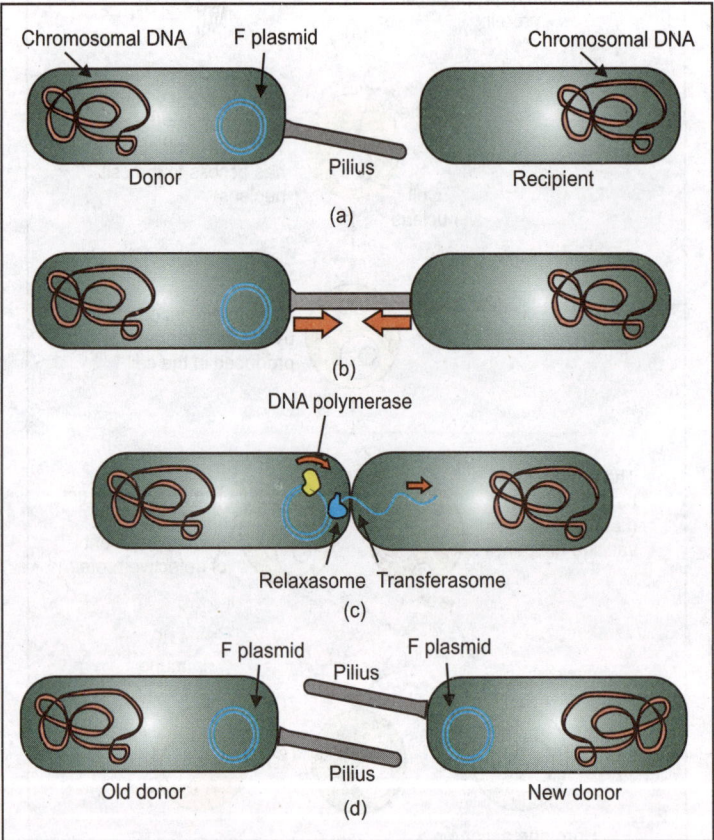

Fig. 2.11. Schematic drawing of bacterial conjugation. Conjugation diagram: (a) donor cell produces pilus, (b) pilus attaches to recipient cell and brings the two cells together, (c) the mobile plasmid is nicked and a single strand of DNA is then transferred to the recipient cell, and (d) both cells synthesise a complementary strand to produce a double stranded circular plasmid and also reproduce pili; both cells are now viable donors.

Among other genetic information the F-plasmid carries a *tra* and *trb* locus, which together are about 33 kb long and consist of about 40 genes.

The *tra* locus includes the *pilin* gene and regulatory genes, which together form pili on the cell surface. The locus also includes the genes for the proteins that attach themselves to the surface of F⁻ bacteria and initiate conjugation. Though there is some debate on the exact mechanism of conjugation it seems that the pili are not the structures through which DNA exchange occurs. This has been shown in experiments where the pilus are allowed to make contact, but then are denatured with SDS and yet DNA transformation still proceeds. Several proteins coded for in the *tra* or *trb* locus seem to open a channel between the bacteria and it is thought that the *traD* enzyme, located at the base of the pilus, initiates membrane fusion.

When conjugation is initiated by a signal the relaxase enzyme creates a nick in one of the strands of the conjugative plasmid at the *oriT*. Relaxase may work alone or in a complex of over a dozen proteins known collectively as a relaxosome. In the F-plasmid system the relaxase enzyme is called *TraI* and the relaxosome consists of *TraI*, *TraY*, *TraM* and the integrated host factor IHF. The nicked strand, or T-strand, is then unwound from the unbroken strand and transferred to the recipient cell in a 5′-terminus to 3′-terminus direction.

The remaining strand is replicated either independent of conjugative action (vegetative replication beginning at the *oriV*) or in concert with conjugation (conjugative replication similar to the rolling circle replication of lambda phage). Conjugative replication may require a second nick before successful transfer can occur. A recent report claims to have inhibited conjugation with chemicals that mimic an intermediate step of this second nicking event.

If the F-plasmid that is transferred has previously been integrated into the donor's genome some of the donor's chromosomal DNA may also be transferred with the plasmid DNA. The amount of chromosomal DNA that is transferred depends on how long the two conjugating bacteria remain in contact. In common laboratory strains of *E. coli* the transfer of the entire bacterial chromosome takes about 100 minutes. The transferred DNA can then be integrated into the recipient genome via homologous recombination.

A cell culture that contains in its population cells with non-integrated F-plasmids usually also contains a few cells that have accidentally integrated their plasmids. It is these cells that are responsible for the low-frequency chromosomal gene transfers that occur in such cultures. Some strains of bacteria with an integrated F-plasmid can be isolated and grown in pure culture. Because such strains transfer chromosomal genes very efficiently they are called *Hfr* (high frequency of recombination). The *E. coli* genome was originally mapped by interrupted mating experiments in which various *Hfr* cells in the process of conjugation were sheared from recipients after less than 100 minutes (initially using a Waring blender). The genes that were transferred were then investigated.

Inter-kingdom transfer

The nitrogen fixing *Rhizobia* are an interesting case of inter-kingdom conjugation. For example, the tumour-inducing (Ti) plasmid of *Agrobacterium* and the root-tumour inducing (Ri) plasmid of *A. rhizogenes* contain genes that are capable of transferring to plant cells. The expression of these genes effectively transforms the plant cells into opine-producing factories. Opines are used by the bacteria as sources of nitrogen and energy. Infected cells form crown gall or root tumours, respectively. The Ti and Ri plasmids are thus endosymbionts of the bacteria, which are in turn endosymbionts (or parasites) of the infected plant.

The Ti and Ri plasmids can also be transferred between bacteria using a system (the *tra*, or transfer, operon) that is different and independent of the system used for inter-kingdom transfer (the *vir*, or virulence, operon). Such transfers create virulent strains from previously avirulent strains.

Genetic engineering applications

Conjugation is a convenient means for transferring genetic material to a variety of targets. In laboratories successful transfers have been reported from bacteria to yeast, plants, mammalian cells and isolated mammalian mitochondria. Conjugation has advantages over other forms of genetic transfer including minimal disruption of the target's cellular envelope and the ability to transfer relatively large amounts of genetic material. In plant engineering, *Agrobacterium*-like conjugation complements other standard vehicles such as tobacco mosaic virus (TMV). While TMV is capable of infecting many plant families, these are primarily herbaceous dicots. *Agrobacterium*-like conjugation is also primarily used for dicots, but monocot recipients are not uncommon.

Chapter 3

Molecular Research Procedures

INTRODUCTION

DNA can be synthesised artificially in a test tube by chemical process instead of using biological synthesis. The process of synthesising a short stretch of DNA by using a chemical reaction is called as chemical DNA method. Machines that automate the chemical reaction involved in DNA synthesis which can synthesise a single strand, when the sequence and chemicals are provided, are called as gene machines or DNA synthesisers. A DNA synthesiser consists of a set of valves and pumps that are programmed to introduce specific nucleotides and the reagents required for the coupling of each consecutive nucleotide to the growing chain. Chemical DNA synthesis does not follow the biological direction of DNA synthesis.

In the chemical process each incoming DNA is added to the 5′-hydroxyl terminus of the growing chain. These processes of adding are controlled by computer and are carried in a single reaction vessel that is a column, so that reagents from one reaction step can be readily washed away before the reagents for the next step are added and the reagents can be used in excess to drive the reactions as close as possible to compilation.

CHEMICAL SYNTHESIS OF GENE

The amino acid sequence of the protein (or the base sequence of mRNA) produced by a gene enables the deduction of base sequence of the concerned gene on the basis of the codons for the various amino acids. However, the degeneracy of genetic code may present some problems but a functional sequence of the gene can nonetheless be worked out. Once the base sequence of a gene is deduced, a polynucleotide of the same base sequence can be synthesised either (i) chemically, or even (ii) enzymatically.

The chemical synthesis of a gene utilises chemical reagents for the various steps of the process. There are three distinct methods, differing mainly in the strategy of protection of OH groups of the phosphate residues: (i) phosphodiester approach, (ii) phosphotriester or phosphate triester approach, and (iii) phosphite triester or phosphoramidite approach.

Phosphodiester Approach

The first significant success was achieved by Smith and coworkers who synthesised the gene for alanine (suppressor) tRNA of yeast in 1970, while Brown and coworkers synthesised the gene for tyrosine (suppressor) tRNA of *E. coli*. In this method, 3′ and 5′ OH groups of the deoxyribose moiety of nucleosides are suitably blocked or protected; they are selectively unblocked for joining of the additional nucleotides.

This approach has now been almost completely replaced by the more convenient approaches (described below) since it presents a variety of solubility problems.

Phosphotriester Approach

Both phosphotriester and the phosphite triester methods utilise deoxyribonucleosides as starting materials, and involve the stepwise addition of mononucleotides and oligonucleotides. The amino groups of nucleosides deoxyadenosine and deoxcytidine are usually benzoylated, and that on deoxyguanosine is protected by an isobutyryl group (Fig. 3.1); thymidine requires no protection. The 5′ OR group is protected by dimethoxytrityl (Fig. 3.2) commonly abbreviated as DMTr or $(MeO)_2$ Tr (Table 3.1). The amino groups of the bases are freed by mild alkaline hydrolysis, while $(MeO)_2$ Tr is removed by gentle acid hydrolysis. These steps are common to both phosphotriester and phosphite triester approaches.

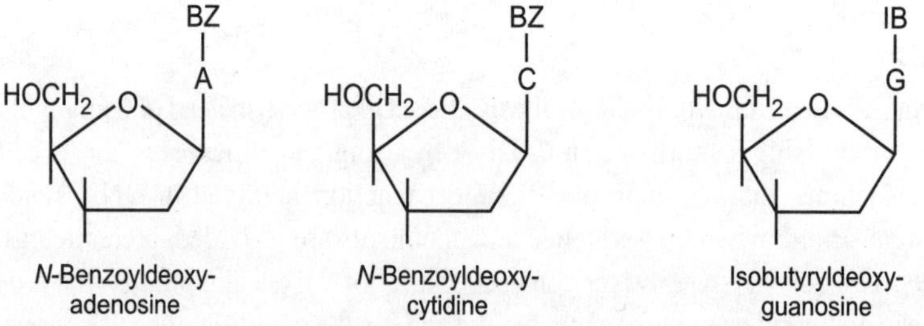

Fig. 3.1. Protection of the amino groups of nucleosides (thymine needs no protection). Bz = Benzoyl group, IB = Isobutyryl group (attached to the free amino groups of DNA bases).

Table 3.1. Agents used for the protection and deprotection of different reactive groups of nucleotides used in chemical synthesis of DNA.

Protected group	Protected by	Ptotecting group removed by
Both phosphotriester and phosphite triester approaches		
The free —NH_2 group of		
Deoxyadenosine	Benzoate	Mild alkaline hydrolysis
Deoxycytidine	Benzoate	Mild alkaline hydrolysis
Deoxyguanosine	Isobutyrate	Mild alkaline hydrolysis
Thymidine	Not required	Not required
Hydroxyl groups of		
Deoxyribose: 5′ OH	Dimethoxytrityl [$(MeO)_2Tr$] or DMTr	Gentle acid hydrolysis by benzene sulphonic acid or $ZnBr_2$
Phosphotriester approach only		
Phosphorylation by OH group of phosphate	p-chlorophenyl- phosphorodichloridate	Not done
	β-cyanoethanol	Triethyl amine

In phosphotriester approach, the 3′ OH is coupled with a suitable phosphorylating agent, say, p-chlorophenylphosphorodichloridate; the phosphate residue has a free OH group (Fig. 3.3) which accepts any nucleotide or oliogonucleotide with a free 5′ OH group. Therefore, such protected nucleotides have phosphodiesters and serve as the 5′-terminus residue in oligonucleotide synthesis.

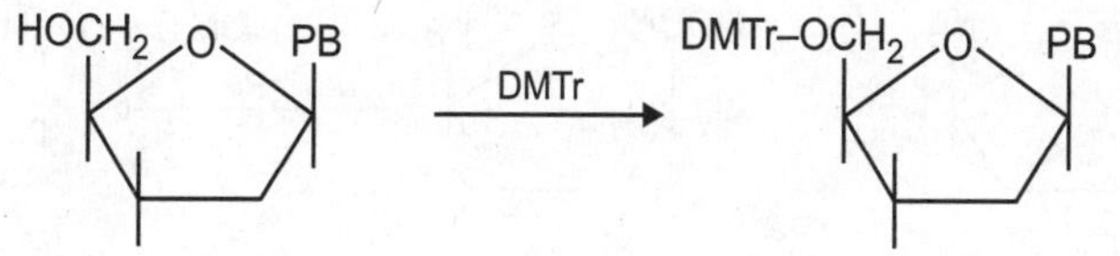

Fig. 3.2. Protection of the 5' OH by addition of dimethoxytrityl (DMTr). PB = amino group protected base.

Such protected and phosphorylated nucleotides are further modified to make them suitable for joining to the OH group of the 3' phosphate residue. The OH group of the 3' phosphate residue of such nucleotides is blocked by a suitable agent, e.g. β-cyanoethanol, following which the 5' OH is freed by mild acid hydrolysis (this removes the $(MeO)_2$ Tr. This yields phosphotriester nucleotides which have a free 5'OH (Fig. 3.3).

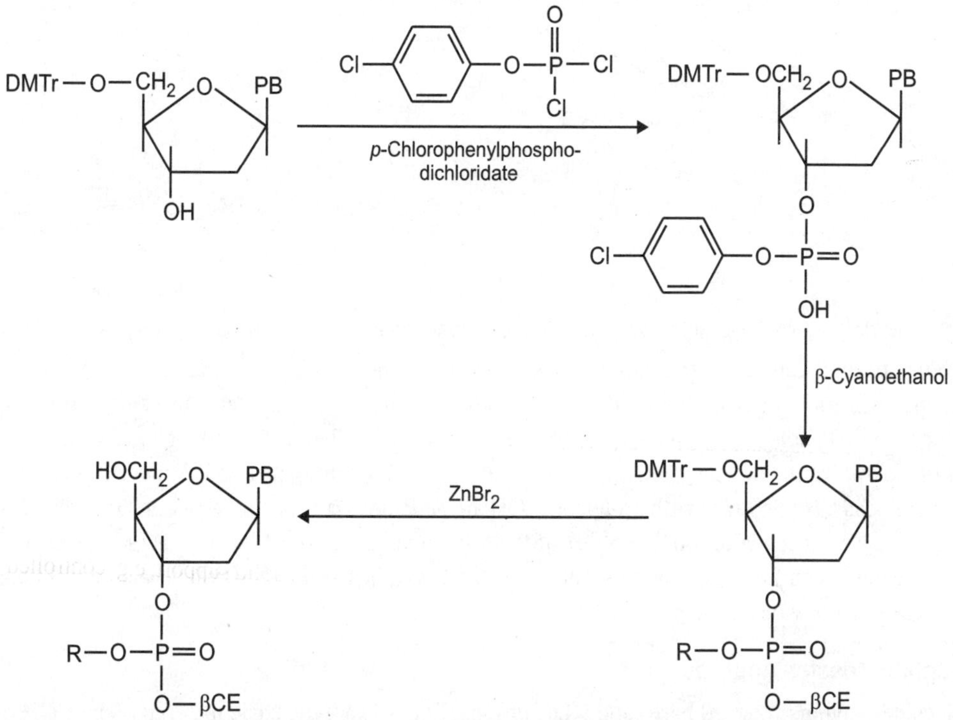

Fig. 3.3. Phosphorylation of the 5' protected nucleoside to yield phosphodiester. β-cyanoethanol (βCE) protects the free OH of phosphate to yield a triester. Finally, the 5' OH is freed by gentle acid hydrolysis.

A desired diester nucleotide (free OH at 3' phosphate residue) is now mixed with the desired triester nucleotide, and agents that promote their coupling are added to the mixture. Coupling is promoted by arylsulfonyl compounds, e.g. tri-isopropyl-benzenesulfonyl chloride (TPS). This reaction yields a fully protected dinucleotide (Fig. 3.4), which can be either fully unprotected, or may be selectively unprotected to be used as the starting material for construction of larger molecules. The 5' OH of a dinucleotide is selectively freed by hydrolysis with an acid like benzenesulfonic acid or $ZnBr_2$, while the OH group of 3' phosphate is freed by preferential removal of the cyanoethyl ester by using triethylamine. Two dinucleotides, one having a free 5' OH and the other having a free OH at the 3' phosphate, may thus be coupled together to yield a tetranucleotide and so on. The DNA chains can be constructed either in 3' → 5' or 5' → 3' direction.

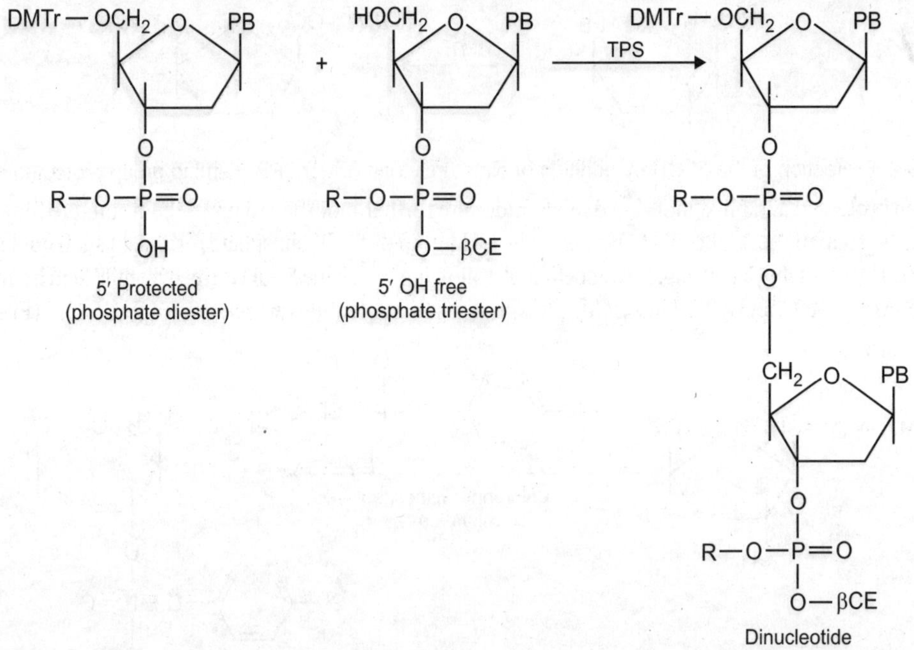

Fig. 3.4. Linking of two nucleotides by TPS (triisopropylbenzenesulphonyl chloride) to yield a dinucleotide.

Tedius purifications are essential after every addition to the growing chain to remove the uncoupled mononucleotides/oligonucleotides. This and some other problems are eliminated by using a solid support to which the first nucleotide is fixed. Somehow fixing the 3'OH is better than fixing the 5'OH; generally, this is done by forming on ester between the 3'OH and a carboxyl group on a solid support, e.g. controlled pore glass beads. Nucleotides with protected 5'OH are added one by one and are coupled to the growing chain. In between each addition, the 5'OH of the growing chain is freed by mild acid hydrolysis. This procedure has been adopted for automated stepwise synthesis; a 10–20 nucleotide long chain is synthesised in a few days.

Phosphite Triester Approach

Nucleosides having protected bases and 5'OH groups (Fig. 3.1) are the basic materials. The 3'OH of the terminal nucleotide is fixed to a solid support and, then, its 5'OH is freed by gentle acid hydrolysis (Fig. 3.5).

The subsequent nucleotides are used as 3'-phosphoramidities, which are readily produced by coupling the nucleotides with di-isopropylammonium tetrazolide. The phosphoramidites are stable and efficient coupling agents, and are readily synthesised.

The desired nucleotide 3'-phosphoramidite is now added and is activated for coupling by the addition of tetrazole; the immediate product is a phosphite, which is oxidised to phosphate by iodine (I_2). This phosphate remains as a triester (Fig. 3.5). The 5'OH of the second nucleotide is now freed, and the third desired nucleotide 3'-phosphoramidite is added and joined to the growing chain. In this manner, the oligo-nucleotide chain is elongated. Finally, the various protective groups are removed and the chain is freed from the solid support by alkaline hydrolysis.

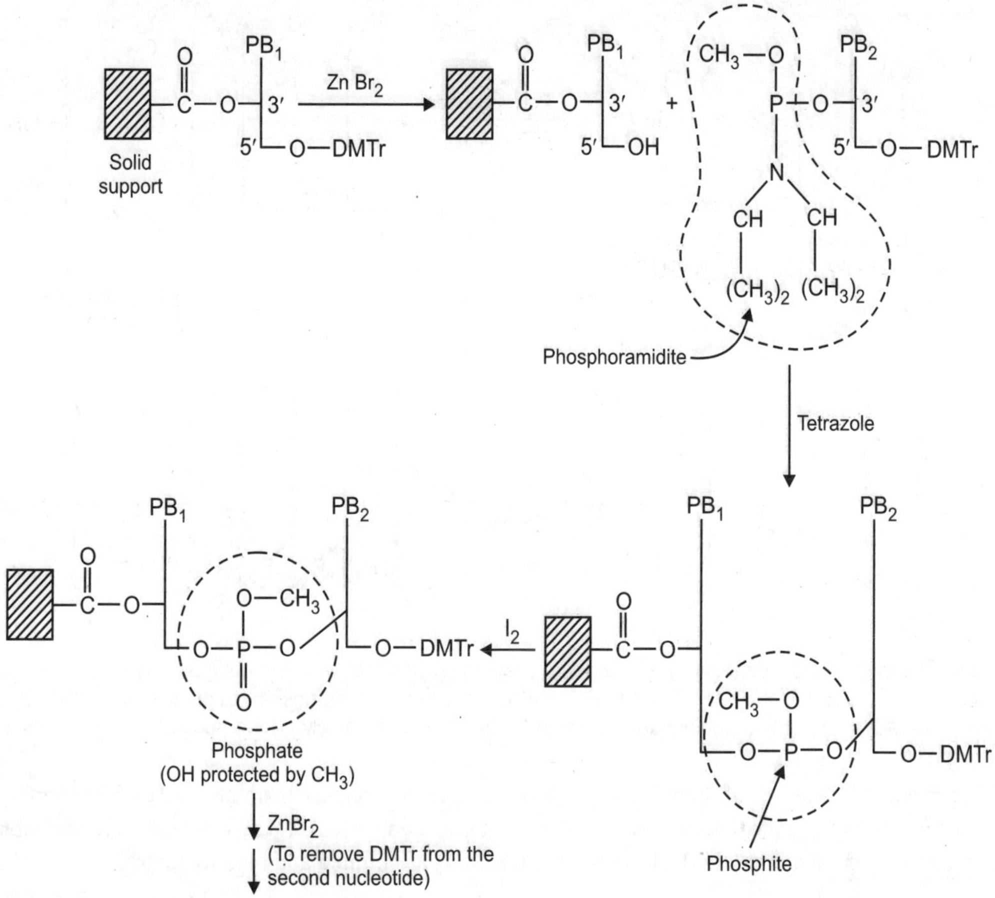

Fig. 3.5. The phosphate triester approach to oligonucleotide synthesis. Phosphoramidite may be depicted as CH_3—O — P—O—for simplicity. DMT$_r$ = dimethoxtrityl, PB_1, PB_2, etc. = protected bases of first, second , etc. nucleotides added to the elongating chain.

This approach using silica based or controlled pore glass beads solid support is used for automated synthesis of oligo-nucleotides. It takes less than 15 minutes for adding one nucleotide to the chain, and chains as long as 50 nucleotides can be prepared in good yields. The automated DNA synthesisers are popularly called gene machines; they are microprocessor controlled and carry out all the operations automatically.

Enzymatic Synthesis of DNA

These methods use the bacterial enzyme polynucleotide phosphorylase, which is specific for ribonucleotides, but polymerises deoxyribonucleotides albeit at a slow rate when Mn^{2+} replaces Mg^{2+} in the reaction mixture. It uses as substrate deoxyribonucleoside diphosphates and does not require a template. But it does need a primer at least 3′ nucleotides long (Fig. 3.6). The enzyme adds one or two nucleotides at a time to the primer (and to the growing chain).

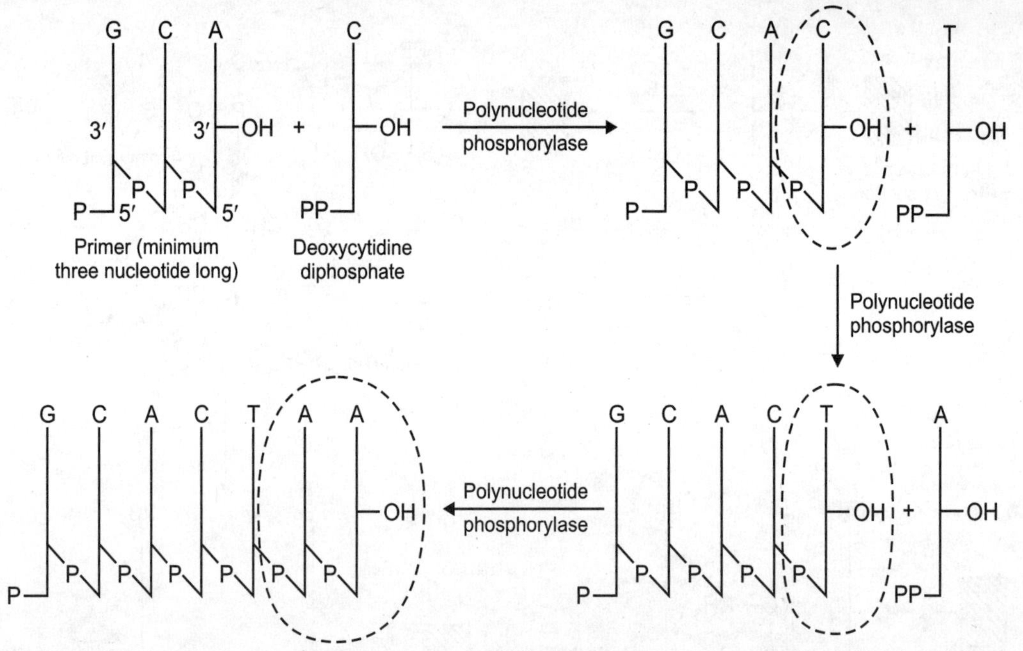

Fig. 3.6. Oligonucleotide synthesis by the bacterial enzyme polynucleotide phosphorylase. A primer of atleast 3′ nucleotides is essential; it is extended in the 5′ → 3′ direction using 5′ diphosphates of the DNA nucleosides. The enzyme adds one or two nucleotides at a time to the chain. The newly added nucleotides are encircled by broken lines.

The enzymatic synthesis of short oligonucleotides of defined sequence is simpler and easier to perform than that by strictly chemical methods, except when automated systems (gene machines) are available. No protective groups are required. However, the reactions are limited and hard to control.

Applications of Chemically Synthesised DNA Molecules or Oligonucleotides

There are immense applications of chemically synthesised DNA molecules or oligonucleotide.
1. Single stranded oligonucleotides are used as probes in medical research, as primers in PCR, in sequencing and *in vitro* mutagenesis.
2. Double stranded oligonucleotides can also be synthesised from single stranded DNA by using DNA polymerase and a short single stranded primer.
3. These double stranded oligonucleotides are usually used as adapters and linkers.
4. Genes with effective set of codons that are better suited to the host organism can be synthesised without changing the true amino acid sequence of the protein.

Drawbacks of chemical DNA synthesis

The major drawback in this method is that the process is time consuming and involves excessive wastage of phosphoroamidite molecule. Secondly, as the length of the oligonucleotide increases the yield falls down.

Gene Synthesis

Commercial gene synthesis services are now available from numerous companies worldwide, some of which have built their business model around this task. Current gene synthesis approaches are most often based on a combination of organic chemistry and molecular biological techniques and entire genes may be synthesised '*de novo*', without the need for precursor template DNA. Gene synthesis has become an important tool in many fields of recombinant DNA technology including heterologous gene expression, vaccine development, gene therapy and molecular engineering. The synthesis of nucleic acid sequences is often more economical than classical cloning and mutagenesis procedures.

Gene optimisation

While the ability to make increasingly long stretches of DNA efficiently and at lower prices is a technological driver of this field, increasingly attention is being focused on improving the design of genes for specific purposes. Early in the genome sequencing era, gene synthesis was used as an (expensive) source of cDNA's that were predicted by genomic or partial cDNA information but were difficult to clone. As higher quality sources of sequence verified cloned cDNA have become available, this practice has become less urgent.

Producing large amounts of protein from gene sequences (or at least the protein coding regions of genes, the open reading frame) found in nature can sometimes prove difficult and is a problem of sufficient impact that scientific conferences have been devoted to the topic. Many of the most interesting proteins sought by molecular biologist are normally regulated to be expressed in very low amounts in wild type cells. Redesigning these genes offers a means to improve gene expression in many cases. Rewriting the open reading frame is possible because of the degeneracy of the genetic code. Thus it is possible to change up to about a third of the nucleotides in an open reading frame and still produce the same protein. The available number of alternate designs possible for a given protein is astronomical. For a typical protein sequence of 300 amino acids there are over 10^{150} codon combinations that will encode an identical protein. Using optimisation methods such as replacing rarely used codons with more common codons sometimes have a dramatic effects. Further optimisations such as removing RNA secondary structures can also be included. At least in the case of *E. coli*, protein expression is maximised by predominantly using codons corresponding to tRNA's that retain amino acid charging during starvation. Computer programmes are written to perform these and other simultaneous optimisations are used to handle the enormous complexity of the task. A well optimised gene can improve protein expression 2 to 10 fold, and in some cases more than 100 fold improvements have been reported. Because of the large numbers of nucleotide changes made to the original DNA sequence, the only practical way to create the newly designed genes is to use gene synthesis.

Standard methods

Chemical synthesis of oligonucleotides

Oligonucleotides are chemically synthesised using nucleotides, called phosphoramidites, normal nucleotides which have protection groups: preventing amine, hydroxyl groups and phosphate groups interacting incorrectly. One phosphoramidite is added at a time, the product's 5' phosphate is deprotected and a new base is added and so on (backwards), at the end, all the protection groups are removed. Nevertheless, being a chemical process, several incorrect interactions occur leading to some defective products. The longer the oligonucleotide sequence that is being synthesised, the more defects there are, thus this process is only practical for producing short sequences of nucleotides. The current practical limit is about 200 bp for an oligonucleotide with sufficient quality to be used directly for a biological application. HPLC can be used to isolate products with the proper sequence. Meanwhile a large number of oligos can be synthesised in parallel on gene chips. For optimal performance in subsequent gene synthesis procedures should be prepared individually and in larger scales.

Annealing based connection of oligonucleotides

Usually, a set of individually designed oligonucleotides is made on automated solid-phase synthesisers, purified and then connected by specific annealing and standard ligation or polymerase reactions. To improve specificity of oligonucleotide annealing, the synthesis step relies on a set of thermostable DNA ligase and polymerase enzymes. To date, several methods for gene synthesis have been described, such as the ligation of phosphorylated overlapping oligonucleotides, the Fok I method and a modified form of ligase chain reaction for gene synthesis. Additionally, several PCR assembly approaches have been described. They usually employ oligonucleotides of 40–50 nt long that overlap each other. These oligonucleotides are designed to cover most of the sequence of both strands, and the full-length molecule is generated progressively by overlap extension (OE) PCR, thermodynamically balanced inside-out (TBIO) PCR or combined approaches. The most commonly synthesised genes range in size from 600 to 1,200 bp. although much longer genes have been made by connecting previously assembled fragments of under 1,000 bp. In this size range it is necessary test several candidate clones confirming the sequence of the cloned synthetic gene by automated sequencing methods.

Limitations

Moreover, because the assembly of the full-length gene product relies on the efficient and specific alignment of long single stranded oligonucleotides, critical parameters for synthesis success include extended sequence regions comprising secondary structures caused by inverted repeats, extraordinary high or low GC-content, or repetitive structures. Usually these segments of a particular gene can only be synthesised by splitting the procedure into several consecutive steps and a final assembly of shorter sub-sequences, which in turn leads to a significant increase in time and labour needed for its production. The result of a gene synthesis experiment depends strongly on the quality of the oligonucleotides used. For these annealing based gene synthesis protocols, the quality of the product is directly and exponentially dependent on the correctness of the employed oligonucleotides. Alternatively, after performing gene synthesis with oligos of lower quality, more effort must be made in downstream quality assurance during clone analysis, which is usually done by time-consuming standard cloning and sequencing procedures. Another problem associated with all current gene synthesis methods is the high frequency of sequence errors because of the usage of chemically synthesised oligonucleotides. The error frequency increases with longer oligonucleotides, and as a consequence the percentage of correct product decreases dramatically as more oligonucleotides are used. The mutation problem could be solved by shorter oligonucleotides used to assemble the gene. However, all annealing based assembly methods require the primers to be mixed together in one tube. In this case, shorter overlaps do not always allow precise and specific annealing of complementary primers, resulting in the inhibition of full length product formation. Manual design of oligonucleotides is a laborious procedure and does not guarantee the successful synthesis of the desired gene. For optimal performance of almost all annealing based methods, the melting temperatures of the overlapping regions are supposed to be similar for all oligonucleotides. The necessary primer optimisation should be performed using specialised oligonucleotide design programmes. Several solutions for automated primer design for gene synthesis have been presented so far.

Error correction procedures

To overcome problems associated with oligonucleotide quality several elaborate strategies have been developed, employing either separately prepared fishing oligonucleotides, mismatch binding enzymes of the mutS family or specific endonucleases from bacteria or phages. Nevertheless, all these strategies increase time and costs for gene synthesis based on the annealing of chemically synthesised oligonucleotides.

DNA SEQUENCING

Determination of nucleotide or base sequence of a DNA molecule/fragment is known as DNA sequencing. At present, DNA sequencing is possible for only one to few hundred bp long DNA fragments. DNA sequencing has become feasible as a result of the following important developments: (i) the availability of restriction endonucleases, (ii) the development of highly sensitive gel electrophoretic techniques which can separate DNA fragments differing by one nucleotide only, (iii) the gene cloning and PCR techniques making available large quantities of individual DNA fragments, and (iv) the development of two reliable, relatively easy and rapid DNA sequencing procedures, called (i) Maxam and Gilbert procedure, and (ii) the enzymatic procedure.

Maxam and Gilbert Procedure

In the first DNA sequencing technique, called maxam and gilbert procedure, the DNA fragment to be sequenced is end-labelled by the addition of ^{32}p-dATP either at the 5-ends (by the enzyme polynucleotide kinase) or at the 3-ends (by the enzyme deoxynucleotidyl transferase) of its two strands. The end-labelled fragment is now (i) digested with a restriction endonuclease which cleaves it into only two fragments of unequal lengths. As a result, only one end of each of the two fragments thus produced will be labelled. The two unequal fragments are separated through gel electrophoresis and they are sequenced separately (Fig. 3.7).

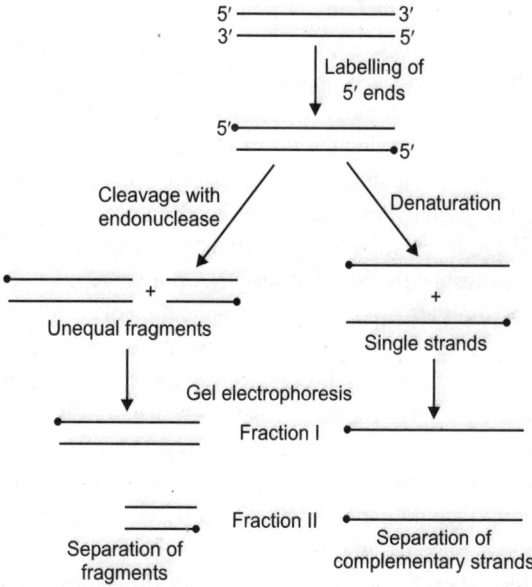

Fig. 3.7. A schematic representation of the production of single-end-labelled DNA molecules/strands for nucleotide sequencing through chemical cleavage procedure.

Alternatively, (ii) the end-labelled fragment is denatured and its two complementary strands are separated through gel electrophoresis. For some unknown reason, the two complementary strands of a DNA molecule generally show different mobilities during gel electrophoresis. The samples of complementary strands thus separated are sequenced separately. It may be noted that each strand will be labelled at one end (either 5′ or 3′) only.

The single-end-labelled double or single-stranded DNA samples thus produced are subjected to base-specific chemical cleavage so that in a reaction mixture cleavage occurs only at one of the following four sites: sites having G, C, G + A or C + T. Each DNA sample is partially digested in four separate reaction mixtures (one each for specific cleavage at the sites of G, C, G + A or C + T). In these reaction mixtures each DNA fragment/strand is expected to be cleaved, on an average only once at anyone of the sites having the particular base for which the reaction mixture is specific, each such site in the DNA fragment/strand being equally likely to be cleaved.

The base-specific cleavage of DNA fragments involves the following steps: (i) modification of the concerned base, (ii) removal of the modified base from the DNA strand, and (iii) induction of strand break (break in the sugar-phosphate backbone) in the position from which the modified base has been removed. Such a cleavage generates a mixture of end-labelled DNA fragments of variable lengths. Digests of double-stranded DNA are denatured before they are subjected to electrophoresis. The digests from the four reaction mixtures are then separately subjected to gel electrophoresis to separate the fragments according to their lengths; the base sequence is determined by sequential reading of the bands developed in the four lanes of the gel through autoradiography (Fig. 3.8).

Enzymatic Procedure

The second technique is an enzymatic procedure developed by F. Sanger and coworkers. In this technique, the DNA fragment to be sequenced is denatured and the complementary strands are separated through electrophoresis. One of the two complementary strands (or often both the strands, but in separate experiments) is used as template for DNA replication catalysed by the larger subunit (called, *Klenow fragment*) of *E. coli* DNA polymerase I. The smaller subunit of the enzyme is not used in view of its 5′ → 3′ exonuclease activity. Single-stranded samples of DNA fragments may also be obtained by cloning DNA fragments in a single-stranded DNA virus, e.g. M13, vector.

In the reaction system for DNA replication, at least one of the four deoxyribonucleotides is radioactive in order to permit the radioautographic development of bands after gel electrophoresis. A small primer sequence with a free 3′ OH group must be provided with the template strand for DNA replication to proceed, since a free 3′ OH is absolutely essential for DNA polymerase I to catalyse DNA replication.

Four different reaction mixtures are prepared for the replication of each DNA strand to be sequenced. In one of the reaction systems, 2′, 3′-dideoxycytidine triphosphate (ddCTP) is added in a concentration about 1/100th of the normal deoxycytidine triphosphate present in the system. ddCTP acts as a terminator of the polynucleotide chain being newly synthesised on the template strand. Chain termination by ddCTP is achieved due to the fact that it (and the other 2′–3′ dideoxynucleotides) does not have a free 3′ OH group as a result of which further nucleotides cannot be added to the new chain. At the concentration used here, ddCTP would terminate the newly synthesised polynucleotide chains at anyone of all the possible sites where cytosine is to be incorporated in the new chain.

In one each of the three other reaction mixtures using the same DNA fragment as template, 2′, 3′-dideoxythymidine triphosphate (ddTTP), 2′, 3′-dideoxyadenosine triphosphate (ddATP), or 2′, 3′-dideoxyguanosine triphosphate (ddGTP) is used as chain terminator to terminate the polynucleotide chains at anyone of all the positions where T, A or G, respectively, are to be incorporated in the new chain (each 2′, 3′-dideoxynucleotide is used in a separate reaction mixture).

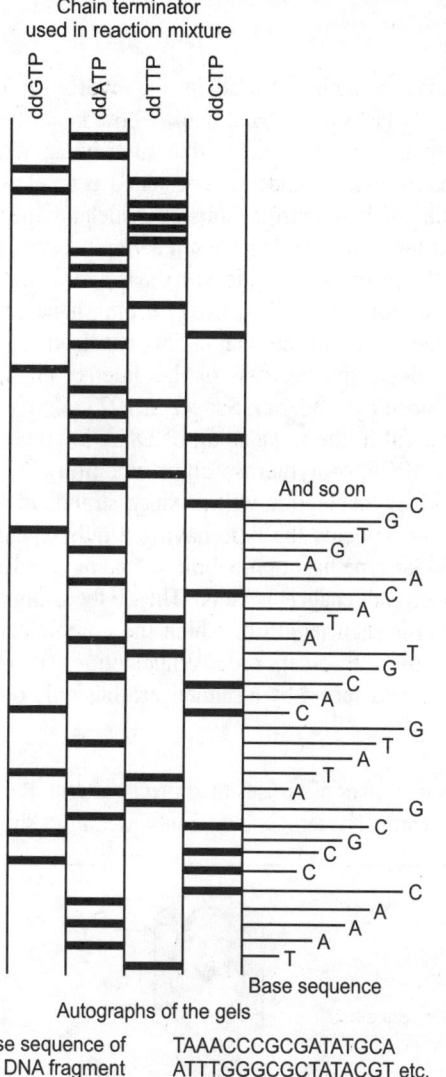

Fig. 3.8. Diagrammatic representation of the bands obtained in a DNA sequencing gel. The single-stranded fragment was used at template for DNA synthesis and chains were terminated using either ddGTP, ddATP, ddTTP or ddCTP. The shortest fragments are the bottom most: only a small segment of the gel is shown.

The partially synthesised (due to chain termination) DNA chains from each of the above four reaction mixtures are separated from the template strand by denaturation. The four single-stranded samples are now separately subjected gel electrophoresis in order to separate the strands according to their size. The bands in the gels are developed onto an X-ray film through autoradiography. The fastest moving fragment will be the smallest one, and each subsequent band will be one nucleotide longer than the previous one. Therefore, by comparing the bands of the four gels thus obtained, nucleotide sequence of the DNA fragment can be determined (Fig. 3.8). The position of a band in the gel from a reaction mixture will indicate the position of the base of which 2′, 3′-dideoxynucleotide triphosphate was used as chain terminator in that mixture.

Dideoxynucleotide

Dideoxynucleotides, or ddNTPs, are nucleotides lacking a 3′-hydroxyl (–OH) group on their deoxyribose sugar. Since deoxyribose already lacks a 2′–OH, dideoxyribose lacks hydroxyl groups at both its 2′ and 3′ carbons. The lack of this hydroxyl group means that, after being added by a DNA polymerase to a growing nucleotide chain, no further nucleotides can be added as no phosphodiester bond can be created based on the fact that deoxyribonucleoside triphosphates (which are the building blocks of DNA) allow DNA chain synthesis to occur through a condensation reaction between the 5′ phosphate (following the cleavage of pyrophospate) of the current nucleotide with the 3′ hydroxyl group of the previous nucleotide. The dideoxyribonucleotides do not have a 3′ hydroxyl group, hence no further chain elongation can occur once this dideoxynucleotide is on the chain. This can lead to the determination of the DNA sequence. Thus, these molecules form the basis of the dideoxy chain-termination method of DNA sequencing, which was developed by Frederick Sanger in 1977.

Dideoxynucleotides are useful in the sequencing of DNA in combination with electrophoresis. A DNA sample that undergoes PCR (polymerase chain reaction) in a mixture containing all four deoxynucleotides and one dideoxynucleotide will produce strands of length equal to the position of each base of the type that complements the type having a dideoxynucleotide present. That is, each nucleotide base of that particular type has a probability of being bonded to not a deoxynucleotide but rather a dideoxynucleotide, which ends chain elongation. Thus, if the sample then undergoes electrophoresis, there will be a band present for each length at which the complement of the dideoxynucleotide is present. It is now common to use fluorescent dideoxynucleotides such that each one of the four has a different fluorescence that can be detected by a sequencer; thus only one reaction is needed.

Bacteriophage

A bacteriophage is any one of a number of viruses that infect bacteria. Bacteriophages are among the most common biological entities on earth. The term is commonly used in its shortened form, *phage* (Fig. 3.9).

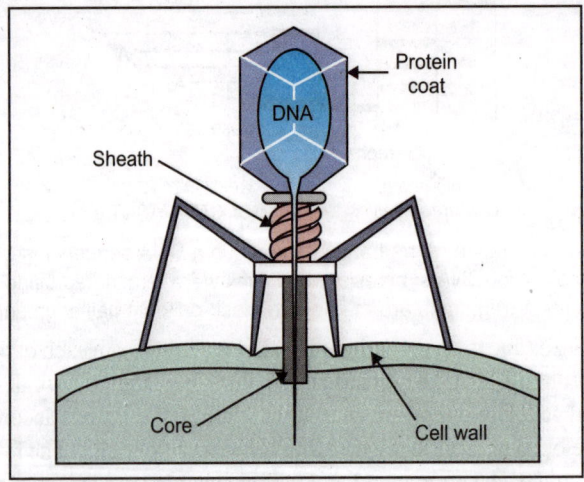

Fig. 3.9. The structure of a typical tailed bacteriophage.

Typically, bacteriophages consist of an outer protein capsid enclosing genetic material. The genetic material can be ssRNA, dsRNA, ssDNA, or dsDNA ('ss-' or 'ds-' prefix denotes single-strand or double-strand) long with either circular or linear arrangement. Bacteriophages are much smaller than the bacteria they destroy.

Phages are estimated to be the most widely distributed and diverse entities in the biosphere. Phages are ubiquitous and can be found in all reservoirs populated by bacterial hosts, such as soil or the intestines of animals. One of the densest natural sources for phages and other viruses is sea water, where up to 9×10^8 virions per milliliter have been found in microbial mats at the surface, and up to 70 per cent of marine bacteria may be infected by phages. They have been used for over 60 years as an alternative to antibiotics in the former Soviet Union and Eastern Europe. They are seen as a possible therapy against multi drug resistant strains of many bacteria.

Classification

The dsDNA tailed phages, or *Caudovirales*, account for 95 per cent of all the phages reported in the scientific literature, and possibly make up the majority of phages on the planet. However, there are other phages that occur abundantly in the biosphere, phages with different virions, genomes and lifestyles. Phages are classified by the International committee on taxonomy of viruses (ICTV) according to morphology and nucleic acid (Table 3.2).

Table 3.2. ICTV classification of phages.

Order	Family	Morphology	Nucleic acid	Examples
	Myoviridae	Non-enveloped, contractile tail	Linear dsDNA	
Caudovirales	*Siphoviridae*	Non-enveloped, long non-contractile tail	Linear dsDNA	λ phage
	Podoviridae	Non-enveloped, short noncontractile tail	Linear dsDNA	T7phage
	Tectiviridae	Non-enveloped, isometric	Linear dsDNA	
	Corticoviridae	Non-enveloped, isometric	Circular dsDNA	
	Lipothrixviridae	Enveloped, rod-shaped	Linear dsDNA	
	Plasmaviridae	Enveloped, pleomorphic	Circular dsDNA	
	Rudiviridae	Non-enveloped, rod-shaped	Linear dsDNA	
Unassigned	*Fuselloviridae*	Non-enveloped, lemon-shaped	Circular dsDNA	
	Inoviridae	Non-enveloped, filamentous	Circular ssDNA	
	Microviridae	Non-enveloped, isometric	Circular ssDNA	
	Leviviridae	Non-enveloped, isometric	Linear ssRNA	
	Cystoviridae	Enveloped, spherical	Segmented dsRNA	

Replication

Bacteriophages may have a lytic cycle or a lysogenic cycle, and a few viruses are capable of carrying out both. With lytic phages such as the T4 phage, bacterial cells are broken open (lysed) and destroyed after immediate replication of the virion. As soon as the cell is destroyed, the new phages can find new hosts. Lytic phages are the kind suitable for phage therapy.

In contrast, the lysogenic cycle does not result in immediate lysing of the host cell. Those phages able to undergo lysogeny are known as temperate phages. Their viral genome will integrate with host DNA and replicate along with it fairly harmlessly, or may even become established as a plasmid. The virus remains dormant until host conditions deteriorate, perhaps due to depletion of nutrients, then the endogenous phages (known as prophages) become active. At this point they initiate the reproductive cycle, resulting in lysis of the host cell. As the lysogenic cycle allows the host cell to continue to survive and reproduce, the virus is reproduced in all of the cell's offspring.

Sometimes prophages may provide benefits to the host bacterium while they are dormant by adding new functions to the bacterial genome in a phenomenon called lysogenic conversion. A famous example is the conversion of a harmless strain of *Vibrio cholerae* by a phage into a highly virulent one, which causes cholera. This is why temperate phages are not suitable for phage therapy.

Attachment and penetration

To enter a host cell, bacteriophages attach to specific receptors on the surface of bacteria, including lipopolysaccharides, teichoic acids, proteins, or even flagella. This specificity means that a bacteriophage can only infect certain bacteria bearing receptors that they can bind to, which in turn determines the phage's host range. Host growth conditions also influence the ability of the phage to attach and invade bacteria. As phage virions do not move independently, they must rely on random encounters with the right receptors when in solution (blood, lymphatic circulation, irrigation, soil water, etc.).

Complex bacteriophages use a hypodermic syringe-like motion to inject their genetic material into the cell. After making contact with the appropriate receptor, the tail fibres bring the base plate closer to the surface of the cell. Once attached completely, the tail contracts, possibly with the help of ATP present in the tail, injecting genetic material through the bacterial membrane (Fig. 3.10).

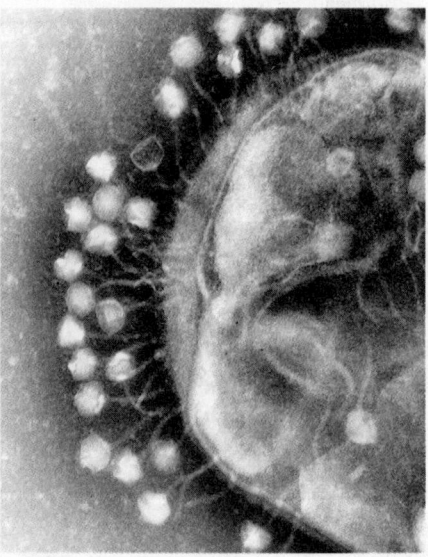

Fig. 3.10. An electron micrograph of bacteriophages attached to a bacterial cell. These viruses are the size and shape of coliphage T1.

Synthesis of proteins and nucleic acid

Within minutes, bacterial ribosomes start translating viral mRNA into protein. For RNA-based phages, RNA replicase is synthesised early in the process. Proteins modify the bacterial RNA polymerase so that it preferentially transcribes viral mRNA. The host's normal synthesis of proteins and nucleic acids is disrupted, and it is forced to manufacture viral products instead. These products go on to become part of new virions within the cell, helper proteins which help assemble the new virions, or proteins involved in cell lysis.

Virion assembly

In the case of the T4 phage, the construction of new virus particles involves the assistance of helper proteins. The base plates are assembled first, with the tails being built upon them afterwards. The head capsids, constructed separately, will spontaneously assemble with the tails. The DNA is packed efficiently within the heads. The whole process takes about 15 minutes.

Release of virions

Phages may be released via cell lysis, by extrusion, or, in a few cases, by budding. Lysis, by tailed phages, is achieved by an enzyme called endolysin, which attacks and breaks down the cell wall peptidoglycan. An altogether different phage type, the filamentous phages, make the host cell continually secrete new virus particles. Released virions are described as free, and, unless defective, are capable of infecting a new bacterium. Budding is associated with certain Mycoplasma phages. In contrast to virion release, phages displaying a lysogenic cycle do not kill the host but, rather, become long-term residents as prophage.

Phage therapy

Phages were discovered to be anti-bacterial agents but the medical trials performed in western countries were sub-standard to the point of not being scientifically viable, this because the early tests were conducted poorly and without an idea of what a phage was. Phage therapy was shortly thereafter ruled out as untrustworthy much because many of the trials were conducted on totally unrelated diseases such as allergies and viral infections. Antibiotics were discovered some years later and marketed widely, popular because of their broad spectrum and easier to manufacture in bulk, store, and prescribe.

In the environment

Metagenomics has allowed the detection of bacteriophages in water that was not possible previously. These investigations revealed that phage are much more abundant in the water column of both freshwater and marine habitats than previously thought and that they can cause significant mortality of bacterioplankton. Methods in phage community ecology have been developed to assess phage-induced mortality of bacterioplankton and its role for food web process and biogeochemical cycles, to genetically fingerprint phage communities or populations and estimate viral biodiversity by metagenomics. The lysis of bacteria by phages releases organic carbon that was previously particulate (cells) into dissolved forms, which makes the carbon more available to other organisms. Phages are not only the most abundant biological entities but probably also the most diverse ones. The majority of the sequence data obtained from phage communities has no equivalent in databases. These data and other detailed analyses indicate that phage-specific genes and ecological traits are much more frequent than previously thought. In order to reveal the meaning of this genetic and ecological versatility, studies have to be performed with communities and at spatiotemporal scales relevant for micro-organisms.

Bacteriophages have also been used in hydrological tracing and modelling in river systems especially where surface water and groundwater interactions occur. The use of phages is preferred to the more conventional dye marker because they are significantly less absorbed when passing through groundwaters and they are readily detected at very low concentrations.

Role in food fermentation

A broad number of food products, commodity chemicals, and biotechnology products are manufactured industrially by large-scale bacterial fermentation of various organic substrates. Because enormous amounts of bacteria are being cultivated each day in large fermentation vats, the risk of bacteriophage contamination could rapidly bring fermentation to a halt. The resulting economical setback is a serious threat in these industries. The relationship between bacteriophages and their bacterial hosts is very important in the context of the food fermentation industry. Sources of phage contamination, measures to control their propagation and dissemination, and biotechnological defense strategies developed to restrain phages are of interest. The dairy fermentation industry has openly acknowledged the problem of phage and has been working with academia and starter culture companies to develop defense strategies and systems to curtail the propagation and evolution of phages for decades.

M13 Bacteriophage

M13 is a filamentous bacteriophage composed of circular single stranded DNA (ssDNA) which is 6407 nucleotides long encapsulated in approximately 2700 copies of the major coat protein P8, and capped with 5 copies of two different minor coat proteins (P9, P6, P3) on the ends. The minor coat protein P3 attaches to the receptor at the tip of the *F* pilus of the host *Escherichia coli*. Infection with filamentous phages is not lethal, however the infection causes turbid plaques in *E. coli*. It is a non-lytic virus. However a decrease in the rate of cell growth is seen in the infected cells. M13 plasmids are used for many recombinant DNA processes, and the virus has also been studied for its uses in nanostructures and nanotechnology.

The phage coat is primarily assembled from a 50 amino acid protein called pVIII (or p8), which is encoded by gene VIII (or g8) in the phage genome. For a wild type M13 particle, it takes about approximately 2700 copies of p8 to make the coat about 900 nm long. The coat's dimensions are flexible though and the number of p8 copies adjusts to accommodate the size of the single stranded genome it packages. For example, when the phage genome was mutated to reduce its number of DNA bases (from 6.4 kb to 221 bp), then the number of p8 copies was decreased to fewer than 100, causing the p8 coat to shrink in order to fit the reduced genome. The phage appear to be limited at approximately twice the natural DNA content. However, deletion of a phage protein (p3) prevents full escape from the host *E. coli*, and phage that are 10–20X the normal length with several copies of the phage genome can be seen shedding from the *E. coli* host.

There are four other proteins on the phage surface, two of which have been extensively studied. At one end of the filament are five copies of the surface exposed pIX (p9) and a more buried companion protein, pVII (p7). If p8 forms the shaft of the phage, p9 and p7 form the 'blunt' end that is seen in the micrographs. These proteins are very small, containing only 33 and 32 amino acids respectively, though some additional residues can be added to the N-terminal portion of each which are then presented on the outside of the coat. At the other end of the phage particle are five copies of the surface exposed pIII (p3) and its less exposed accessory protein, pVI (p6). These form the rounded tip of the phage and are the first proteins to interact with the *E. coli* host during infection. p3 is also the last point of contact with the host as new phage bud from the bacterial surface.

Phage life-cycle

The general stages to a viral life cycle are: infection, replication of the viral genome, assembly of new viral particles and then release of the progeny particles from the host. Filamentous phage use a bacterial structure known as the F pilus to infect *E. coli*, with the M13 p3 tip contacting the TolA protein on the bacterial pilus. The phage genome is then transferred to the cytoplasm of the bacterial cell where resident proteins convert the single stranded DNA genome to a double stranded replicative form ('RF'). This DNA then serves as a template for expression of the phage genes.

Two phage gene products play critical roles in the next stage of the phage life cycle, namely amplification of the genome. pII (aka p2) nicks the double stranded form of the genome to initiate replication of the + strand. Without p2, no replication of the phage genome can occur. Host enzymes copy the replicated + strand, resulting in more copies of double stranded phage DNA. pV (aka p5) competes with double stranded DNA formation by sequestering copies of the + stranded DNA into a protein/DNA complex destined for packaging into new phage particles. Interestingly there is one additional phage-encoded protein, pX (p10), that is important for regulating the number of double stranded genomes in the bacterial host. Without p10 no + strands can accumulate. What's particularly interesting about p10 is that it's identical to the C-terminal portion of p2 since the gene for p10 is within the gene for p2 and the protein arises from transcription initiation within gene 2. This makes the manipulation of p10 inextricably linked to manipulation of p2 (an engineering headache) but it also makes for a compact and efficient phage in nature.

Phage maturation requires the phage-encoded proteins pIV (p4), pI (p1) and its translational restart product pXI (p11). Multiple copies (on the order of 12 or 14) of p4 assemble in the outer membrane into a stable, i.e. detergent resistant, barrel-shaped structure. Similarly a handful of the p1 and p11 proteins (5 or 6 copies of each) assemble in the bacterial inner membrane, and genetic evidence suggests C-terminal portions of p1 and p11 interact with the N-terminal portion of p4 in the periplasm. Together the p1, p11, p4 complex forms channels through which mature phage are secreted from the bacterial host.

To initiate phage secretion, two of the minor phage coat proteins, p9 and p7, are thought to interact with the p5-single stranded DNA complex at a region of the DNA called the packaging sequence (aka PS). The p5 proteins covering the single stranded DNA are then replaced by p8 proteins that are embedded in the bacterial membrane and the growing phage filament is threaded through the p1, p11, p4 channel. This replacement of p5 by p8 explains the microphage data presented earlier indicate how the size of the phage particle is determined by the number of bases the phage packages. Once the phage DNA has been fully coated with p8, the secretion terminates by adding the p3/p6 cap, and the new phage detaches from the bacterial surface. How long does all this take? Amazingly, new M13 phage particles are secreted within 10 minutes from a newly infected host and can arise at a rate of 1000/cell within the first hour of infection. The bacterial host can continue to grow and divide, allowing this process to continue indefinitely.

Replication in E. coli

Below are steps involved with replication of M13 in *E. coli*.

1. Viral (+) strand DNA enters cytoplasm.
2. Complementary (–) strand is synthesised by bacterial enzymes.
3. DNA Gyrase, a type II topoisomerase, acts on double-stranded DNA and catalyses formation of negative supercoils in double-stranded DNA.
4. Final product is parental replicative form (RF) DNA.
5. A phage protein, pII, nicks the (+) strand in the RF.
6. 3′-hydroxyl acts as a primer in the creation of new viral strand.
7. pII circulises displaced viral (+) strand DNA.
8. Pool of progeny double-stranded RF molecules produced.

9. Negative strand of RF is template of transcription.
10. mRNAs are translated into the phage proteins.

Phage proteins in the cytoplasm are pII, pX, and pV, and they are part of the replication process of DNA. The other phage proteins are synthesised and inserted into the cytoplasmic or outer membranes.

1. pV dimers bind newly synthesised single-stranded DNA and prevent conversion to RF DNA.
2. RF DNA synthesis continues and amount of pV reaches critical concentration.
3. DNA replication switches to synthesis of single-stranded (+) viral DNA.
4. pV-DNA structures from about 800 nm long and 8 nm in diamter.
5. pV-DNA complex is substrate in phage assembly reaction.

Primer Walking

Primer walking is a sequencing method of choice for sequencing DNA fragments between 1.3 and 7 kilobases. Such fragments are too long to be sequenced in a single sequence read using the chain termination method. This method works by dividing the long sequence into several consecutive short ones. The DNA of interest may be a plasmid insert, a PCR product or a fragment representing a gap when sequencing a genome. The term 'primer walking' is used where the main aim is to sequence the genome. The term 'chromosome walking' is used instead when we know the sequence but don't have a clone of a gene. For example the gene for a disease may be located near a specific marker such as an RFLP on the sequence.

The fragment is first sequenced as if it were a shorter fragment—sequencing will be performed from each end using either universal primers or primers designated by the customer. This should identify the first 1000 (approx.) bases. In order to completely sequence the region of interest, design and synthesis of new primers—complementary to the final 20 bases of the known sequence—is necessary to obtain contiguous sequence information.

The basic technique is as follows:

1. A primer that matches the beginning of the DNA to sequence is used to synthesise a short DNA strand adjacent to the unknown sequence, starting with the primer (see PCR).
2. The new short DNA strand is sequenced using the chain termination method.
3. The end of the sequenced strand is used as a primer for the next part of the long DNA sequence.

That way, the short part of the long DNA that is sequenced keeps 'walking' along the sequence. The method can be used to sequence entire chromosomes (thus, *chromosome walking*). A different method with the same purpose which becomes more popular for large-scale sequencing (e.g. the Human genome project) is shotgun sequencing.

POLYMERASE CHAIN REACTION

The polymerase chain reaction (PCR) is a technique in molecular biology to amplify a single or few copies of a piece of DNA across several orders of magnitude, generating thousands to millions of copies of a particular DNA sequence. The method relies on thermal cycling, consisting of cycles of repeated heating and cooling of the reaction for DNA melting and enzymatic replication of the DNA. Primers (short DNA fragments) containing sequences complementary to the target region along with a DNA polymerase (after which the method is named) are key components to enable selective and repeated amplification. As PCR progresses, the DNA generated is itself used as a template for replication, setting in motion a chain reaction in which the DNA template is exponentially amplified. PCR can be extensively modified to perform a wide array of genetic manipulations.

Almost all PCR applications employ a heat-stable DNA polymerase, such as Taq polymerase, an enzyme originally isolated from the bacterium *Thermus aquaticus*. This DNA polymerase enzymatically assembles a new DNA strand from DNA building blocks, the nucleotides, by using single-stranded DNA as a template and DNA oligonucleotides (also called DNA primers), which are required for initiation of DNA synthesis.

The vast majority of PCR methods use thermal cycling, i.e. alternately heating and cooling the PCR sample to a defined series of temperature steps. These thermal cycling steps are necessary first to physically separate the two strands in a DNA double helix at a high temperature in a process called DNA melting. At a lower temperature, each strand is then used as the template in DNA synthesis by the DNA polymerase to selectively amplify the target DNA. The selectivity of PCR results from the use of primers that are complementary to the DNA region targeted for amplification under specific thermal cycling conditions.

PCR is now a common and often indispensable technique used in medical and biological research labs for a variety of applications. These include DNA cloning for sequencing, DNA-based phylogeny, or functional analysis of genes; the diagnosis of hereditary diseases; the identification of genetic fingerprints (used in forensic sciences and paternity testing); and the detection and diagnosis of infectious diseases.

PCR Principles and Procedure

PCR is used to amplify a specific region of a DNA strand (the DNA target). Most PCR methods typically amplify DNA fragments of up to ~10 kilo base pairs (kb), although some techniques allow for amplification of fragments up to 40 kb in size.

A basic PCR set up requires several components and reagents. These components include:

1. DNA template that contains the DNA region (target) to be amplified.
2. Two primers that are complementary to the 3′ (three prime) ends of each of the sense and anti-sense strand of the DNA target.
3. Taq polymerase or another DNA polymerase with a temperature optimum at around 70°C.
4. Deoxynucleoside triphosphates (dNTPs; also very commonly and erroneously called deoxynucleotide triphosphates), the building blocks from which the DNA polymerases synthesises a new DNA strand.
5. Buffer solution, providing a suitable chemical environment for optimum activity and stability of the DNA polymerase.
6. Divalent cations, magnesium or manganese ions; generally Mg^{2+} is used, but Mn^{2+} can be utilised for PCR-mediated DNA mutagenesis, as higher Mn^{2+} concentration increases the error rate during DNA synthesis.
7. Monovalent cation potassium ions.

The PCR is commonly carried out in a reaction volume of 10–200 µl in small reaction tubes (0.2–0.5 ml volumes) in a thermal cycler. The thermal cycler heats and cools the reaction tubes to achieve the temperatures required at each step of the reaction. Many modern thermal cyclers make use of the Peltier effect which permits both heating and cooling of the block holding the PCR tubes simply by reversing the electric current. Thin-walled reaction tubes permit favourable thermal conductivity to allow for rapid thermal equilibration. Most thermal cyclers have heated lids to prevent condensation at the top of the reaction tube. Older thermocyclers lacking a heated lid require a layer of oil on top of the reaction mixture or a ball of wax inside the tube.

Procedure

Typically, PCR consists of a series of 20–40 repeated temperature changes, called cycles, with each cycle commonly consisting of 2–3 discrete temperature steps. Most protocols call for cycles that have three temperature steps (Fig. 3.11). The cycling is often preceded by a single temperature step (called *hold*) at a high temperature (>90°C), and followed by one hold at the end for final product extension or brief storage. The temperatures used and the length of time they are applied in each cycle depend on a variety of parameters. These include the enzyme used for DNA synthesis, the concentration of divalent ions and dNTPs in the reaction, and the melting temperature (Tm) of the primers.

1. Initialisation step: This step consists of heating the reaction to a temperature of 94°–96°C (or 98 °C if extremely thermostable polymerases are used), which is held for 1–9 minutes. It is only required for DNA polymerases that require heat activation by hot-start PCR.

2. Denaturation step: This step is the first regular cycling event and consists of heating the reaction to 94°–98°C for 20–30 seconds. It causes DNA melting of the DNA template by disrupting the hydrogen bonds between complementary bases, yielding single-stranded DNA molecules.

3. Annealing step: The reaction temperature is lowered to 50°–65°C for 20–40 seconds allowing annealing of the primers to the single-stranded DNA template. Typically the annealing temperature is about 3–5 degrees Celsius below the Tm of the primers used. Stable DNA-DNA hydrogen bonds are only formed when the primer sequence very closely matches the template sequence. The polymerase binds to the primer-template hybrid and begins DNA synthesis.

4. Extension/elongation step: The temperature at this step depends on the DNA polymerase used; Taq polymerase has its optimum activity temperature at 75°–80°C, and commonly a temperature of 72°C is used with this enzyme. At this step the DNA polymerase synthesises a new DNA strand complementary to the DNA template strand by adding dNTPs that are complementary to the template in 5′ to 3′ direction, condensing the 5′-phosphate group of the dNTPs with the 3′-hydroxyl group at the end of the nascent (extending) DNA strand. The extension time depends both on the DNA polymerase used and on the length of the DNA fragment to be amplified. As a rule-of-thumb, at its optimum temperature, the DNA polymerase will polymerise a thousand bases per minute. Under optimum conditions, i.e. if there are no limitations due to limiting substrates or reagents, at each extension step, the amount of DNA target is doubled, leading to exponential (geometric) amplification of the specific DNA fragment.

5. Final elongation: This single step is occasionally performed at a temperature of 70°–74°C for 5–15 minutes after the last PCR cycle to ensure that any remaining single-stranded DNA is fully extended.

6. Final hold: This step at 4°–15°C for an indefinite time may be employed for short-term storage of the reaction.

To check whether the PCR generated the anticipated DNA fragment (also sometimes referred to as the amplimer or amplicon), agarose gel electrophoresis is employed for size separation of the PCR products. The size(s) of PCR products is determined by comparison with a DNA ladder (a molecular weight marker), which contains DNA fragments of known size, run on the gel alongside the PCR products.

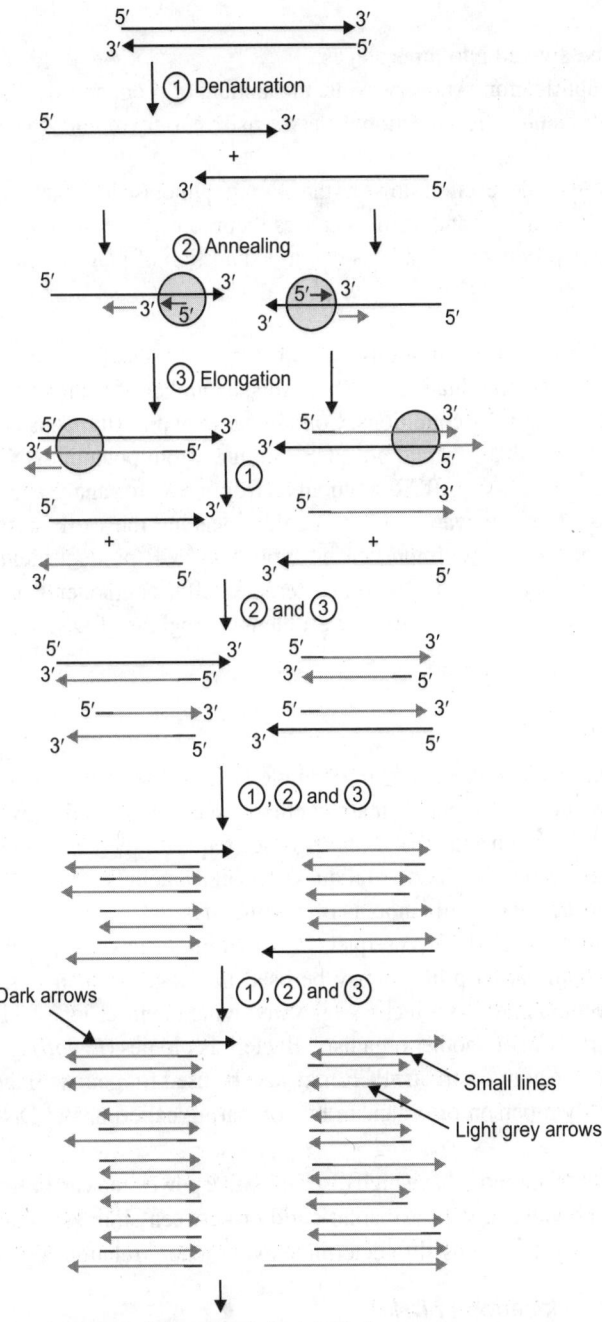

Fig. 3.11. Schematic drawing of the PCR cycle. (1) Denaturing at 94°–96°C. (2) Annealing at ~65°C. (3) Elongation at 72°C. Four cycles are shown here. The dark arrows represent the DNA template to which primers (smal lines) anneal that are extended by the DNA polymerase (light grey circles), to give shorter DNA products (light grey arrows), which themselves are used as templates as PCR progresses.

PCR Stages

The PCR process can be divided into three stages:

1. Exponential amplification: At every cycle, the amount of product is doubled (assuming 100 per cent reaction efficiency). The reaction is very sensitive: only minute quantities of DNA need to be present.
2. Levelling off stage: The reaction slows as the DNA polymerase loses activity and as consumption of reagents such as dNTPs and primers causes them to become limiting.
3. Plateau: No more product accumulates due to exhaustion of reagents and enzyme.

PCR optimisation

In practice, PCR can fail for various reasons, in part due to its sensitivity to contamination causing amplification of spurious DNA products. Because of this, a number of techniques and procedures have been developed for optimising PCR conditions. Contamination with extraneous DNA is addressed with lab protocols and procedures that separate pre-PCR mixtures from potential DNA contaminants. This usually involves spatial separation of PCR-setup areas from areas for analysis or purification of PCR products, use of disposable plasticware, and thoroughly cleaning the work surface between reaction setups. Primer-design techniques are important in improving PCR product yield and in avoiding the formation of spurious products, and the usage of alternate buffer components or polymerase enzymes can help with amplification of long or otherwise problematic regions of DNA.

Application of PCR

Selective DNA isolation

PCR allows isolation of DNA fragments from genomic DNA by selective amplification of a specific region of DNA. This use of PCR augments many methods, such as generating hybridisation probes for southern or northern hybridisation and DNA cloning, which require larger amounts of DNA, representing a specific DNA region. PCR supplies these techniques with high amounts of pure DNA, enabling analysis of DNA samples even from very small amounts of starting material.

Other applications of PCR include DNA sequencing to determine unknown PCR-amplified sequences in which one of the amplification primers may be used in Sanger sequencing, isolation of a DNA sequence to expedite recombinant DNA technologies involving the insertion of a DNA sequence into a plasmid or the genetic material of another organism. Bacterial colonies (*E. coli*) can be rapidly screened by PCR for correct DNA vector constructs. PCR may also be used for genetic fingerprinting; a forensic technique used to identify a person or organism by comparing experimental DNAs through different PCR-based methods.

Some PCR 'fingerprints' methods have high discriminative power and can be used to identify genetic relationships between individuals, such as parent-child or between siblings, and are used in paternity testing. This technique may also be used to determine evolutionary relationships among organisms.

Amplification and quantification of DNA

Because PCR amplifies the regions of DNA that it targets, PCR can be used to analyse extremely small amounts of sample. This is often critical for forensic analysis, when only a trace amount of DNA is available as evidence. PCR may also be used in the analysis of ancient DNA that is tens of thousands of years old. These PCR-based techniques have been successfully used on animals, such as a forty-thousand-year-old mammoth, and also on human DNA, in applications ranging from the analysis of Egyptian mummies to the identification of a Russian tsar.

Quantitative PCR methods allow the estimation of the amount of a given sequence present in a sample — a technique often applied to quantitatively determine levels of gene expression. Real-time PCR is an established tool for DNA quantification that measures the accumulation of DNA product after each round of PCR amplification.

PCR in diagnosis of diseases

PCR permits early diagnosis of malignant diseases such as leukemia and lymphomas, which is currently the highest developed in cancer research and is already being used routinely. PCR assays can be performed directly on genomic DNA samples to detect translocation-specific malignant cells at a sensitivity which is at least 10,000 fold higher than other methods.

PCR also permits identification of non-cultivatable or slow-growing micro-organisms such as mycobacteria, anaerobic bacteria, or viruses from tissue culture assays and animal models. The basis for PCR diagnostic applications in microbiology is the detection of infectious agents and the discrimination of non-pathogenic from pathogenic strains by virtue of specific genes.

Viral DNA can likewise be detected by PCR. The primers used need to be specific to the targeted sequences in the DNA of a virus, and the PCR can be used for diagnostic analyses or DNA sequencing of the viral genome. The high sensitivity of PCR permits virus detection soon after infection and even before the onset of disease. Such early detection may give physicians a significant lead in treatment. The amount of virus ('viral load') in a patient can also be quantified by PCR-based DNA quantitation techniques.

Variations on the Basic PCR Technique

1. Allele-specific PCR: A diagnostic or cloning technique which is based on single-nucleotide polymorphisms (SNPs) (single-base differences in DNA). It requires prior knowledge of a DNA sequence, including differences between alleles, and uses primers whose 3′ ends encompass the SNP. PCR amplification under stringent conditions is much less efficient in the presence of a mismatch between template and primer, so successful amplification with an SNP-specific primer signals presence of the specific SNP in a sequence.

2. Assembly PCR or polymerase cycling assembly (PCA): Artificial synthesis of long DNA sequences by performing PCR on a pool of long oligonucleotides with short overlapping segments. The oligonucleotides alternate between sense and antisense directions, and the overlapping segments determine the order of the PCR fragments, thereby selectively producing the final long DNA product.

3. Asymmetric PCR: Preferentially amplifies one DNA strand in a double-stranded DNA template. It is used in sequencing and hybridisation probing where amplification of only one of the two complementary strands is required. PCR is carried out as usual, but with a great excess of the primer for the strand targeted for amplification. Because of the slow (arithmetic) amplification later in the reaction after the limiting primer has been used up, extra cycles of PCR are required. A recent modification on this process, known as Linear-after-the-exponential-PCR (LATE-PCR), uses a limiting primer with a higher melting temperature (Tm) than the excess primer to maintain reaction efficiency as the limiting primer concentration decreases mid-reaction.

4. Helicase-dependent amplification: Similar to traditional PCR, but uses a constant temperature rather than cycling through denaturation and annealing/extension cycles. DNA helicase, an enzyme that unwinds DNA, is used in place of thermal denaturation.

5. Hot-start PCR: A technique that reduces non-specific amplification during the initial set up stages of the PCR. It may be performed manually by heating the reaction components to the melting temperature (e.g. 95°C) before adding the polymerase. Specialised enzyme systems have been developed that inhibit the polymerase's activity at ambient temperature, either by the binding of an antibody or by the presence of covalently bound inhibitors that only dissociate after a high-temperature activation step. Hot-start/cold-finish PCR is achieved with new hybrid polymerases that are inactive at ambient temperature and are instantly activated at elongation temperature.

6. Intersequence-specific PCR (ISSR): A PCR method for DNA fingerprinting that amplifies regions between simple sequence repeats to produce a unique fingerprint of amplified fragment lengths.

7. Inverse PCR: Inverse PCR is commonly used to identify the flanking sequences around genomic inserts. It involves a series of DNA digestions and self ligation, resulting in known sequences at either end of the unknown sequence.

8. Ligation-mediated PCR: Uses small DNA linkers ligated to the DNA of interest and multiple primers annealing to the DNA linkers; it has been used for DNA sequencing, genome walking, and DNA footprinting.

9. Methylation-specific PCR (MSP): Developed by Stephen Baylin and Jim Herman at the Johns Hopkins School of Medicine, and is used to detect methylation of CpG islands in genomic DNA. DNA is first treated with sodium bisulphite, which converts unmethylated cytosine bases to uracil, which is recognised by PCR primers as thymine. Two PCRs are then carried out on the modified DNA, using primer sets identical except at any CpG islands within the primer sequences. At these points, one primer set recognises DNA with cytosines to amplify methylated DNA, and one set recognises DNA with uracil or thymine to amplify unmethylated DNA. MSP using qPCR can also be performed to obtain quantitative rather than qualitative information about methylation.

10. Miniprimer PCR: Uses a thermostable polymerase (S-Tbr) that can extend from short primers ('smalligos') as short as 9 or 10 nucleotides. This method permits PCR targeting to smaller primer binding regions, and is used to amplify conserved DNA sequences, such as the 16S (or eukaryotic 18S) rRNA gene.

11. Multiplex ligation-dependent probe amplification (MLPA): Permits multiple targets to be amplified with only a single primer pair, thus avoiding the resolution limitations of multiplex PCR.

12. Multiplex-PCR: Consists of multiple primer sets within a single PCR mixture to produce amplicons of varying sizes that are specific to different DNA sequences. By targeting multiple genes at once, additional information may be gained from a single test run that otherwise would require several times the reagents and more time to perform. Annealing temperatures for each of the primer sets must be optimised to work correctly within a single reaction, and amplicon sizes, i.e. their base pair length, should be different enough to form distinct bands when visualised by gel electrophoresis.

13. Nested PCR: Increases the specificity of DNA amplification, by reducing background due to non-specific amplification of DNA. Two sets of primers are used in two successive PCRs. In the first reaction, one pair of primers is used to generate DNA products, which besides the intended target, may still consist of non-specifically amplified DNA fragments. The product(s)

are then used in a second PCR with a set of primers whose binding sites are completely or partially different from and located 3′ of each of the primers used in the first reaction. Nested PCR is often more successful in specifically amplifying long DNA fragments than conventional PCR, but it requires more detailed knowledge of the target sequences.

14. Overlap-extension PCR: A genetic engineering technique allowing the construction of a DNA sequence with an alteration inserted beyond the limit of the longest practical primer length.

15. Quantitative PCR (Q-PCR): Used to measure the quantity of a PCR product (commonly in real-time). It quantitatively measures starting amounts of DNA, cDNA or RNA. Q-PCR is commonly used to determine whether a DNA sequence is present in a sample and the number of its copies in the sample. Quantitative real time PCR has a very high degree of precision. QRT-PCR methods use fluorescent dyes, such as Sybr Green, EvaGreen or fluorophore-containing DNA probes, such as TaqMan, to measure the amount of amplified product in real time. It is also sometimes abbreviated to RT-PCR (real time PCR) or RQ-PCR. QRT-PCR or RTQ-PCR are more appropriate contractions, since RT-PCR commonly refers to reverse transcription PCR, often used in conjunction with Q-PCR.

16. Reverse transcription PCR (RT-PCR): For amplifying DNA from RNA. Reverse transcriptase reverse transcribes RNA into cDNA, which is then amplified by PCR. RT-PCR is widely used in expression profiling, to determine the expression of a gene or to identify the sequence of an RNA transcript, including transcription start and termination sites. If the genomic DNA sequence of a gene is known, RT-PCR can be used to map the location of exons and introns in the gene. The 5′ end of a gene (corresponding to the transcription start site) is typically identified by RACE-PCR (Rapid Amplification of cDNA Ends).

17. Solid phase PCR: Encompasses multiple meanings, including Polony Amplification (where PCR colonies are derived in a gel matrix, for example), Bridge PCR (primers are covalently linked to a solid-support surface), conventional Solid Phase PCR (where Asymmetric PCR is applied in the presence of solid support bearing primer with sequence matching one of the aqueous primers) and enhanced solid phase PCR (where conventional Solid Phase PCR can be improved by employing high T_m and nested solid support primer with optional application of a thermal 'step' to favour solid support priming).

18. Thermal asymmetric interlaced PCR (TAIL-PCR): For isolation of an unknown sequence flanking a known sequence. Within the known sequence, TAIL-PCR uses a nested pair of primers with differing annealing temperatures; a degenerate primer is used to amplify in the other direction from the unknown sequence.

19. Touchdown PCR (Step-down PCR): A variant of PCR that aims to reduce nonspecific background by gradually lowering the annealing temperature as PCR cycling progresses. The annealing temperature at the initial cycles is usually a few degrees (3°–5°C) above the T_m of the primers used, while at the later cycles, it is a few degrees (3°–5°C) below the primer T_m. The higher temperatures give greater specificity for primer binding, and the lower temperatures permit more efficient amplification from the specific products formed during the initial cycles.

20. PAN-AC: Uses isothermal conditions for amplification, and may be used in living cells.

21. Universal fast walking: For genome walking and genetic fingerprinting using a more specific 'two-sided' PCR than conventional 'one-sided' approaches (using only one gene-specific primer and one general primer-which can lead to artefactual 'noise') by virtue of a mechanism involving lariat structure formation. Streamlined derivatives of UFW are LaNe RAGE (lariat-dependent nested PCR for rapid amplification of genomic DNA ends), 5′RACE LaNe and 3′RACE LaNe.

MONOCLONAL ANTIBODIES

Monoclonal antibodies (mAb or moAb) are monospecific antibodies that are the same because they are made by identical immune cells that are all clones of a unique parent cell. Given almost any substance, it is possible to create monoclonal antibodies that specifically bind to that substance; they can then serve to detect or purify that substance. This has become an important tool in biochemistry, molecular biology and medicine. When used as medications, the non-proprietary drug name ends in-mab. A general representation of the methods used to produce monoclonal antibodies is shown in Fig 3.12.

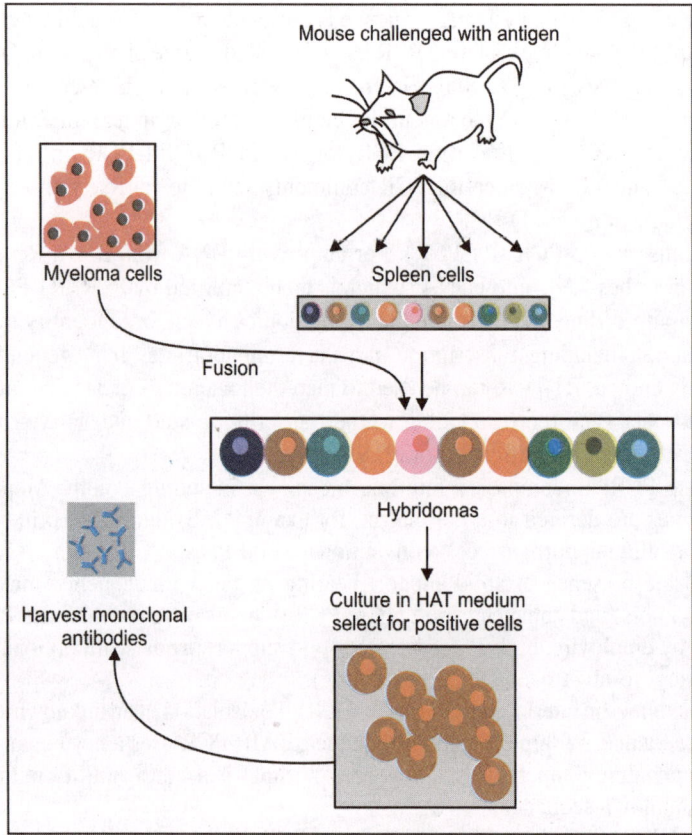

Fig. 3.12. A general representation of the methods used to produce monoclonal antibodies.

Antibodies are special types of proteins, ordinarily glycosylated, called immunoglobulins (*Ig*) produced in response to antigens; an antibody specifically interacts with the antigen which induced its production. The antigen-antibody interaction is highly specific, but some cases of cross-reaction (interaction of an antibody induced by one antigen with another antigen) are known possibly due to a similarity between the epitopes of the two antigens. Epitope or antigenic determinant is that portion of an antigen molecule which is involved in antigen-antibody interaction. Interaction with an antibody renders the antigen molecule nonfunctional; this is the basis for protection or immunity produced by antibodies against their antigens. Therefore, production of antibodies by an animal in response to an antigen is known as immune response, and this activity of the antigen is called immunogenicity. In contrast, the ability of antigens to interact with antibodies is referred to as antigenicity.

In general, antigens are also immunogenic, and the same antigen epitope functions in both the phenomena. However, some small molecules show antigenicity but by themselves they are unable to produce immune response; such molecules are called haptens. However, when a hapten is linked to a large molecule, called carrier, it elicits, immunogenic response as well, i.e. is able to induce antibody production against itself. The carrier molecule may itself be either non-immunogenic or immunogenic (in which case antibodies will be produced against the carrier as well).

Antibody Structure

An antibody molecule consists of two identical light chains (220 amino acids each) and two identical heavy chains (about 440–450 amino acids each) held together by disulphide bridges; this constitutes the monomeric form of an antibody (Fig. 3.13). Enzyme papain cleaves each monomeric form into two fragments that bind to the antigen (designated as F_{AB}; fragment with antigen binding) and one fragment which does not bind to antigen but forms crystals (hence called Fc, crystal forming fragment).

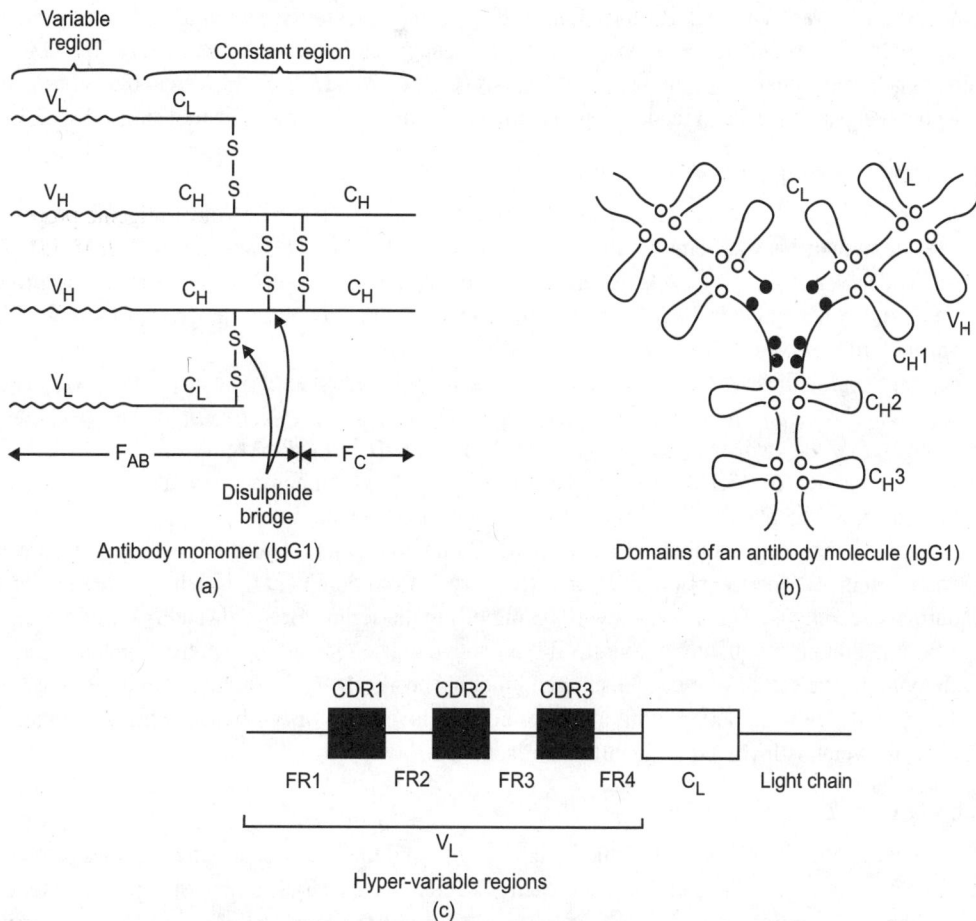

Fig. 3.13. Organisation of an antibody (*IgG1*) molecule and its domains. V_L and V_H, variable region of light and heavy chains, respectively; C_L and C_H constant regions of light and heavy chains, respectively; F_{AB}, fragment with antigen binding; F_c, fragment forming crystal; CDR, complementarity determining region; FR, Framework Region; o o intrachain disulphide bridge; ● ●, interchain disulphide bridge.

About 100 amino acid long amino-terminal ends of both light and heavy chains constitute their variable region denoted as V_L and V_H, respectively; the amino acid sequence of this region varies among antibodies specific to different antigens. The remaining regions of the heavy and light chains are called constant region (designated as C_H and C_L, respectively) since there is little variation in the amino acid sequence of this region among the antibodies belonging to the same class.

Each antibody molecule has two antigen-binding sites or domains, each domain being constituted by the variable regions of one light and one heavy chain (Fig. 3.13). The constant regions of two heavy chains of an antibody molecule form its effector function domain, which determines its interaction with the other components of the immune system. The light chains are of two types: kappa (κ) and lambda (λ); the type of a light chain is determined by its constant region. An antibody molecule contains only either two kappa or two lambda light chains. Separate genes encode the kappa (located in human chromosome 2) and lambda (chromosome 22) light chains, and the heavy chain (chromosome 14).

The variable region of each chain, in fact, contains 3 highly variable regions, called hyper variable regions and denoted as CDR1, CDR2 and CDR3 (CDR = complementarity-determining region) separated by 4 invariant regions called framework regions (designated as FR1, FR2, FR3, FR4). The constant region of each heavy chain has 3 homologous regions (C_H1, C_H2 and C_H3) which most likely originated from a common parental gene (3 tandem repeats of the parental gene, followed by mutations) (Fig. 3.13).

Classes of Immunoglobulins

Immunoglobulins (antibodies) are grouped into five classes based on their unique antigenic properties, which reside in their heavy chains (in the constant region). These five classes are: *IgG, IgM, IgA, IgD* and *IgE*. The heavy chains of an *Ig* class are designated by the small Greek letter corresponding to the class of *Ig*, i.e. γ heavy chain in *IgG*, μ in *IgM*, α in *IgA*, δ in *IgD* and ε in *IgE*. An individual has antibodies of all the five classes of *Ig*.

The immunoglobulins are further divided into subclasses based on antigenic differences within each of the different classes. In human, *IgG* has four subclasses (*IgG1, IgG2, IgG3, IgG4*), *IgA* has to subclasses (*IgA1, IgA2*), *IgM* has two subclasses (*IgM1, IgM2*), while *IgD* and *IgE* have no subclasses.

IgG is a monomer (Fig. 3.13), makes up Ca 75 per cent of the total human *Ig*, and is the only class of *Ig* which can cross the placenta and protect the newborn. *IgM* constitutes 10 per cent of human *Ig*, is a pentamer of the monomeric units and has a fourth C_H domain (C_H4). *IgA* is of two types: serum *IgA* (present in serum at 20 per cent of total *Ig*) and secretary *IgA* (predominant *Ig* in saliva, colostrum, milk, genitourinary secretions). *IgD* is very low (0.03 mg/ml) in the serum. Both *IgD* and *IgM* are present on the surface membranes of mature but virgin B lymphocytes. The *IgD* and *IgM* present on the surface of a single lymphocyte cell have the same antigen binding specificity. *IgE* is involved in hypersensitivity and allergy, and is only 0.00005 mg/ml in the serum. The Fc portion of *IgE* binds strongly to a receptor on mast cells which is involved in the allergic reaction.

Antibody Genes

The three genes encoding kappa and lambda light chains, and the heavy chain of antibodies present an interesting organisation. In the germline cells, each gene consists of a large number of segments belonging to V (variable), J (joining) and C (constant) types (in case of the light chains) or to V, D (deversity), J and C types (in the case of heavy chain). For example, the kappa light chain gene has 300 different V segments, five different J segments and a single C segment. During lymphocyte maturation, anyone of the V segments joins with any of the J segments; the rest of *V* and *J* segments are deleted. The mature lymphocyte, therefore, has the light chain gene rearranged as V–J–C segments. The lambda light chain gene undergoes a similar reorganisation. A given lymphocyte expresses either the kappa or the lambda light chain gene.

Similarly, the heavy chain gene is reorganised by joining together any one V segment, with anyone D segment and a single J segment; these are brought into association with one C segment, usually the C_μ segment. It should be noted that while the light chains have a single C segment, the heavy chain has 9–10 different C segments, each C segment representing a distinct class/subclass of *Ig*. In human, the sequence of C_H segments is as follows 5′C_μ–$C\delta$–$C\gamma3$–$C\gamma1$–$C\epsilon2$–$C\gamma1$–$C\alpha2$–$C\gamma4$–$C\alpha1$ 3′. Therefore, during lymphocyte proliferation, the first antibodies produced are *IgM*, but subsequently, antibodies of different classes begin to be produced; this phenomenon is known as class switching. Class switching occurs when the V–D–J segments of heavy chain gene become associated by a gene segment rearrangement with another C_H segment, e.g. $C\gamma1$ or $C\alpha1$, in place of the original $C\mu$ segment. In class switching, there is a change only in the C-region (constant region) of heavy chain, while its V region (variable region) remains the same; therefore, class switching does not affect the specificity of antibodies produced by a lymphocytes.

Lymphocytes

Lymphocytes are specialised cells which are responsible for the immune response of an animal. Lymphocytes originate from multi potent stem cells present in bone marrow; these stem cells give rise to both lymphoid stem cells (giving rise to lymphocytes) and to those that produce the various blood cells (myeloid stem cells). The lymphoid stem cells, in turn give rise to lymphocyte progenitor cells, Pre-B and Pre-T cells, which are further processed in lymphoid inducing microenvironments of bone marrow and thymus. Bone marrow processed cells mature into B-lymphocytes while those processed in thymus develop into *T*-lymphocytes (Fig. 3.14). Bone marrow and thymus provide the sites for lymphocyte differentiation, and are called primary lymphoid organs. The mature lymphocytes migrate to spleen and lymph nodes, which constitute the secondary lymphoid tissues; the B-lymphocytes and T-lymphocytes are present in discrete areas of these organs.

B-lymphocytes are antibody producing cells, while T-cells act as effector, helper or suppresser cells. The characteristic feature of B-lymphocytes is that they possess cell surface immunoglobulin (*sIg*), while T-lymphocytes express on their surface a differentiation antigen, viz. Thy 1. The differentiation of Pre-*T* cells is brought about by inducing factors secreted by thymus epithelial cells; the factors that have been identified are: Thymosin (induces expression of Thy 1), Thymopoietin and Thymic Humoral Factor. The factors associated with B-cell differentiation are not well known.

Lymphocytes are the major cell type of the lymph nodes, and they lie in a fine meshwork called reticulum. Lymphocytes circulate through body, passing between blood and lymphatic vascular systems at the lymph nodes. In antibody production, some T-cells act as helper cells to enable B-cells to produce antibody (B-cells are called effector cells). The helper T-cells and the effector B-cells interact with different parts of the immunogen (the antigen inducing immune response). Therefore, an immunogenic molecule must have one recognition site for the helper T-cells and another for effector B-cells to be able to induce antibody production.

The surface immunoglobulin (*sIg*) present on a B-cell has the same specificity as the antibody secreted by it. Thus the *sIg* molecules on a B-cell surface act as antigen-specific receptors. However, the nature of T-cell receptor is not clearly understood, but the T-cells react to the antigens in a specific manner. Binding of the antigen to *sIg* is necessary for the activation of B-lymphocytes; however, it is also essential that the antigen must cause cross-linking of the receptor molecules for activation to occur.

Once this has happened, proliferation and differentiation of the activated B-cells is induced by Interleukin-4 (IL-4) produced by T-lymphocytes. The differentated B-cell (plasma cells) produce and secrete the antibody (Fig. 3.15).

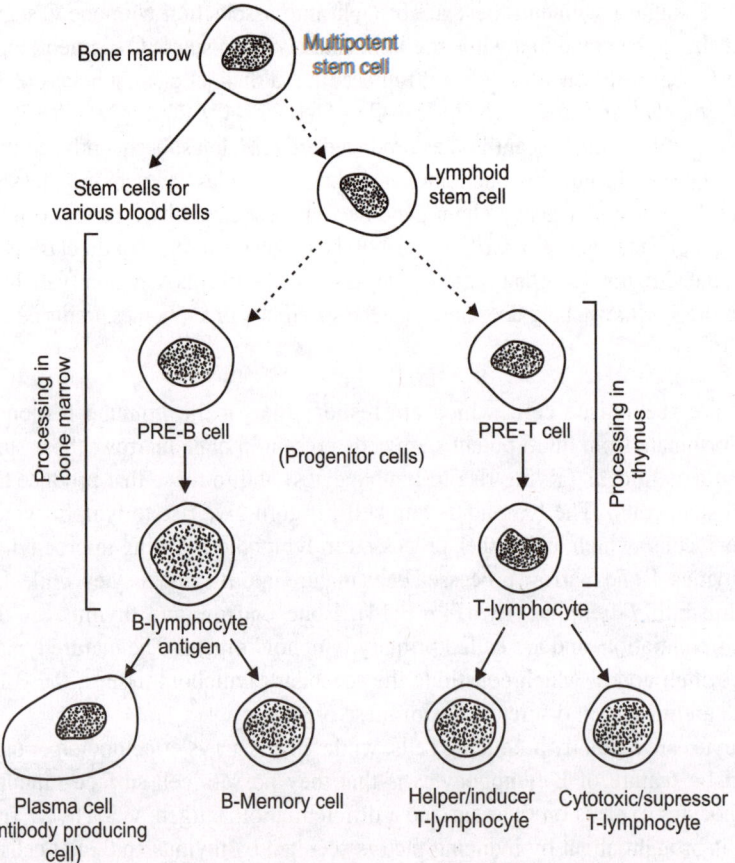

Fig. 3.14. A schematic representation of lymphocyte differentiation.

Monoclonal and Polyclonal Antibodies

In general, an antigen molecule has antigenic determinants of more than one specificity, i.e. different determinants will interact with different antibodies. In Fig. 3.15, the antigen has determinants specific for two antibodies. Each distinct antigenic determinant of the antigen will bind to a distinct mature B-cell whose *sIg* matches the specificity presented by the concerned determinant. As a result, such a single antigen will activate B-cells of more than one *sIg* specificity. Activated B-cells of each *sIg* specificity will divide and differentiate to give rise to clones of plasma cells producing antibodies of the same specificity. Thus a single antigen would induce more than one distinct clones of plasma cells which will produce antibodies of different specificities. Therefore, the serum of an animal immunised by a single antigen will contain antibodies of different specificities but reacting to the same antigen; these are called polyclonal antibodies since they are produced by several different plasma cell clones.

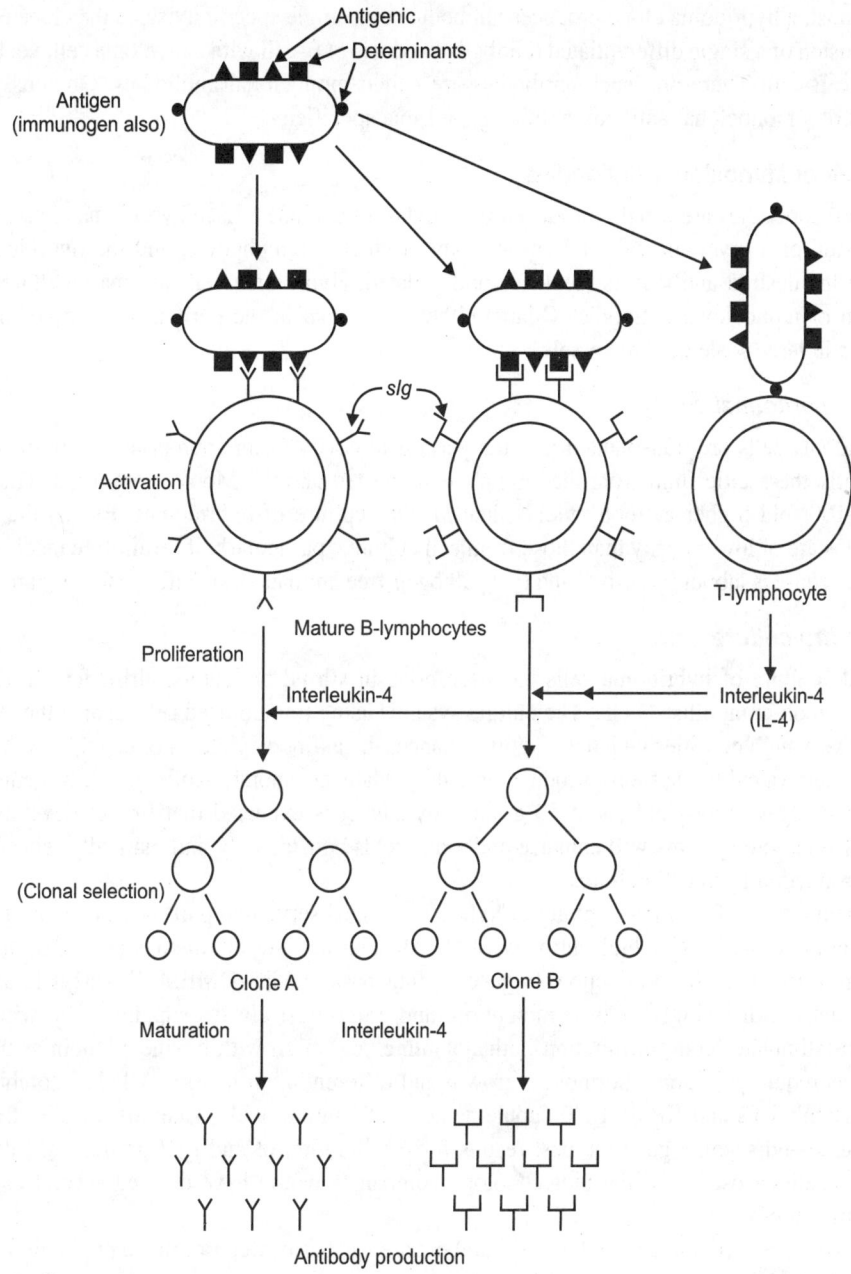

Fig. 3.15. A schematic representation of activation of mature B-lymphocytes leading to their proliferation and differentiation into antibody producing plasma cells. B-cells are activated when an antigen binds to and cross-links their *sIg* receptors. T-cells also interact with the antigen in a antigen-specific manner and produce Interleukln-4 which induces proliferation and differentiation of activated B-cells- Each B-cell divides to produce a clone of identical cells which produce antibodies having the same specificity as its *sIg* with which the antigen interacted. ▲ and ■, antigenic determinants having different specificities.

In contrast, a hybridoma clone produces antibodies of a single specificity since the clone is derived from the fusion of a single differentiated (antibody producing) B-cell with a myeloma cell, i.e. is a clone of a single B-cell. Therefore, such antibodies are called monoclonal antibodies. Obviously, all the molecules of a monoclonal antibody will have the same specificity.

Production of Monoclonal Antibodies

Monoclonal antibodies are usually produced from hybridoma clones. Each hybridoma clone is derived by the fusion of a myeloma cell and an antibody producing lymphocyte, and the hybridoma clone producing the desired antibody is identified and isolated. Hybridoma cells are mass cultured for the production of monoclonal antibodies (Mabs) either (i) *in vivo* in the peritoneal cavity of mice, and (ii) *in vitro* in large scale culture vessels.

Culture in peritoneal cavity

The hybridoma cells are transplanted into the peritoneal cavity of an appropriate strain of mice, and subsequently the ascitic fluid from the animals is harvested and the Moos are purified. This method gives 50–100 fold higher antibody yields than *in vitro* culture of hybridomas. But (i) the antibody preparations are of lower purity than those from cell cultures, particularly if serum-free media are used, (ii) the procedure is labour intensive, and (iii) pathogen-free animals of specific genotypes are required.

Mass in vitro culture

Large-scale culture of hybridoma cells has been done in stirred bioreators, airlift fermenters and in vessels based on immobilised cells. The culture systems using immobilised cells enable the cultivation of cells at very high densities which markedly enhances the antibody yields. For example, some hollow fibre cartridges (a culture system), produce upto 40 g Mabs per month, while opticle systems (special ceramic cartridges) may yield about 50 g antibody/day. It is expected that further developments in immobilised culture systems will enhance antibody yields considerably and markedly reduce the cost of their production from cell cultures.

The medium used for *in vitro* culture of hybridomas must serve two purposes: (i) support adequate cell proliferation, and (ii) give high antibody yields. Most basal tissue culture media have been designed for cell proliferation or for production. In general, four basal media (DMEM, IMDM, F12 and RPMI 1640) are used either singly or in combination, and are almost always supplemented with insulin, transferrin (stimulates cell proliferation), ethanolamine, and often with bovine albumin serum. Many hybridomas require additional hormones, growth and differentiation factors. A 1 : 1 : 2 combination of DMEM, Ham's F12 and RPMI 1640 supplemented with amino acids, vitamins, insulin, transferrin, ethanolamine and selenite gave the best results for proliferation of and *IgM* production from human hybridoma cells. Most likely, the biotechnology companies would have devised several undisclosed media formulations.

It is fairly easy to produce rodent Mabs, but there are various difficulties in the production of human Mabs. Rodent Mabs are good enough for diagnostic and separation procedures, but for therapeutic purposes human Mabs are far more desirable. Since antibodies are themselves immunogenic (and antigenic), human Mabs are likely to be much better tolerated by patients than rodent Mabs. In addition, human Mabs can be prepared against those antigens as well which are non-immunogenic in rodents.

The chief problem with the production of human hybridoma clones relates to the collection of lymphocytes producing specific antibodies since human beings cannot be immunised at will and their spleen (or lymph node) cannot be excised (the normal practices in rodent hybridoma production). Human lymphocytes are usually collected from blood of volunteers who have been immunised with some antigen, e.g. tetanus toxoid. The antibody producing lymphocytes are then immortalised in one of the following three ways.

1. The B-lymphocytes are transfected with DNA from a tumour; this transforms the lymphocytes making them capable of indefinite proliferation.

2. Fusion of the B-lymphocytes with suitable lymphoid tumour cells to produce hybridoma clones. The tumour cell line must be antibody non-producing (Ig^-).

3. Transformation of B-lymphocytes following their infection with Epstein Barr virus to lymphoblastoid cell lines. These lymphoblastoid cell lines can either themselves be used for Mab production or may be used to produce hybridoma clones (they are used in place of the B-lymphocytes).

At present, the second and third approaches of producing human-human hybridoma clones are being most commonly used. Several human Mabs are available commercially, e.g. against lung carcinoma, breast carcinoma, tetanus toxoid (human-mouse hybridoma), against glioma, measles virus (human-human hybridoma), against RhD, hepatitis B surface antigen (Eptein-Barr virus transformed B-lymphocytes), find against tetanus toxoid (hybridoma involving fusion of Epstein-Barr induced transformed lymphocytes in place of normal-B lymphocytes).

Applications of Monoclonal Antibodies

The chief advantage of monoclonal antibodies (Mabs) is that all the antibody molecules in a single preparation react with a single epitope or antigenic determinant. As a consequence, the results obtained by using Mabs are clear-cut as there is no background confusion that arises due to the presence of antibodies of other specificities in the case of conventionally used antisera. The multitude of various applications of Mabs may be grouped into the following 3 categories: (i) diagnostic, (ii) therapeutic, and (iii) purification.

Diagnostic applications

When Mabs are used to detect the presence of a specific antigen or of antibodies specific to an antigen in a sample or samples, this constitutes a diagnostic application. The presence of antigen is detected by assaying the formation of antigen-antibody complex (Ag-Ab complex) for which a number of assay techniques have been devised. These assays are highly precise, extremely efficient (some can detect picogram, pg, i.e. 10^{-12} g, quantities), fairly rapidly, and surprisingly versatile for a large variety of applications. Some examples of diagnostic applications are as follows.

1. Mabs are available for unequivocal classification of blood groups, e.g. ABO, Rh, etc.

2. Mabs are applied for a clear and decisive detection of pathogens involved in diseases (disease diagnosis). The principle in simple terms is as follows. An antigen specific to the pathogen to be detected is isolated and Mabs specific to the antigen are produced. This Mab preparation is applied to the tissue/fluid in which the presence of the above pathogen is to be detected. Ag-Ab complex will form only if the pathogen is present in the test sample since the antigen in question is present only in association with this pathogen. The formation of Ag-Ab complex is assayed using one of the immune assay procedures, of which the most commonly used is the ELISA. ELISA is widely used for the detection of specific viruses in plants, especially in germplasm being imported from outside.

3. Tumours contain several antigens that are associated with tumour cell differentiation, tumour growth and tumour immunology. An important marker antigen present in most tumours is the carcinoembryonic antigen (CEA). Mabs have been produced for CEA and some other tumour-associated antigens. Use of such Mabs in histochemical assays permits the identification of (i) tumour cell type, (ii) benign and malignant nature of tumours, and (iii) early cases of metastasis. Immunological assays enable a very early and accurate detection of cancer which is an important advantage in cancer therapy. Radioimmune assays can detect tumours as small as 0.5 cm which are otherwise not detectable.

4. Mabs can be used for an accurate detection of specific chromosomes of a given species. This is done by raising Mabs against specific proteins encoded by the genes present in different chromosomes of a species, e.g. for amylase inhibitors encoded by genes in chromosomes and 6 of wheat. The amount of Ag-Ab formation in the tissues, e.g. seed, extracts, from the different individuals can be used to determine if an individual is nullismic (no Ag-Ab formed), monosomic (low amount of Ag-Ab), normal disomic (intermediate amount of Ag-Ab) or trisomic (high amount of Ag-Ab) for the concerned chromosome.

Therapeutic applications

Such an application involves the use of Mabs for either the treatment of or protection from a disease. Some important developments in this area are briefly listed below:

1. Antibodies specific to a cell type, say, tumour cells, can be linked with a toxin polypeptide to yield a conjugate molecule called immunotoxin. The antibody component of immunotoxin will ensure its binding specifically and only to the target cells and the attached toxin will kill such cells. Immunotoxins having 'Ricin' have been prepared and evaluated for killing of tumour cells with considerable success. 'Ricin' is a natural toxin found in the endosperm of castor (*Ricinus communis*). It has two polypeptides called A (toxin peptide) and B (a cell binding polypeptide, lectin). Ricin A polypeptide enzymatically and irreversibly modifies the larger subunit of ribosomes (in fact, their EF2 binding site) making them incapable of protein synthesis. This toxin is effective against both dividing and nondividing cells as it inhibits protein synthesis. Antibody-Ricin A conjugate has been shown to reduce protein synthesis in mouse B-cell tumours; the antibody used in the conjugate was specific to the antigen molecules present on the surface of target tumour cells. It is noteworthy that this immunotoxin did not bind to either other tumour cells or the normal cells (Fig. 3.16).

   The same principle has been used to deliver radioactivity specificially to target tumour cells. In such cases, radioactivity due to ^{131}I (iodine), ^{90}Y (yitrium), ^{67}Cu, ^{212}Pb, etc. is incorporated into the tumour specific antibody (toxin is not used). The radioactive antibody specifically binds to the tumour cells that express the specific antigen, and the radiation emitted by the isotopes kills the tumour cells as well as their neighbour cells. This approach is also used for radioimaging to detect tumour cells for which the antibodies are specific. Radio labelled antibodies have been used in patients having hepatoma, HTLV-l (human T-Cell leukemia/lymphoma virus-1), ATL (adult-T cell leukemia), etc.

2. B-lymphocyte proliferation, maturation and antibody secretion are dependent on Interleukin-4 produced by activated T-lymphocytes. This would explain the observations that tissue and bone marrow explant rejections are mediated, by T-lymphocytes. Thus an effective strategy to minimise the rejection of grafts from other individuals (allografts) would be to eliminate the T-cells from their bone marrow/circulatory system (blood stream) by using T-cell specific Mabs. T-cells

exhibit several antigens of which CD3, CD4, CD8, etc. have been the preferred targets for Mab development.

In bone marrow transplantation, the bone marrow cells of the recipient are inactivated by appropriate irradiation. The donor bone marrow cells are treated with T-cell specific antibodies to destroy the T-cells present in them; the remaining cells are then transplanted into the recipient. Experiments with mice have shown remarkable success.

In order to minimise tissue-graft rejection, the T-cells present in circulatory system of the recipient are eliminated prior to the transplant by an administration of T-cell specific Mabs. This treatment abolishes, though temporarily, the ability of recipient to generate antibodies against any foreign antigen, including those present in the graft tissue. Mab OKT3 is the most widely used for treatment of acute cases of rejection of kidney transplants.

3. Mabs can be administered to provide passive immunity against diseases. In active immunity the immunised individual itself produces the antibodies against the concerned pathogen, while in case of passive immunity antibodies produced elsewhere are introduced into the body of an individual to provide immunity against the concerned pathogens.

4. Mabs are very useful in the purification of antigens specific to pathogens; these purified antigens are used as vaccines.

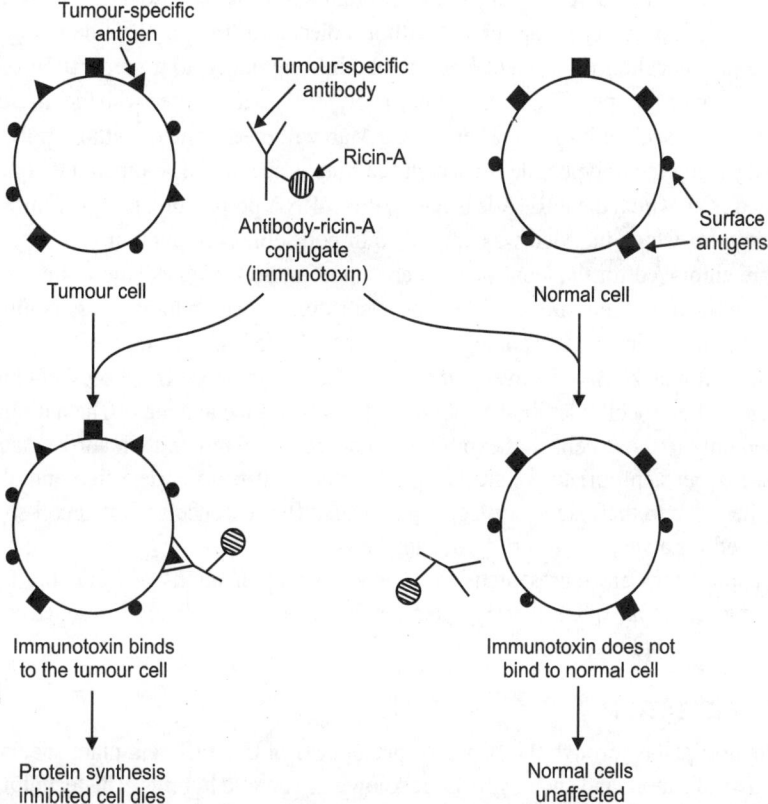

Fig. 3.16. A schematic representation of the principle of action of an immunotoxin containing the A polypeptide (toxin polypeptide) of Ricin, a seed protein from castor (Ricinus communis).

Immunopurification

The highly specific interaction of an antibody to the antigen is used to purify antigens present in small quantities as a mixture with several types of molecules; this is known as immunopurification. The different types of immunopurification are briefly described below:

1. A Mab specific to the antigen to be purified is fixed to an insoluble matrix, e.g. dextran or agarose beads, by a cross-linking agent like cyanogen bromide in such a way that its antigen binding is not affected. The beads are packed in a column through which the solution containing the antigen is passed. The antibody molecules interact with the antigen molecules forming Ag-Ab complex which is retained in the column while the remaining molecules freely pass through. Suitable washing procedures allow collection of the purified antigen held as Ag-Ab complex in the column. This technique, called affinity chromatography, is extremely specific and highly efficient. Examples of proteins purified in this manner are α-fetoprotein, interferon etc.

   The reverse of this approach may be employed for the purification of monoclonal antibodies. In this case, the purified antigen is fixed to the beads packed in a column through which the antibodies are passed. The antibodies form Ag-Ab complex and are subsequently recovered in a purified form.

2. Mabs have been used to isolate mRNA encoding the protein to which the Mabs are specific. Each mRNA molecule supporting active protein synthesis is associated with upto a dozen ribosomes each of which is associated with a molecule of the polypeptide being synthesised; this structure is called polysome. When antibodies are added to a preparation of polysomes, they interact with the specific nascent (young) polypeptides associated with the ribosomes causing precipitation of such polysomes. Therefore, a Mab will precipitate only those polysomes which are synthesising the polypeptide for which the Mab is specific. The precipitated polysomes are recovered from which the mRNA is isolated; this mRNA preparation is highly pure and encodes the protein for which the Mab was employed in polysome precipitation.

3. Mabs are employed for the identification and, more importantly, isolation of cells displaying a specific antigen on their surface. Mab specific to the concerned antigen is conjugated with a fluorescent molecule, and this conjugate is added to the cell suspension to allow Ag-Ab complex formation. (It may be more convenient to use a second non-specific fluorescent anti-*Ig* to bind to the unlabelled specific antibodies bound to the tell surface antigens). The antibody conjugate will bind only to those cells that exhibit the concerned antigen on their surface; such cells will fluoresce under appropriate conditions. Such cells are therefore identified and also separated from others due to their fluorescence; sophisticated fluorescence activated cell sorters (FACS) can be used for a very rapid sorting of such cells.

The above applications are representative of the various applications of Mabs the technology of which is advancing very rapidly. It is, therefore, neither desirable nor practical to present a comprehensive review of their various applications.

SOMATIC HYBRIDISATION

Production of hybrid plants through the fusion of protoplasts of two different plant species/varieties is called somatic hybridisation, and such hybrids are known as somatic hybrids. The technique of somatic hybridisation involves the following four steps: (i) isolation of protoplasts, (ii) fusion of the protoplasts of desired species/varieties, (iii) selection of somatic hybrid cells, and (iv) culture of the hybrid cells and regeneration of hybrid plants from them. A brief, elementary consideration of these steps is presented below (Fig. 3.17).

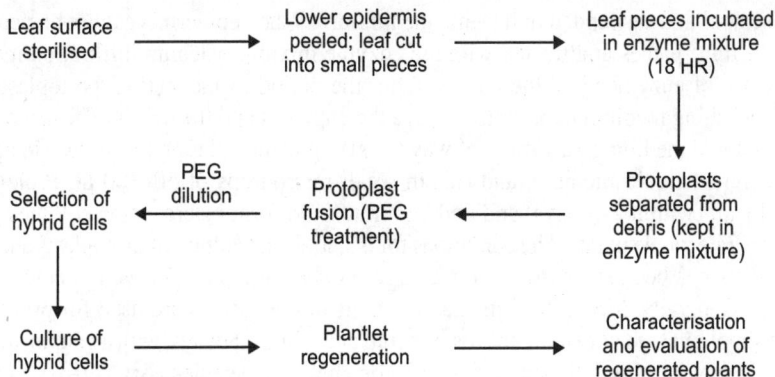

Fig. 3.17. A schematic representation of the various steps in somatic hybridisation.

Protoplast Isolation

Isolation of protoplasts Fig. 3.18 is readily achieved by treating cells/tissues with a suitable mixture of cell wall degrading enzymes. Usually a mixture of pectinase or macerozyme (0.1–1.9 per cent) and cellulase (1–2 per cent) is appropriate for most plant materials.

Hemicellulase may be necessary for some tissues. Generally, crude commercial preparations of enzymes are used. The pH of enzyme solution is adjusted between 4.7 and 6.0 and the temperature is kept at 25°–30°C. The osmotic concentration of enzyme mixture and of subsequent media is elevated (usually by adding 500–800 m mol 1^{-1} sorbitol or mannitol) to stabilise the protoplasts and to prevent them from bursting. Usually, 50–100 m mol 1^{-1} $CaCl_2$ is added to the osmoticum as it improves plasma membrane stability. The cells and tissues are incubated in the enzyme mixture for few to several (generally, 16–18) hours; naked protoplasts devoid of cell wall are gradually released in the enzyme mixture.

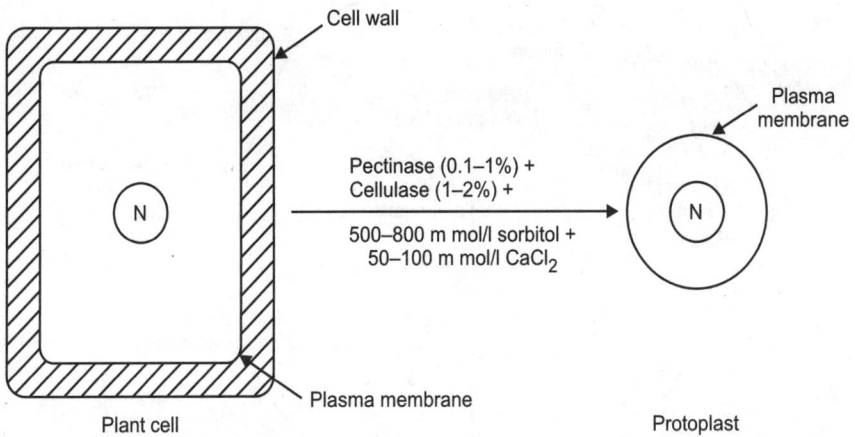

Fig. 3.18. Production of protoplasts by enzyme treatment (enzymes are depicted above the arrow). Osmoticum (shown below the arrow) is added to stabilise the protoplasts and prevent them from bursting. N, nucleus.

Protoplasts have been isolated from virtually all plant parts, but leaf mesophyll is the most preferred tissue, at least in case of dicots, for this purpose. In general, fully expanded leaves are surface sterilised, their lower epidermis is peeled off with a pair of forceps and the peeled areas are cut into small (ca. 1 cm^2) pieces with a scalpel and suspended in the enzyme mixture. When epidermis cannot be peeled, leaf may be cut into ca. 1 mm^2 pieces and treated with the enzyme mixture; vacuum infiltration may be used to facilitate the entry of enzymes into the tissues. After the period of incubation, protoplasts are washed with a suitable washing medium in order to remove the enzymes and the debris. The protoplasts may be cultured on a suitable medium in a variety of ways: (i) Bergmann's plating technique (in agar medium), (ii) in a thin layer of liquid medium, and (iii) in small microdrops of 50–100 µl. Protoplasts readily regenerate cell wall (within 2–4 days) and undergo mitosis to form macroscopic colonies which can be induced to regenerate whole plants. The conditions for isolation and culture of protoplasts and regeneration of complete plants has been standardised for a large number of plant species, but cereals still present some problems. Generally, MS and B5 media, and their modifications are used for protoplast culture. The media are supplemented with a suitable osmoticum and, almost always, with an auxin and a cytokinin, their types and concentrations depending mainly on the plant species. After 7–10 days of culture, protoplasts regenerate cell wall and the osmolarity of medium is gradually reduced to that of normal medium. The macroscopic colonies are transferred onto normal tissue culture media. Protoplasts are very sensitive to light; therefore, they are cultured in diffuse light or dark for the first 4–7 days.

Protoplast Fusion

A number of strategies have been used to induce fusion between protoplasts of different strains/species; of these the following three (Fig. 3.19) have been relatively more successful. Protoplasts of desired strains/species are mixed in almost equal proportion; generally they are mixed while still suspended in the enzyme mixture. The protoplast mixture is then subjected to a high pH (10.5) and high Ca^{2+} concentration (50 m mol 1^{-1}) at 37°C for about 30 min (high pH– high Ca^{2+} treatment). This technique is quite suitable for some species, while for some others it may be toxic.

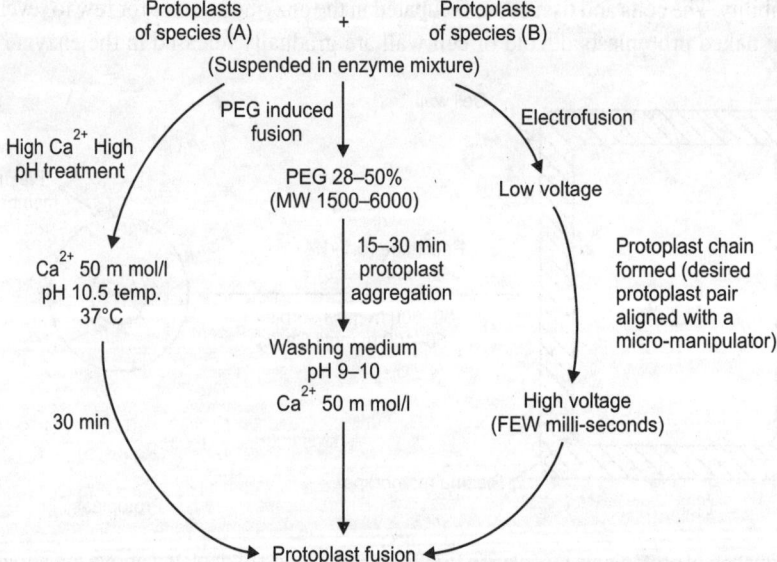

Fig. 3.19. A schematic representation of the 3 most successful protoplast fusion strategies.

Polyethylene glycol (PEG) induced protoplast fusion is the most commonly used as it induces reproducible high frequency fusion accompanied with low toxicity to most cell types. The protoplast mixture is treated with 28–50 per cent PEG (MW 1500–6000) for 15–30 min followed by gradual washing of the protoplasts to remove PEG; protoplast fusion occurs during the washing. The washing medium may be alkaline, (pH 9–10) and contain a high Ca^{2+} ion concentration (50 m mol 1^{-1}); this approach is a combination of PEG and high pH^- high Ca^{2+} treatments, and is usually more effective than either treatment alone. PEG is negatively charged and may bind to cation like Ca^{2+} which, in turn, may bind to the negatively charged molecules present in plasma lemma; they can also bind to cationic molecules of plasma membrane. During the washing process, PEG molecules may pull out the plasma lemma components bound to them. This would disturb plasma lemma organisation and may lead to the fusion of protoplasts located close to each other (Fig. 3.20).

The above fusion techniques are nonselective in that they induce fusion between any two or more protoplasts. A more selective and less drastic approach is the electrofusion technique which utilises low voltage electric current pulses to align the protoplasts in a single row like a pearl-chain. The aligned protoplasts are pushed, with a micromanipulator; at a gentle pace through the narrow gap between the two electrodes. When two protoplasts that are to be fused are appropriately oriented opposite the electrodes, a short pulse of high voltage is released which induces the protoplasts to fuse. The high voltage creates transient disturbances in the organisation of plasma lemma, which leads to the fusion of neighbouring protoplasts. The entire operation is carried out manually in a specially designed equipment, called electroporator, under a microscope. Many workers feel that this fusion technique is more desirable than the others for a number of important reasons. The techniques for protoplast fusion are pretty well refined and highly effective for almost all the systems.

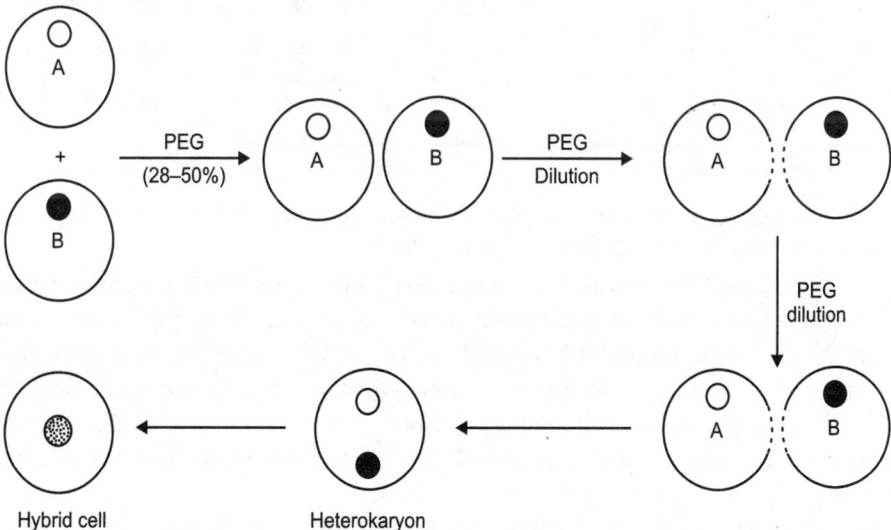

Fig. 3.20. PEG induced protoplast fusion. Protoplasts are first brought close together (aggregation) by PEG. Fusion occurs during PEG dilution due to disturbances created in plasma membrane.

Selection of Hybrid Cells

The protoplast suspension recovered after a treatment with a fusion inducing agent (fusogen) consists of the following cell types: (i) unfused protoplasts of the two species/strains, (ii) products of fusion between two or more protoplasts of the same species (homokaryons), and (iii) 'hybrid' protoplasts produced by fusion between one (or more) protoplast(s) of each of the two species (heterokaryons) (Fig. 3.21). In somatic hybridisation experiments, only the heterokaryotic or hybrid protoplasts, particularly those resulting from fusion between one protoplast of each of the two species, are of interest. However, they form only a small proportion of the population (usually 0.5–10 per cent). Therefore, an effective strategy has to be employed for their identification and isolation. This step is called the selection of hybrid cells, and is the most critical, and is still an active area of investigation.

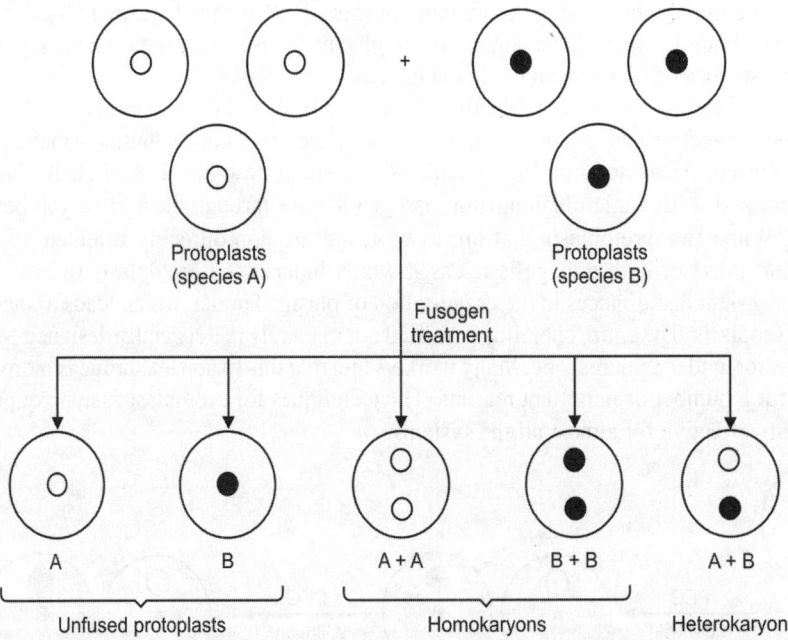

Fig. 3.21. Different types of products recovered after fusogen, (fusion agent) treatment of protoplasts of two different species (A and B) mixed together (usually in 1 : 1 ratio).

A number of strategies have been used for the selection of hybrid protoplasts: (i) some visual markers, e.g. pigmentation, of the parental protoplasts may be used for the identification of hybrid cells under a microscope; these are then mechanically isolated and cultured. For example, the protoplasts of one species may be green and vacuolated (from mesophyll cells), while those of the other may be nonvacuolated and nongreen (from cell cultures). Where such features are not available, the protoplasts of two parental species may be separately labelled with different fluorescent agents. This approach is time consuming, and requires considerable skill and effort.

Several workers have attempted to devise systems which specifically select for hybrid cells. In simple words (ii) these systems exploit some properties (usually, deficiencies) of the parental species which are not expressed in the hybrid cells due to complementation between their genetic systems. These properties may be sensitivity to culture medium constituents, antimetabolites, temperature, etc. inability to produce an essential biochemical (auxotrophic mutants), chlorophyll or some other pigmentation, etc. These properties may be naturally present in the parental species or may be artificially induced through mutagenesis.

The following example should be enough to clearly bring out the essential features of the above approach. Protoplasts of *Petunia hybrida* form calli on the MS medium, while those of *P. parodii* produce only small cell colonies. Further, actinomycin D (1 μg ml⁻¹) inhibits cell division of *P. hybrida* protoplasts, but it has no effect on those of *P. parodii*. Thus protoplasts of both these *Petunia* species fail to produce macroscopic colonies (calli) on MS medium supplemented with 1 μg ml⁻¹ actinomycin D. *However*, their hybrid cells (*P. hybrida* + *P. parodii*; it may be noted that somatic hybrids are denoted by a + sign as against the sexual hybrids being designated by a × symbol) divide normally on this medium to produce macroscopic colonies. This selection strategy exploits those natural properties of the two parental species which show complementation in the hybrid cells and, at the same time, permit their selection. These strategies are simple, highly effective and the least demanding, but their application is drastically limited by the nonavailability of suitable properties (both natural and induced) in most of the parental species of interest to the experimenters.

A more general and widely applicable strategy, but demanding more work than the previous approach is (iii) to culture the entire protoplast population without applying any selection for the hybrid cells. All the types of protoplasts form calli; the hybrid calli are later identified on the basis of callus morphology, chromosome constitution, protein and enzyme banding patterns, etc. In some cases, the identification may be delayed till plants are regenerated. In such an approach it will be desirable to culture the protoplasts in very low densities since neighbouring colonies are likely to fuse at higher densities; ideally, they should be cultured in microdrops, each drop containing but a single cell. Many workers tend to favour this approach since it does not depend the presence of appropriate but difficult to find markers in the parental species.

Regeneration of Hybrid Plants

Once hybrid calli are obtained, plants are induced to regenerate from them since this is a prerequisite for their exploitation in crop improvement. Further, the hybrid plants must be at least partially fertile, in addition to having some useful property, to be of any use in breeding schemes. The culture techniques have been refined to a state where plant regeneration has been obtained in a number of somatic hybrids Table 3.3. But even today, it has not been possible to recover hybrid plants and/or calli from a number of somatic combinations; this phenomenon is called 'somatic incompatibility'. The reasons for somatic incompatibility are not clearly understood.

Table 3.3. A list of some distant somatic hybrid plants.

Symmetric or near-symmetric Hybrids
Salanun tuberosum + Lycopersicon esculentum*
Datura innoxia + Atropa belladona
Arabidopsis thaliana + Brassica campestris
Atropa belladona + Nicotiana chinensis
Asymmetric Hybrids
Daucus carota + Aegopodium podagraria
Daucus carota + Petroselinum hortense
Hyoscyamus muticus + Nicotiana tabacum
Datura innoxia + Physalis minima
Nicotiana tabacum + Daucus carota

* The + symbol indicates that the hybrid was obtained through protoplast fusion.

Symmetric hybrids

Some somatic hybrid plants retain the full or nearly full somatic complements of the two parental species; these are called symmetric hybrids. Such hybrids provide unique opportunities for synthesising novel species which may be of theoretical and/or practical interest.

Frequently, somatic hybrids (symmetric) between distantly related sexually incom-patible species are sterile, precluding their incorporation in a breeding programme. This may be circumvented by producing $3n$ somatic hybrids by fusing somatic $(2n)$ cells of one species with haploid (n) cells of the other species; such $3n$ plants may be expected to be partially fertile. These somatic hybrids can now be used in breeding programmes for limited gene/chromosome introgression from the species contributing the haploid protoplast. An approach to the improvement of apparently useless somatic hybrids, e.g. nonflowering somatic hybrid Daucus carota + Aegopodium podagraria, is to fuse protoplasts from the hybrid with those of one of the parental species. The fusion of a somatic hybrid protoplast with that from one of its parents is called somatic back hybridisation. When protoplasts from the above somatic hybrid were fused with carrot protoplasts, the resulting somatic hybrid produced flowers. Such hybrids can now be ordered into breeding programmes with the aim of gene/chromosome introgression.

Asymmetric hybrids

Many somatic hybrids exhibit the full somatic complement of one parental species, while all or nearly all chromosomes of the other parental species are lost during the preceding mitotic divisions; such hybrids are referred to as asymmetric hybrids. The available evidence suggests that such hybrids are likely to show a limited introgression of chromosome segments from the eliminated genome(s) due to drastically enhanced chromosomal aberrations and/or mitotic crossing over *in vitro*. Asymmetric hybrids can be obtained even from those combinations which normally produce symmetric hybrids by the following approach: protoplasts of one of the parental species are irradiated with a suitable dose of X-rays or gamma-rays to induce extensive chromosome breakage. In such cases, chromosome segment introgression may be markedly enhanced. It may be pointed out that asymmetric hybrids are essentially cytoplasmic hybrids or cybrids except for the introgressed genes.

Fate of plasma genes

In contrast to sexual hybrid cells, i.e. zygotes, which contain the cytoplasmic genes (plasmon) from the female parent only, somatic hybrid cells contain cytoplasmic complements from both the parental species. The cytoplasmic genes (generally studied in terms of chloroplast types or chloroplast DNA, cp-DNA) appear to be distributed randomly during the mitotic cell divisions. As a result, some cells receive chloroplasts of one parental species, some others of the other species and a small proportion retain the chloroplasts of both the species. This is reflected in the plants regenerated from these cells. The same applies to mitochondria as well. In addition, the distribution of chloroplasts is independent from that of mitochondria. Therefore, a somatic hybrid plant may contain chloroplasts from one parental species and mitochondria from the other fusion parent. There is considerable evidence that the genomes of both chloroplasts and mitochondria, particularly the latter, undergo recombination in the hybrid cells; this produces recombinant organelles in the progeny.

Cybrids

Cybrids or cytoplasmic hybrids are cells or plants containing nucleus of one species but cytoplasm from both the parental species. They are produced in variable frequencies in normal protoplast fusion experiments due to one of the following: (i) fusion of a normal protoplast of one species with an enucleate protoplast or a protoplast having an inactivated nucleus of the other species, (ii) elimination of the nucleus of one species from a normal heterokaryon, and (iii) gradual elimination of the chromosomes of one species from a hybrid cell during the subsequent mitotic divisions. Cybrids may be produced in relatively high frequency by (i) irradiating (with X-rays or gamma-rays) the protoplasts of one species prior to fusion in order to inactivate their nuclei, or (ii) by preparing enucleate protoplasts (cytoplasts) of one species and fusing them with normal protoplasts of the other species.

The objective of cybrid production is to combine the cytoplasmic genes of one species with the nuclear and cytoplasmic genes of another species. But the mitotic segregation of plasma genes, as evidenced by the distribution of chloroplasts, leads to the recovery of plants having plasma genes of one or the other species only; only a small proportion of the plants remain 'cybrid' which would further segregate into the two parental types.

This provides the following unique opportunities: (i) transfer of plasma genes of one species into the nuclear background of another species in a single generation and even in, (ii) sexually incompatible combinations, (iii) recovery of recombinants between the parental mitochondrial or chloroplast DNAs (genomes), and (iv) production of a wide variety of combinations of the parental and recombinant chloroplasts with the parental or recombinant mitochondria. When cybrids are produced by irradiating the protoplasts of one species prior to fusion, they provide the additional opportunity for (v) recovery; of chromosome segment introgressions from the lost genome, in combination with variations in the plasmon. The cybrid approach has been used for the transfer of cytoplasmic male sterility from *Nicotiana tabacum* to *N. sylvestris*, from Petunia hybrida to *P. axillaris*, etc. (vi) in addition, mitochondria from one parental species may be combined with the chloroplasts of the other parental species.

Hybrid Antibodies

When antibody molecules are modified or designed using recombinant DNA technology to suit specific applications, such antibodies are called recombinant or hybrid antibodies, and the approach itself is termed as antibody engineering.

The essential steps in antibody engineering are:

1. To develop the antibody design to serve the specific purpose.
2. To bring together the DNA sequences that would generate this antibody molecule into a suitable expression vector.
3. To introduce this recombinant DNA into a myeloma cell line where the recombinant antibody gene expresses itself.
4. To mass culture the transfected (i.e. containing the recombinant antibody gene) clones of myeloma cell line.
5. To harvest the recombinant antibodies produced. It is essential that the myeloma cell line used for transfection is *Ig*- (immunoglobulin negative), i.e. does not produce any antibody of its own.

A recombinant antibody could be constructed so that the constant end of its heavy chain is fused to a polypeptide chain having an enzymatic function. The enzymatic polypeptide chain could replace the CH2 and CH3 regions of the heavy chain and be fused to the CH1 segment.

Such an antibody will be extremely useful for ELISA as there will be no need for a second antibody. A gene producing such an antibody can be produced by fusing the heavy chain gene having the appropriate L-V-D-J and yl sequences with the sequence coding for the selected enzyme function.

The heavy chain gene of an antibody specific to a tumour-specific antigen may be fused with a gene encoding a toxin polypeptide. Such hybrid antibodies will carry the toxin specifically to the tumour cells and, thereby, kill them.

Gene segments encoding the variable region or V-region (involved in antigen-antibody interaction) of an antibody have been fused with the constant region or C-region of another antibody to yield a hybrid antibody. A hybrid antibody has the antigen specificity of the first antibody (which contributed the V-region segments), but its other properties are due to the second antibody (contributing the C-region segments). This approach has been used to produce hybrid antibodies with their antigen-binding portion from a mouse antibody gene, and their C-region from the human antibody gene. Such antibodies are often known as humanised rodent antibodies. This is very useful in cases where it is not possible to either immunise humans or to induce antibody production in cultured human cells.

The knowledge of three dimensional structures of antigens and antibody regions involved in antigen binding can be used to predict the amino acid sequence of V-region of the antibody specific to the given antigen. This involves a detailed computer modelling using the data on molecular organisation of the antigen to predict the corresponding organisation of the specific antibody. The gene encoding an antibody having the given amino acid sequence can now be synthesised and expressed in a suitable host cell. The hybrid antibodies are monoclonal in nature since each preparation has antibodies of a single specificity.

Selection of somatic hybrids and cybrids

Proper selection of the hybrid cells or fusion products after fusion treatment is necessary since the protoplast populations consist of a heterogeneous mixture of unfused parental types, homokaryons, and heterokaryons. This is because the fusion induced by various methods is random and uncontrolled. Generally, 20–25 per cent protoplasts may be involved in a fusion event although heterokaryon formation as high as 50–100 per cent has been reported. The low number of true hybrid cells formed may get lost in the population of actively dividing homokaryotic fusion products and unfused parental protoplasts.

Hence, selective recovery of the few hybrid cells formed from the mixed population of regenerating protoplasts is a key factor in successful somatic hybridisation. Many selection procedures are employed.

Chapter 4

Regulation of Gene Expression in Prokaryotes

INTRODUCTION

Regulation of gene expression (or gene regulation) includes the processes that cells and viruses use to regulate the way that the information in genes is turned into gene products. Although a functional gene product may be an RNA or a protein, the majority of known mechanisms regulate protein coding genes. Any step of the gene's expression may be modulated, from DNA-RNA transcription to the post-translational modification of a protein.

Gene regulation is essential for viruses, prokaryotes and eukaryotes as it increases the versatility and adaptability of an organism by allowing the cell to express protein when needed. The first discovered example of a gene regulation system was the *lac* operon, discovered by Jacques Monod, in which protein involved in lactose metabolism are expressed by *E. coli* only in the presence of lactose and absence of glucose.

Furthermore, gene regulation drives the processes of cellular differentiation and morphogenesis, leading to the creation of different cell types in multicellular organisms where the different types of cells may possess different gene expression profiles though they all possess the same genome sequence.

REGULATED STAGES OF GENE EXPRESSION

Any step of gene expression may be modulated, from the DNA-RNA transcription step to post-translational modification of a protein. The following is a list of stages where gene expression is regulated, the most extensively utilised point is transcription initiation:

1. Chromatin domains.
2. Transcription.
3. Post-transcriptional modification.
4. RNA transport.
5. Translation.
6. mRNA degradation.

Modification of DNA

In eukaryotes, the accessibility of large regions of DNA can depend on its chromatin structure which can be altered as a result of histone modifications which are directed by DNA methylation, ncRNA or DNA binding protein. Methylation of DNA is a common method of gene silencing. DNA is typically methylated by methyltransferase enzymes on cytosine nucleotides in a CpG dinucleotide sequence (also called 'CpG islands' when densely clustered). Analysis of the pattern of methylation in a given region of DNA (which can be a promoter) can be achieved through a method called bisulphite mapping. Methylated cytosine residues are unchanged by the treatment, whereas unmethylated ones are changed to uracil. The differences are analysed by DNA sequencing or by methods developed to quantify SNPs, such as pyrosequencing (biotage) or MassArray (Sequenom), measuring the relative amounts of C/T at the CG dinucleotide. Abnormal methylation patterns are thought to be involved in carcinogenesis.

Structural

Transcription of DNA is dictated by its structure. In general, the density of its packing is indicative of the frequency of transcription. Octameric protein complexes called nucleosomes are responsible for the amount of supercoiling of DNA, and these complexes can be temporarily modified by processes such as phosphorylation or more permanently modified by processes such as methylation. Such modifications are considered to be responsible for more or less permanent changes in gene expression levels.

Histone acetylation is also an important process in transcription. Histone acetyltransferase enzymes (HATs) such as CREB binding protein also dissociate the DNA from the histone complex, allowing transcription to proceed. Often, DNA methylation and histone deacetylation work together in gene silencing. The combination of the two seems to be a signal for DNA to be packed more densely, lowering gene expression.

REGULATION OF TRANSCRIPTION

Regulation of transcription controls when transcription occurs and how much RNA is created. Transcription of a gene by RNA polymerase can be regulated by at least five mechanisms:
1. Specificity factors alter the specificity of RNA polymerase for a given promoter or set of promoters, making it more or less likely to bind to them (i.e. sigma factors used in prokaryotic transcription).
2. Repressors bind to non-coding sequences on the DNA strand that are close to or overlapping the promoter region, impeding RNA polymerase's progress along the strand, thus impeding the expression of the gene.
3. General transcription factors: These transcription factors position RNA polymerase at the start of a protein-coding sequence and then release the polymerase to transcribe the mRNA.
4. Activators enhance the interaction between RNA polymerase and a particular promoter, encouraging the expression of the gene. Activators do this by increasing the attraction of RNA polymerase for the promoter, through interactions with subunits of the RNA polymerase or indirectly by changing the structure of the DNA.
5. Enhancers are sites on the DNA helix that are bound to by activators in order to loop the DNA bringing a specific promoter to the initiation complex. Enhancers are much more common in eukaryote than prokaryotes, where only a few examples exist (to date).

Post-transcriptional Regulation

After the DNA is transcribed and mRNA is formed there must be some sort of regulation on how much the mRNA is translated into proteins. Cells do this by modulating the capping, splicing, addition of a Poly(A) Tail, the sequence-specific nuclear export rates and in several contexts sequestration of the RNA transcript. These processes occur in eukaryotes but not in prokaryotes. This modulation is a result of a protein or transcript which in turn is regulated and may have an affinity for certain sequences.

1. Capping changes the five prime end of the mRNA to a three prime end by 5′–5′ linkage, which protects the mRNA from 5′ exonuclease, which degrades foreign RNA. The cap also helps in ribosomal binding.
2. Splicing removes the introns, noncoding regions that are transcribed into RNA, in order to make the mRNA able to create proteins. Cells do this by spliceosomes binding on either side of an intron, looping the intron into a circle and then cleaving it off. The two ends of the exons are then joined together.
3. Addition of poly(A) tail otherwise known as poly-adenylation. Junk RNA is added to the 3′ end, and acts as a buffer to the 3′ exonuclease in order to increase the half life of mRNA.

Regulation of Translation

The translation of mRNA can also be controlled by a number of mechanisms, mostly at the level of initiation. Recruitment of the small ribosomal subunit can indeed be modulated by mRNA secondary structure, antisense RNA binding or protein binding. In both prokaryotes and eukaryotes a large number of RNA binding proteins exist, which often are directed to their target sequence by the secondary structure of the transcript, which may change depending on certain conditions, such as temperature or presence of a ligand (aptamer), some transcripts act as ribozymes and self-regulate their expression.

Examples of gene regulation

1. Enzyme induction is a process in which a molecule (e.g. a drug) induces (i.e. initiates or enhances) the expression of an enzyme.
2. The induction of heat shock proteins in the fruit fly *Drosophila melanogaster*.
3. The *lac* operon is an interesting example of how gene expression can be regulated.
4. Viruses despite having only a few genes, possess mechanisms to regulate their gene expression, typically into an early and late phase, using collinear systems regulated by anti-terminators (lambda phage) or splicing modulators (HIV).

Circuitry

Up-regulation and down-regulation

Up-regulation is a process which occurs within a cell triggered by a signal (originating internal or external to the cell) which results in increased expression of one or more genes and as a result the protein(s) encoded by those genes. Conversely down-regulation is a process resulting in decreased gene and corresponding protein expression.

1. Up-regulation occurs for example when a cell is deficient in some kind of receptor. In this case, more receptor protein is synthesised and transported to the membrane of the cell and thus the sensitivity of the cell is brought back to normal reestablishing homeostasis.
2. Down-regulation occurs for example when a cell is overly stimulated by a neurotransmitter, hormone, or drug for a prolonged period of time and the expression of the receptor protein is decreased in order to protect the cell.

Inducible vs. repressible systems

Gene regulation can be summarised as how they respond:

1. Inducible systems: An inducible system is off unless there is the presence of some molecule (called an inducer) that allows for gene expression. The molecule is said to 'induce expression'.

The manner in which this happens is dependent on the control mechanisms as well as differences between prokaryotic and eukaryotic cells.

2. Repressible systems: A repressible system is on except in the presence of some molecule (called a corepressor) that suppresses gene expression. The molecule is said to 'repress expression'. The manner in which this happens is dependent on the control mechanisms as well as differences between prokaryotic and eukaryotic cells.

Developmental biology

A large number of studied regulatory systems come from developmental biology. Examples include:

1. The colinearity of the Hox gene cluster with their nested antero-posterior patterning.
2. It has been speculated that pattern generation of the hand (digits – interdigits). The gradient of Sonic hedgehog (secreted inducing factor) from the zone of polarising activity in the limb which creates a gradient of active Gli3 which activates Gremlin which inhibits BMPs also secreted in the limb resulting in the formation of an alternating pattern of activity as a result of this reaction-diffusion system.
3. Somitogenesis is the creation of segments (somites) from a uniform tissue (Pre-somitic Mesoderm, PSM). They are formed sequentially from anterior to posterior, this is achieved in amniotes possibly by means of two opposing gradients, Retinoic acid in the anterior (wavefront) and Wnt and Fgf in the posterior, coupled to an oscillating pattern (segmentation clock) composed of FGF + Notch and Wnt in antiphase.
4. Sex determination in the soma of a Drosophila requires the sensing of the ratio of autosomal genes to sex chromosome encoded genes, which results in the production of sexless splicing factor in females resulting in the female isoform of doublesex.

Theoretical circuits

1. Repressor/Inducer: an activation of a sensor results in the change of expression of a gene.
2. Negative feedback: the gene product down-regulates its own production directly or indirectly, which can result in:
   (a) Keeping transcript levels constant/proportional to a factor.
   (b) Inhibition of runaway reactions when coupled with a positive feedback loop.
   (c) Creating an oscillator by taking advantage in the time delay of transcription and translation, given that the mRNA and protein half-life is shorter.
3. Positive feedback: the gene product upregulates its own production directly or indirectly, which can result in:
   (a) Signal amplification.
   (b) Bistable switches when two genes inhibit each other and have both positive feedback.
   (c) Pattern generation.

Methods

Generally, most experiments investigating differential expression used whole cell extracts of RNA, called steady-state levels, to determine which genes changed and by how much they did. These are however not informative of where the regulation has occurred and may actually mask conflicting regulatory processess, but it is still the most commonly analysed (QPCR and DNA microarray). When studying gene expression there are several methods to look at the various stages.

In eukaryotes these include:

1. The chromatin conformation of the region can be determined by ChIP-chip analysis by pulling down RNA Polymerase II, histone 3 modifications, trithorax-group protein, polycomb-group protein or any other DNA binding element to which a good antibody is available.

2. Epistatic interactions can be investigated by synthetic genetic array analysis.

3. Due to post-transcriptional regulation, transcription rates and total RNA levels differ significantly, to measure the transcription rates nuclear run-on assays can be done and newer high-throughput methods are being developed, using thiol labelling instead of radioactivity.

4. Only 5 per cent of the RNA polymerised in the nucleus actually exists and not only introns, abortive products and nonsense transcripts are degradated therefore the differences in nuclear and cytoplasmic levels can be seen by separating the two fractions by gentle lysis.

5. Alternative splicing can be analysed with a splicing array or with a tiling array.

6. All *in vivo* RNA is complexed as RNPs. The quantity of transcripts bound to specific protein can be also analysed by RIP-chip, for example DCP2 will give an indication of sequestered protein, ribosome bound gives and indication of transcripts active in transcription (although it should be noted that a more dated method, called polysome fractionation, is still popular in some labs).

7. Protein levels can be analysed by mass spectrometry, which can only be compare to QPCR data as microarray data is relative and not absolute.

8. RNA and protein degradation rates are measured by means of transcription inhibitors (actinomycin D or α-amanitin) or translation inhibitors (cycloheximide) respectively.

GENE CONTROL IN PROKARYOTES

The controls that act on gene expression (i.e. the ability of a gene to produce a biologically active protein) are much more complex in eukaryotes than in prokaryotes. A major difference is the presence in eukaryotes of a nuclear membrane, which prevents the simultaneous transcription and translation that occurs in prokaryotes. Whereas, in prokaryotes, control of transcriptional initiation is the major point of regulation, in eukaryotes the regulation of gene expression is controlled nearly equivalently from many different points.

In bacteria, genes are clustered into operons: gene clusters that encode the proteins necessary to perform coordinated function, such as biosynthesis of a given amino acid. RNA that is transcribed from prokaryotic operons is polycistronic a term implying that multiple proteins are encoded in a single transcript.

In bacteria, control of the rate of transcriptional initiation is the predominant site for control of gene expression. As with the majority of prokaryotic genes, initiation is controlled by two DNA sequence elements that are approximately 35 bases and 10 bases, respectively, upstream of the site of transcriptional initiation and as such are identified as the –35 and –10 positions. These two sequence elements are termed promoter sequences, because they promote recognition of transcriptional start sites by RNA polymerase. The consensus sequence for the –35 position is TTGACA, and for the –10 position, TATAAT. (The –10 position is also known as the Pribnow-box.) These promoter sequences are recognised and contacted by RNA polymerase.

The activity of RNA polymerase at a given promoter is in turn regulated by interaction with accessory proteins, which affect its ability to recognise start sites. These regulatory proteins can act both positively (activators) and negatively (repressors). The accessibility of promoter regions of prokaryotic DNA is in many cases regulated by the interaction of proteins with sequences termed operators. The operator region is adjacent to the promoter elements in most operons and in most cases the sequences of the operator bind a repressor protein. However, there are several operons in *E. coli* that contain overlapping sequence elements, one that binds a repressor and one that binds an activator.

As indicated above, prokaryotic genes that encode the proteins necessary to perform coordinated function are clustered into operons. Two major modes of transcriptional regulation function in bacteria (*E. coli*) to control the expression of operons. Both mechanisms involve repressor proteins. One mode of regulation is exerted upon operons that produce gene products necessary for the utilisation of energy; these are catabolite-regulated operons. The other mode regulates operons that produce gene products necessary for the synthesis of small biomolecules such as amino acids. Expression from the latter class of operons is attenuated by sequences within the transcribed RNA.

A classic example of a catabolite-regulated operon is the *lac* operon, responsible for obtaining energy from β-galactosides such as lactose. A classic example of an attenuated operon is the *trp* operon, responsible for the biosynthesis of tryptophan.

lac Operon

The *lac* operon (Fig. 4.1) consists of one regulatory gene (the *i* gene) and three structural genes (*z*, *y*, and *a*). The *i* gene codes for the repressor of the *lac* operon. The *z* gene codes for β-galactosidase (β-gal), which is primarily responsible for the hydrolysis of the disaccharide, lactose into its monomeric units, galactose and glucose. The *y* gene codes for permease, which increases permeability of the cell to β-galactosides. The *a* gene encodes a transacetylase. During normal growth on a glucose-based medium, the *lac* repressor is bound to the operator region of the *lac* operon, preventing transcription. However, in the presence of an inducer of the *lac* operon, the repressor protein binds the inducer and is rendered incapable of interacting with the operator region of the operon. RNA polymerase is thus able to bind at the promoter region, and transcription of the operon ensues. The *lac* operon is repressed, even in the presence of lactose, if glucose is also present. This repression is maintained until the glucose supply is exhausted. The repression of the *lac* operon under these conditions is termed catabolite repression and is a result of the low levels of cAMP that result from an adequate glucose supply. The repression of the *lac* operon is relieved in the presence of glucose if excess cAMP is added. As the level of glucose in the medium falls, the level of cAMP increases. Simultaneously there is an increase in inducer binding to the *lac* repressor. The net result is an increase in transcription from the operon. The ability of cAMP to activate expression from the *lac* operon results from an interaction of cAMP with a protein termed CRP (for cAMP receptor protein).

The protein is also called CAP (for catabolite activator protein). The cAMP-CRP complex binds to a region of the *lac* operon just upstream of the region bound by RNA polymerase and that somewhat overlaps that of the repressor binding site of the operator region. The binding of the cAMP-CRP complex to the *lac* operon stimulates RNA polymerase activity 20-to-50-fold.

Regulation of the *lac* operon in *E. coli*. The repressor of the operon is synthesised from the *i* gene. The repressor protein binds to the operator region of the operon and prevents RNA polymerase from transcribing the operon. In the presence of an inducer (such as the natural inducer, allolactose) the repressor is inactivated by interaction with the inducer. This allows RNA polymerase access to the operon and transcription proceeds. The resultant mRNA encodes the β-galactosidase, permease and transacetylase activities necessary for utilisation of β-galactosides (such as lactose) as an energy source. The *lac* operon is additionally regulated through binding of the cAMP-receptor protein, CRP (also termed the catabolite activator protein, CAP) to sequences near the promoter domain of the operon. The result is a 50 fold enhancement of polymerase activity.

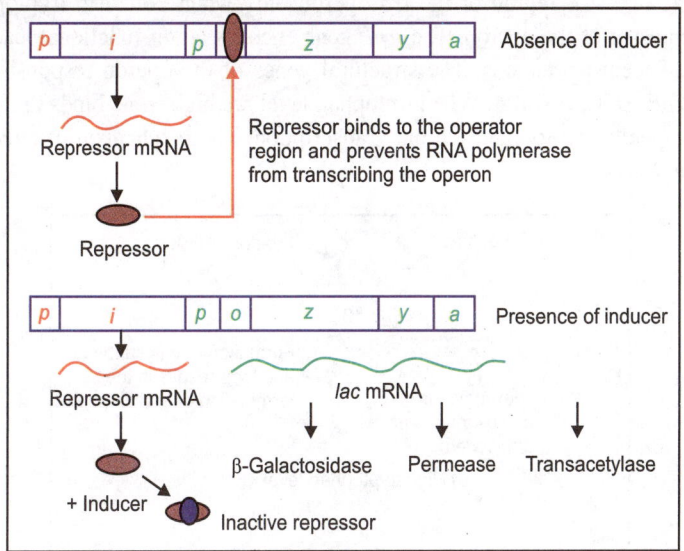

Fig. 4.1. The *lac* operon.

trp Operon

The *trp* operon (Fig. 4.2) encodes the genes for the synthesis of tryptophan. This cluster of genes, like the *lac* operon, is regulated by a repressor that binds to the operator sequences. The activity of the *trp* repressor for binding the operator region is enhanced when it binds tryptophan; in this capacity, tryptophan is known as a corepressor. Since the activity of the *trp* repressor is enhanced in the presence of tryptophan, the rate of expression of the *trp* operon is graded in response to the level of tryptophan in the cell.

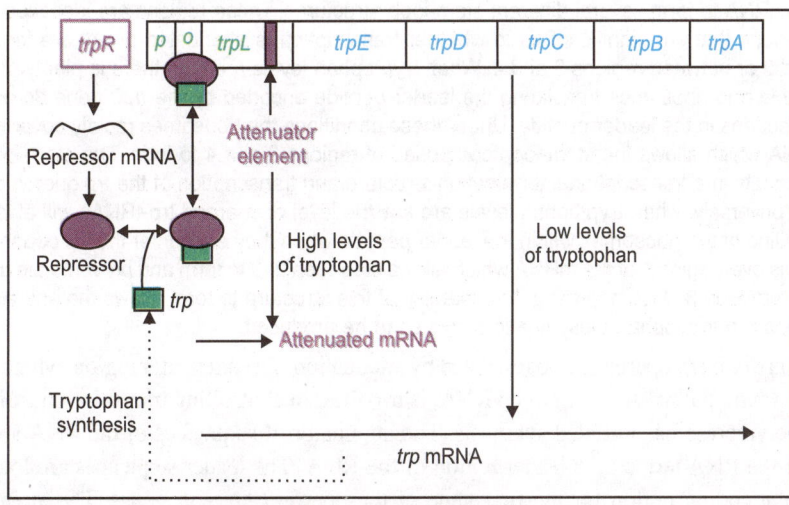

Fig. 4.2. Structure of the *trp* operon.

Regulation of the *trp* operon in *E. coli*: The *trp* operon is controlled by both a repressor protein binding to the operator region as well as by translation-induced transcriptional attenuation. The *trp* repressor binds the operator region of the *trp* operon only when bound to tryptophan. This makes tryptophan a corepressor of the operon. The *trpL* gene encodes a non-functional leader peptide which contains several adjacent trp codons. The structural genes of the operon responsible for tryptophan biosynthesis are *trpE, D, C, B* and *A*. When trptophan level are high some binds to the repressor which then binds to the operator region and inhibits transcription. The mechanism of attenuation of the *trp* operon is shown in Fig. 4.3.

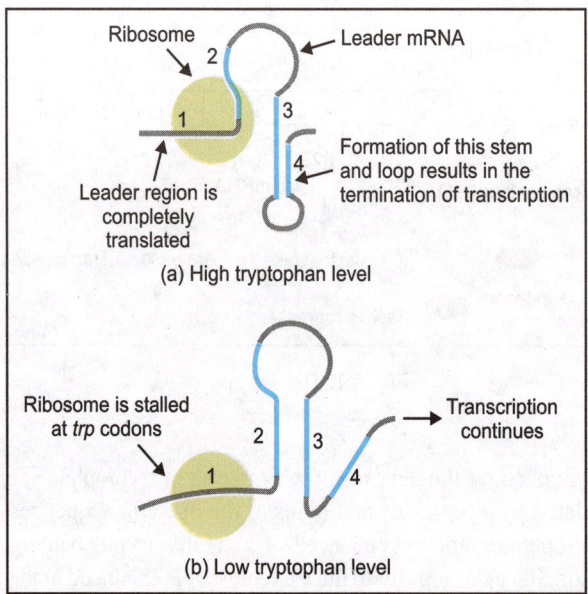

Fig. 4.3. Attenuation of the *trp* operon. The attenuation region of the *trp* operon contains sequences that allow the resulting mRNA to form several different stem-loop structures. These regions are identified as 1 through 4. The stem-loops that are significant as to whether transcription is attenuated or not are formed between regions 2 and 3 or between regions 3 and 4. When tryptophan levels are high there is plenty of charged *trp-tRNAs* available and ribosomes translating the leader peptide encoded by the *trpL* gene do not stall at the repeated trp codons in the leader peptide. Under these conditions the ribosomes rapidly cover regions 1 and 2 of the mRNA which allows the stem-loop composed of regions 3 and 4 to form. The stem-loop formed by regions 3-4 results in a transcriptional termination structure and transcription of the *trp* operon ceases, i.e. is attenuated. Conversely, when tryptophan levels are low the level of charged trp-tRNAs will also be low. This leads to a stalling of the ribosomes within the leader peptide when they encounter the trp codon repeats. The ribosome stalls over region 1 of the mRNA which allows step-loop 2-3 to form and prevents the transcriptional termination stem-loop 3-4 from forming. The inability of this structure to form allows the entire operon to be transcribed and the tryptophan biosynthetic enzymes to be produced.

Expression of the *trp* operon is also regulated by attenuation. The attenuator region, which is composed of sequences found within the transcribed RNA, is involved in controlling transcription from the operon after RNA polymerase has initiated synthesis. The attenuator of sequences of the RNA are found near the 5′ end of the RNA termed the leader region of the RNA. The leader sequences are located prior to the start of the coding region for the first gene of the operon (the *trpE* gene). The attenuator region contains codons for a small leader polypeptide, that contains tandem tryptophan codons. This region of the RNA is also capable of forming several different stable stem-loop structures. Depending on the level of tryptophan in the cell and hence the level of charged *trp*-tRNAs, the position of ribosomes on the leader polypeptide and the rate at which they are translating allows different stem-loops to form. If tryptophan is abundant, the ribosome prevents stem-loop 1–2 from forming and thereby favours stem-loop 3–4. The latter is found near a region rich in uracil and acts as the transcriptional terminator loop as described in the RNA synthesis page. Consequently, RNA polymerase is dislodged from the template. The operons coding for genes necessary for the synthesis of a number of other amino acids are also regulated by this attenuation mechanism. It should be clear, however, that this type of transcriptional regulation is not feasible for eukaryotic cells.

GENE CONTROL IN EUKARYOTES

In eukaryotic cells, the ability to express biologically active proteins comes under regulation at several points:

1. Chromatin structure: The physical structure of the DNA, as it exists compacted into chromatin, can affect the ability of transcriptional regulatory proteins (termed transcription factors) and RNA polymerases to find access to specific genes and to activate transcription from them. The presence modifications of the histones and of CpG methylation mostly affect accessibility of the chromatin to RNA polymerases and transcription factors.

2. Epigenetic control: Epigenesis refers to changes in the pattern of gene expression that are not due to changes in the nucleotide composition of the genome. Literally 'epi' means 'on' thus, epigenetics means 'on' the gene as opposed to 'by' the gene.

3. Transcriptional initiation: This is the most important mode for control of eukaryotic gene expression. Specific factors that exert control include the strength of promoter elements within the DNA sequences of a given gene, the presence or absence of enhancer sequences (which enhance the activity of RNA polymerase at a given promoter by binding specific transcription factors), and the interaction between multiple activator proteins and inhibitor proteins.

4. Transcript processing and modification: Eukaryotic mRNAs must be capped and polyadenylated, and the introns must be accurately removed. Several genes have been identified that undergo tissue-specific patterns of alternative splicing, which generate biologically different proteins from the same gene.

5. RNA transport: A fully processed mRNA must leave the nucleus in order to be translated into protein.

6. Transcript stability: Unlike prokaryotic mRNAs, whose half-lives are all in the range of 1 to 5 minutes, eukaryotic mRNAs can vary greatly in their stability. Certain unstable transcripts have sequences (predominately, but not exclusively, in the 3'-nontranslated regions) that are signals for rapid degradation.

7. Translational initiation: Since many mRNAs have multiple methionine codons, the ability of ribosomes to recognise and initiate synthesis from the correct AUG codon can affect the expression of a gene product. Several examples have emerged demonstrating that some eukaryotic proteins initiate at non-AUG codons. This phenomenon has been known to occur in *E. coli* for quite some time, but only recently has it been observed in eukaryotic mRNAs.

8. Small RNAs and control of transcript levels: Within the past several years a new model of gene regulation has emerged that involves control exerted by small noncoding RNAs. This small RNA-mediated control can be exerted either at the level of the translatability of the mRNA, the stability of the mRNA or via changes in chromatin structure.

9. Post-translational modification: Common modifications include glycosylation, acetylation, fatty acylation, disulphide bond formations, etc.

10. Protein transport: In order for proteins to be biologically active following translation and processing, they must be transported to their site of action.

11. Control of protein stability: Many proteins are rapidly degraded, whereas others are highly stable. Specific amino acid sequences in some proteins have been shown to bring about rapid degradation.

CHROMATIN STRUCTURE AND CONTROL OF GENE EXPRESSION

In a broad consideration of chromatin structure there are two forms: heterochromatin and euchromatin which were originally designated based on cytological observations of how darkly the two regions were stained. Heterochromatin is more densely packed than euchromatin and is often found near the centromeres of the chromosomes. Heterochromatin is generally transcriptionally silent. Euchromatin on the other hand is more loosely packed and is where active gene transcription will be found to be taking place.

Although it is possible to predict transcriptionally active regions of chromatin based on cytological assays, research over the past few decades have begun to define the molecular basis for chromatin structure in the context of regulation of gene expression. Two primary mechanisms exist that alter chromatin structure and as a consequence effect alterations in gene expression. These mechanisms are methylation of cytidine residues in the DNA that are found in the dinucleotide, CG (most often written as a CpG dinucleotide) and histone modification. Methylation as a modification of DNA was addressed in the DNA metabolism page, however, here discussion will expand to define how this modification alters the pattern of gene expression.

When determining which C residues in DNA are targets for methylation it was discovered that greater than 90 per cent of methyl-C is found in the dinucleotide, CpG. This is not to say that all CpG dinucleotides contain a methylated C residue. When examining the structure of eukaryotic genes and identifying regions of CpG dinucleotides it is the case that the promoter regions of genes contain 10–20 times as many CpGs when compared to the rest of the genome. In a general sense what is known about DNA methylation and transcriptional status is that when regions of a gene that can be methylated are, the associated gene is transcriptionally silent and when the region is under methylated the gene is transcriptionally active or can be activated. When cells undergo differentiation it has been observed that genes that become transcriptionally activated exhibit a reduction in methylation status relative to the level prior to activation and that this under-methylation remains even after transcription ceases. The role of DNA methylation in controlling transcriptionally activity was first demonstrated by treating cells in culture with the cytidine analog, 5-azacytidine (5-azaC) which has a nitrogen at position 5 of the pyrimidine ring instead of a carbon and thus cannot serve as a substrate for methylation. When fibroblasts were grown in the presence of 5-azaC they differentiated into myoblasts. This differentiation was shown to be the result of under-methylation and activation of the MyoD gene (a master regulator of muscle differentiation).

The methylation of DNA is catalysed by several different DNA methyltransferases (abbreviated Dnmt). The critical role of DNA methylation in controlling developmental fates was demonstrated in mice by inactivating either Dnmt3a or Dnmt3b. Loss of either gene resulted in death shortly after birth. When cells divide the DNA contains one strand of parental DNA and one strand of the newly replicated DNA (the daughter strand). If the DNA contains methylated cytidines in CpG dinucleotides the daughter strand must undergo methylation in order to maintain the parental pattern of methylation. This 'maintenance' methylation is catalysed by Dnmt1 and thus, this enzyme is called the maintenance methylase.

The correlation between DNA methylation and chromatin structure as it relates to transcriptional activity is demonstrated by the observation that there are several proteins that bind to methylated CpGs but not to unmethylated CpGs. One such protein is MeCP2 (methyl CP binding protein 2). When MeCP2 binds to methylated CpG dinucleotides the DNA takes on a closed chromatin structure and leads to transcriptional repression. The ability of MeCP2 to bind methylated CpGs is in turn controlled by its' state of phosphorylation. When MeCP2 is phosphorylated it binds with less affinity and the DNA acquires a more open chromatin state. The importance of MeCP2 in regulating chromatin structure and consequently transcription is demonstrated by the fact that deficiencies in this protein result in the Rett syndrome. Rett syndrome is a neurodevelopmental disorder that occurs almost exclusively in females manifesting as mental retardation, seizures, microcephaly, arrested development, and loss of speech.

As described in the DNA metabolism page, histone proteins are subjected to number of modifications and these modifications are known to affect the structure of chromatin. Histone acetylation is known to result in a more open chromatin structure and these modified histones are found in regions of the chromatin that are transcriptionally active. Conversely, underacetylation of histones is associated with closed chromatin and transcriptional inactivity. A direct correlation between histone acetylation and transcriptional activity was demonstrated when it was discovered that protein complexes, previously known to be transcriptional activators, were found to have histone acetylase activity. And as expected, transcriptional repressor complexes were found to contain histone deacetylase activity. Linkage between DNA methylation and transcriptional silencing was demonstrated by the observation that proteins that bind to methyl CpG dinucleotides can recruit histone deacetylases to the DNA. Proteins are known to interact with acetylated lysines in histones that together lead to a more open chromatin structure. Proteins that bind to acetylated histones contain a domain called a bromodomain. The bromodomain is composed of a bundle of four α-helices and is a domain involved in protein-protein interactions in a number of cellular systems in addition to acetylated histone binding and chromatin structure modification.

Another histone modification known to affect chromatin structure is methylation. However, with histone methylation there is not a direct correlation between the modification and a specific effect on transcription. The methylation of histone H4 on R4 (arginine at position 4) promotes an open chromatin structure and thereby, leads to transcriptional activation. Methylation of histone H3 on K4 and K79 (lysines 4 and 79) has been shown to act similarly to histone H4 R4 methylation. However, methylation of histone H3 on K9 and K27 is known to be associated with transcriptionally inactive genes. The methylation of histones provides a site for the binding of other proteins which then leads to alteration of chromatin structure to a more compacted state. Proteins that bind to methylated lysines present in histones (as well as other proteins) contain a domain called chromodomain. The chromodomain consists of a conserved stretch of 40–50 amino acids and is found in many proteins involved in chromatin remodelling complexes. In addition, chromodomain proteins are found in the RNA-induced transcriptional silencing (RITS) complex which involves small interfering RNA (siRNA) and microRNA (miRNA)-medicated down-regulation of transcription.

Histone proteins can also be modified by addition of the small protein ubiquitin. With respect to the histones, ubiquitin is found only on histones H2A and H2B and only a small percentage of histone H2A is found ubiquitinated. However, when ubiquitinated, H2A is associated with repression of transcription. The exact opposite effect is observed when histone H2B is ubiquitinated, leading to a stimulation of gene activity. The reason that ubiquitinated histone H2B is associated with transcriptional activity is that this modification promotes the methylation of histone H3 at K4 and K79.

Phosphorylation of histones occurs primarily in response to outside signals such as growth factor stimulation or stress inducers such as heat shock. Phosphorylated histone are localised to genes that become transcriptionally active as a consequence of these outside signals. The importance of histone phosphorylation in control of gene expression can be demonstrated in patients with Coffin-Lowry syndrome. This disease results from defects in the RSK2 gene which encodes the histone phosphorylating enzyme. Coffin-Lowry syndrome is a rare form of X-linked mental retardation characterised by skeletal malformations, growth retardation, hearing deficit, paroxysmal movement disorders, and cognitive impairment in affected males.

EPIGENETIC CONTROL OF GENE EXPRESSION

The term epigenetics was first coined by Conrad Waddington in 1939 to define the unfolding of the genetic program during development. In addition, he coined the term epigenotype to define 'the total developmental system consisting of interrelated developmental pathways through which the adult form of an organism is realised'. Clearly this definition encompasses a broad range of concepts dealing with genetics, inheritance and development. Today the term epigenetics is used to define the mechanism by which changes in the pattern of inherited gene expression occur in the absence of alterations or changes in the nucleotide composition of a given gene. A literal interpretation is that epigenetics mean 'in addition to changes in genome sequence'.

The easiest way to understand this concept is to think about the fertilised egg: at the moment of fertilisation that single cell is totipotent, i.e. as it divides the daughter cells ultimately differentiate into all the different cells of the organism. The only difference between the various cells of the resultant organism are the consequences of differential gene expression, not due to differences in the sequences of the genes themselves. Evidence indicates that most of the epigenetic modifications are erased during gametogenesis and/or following fertilisation.

Several different types of epigenetic events have been identified. As described in the section above relating to chromatin structure as a means to control gene expression and the role of DNA methylation in these structural changes, DNA methylation is likely to be the most important epigenetic event controlling and importantly maintaining the pattern of gene expression during development. Other DNA modification events are also known to effect epigenetic phenomena including acetylation, methylation phosphorylation, ubiquitylation and sumoylation of histone proteins. Thus, it should be clear that the same events that affect chromatin structure can be defined as epigenetic events. An additional process that affects chromatin structure and therefore gene expression is considered an epigenetic event and this involves the small interfering RNAs (siRNAs).

Whereas, epigenesis plays a vital role in the regulation, control, and maintenance of gene expression leading to the many differentiation states of cells in an organism, recent evidence has identified a linkage between epigenetic processes and disease. Most significant is the link between epigenesis and cancer which has been suggested to be a contributing factor in nearly half of all cancers. A clear demonstration has been made between changes in the methylation status of tumour suppressor genes and the development of many types of cancers. Epigenetic effects on immune system function have also been identified. In addition, there is evidence suggesting a link between epigenetic processes and mental health.

CONTROL OF EUKARYOTIC TRANSCRIPTION INITIATION

Transcription of the different classes of RNAs in eukaryotes is carried out by three different polymerases. RNA *pol*I synthesises the rRNAs, except for the 5*S* species. RNA *pol*II synthesises the mRNAs and some small nuclear RNAs (snRNAs) involved in RNA splicing. RNA *pol*III synthesises the 5*S* rRNA and the tRNAs. The vast majority of eukaryotic RNAs are subjected to post-transcriptional processing.

The most complex controls observed in eukaryotic genes are those that regulate the expression of RNA *pol*II-transcribed genes, the mRNA genes. Almost all eukaryotic mRNA genes contain a basic structure consisting of coding exons and noncoding introns and basal promoters of two types and any number of different transcriptional regulatory domains (Fig. 4.4). The basal promoter elements are termed CCAAT-boxes and TATA-boxes because of their sequence motifs. The TATA-box resides 20 to 30 bases upstream of the transcriptional start site and is similar in sequence to the prokaryotic Pribnow-box (consensus TATA$^T/_A$A$^T/_A$, where, $^T/_A$ indicates that either base may be found at that position).

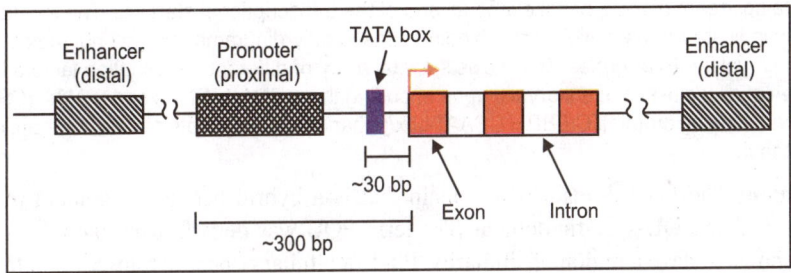

Fig. 4.4. Typical structure of a eukaryotic mRNA gene.

Numerous proteins identified as TFIIA, B, C, etc. (for transcription factors regulating RNA pol II), have been observed to interact with the TATA-box. The CCAAT-box (consensus GG$^T/_C$CAATCT) resides 50 to 130 bases upstream of the transcriptional start site. The protein identified as C/EBP (for CCAAT-box/Enhancer binding protein) binds to the CCAAT-box element.

There are many other regulatory sequences in mRNA genes, as well, that bind various transcription factors (Fig. 4.5). Theses regulatory sequences are predominantly located upstream (5′) of the transcription initiation site, although some elements occur downstream (3′) or even within the genes themselves. The number and type of regulatory elements to be found varies with each mRNA gene. Different combinations of transcription factors also can exert differential regulatory effects upon transcriptional initiation. The various cell types each express characteristic combinations of transcription factors; this is the major mechanism for cell-type specificity in the regulation of mRNA gene expression.

STRUCTURAL MOTIFS IN EUKARYOTIC TRANSCRIPTION FACTORS

Homeodomain: The homeodomain is a highly conserved domain of 60 amino acids found in a large family of transcription factors. This family was first identified in *Drosophila* as a group of genes that, when altered, would cause transformations of one body part for another (e.g. legs for antenna), so called homeotic transformations.

This class of genes has been identified in both invertebrate and vertebrate organisms. The homeodomain itself forms a structure highly similar to the bacterial helix-turn-helix proteins. The principal function of all homeodomain containing proteins is in the establishment of pattern in an organism such as that of the spinal column in vertebrates.

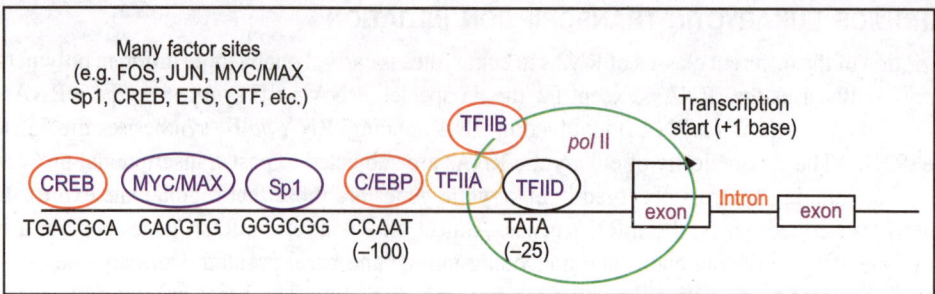

Many factor sites
(e.g. FOS, JUN, MYC/MAX
Sp1, CREB, ETS, CTF, etc.)

Fig. 4.5. Structure of the upstream region of a typical eukaryotic mRNA gene that hypothetically contains 2 exons and a single intron. The diagram indicates the TATA-box and CCAAT-box basal elements reside near nucleotide positions -25 and -100, respectively. The transcription factor TFIID has been shown to be the TATA-box binding protein, TBP. Several additional transcription factor binding sites have been included and shown to reside upstream of the 2 basal elements and of the transcriptional start site. The location and order of the variously indicated transcription factor-binding sites is only diagrammatic and not indicative as being typical of all eukaryotic mRNA genes. There exists a vast array of different transcription factors that regulate the transcription of all 3 classes of eukaryotic gene encoding the mRNAs, tRNAs and rRNAs. [CREB = cAMP response element binding protein] [C/EBP = CCAAT-box/enhancer binding protein]. The large circle represents RNA polymerase II.

POU domain: The POU domain is a domain that is a hybrid between a domain related to the homeodomain and an POU-specific domain. The term POU was derived from the names of the first three factors shown to have a region of similarity, Pit-1 (a pituitary-specific transcription factor), Oct-1 (an octamer binding protein first shown to regulate immunoglobulin gene transcription) and unc-86 (a nematode gene).

Helix-Loop-Helix (HLH): The HLH domain is involved in protein dimerisation. The HLH motif is composed of two regions of a-helix separated by a region of variable length which forms a loop between the 2 α-helices. This motif is quite similar to the Helix-turn-helix motif found in several prokaryotic transcription factors such as the CRP protein involved in the regulation of the *lac* operon. The α-helical domains are structurally similar and are necessary for protein interaction with sequence elements that exhibit a twofold axis of symmetry. This class of transcription factor most often contains a region of basic amino acids located on the N-terminal side of the HLH domain (termed bHLH proteins) that is necessary in order for the protein to bind DNA at specific sequences. The HLH domain is necessary for homo- and heterodimerisation. Examples of bHLH proteins include MyoD (a myogenesis inducing transcription factor) and MYC (originally identified as a retroviral oncogene). Several HLH proteins that do not contain the basic region act as repressors because of this lack. These HLH proteins repress the activity of other bHLH proteins by forming heterodimers with them and preventing DNA binding.

Zinc fingers: The zinc finger domain is a DNA-binding motif consisting of specific spacings of cysteine and histidine residues that allow the protein to bind zinc atoms. The metal atom coordinates the sequences around the cysteine and histidine residues into a finger-like domain. The finger domains can interdigitate into the major groove of the DNA helix. The spacing of the zinc finger domain in this class of transcription factor coincides with a half-turn of the double helix. The classic example is the RNA pol III transcription factor, TFIIIA. Proteins of the steroid/thyroid hormone family of transcription factors also contain zinc fingers.

Leucine zipper: The leucine zipper domain is necessary for protein dimerisation. It is a motif generated by a repeating distribution of leucine residues spaced 7 amino acids apart within α-helical regions of the protein. These leucine residues end up with their R-groups protruding from the α-helical domain in which the leucine residues reside. The protruding R-groups are thought to interdigitate with leucine R groups of another leucine zipper domain, thus stabilising homo- or heterodimerisation. The leucine zipper domain is present in many DNA-binding proteins, such as MYC, and C/EBP.

Winged helix: The winged helix is a DNA-binding motif composed of an α/β structure. This structure contains 3 N-terminal α-helices and a 3-stranded antiparallel β-sheet. The folding of the β-sheet region about the α-helices give the appearance of wings on the helices, hence the term winged-helix. This motif was first identified in the transcription factor HNF-3γ. HNF-3γ is a member of a large family of transcription factors that are related to the *Drosophila* gene forkhead, hence the gene family is termed the fork head (FKH) family. The nomenclature of the fork head family of transcription factors has been changed so that all members have names that initiate with Fox. Table 4.1 given representative transcription factors.

Table 4.1. Representative transcription factors

Factor	*Sequence motif*	*Comments*
MYC and MAX	CACGTG	MYC first identified as retroviral oncogene; MAX specifically associates with MYC in cells
FOS and JUN	TGA$^C/_G$T$^C/_A$A	Both first identified as retroviral oncogenes; associate in cells, also known as the factor AP-1
CREB	TGACG$^C/_T$$^C/_A$$^G/_A$	Binds to the cAMP response element (CRE); family of at least 10 factors resulting from different genes or alternative splicing; can form dimers with JUN
ERBA; also TR) (thyroid hormone receptor)	GTGTCAAAGGTCA	First identified as retroviral oncogene; member of the steroid/thyroid hormone receptor superfamily; binds thyroid hormone
ETS	$^G/_C$$^A/_CGGA^A/_TG^T/_C$	First identified as retroviral oncogene; predominates in B- and T-cells
GATA	$^T/_A$GATA	Family of erythroid cell-specific factors, GATA-1 to -6.
MYB	$^T/_C$AAC$^G/_T$G	First identified as retroviral oncogene; hematopoietic cell-specific factor
MYOD	CAACTGAC	Master control of muscle cell differentiation
NFkB and REL	GGGA$^A/_C$TN$^T/_C$CC$^{(1)}$	Both factors identified independently; REL first identified as retroviral oncogene; predominate in B- and T-cells
RAR (retinoic acid receptor)	ACGTCATGACCT	Binds to elements termed RAREs (retinoic acid response elements) also binds to JUN/FOS site
SRF (serum response factor)	GGATGTCCATATTAGGACATCT	Exists in many genes that are inducible by the growth factors present in serum

The list is only representative of the hundreds of identified factors, some emphasis is placed on several factors that exhibit oncogenic potential.

$^{(1)}$N signifies that any base can occupy that position.

SMALL RNAs AND POST-TRANSCRIPTIONAL REGULATION

As recently as 15 years ago it was believed that the only noncoding RNAs were the tRNAs and the rRNAs of the translational machinery. However, in a landmark study published in 1993 on the control of developmental timing in the roundworm *Caenorhabditis elegans* it was shown that the control of one gene was exerted by the small noncoding RNA product of another gene. This regulatory gene is identified as lin-4 (lin-4 controls the activity of the lin-14 gene product) and it codes for two RNAs, one is approximately 22 nucleotides (nt) and the other is approximately 61 nt. Examination of the sequences of the larger RNA revealed that it could form a stem-loop structure which then serves as the precursor for the shorter RNA. The shorter lin-4 RNA is considered the founding member of class of small regulatory RNAs called microRNAs or miRNAs that consist of approximately 22 nt. It is predicted that at least 250 miRNA genes are present in the human genome.

The processing and functioning of miRNAs is similar to that of the RNA silencing pathway identified in plants known as the posttranscriptional gene silencing (PTGS) pathway and the RNA inhibitory (RNAi) pathway in mammals. The RNAi pathway involves the enzymatic processing of double-stranded RNA into small interfering RNAs (siRNAs) of approximately 22–25 nt that may have evolved as a means to degrade the RNA genomes of RNA viruses such as retroviruses. The pathway of processing both miRNAs and siRNAs is shown in the Fig. 4.6. The stem-loop of the primary miRNA gene transcript (pri-miRNA) is first cleaved through the action of the RNase III-related activity called Drosha which takes place in the nucleus and generates the precursor miRNA (pre-miRNA). In the siRNA pathway the duplex RNAs are cleaved into 22–25 nt pieces through the action of the enzyme Dicer in the cytosol. Processed miRNA stem-loop structures are transported from the nucleus to the cytosol via the activity of exportin5. In the cytosol the processed miRNA stem-loop is targeted by Dicer which removes the loop portion. The nomenclature of the mature miRNA duplex is miRNA:miRNA*, where the miRNA* strand is the nonfunctional half of the duplex. Ultimately, fully processed miRNAs and siRNAs are engaged by the RNA-induced silencing complex (RISC) which separates the two RNA strands. The active strand of RNA derived either from the miRNA or siRNA pathway is antisense to a region of the target mRNA. Two models exist for how siRNAs and miRNAs interfere with the expression of target genes. These models include directed degradation of the target mRNA or interference with the translation of a target mRNA. In the case of miRNA-directed mRNA degradation the proposed model involves the complimentary interaction of the miRNA with the mRNA and then the recruitment of the RISC which ultimately leads to degradation of the target mRNA. In the translation repression model it is believed that either the interaction of the miRNA and the RISC with the mRNA inhibits the progression of the ribosomal machinery along the mRNA without leading to mRNA degradation. This latter model was hypothesised because in the example of lin-4 the amount of lin-14 mRNA does not decrease but the protein product of the lin-14 mRNA is reduced.

Regardless of the mechanism of action the effect is post-transcriptional regulation of gene expression. To date numerous examples of miRNA-mediated gene regulation have been identified in development, cell survival and metabolic pathways. In addition, the involvement of miRNA processes in human disease have been elucidated or inferred. In the case of cancer it is speculated that some miRNAs can be classified as tumour suppressors since the loss of their activity is associated with cancer progression. A role for miRNAs in neurodegenerative diseases is also suggested by the example of the fragile X syndrome. Fragile X syndrome is caused by expansion of a trinucleotide repeat in the FMR1 gene and the product of the FMR1 gene, FMRP, is an RNA-binding protein that associates with miRNAs.

E. coli Plasmid *p*BR316

The plasmid *p*BR316 was used to isolate several promoter sequences. An examination of this protocol provides insights into how this type of research is typically conducted.

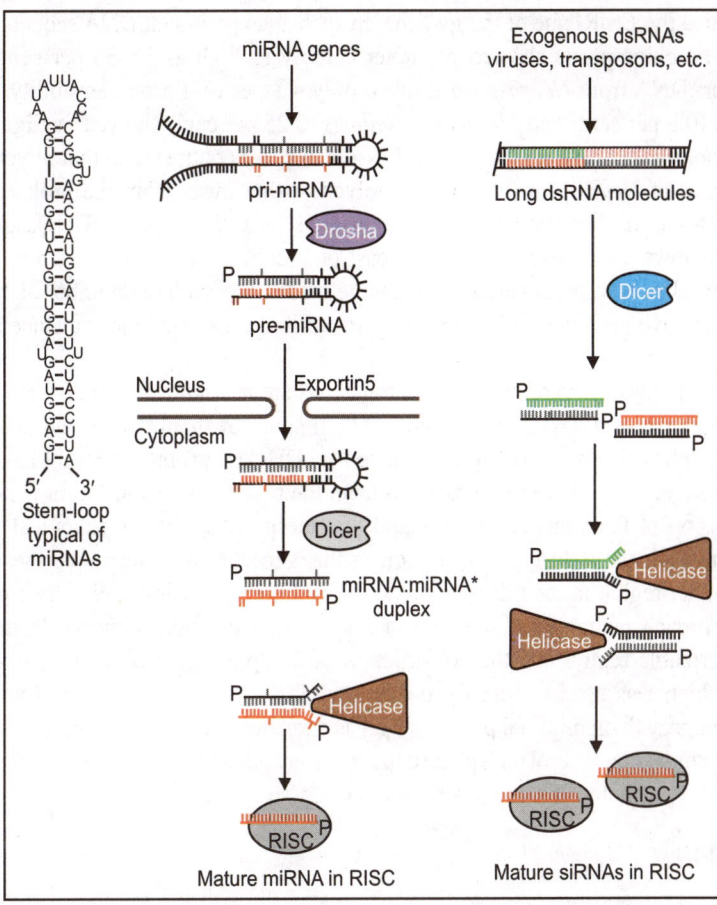

Fig. 4.6. Model for processing miRNAs and siRNAs.

Characterisation of the promoter sequences from a variety of organisms can provide a better insight into the mechanism of transcription, which represents the first step in the gene expression of all organisms. An attempt has been made to isolate promoters from a group of evolutionarily divergent organisms by their ability to facilitate the expression of a gene conferring tetracycline (*tet*) resistance by a hybrid plasmid in *E. coli*. These investigators first modified a hybrid plasmid *p*BR316 [containing the genes for resistance to ampicillin (*amp*) and tetracycline (*tet*)] by inserting a chemically synthesised *Eco*RI linker at the promoter (RNA binding site) of the *tet* gene, thereby decreasing the efficiency of transcription of the *tet* gene and consequently reducing the level of resistance to tetracycline present in the growth medium. In a second step, they inserted small eukaryotic DNA sequences (obtained by restriction endonuclease digestion of the eukaryotic DNA) at the *Eco*RI site within the *tet* gene and then examined the hybrid plasmid for its ability to restore antibiotic resistance. Bacterial colonies not able to grow on plates containing 5 µg/ml of tetracycline were scored as *tet*-sensitive; those able to grow on plates containing 5 µg/ml of tetracycline but not higher drug concentrations were scored as containing a nonrecombinant plasmid, whereas those able to grow on plates containing tetracycline concentrations higher than 5 µg/ml were considered as harbouring a recombinant plasmid with restored promoter activity. Thus the level of drug resistance was taken as a measure of the efficiency of the eukaryotic promoter inserted at the *Eco*RI site of the *tet* gene. In such an experiment, DNA sequences from *E. coli*, yeast, and *Euglena* chloroplasts showed promoter activity as high as 25–30 per cent of the original plasmid promoter; DNA from *Neurospora* showed only 4.5 per cent promoter ability. DNA segments from *Drosophila* (0.8 per cent) and *Magasihia scalaris* (0.25 per cent) showed negligible activity. The fact that the promoter efficiency of *Neurospora* DNA is in sharp contrast with that of yeast suggests that promoter sequences of *Neurospora* may have evolved further away from the prokaryotic DNA than those of yeast. This is further supported by the analysis of a *Neurospora* cDHQase structural gene promoter, which shows no similarity with the yeast or bacterial promoter or even with promoters of higher eukaryotes. However, no generalisation can be made unless a large number of *Neurospora* and/ or yeast promoters have been isolated and fully characterised for nucleotide sequence and *in vitro* and *in vivo* activities.

The promoter regions of several yeast structural genes are now known. All of them seem to contain the canonical sequence of a TATA box, besides which some of them contain an addition sequence, ACACACA, which has also been found in *Neurospora* cDHQase promoter. Struhl has recently shown that a nucleotide sequence 113–155 bp unstream from the transcription start point is necessary for the wild-type expression of the yeast *his-3* gene and that the presence of the canonical TATA sequence alone is not enough for the wild-type expression of this gene. He has elucidated the role of different parts of the promoter region in the mRNA production and the expression of the *his-3* gene by deletion mapping. *His* approach included the deletion of a specific nucleotide sequence from the *his-3* gene before the transcribable region and the construction of an appropriate plasmid (containing the *his-3* deleted gene), which was used to transform auxotrophic (*his⁻*) yeast cells. The transformants were examined for their growth on minimal plates as well as on plates containing aminotriazoe (a competitive inhibitor of yeast imidazoleglycerol phosphate dehydrates encoded by the *his-3⁺* gene). The transformants containing the *his-3* promoter deletions were found to posses three distinct classes of phenotypes.

FUSION PROTEIN

Fusion proteins or chimeric proteins are proteins created through the joining of two or more genes which originally coded for separate proteins. Translation of this fusion gene results in a single polypeptide with functional properties derived from each of the original proteins. Recombinant fusion proteins are created artificially by recombinant DNA technology for use in biological research or therapeutics.

Naturally Occurring Fusion Proteins

Naturally occurring fusion genes are most commonly created when a chromosomal translocation replaces the terminal exons of one gene with intact exons from a second gene. This creates a single gene which can be transcribed, spliced, and translated to produce a functional fusion protein. Many important cancer-promoting oncogenes are fusion genes produced in this way.

Examples include:

1. Gag-onc fusion protein.
2. Bcr-abl fusion protein.
3. Tpr-met fusion protein.

Antibodies are fusion proteins produced by VDJ recombination.

The **gag-onc fusion protein** is a protein formed from a group-specific antigen ('gag') and that of an oncovirus ('onc'), such as C-jun.

Bcr-abl fusion protein is an oncogene fusion protein consisting of BCR and ABL. It is associated with Philadelphia chromosome. Bcr-abl fusion protein comes in three forms: P190, P210 and P230 depending on the breakpoint on the Bcr fragment. The P190 isoform can be produced by alternative splicing from the P210 isoform. It is generally associated with chronic myeloid leukemia but it can also be associated with acute lymphoblastic leukemia.

Tpr-met fusion protein is an oncogene fusion protein consisting of TPR and MET.

Tandem Genes and Clustered Genes

Tandemly arrayed genes reside within segments of DNA that are repeated head-to-tail a number of times. Clustered genes are linked but irregularly spaced, are often mutually inverted in an unpredictable pattern and are connected by non-conserved DNA. Tandem arrays are homogenised by both unequal recombination and gene conversion, are necessary for the maintenance of large gene families, can expand and contract rapidly in response to changing demand, can keep functionally related genes equal in number, and do not engender increased genetic complexity. Gene clusters are homogenised by conversion only, seldom if ever contain more than 50 members, are stable in number, and often engender increased genetic complexity. Tandem gene arrays can evolve into gene clusters. It is suggested that this occurs when some change in the array inhibits unequal recombination but not gene conversion. The most common such change is inversion of part of the tandem array with respect to the rest; however, arrays can evolve into clusters without inversion. Clustered genes are sometimes re-amplified into new tandem arrays. Clustered genes are probably more durable than tandemly arrayed genes during periods of relaxed selection, and in the case of fish antifreeze protein genes, seem to behave as a genetic memory.

PROTEIN STABILITY AND STORAGE

Proteins comprise an extremely heterogeneous class of biological macromolecules. They are often unstable when not in their native environments, which can vary considerably among cell compartments and extracellular fluids. If certain buffer conditions are not maintained, extracted proteins may not function properly or remain soluble. Proteins can lose activity as a result of proteolysis, aggregation and suboptimal buffer conditions. Purified proteins often need to be stored for an extended period of time while retaining their original structural integrity and/or activity. The extent of storage 'shelf-life' can vary from a few days to more than a year and is dependent on the nature of the protein and the storage conditions used. Optimal conditions for storage are distinctive to each protein; nevertheless, it is possible to suggest some general guidelines for protein storage and stability. Common conditions for protein storage are summarised and compared in Table 4.2.

Generally, there are tradeoffs associated with each method. For example, proteins stored in solution at 4°C can be dispensed conveniently as needed but require more diligence to prevent microbial or proteolytic degradation; such proteins may not be stable for more than a few days or weeks. By contrast, lyophilisation allows for long-term storage of protein with very little threat of degradation, but the protein must be reconstituted before use and may be damaged by the lyophilisation process.

General Considerations for Protein Storage

Temperature

Generally, proteins are best stored at 4°C in clean, autoclaved glassware or polypropylene tubes. Storage at room temperature often leads to protein degradation and/or inactivity, commonly as a result of microbial growth. For short term storage (1 day to a few weeks), many proteins may be stored in simple buffers at

4°C. Protein stabilising cocktail (Product No. 89806) is a 4X solution that helps to extend the shelf-life of most proteins for storage at 4° C or –20°C compared to storage in simple phosphate or *tris* buffers.

Table 4.2. Comparison of protein storage conditions.

Characteristics	Storage condition			
	Solution at 4°C	Solution in 25–50% glycerol or ethylene glycol at –20°C	Frozen at –20° to –80°C or in liquid nitrogen	Lyophilised (usually also frozen)
Typical shelf life	1 month	1 year	Years	Years
Requires sterile conditions or addition of antibacterial agent	Yes	Usually	No	No
Number of times a sample may be removed for use	Many	Many	Once; repeated freeze-thaw cycles generally degrade proteins	Once; it is impractical to lyophilise a sample multiple times

For long term storage for 1 month to 1 year, some researchers choose to bead single-use aliquots of the protein in liquid nitrogen for storage in clean plastic containers under liquid nitrogen. This method involves adding the protein solution drop-wise (about 100 μl each) into a pool of liquid nitrogen, then collecting the drop-sized frozen beads and storing them in cryovials under liquid nitrogen.

Frozen at –20°C or –80°C is the more common form of cold protein storage. Because freeze-thaw cycles decrease protein stability, samples for frozen storage are best dispensed and prepared in single-use aliquots so that, once thawed, the protein solution will not have to be refrozen. Alternatively, addition of 50 per cent glycerol or ethylene glycol will prevent solutions from freezing at –20°C, enabling repeated use from a single stock without warming (i.e. thawing).

Protein concentration

Dilute protein solutions (< 1 mg/ml) are more prone to inactivation and loss as a result of low-level binding to the storage vessel. Therefore, it is common practice to add 'carrier' or 'filler' protein, such as purified bovine serum albumin (BSA) to 1–5 mg/ml (0.1–0.5 per cent), to dilute protein solutions to protect against such degradation and loss.

Additives

Many compounds may be added to protein solutions to lengthen shelf-life:

1. Protein stabilising cocktail (Product No. 89806) is a 4X solution that helps to extend the shelf-life of most proteins for storage at 4°C or –20°C.
2. Cryoprotectants such as glycerol or ethylene glycol to a final concentration of 25–50 per cent help to stabilise proteins by preventing the formation of ice crystals at –20°C that destroy protein structure.
3. Protease inhibitors prevent proteolytic cleavage of proteins (Table 4.3).
4. Antimicrobial agents such as sodium azide (NaN_3) at a final concentration of 0.02–0.05 per cent (w/v) or thimerosal at a final concentration of 0.01 per cent (w/v) inhibit microbial growth.
5. Metal chelators such as EDTA at a final concentration of 1–5 mM avoid metal-induced oxidation of –SH groups and helps to maintain the protein in a reduced state.

6. Reducing agents such a dithiothreitol (DTT) and 2-mercaptoethanol (2-ME) at final concentrations of 1–5 mM also help to maintain the protein in the reduced state by preventing oxidation of cysteines.

Table 4.3. Common protease inhibitors.

Protease inhibitor	Target protease	Working concentration
PMSF (Phenylmethylsulphonyl fluoride)	Serine proteases	0.1–1 mM
Benzamidine	Serine proteases	1 mM
Pepstatin A	Acid proteases	1 µg/ml
Leupeptin	Thiol proteases	1 µg/ml
Aprotinin	Serine proteases	5 µg/ml
Antipain	Thiol proteases	1 µg/ml
EDTA and EGTA	Metallo proteases	0.1–1 mM

Storage Conditions for Antibodies and Antibody—Enzyme Conjugates

Antibody stock solutions (e.g. 1 mg/ml) often may be stored at 4°C for days to weeks without significant loss in activity. For increased stability, glycerol or ethylene glycol may be added to a final concentration of 50 per cent and the antibody stored at –20°C. Alternatively, the antibody solution may be stored in small working aliquots at –20°C to avoid repeated freeze-thaw cycles. Antimicrobial agents such as sodium azide or thimerosal may be added to avoid microbial growth. Generally, antibody conjugates are best stored at –20°C with glycerol or ethylene glycol added at a final concentration of 50 per cent. Although some enzyme conjugates may be stored at –20°C without cryoprotectant, frozen stocks must be as single use aliquots to prevent repeated freeze-thaw cycles; alkaline phosphatase conjugates are particularly sensitive to freezing.

Conjugates typically maintain good activity for 1–2 years if stored at –20°C with glycerol or ethylene glycol. However, contaminants in cryoprotectants may affect enzyme activity, and few researchers take steps to ensure the purity of the cryoprotectant used. Pierce offers ethylene glycol (Product No. 29810) that is suitable for enzyme storage because impurities have been removed during the manufacturing process. Ethylene glycol does not support microbial growth, making it preferable to glycerol.

SECRETION

Secretion is the process of elaborating, releasing, and oozing chemicals, or a secreted chemical substance from a cell or gland. In contrast to excretion, the substance may have a certain function, rather than being a waste product. Secretion in bacterial species means the transport or translocation of effect or molecules for example proteins, enzymes or toxins (such as cholera toxin in pathogenic bacteria for example *Vibrio cholerae*) from across the interior (cytoplasm or cytosol) of a bacterial cell to its exterior. Secretion is a very important mechanism in bacterial functioning and operation in their natural surrounding environment for adaptation and survival.

Secretion in Eukaryotic Cells

Mechanism

Eukaryotic cells, including human cells, have a highly evolved process of secretion. Proteins targeted for the outside are synthesised by ribosomes docked to the rough endoplasmic reticulum (ER). As they are synthesised, these proteins translocate into the ER lumen, where they are glycosylated and where molecular chaperones aid protein folding. Misfolded proteins are usually identified here and retrotranslocated by ER-associated degradation to the cytosol, where they are degraded by a proteasome. The vesicles containing the properly-folded proteins then enter the Golgi apparatus. In the Golgi apparatus, the glycosylation of the proteins is modified and further post-translational modifications, including cleavage and functionalisation, may occur.

The proteins are then moved into secretory vesicles which travel along the cytoskeleton to the edge of the cell. More modification can occur in the secretory vesicles (for example insulin is cleaved from proinsulin in the secretory vesicles). Eventually, there is vesicle fusion with the cell membrane at a structure called the porosome, in a process called exocytosis, dumping its contents out of the cell's environment.

Strict biochemical control is maintained over this sequence by usage of a pH gradient: the pH of the cytosol is 7.4, the ER's pH is 7.0, and the *cis*-golgi has a pH of 6.5. Secretory vesicles have pHs ranging between 5.0 and 6.0; some secretory vesicles evolve into lysosomes, which have a pH of 4.8.

Nonclassical secretion

There are many proteins like FGF1 (aFGF), FGF2 (bFGF), interleukin1 (IL1), etc. which do not have a signal sequence. They do not use the classical ER-golgi pathway. These are secreted through various nonclassical pathways.

Secretion in human tissues

Many human cell types have the ability to be secretory cells. They have a well developed endoplasmic reticulum and Golgi apparatus to fulfil their function. Tissues in humans that produce secretions include the gastrointestinal tract which secretes digestive enzymes and gastric acid, the lung which secretes surfactants, and sebaceous glands which secrete sebum to lubricate the skin and hair. Meibomian glands in the eyelid secrete sebum to lubricate and protect the eye.

Secretion in Gram-negative Bacteria

Secretion is not unique to eukaryotes alone, it is present in bacteria and archaea as well. ATP binding cassette (ABC) type transporters are common to all the three domains of life. The *Sec* system is also another conserved secretion system which is homologous to the translocon in the eukaryotic endoplasmic reticulum consisting of *Sec* 61 translocon complex in yeast and *Sec* Y-E-G complex in bacteria. Secretion via the *Sec* pathway generally requires the presence of an N-terminal signal peptide on the secreted protein. Gram negative bacteria have two membranes, thus making secretion topologically more complex. There are at least six specialised secretion systems in Gram negative bacteria.

Type I secretion system (T1SS or TOSS)

It is similar to the ABC transporter, however it has additional proteins that, together with the ABC protein, form a contiguous channel traversing the inner and outer membranes of Gram-negative bacteria. It is a simple system, which consists of only three protein subunits: the ABC protein, membrane fusion protein (MFP), and outer membrane protein (OMP). Type I secretion system transports various molecules, from ions, drugs, to proteins of various sizes (20–900 kDa). The molecules secreted vary in size from the small *Escherichia coli* peptide colicin V, (10 kDa) to the *Pseudomonas fluorescens* cell adhesion protein LapA of 900 kDa. The best characterised are the RTX toxins and the lipases. Type I secretion is also involved in export of nonproteinaceous substrates like cyclic β-glucans and polysaccharides. Many secreted proteins are particularly important in bacterial pathogenesis (Fig. 4.7).

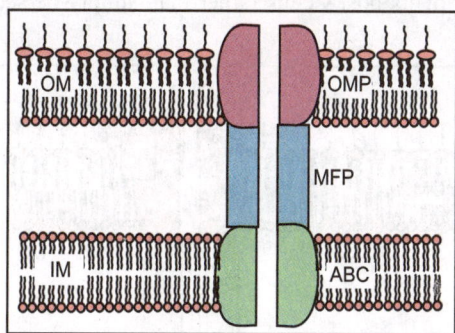

Fig. 4.7. Type I secretion system (T1SS or TOSS).

Type II secretion system (T2SS)

Proteins secreted through the type II system, or main terminal branch of the general secretory pathway, depend on the Sec or Tat system for initial transport into the periplasm. Once there, they pass through the outer membrane via a multimeric (12–14 subunits) complex of pore forming secretin proteins. In addition to the secretin protein, 10–15 other inner and outer membrane proteins compose the full secretion apparatus, many with as yet unknown function. Gram-negative type IV pili use a modified version of the type II system for their biogenesis, and in some cases certain proteins are shared between a pilus complex and type II system within a single bacterial species (Fig. 4.8).

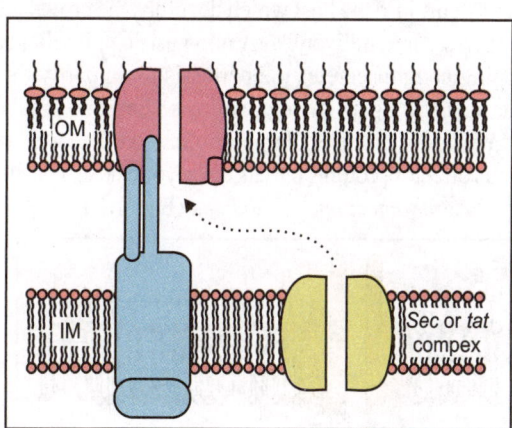

Fig. 4.8. Type II secretion system (T2SS).

Type III secretion system (T3SS or TTSS)

It is homologous to bacterial flagellar basal body. It is like a molecular syringe through which a bacterium (e.g. certain types of *Salmonella*, *Shigella*, *Yersinia*, *Vibrio*) can inject proteins into eukaryotic cells. The low Ca^{2+} concentration in the cytosol opens the gate that regulates T3SS. One such mechanism to detect low calcium concentration has been illustrated by the lcrV (low calcium response) antigen utilised by *Y. pestis*, which is used to detect low calcium concentrations and elicits T3SS attachment. The Hrp system in plant pathogens inject harpins through similar mechanisms into plants. This secretion system was first discovered in *Y. pestis* and showed that toxins could be injected directly from the bacterial cytoplasm into the cytoplasm of its host's cells rather than simply be secreted into the extracellular medium (Fig. 4.9).

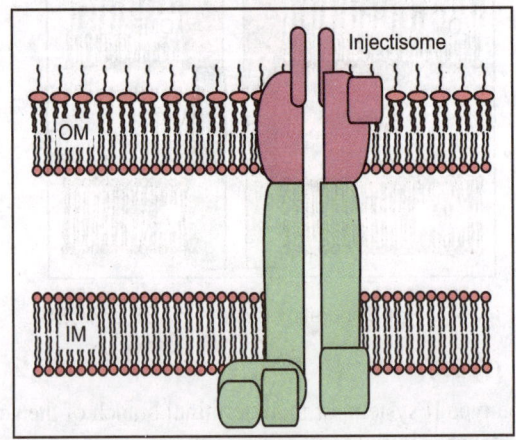

Fig. 4.9. Type III secretion system (T3SS or TTSS).

Type IV secretion system (T4SS or TFSS)

It is homologous to conjugation machinery of bacteria (and archaeal flagella). It is capable of transporting both DNA and proteins. It was discovered in *Agrobacterium tumefaciens*, which uses this system to introduce the Ti plasmid and proteins into the host which develops the crown gall (tumour). *Helicobacter pylori* uses a type IV secretion system to deliver CagA into gastric epithelial cells. *Bordetella pertussis*, the causative agent of whooping cough, secretes the pertussis toxin partly through the type IV system. *Legionella pneumophila*, the causing agent of legionellosis (Legionnaires' disease) utilises type IV secretion system, known as the icm/dot (intracellular multiplication/defect in organelle trafficking genes) system, to translocate numerous effector proteins into its eukaryotic host. The prototypic Type IV secretion system is the VirB complex of *Agrobacterium tumefaciens* (Fig. 4.10).

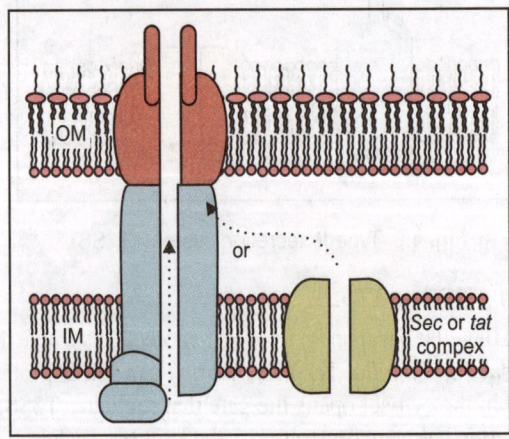

Fig. 4.10. Type IV secretion system (T4SS or TFSS).

Type V secretion system (T5SS)

Also called the autotransporter system, type V secretion involves use of the *Sec* system for crossing the inner membrane. Proteins which use this pathway have the capability to form a beta-barrel with their C-terminus which inserts into the outer membrane, allowing the rest of the peptide (the passenger domain) to reach the outside of the cell. Often, autotransporters are cleaved, leaving the beta-barrel domain in the outer membrane and freeing the passenger domain. Some people believe remnants of the autotransporters gave rise to the porins which form similar beta-barrel structures (Fig. 4.11).

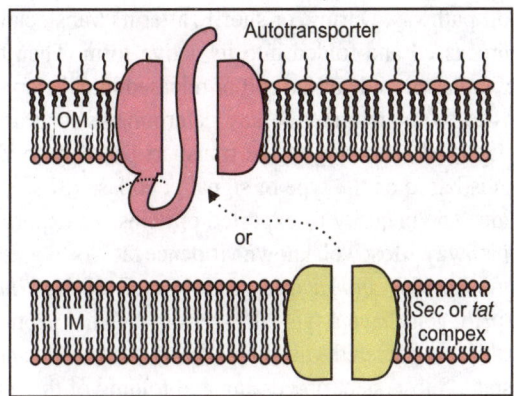

Fig. 4.11. Type V secretion system (T5SS).

Type VI secretion system (T6SS)

Type VI secretion systems have been identified in 2006 by the group of John Mekalanos at the Harvard Medical School (Boston, USA) in two bacterial pathogens, *Vibrio cholerae* and *Pseudomonas aeruginosa*. Since then, Type VI secretion systems have been found in most genomes of proteobacteria, including animal, plant, human pathogens, as well as soil, environmental or marine bacteria. Several studies have shown the involvement of Type VI secretion systems in several processes related to pathogenesis; however, recent studies suggested a broader role for these systems in participating in stress sensing. The Type VI secretion systems are composed of several components, and two proteins, Hcp and VgrG, are regularly found in culture supernatant, suggesting that they are secreted proteins; however, the recent crystal structure of these two proteins suggest that Hcp and VgrG are part of an extracellular appendage. Proteins secreted by the type VI system lack N-terminal signal sequences and therefore presumably do not enter the *Sec* pathway.

Twin-arginine translocation (Tat)

Bacteria as well as mitochondria and chloroplasts also use many other special transport systems such as the twin-arginine translocation pathway which, in contrast to *Sec*-dependent export, transports fully folded proteins across the membrane. The name of the system comes from the requirement for two consecutive arginines in the signal sequence required for targeting to this system.

Release of outer membrane vesicles

In addition to the use of the multiprotein complexes listed above, Gram-negative bacteria possess another method for release of material: the formation of outer membrane vesicles. Portions of the outer membrane pinch off, forming spherical structures made of a lipid bilayer enclosing periplasmic materials. Vesicles from a number of bacterial species have been found to contain virulence factors, some have immunomodulatory effects, and some can directly adhere to and intoxicate host cells. While release of vesicles has been demonstrated as a general response to stress conditions, the process of loading cargo proteins seems to be selective.

Secretion in Gram-positive Bacteria

Proteins with appropriate N-terminal targeting signals are synthesised in the cytoplasm and then directed to a specific protein transport pathway. During, or shortly after its translocation across the cytoplasmic membrane, the protein is processed and folded into its active form. Then the translocated protein is either retained at the extracytoplasmic side of the cell or released into the environment. Since the signal peptides that target proteins to the membrane are key determinants for transport pathway specificity, these signal peptides are classified according to the transport pathway to which they direct proteins. Signal peptide classification is based on the type of signal peptidase (SPase) that is responsible for the removal of the signal peptide. The majority of exported proteins are exported from the cytoplasm via the general Secretory (Sec) pathway. Most well known virulence factors (e.g. exotoxins of *Staphylococcus aureus*, protective antigen of *Bacillus anthracis*, lysteriolysin O of *Listeria monocytogenes*) that are secreted by Gram-positive pathogens have a typical N-terminal signal peptide that would lead them to the Sec-pathway. Proteins that are secreted via this pathway are translocated across the cytoplasmic membrane in an unfolded state. Subsequent processing and folding of these proteins takes place in the cell wall environment on the *trans*-side of the membrane. In addition to the Sec system, some Gram-positive bacteria also contain the Tat-system that is able to translocate folded proteins across the membrane. This is especially appropriate for proteins that need co-factors, such as iron-sulphur clusters and molybdopterin, which are incorporated in the cytoplasm. Pathogenic bacteria may contain certain special purpose export systems that are specifically involved in the transport of only a few proteins. For example, several gene clusters have been identified in mycobacteria that encode proteins that are secreted into the environment via specific pathways (ESAT-6) and are important for mycobacterial pathogenesis. Specific ATP-binding cassette (ABC) transporters direct the export and processing of small antibacterial peptides called bacteriocins. Genes for endolysins that are responsible for the onset of bacterial lysis are often located near genes that encode for holin-like proteins, suggesting that these holins are responsible for endolysin export to the cell wall.

Chapter 5

Production of Heterologous Proteins in Eukaryotic Cells

INTRODUCTION

Advances in genetic engineering have made possible the production of therapeutics and vaccines for human and animals in the form of recombinant proteins. These biotechnology-derived recombinant proteins form a new class of drugs for many ailments like genetic disorders, cancer, hypertension and AIDS for which we have no better treatment or cure. Unlike chemical drugs, biologicals are our own molecules and hence more compatible with biological systems. At present there are more than 100 biotechnology-derived therapeutics and vaccines approved by US FDA for medical use and over 1000 additional drugs and vaccines are in various phases of clinical trials. In addition, use of DNA, proteins and enzymes in diagnostics is increasing exponentially. Industrial uses of enzymes in food, textile, leather, detergent, medicinal chemistry sectors are also increasing rapidly. The growing need of therapeutic and other applications of enzymes and proteins could only be met by heterologous synthesis of recombinant proteins.

In this chapter we outline steps involved in the production of heterologous proteins and then evaluate in detail available expression systems and factors affecting heterologous protein expression.

HETEROLOGOUS PRODUCTION OF PROTEINS

Protein over-expression refers to the directed synthesis of large amounts of desired proteins. The heterologous production of proteins and enzymes involves two major steps:

1. Introduction of foreign DNA into the host cells. This step has three major considerations: (a) identification and isolation of the DNA to be introduced, (b) identification of the vector and construction of recombinant vector, and (c) identification of the suitable expression system to receive rDNA.
2. Factors affecting the expression of foreign DNA for protein synthesis in the chosen expression system.

Points 1(a) and 1(b) are topics in themselves and will not be dealt with in this review. Briefly, at present a variety of vectors are available to ferry DNA in and out of cells: plasmids, lambda phage, cosmids, phagmids, artificial chromosomes from bacteria, yeast or human origin (BAC, YAC and HAC respectively). The vectors could either be integrating (becomes part of the host's chromosomes) or extrachromosomal. They could be in copies varying from one to several hundreds. In general, expression vectors have the following attributes as shown in Fig. 5.1.

117

1. Ori: Sequences that allow their autonomous replication within the cell.
2. Promoter: A tightly regulated promoter, i.e. one which can be switched on and off easily, is desirable.
3. Selection marker(s): Sequences encoding a selectable marker that assures maintenance of the vector in the host.
4. Terminator: A strong transcriptional terminator should be used with a strong promoter to ensure that the RNA polymerase disengages and does not continue to transcribe downstream genes.
5. Polylinker: To simplify the insertion of the heterologous gene in the correct orientation within the vector.

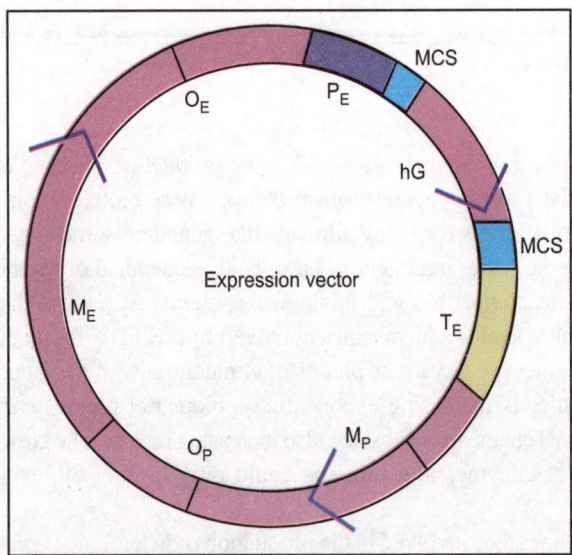

Fig. 5.1. Design of typical shuttle vector for heterologous gene expression. MCS = multiple cloning sequence; O_p = bacterial origin of replication; M_p = marker gene for selection in bacteria; M_E = marker gene for selection in eukaryotes; O_E = eukaryotic origin of replication; P_E = eukaryotic promoter sequence; T_E = eukaryotic terminator sequence; hG = heterologous gene for expression.

In addition, artificial chromosomes have centromeric and telomeric sequences which are host-specific (Fig. 5.2). These attributes permit artificial chromosome vectors to be faithfully replicated and distributed to daughter cells during cell division. Use of artificial chromosomes in commercial production of heterologous proteins remains unexplored.

Available Expression System

Prokaryotic and eukaryotic systems are the two general categories of expression systems. Prokaryotic systems are generally easier to handle and are satisfactory for most purposes. However, there are serious limitations in using prokaryotic cells for the production of eukaryotic proteins. For example, many of the eukaryotic proteins undergo a variety of post-translational modifications like proper folding, glycosylation, phosphorylation, formation of disulphide bridges, etc. There is no universal expression system for heterologous proteins. All expression systems have some advantages as well as some disadvantages that should be considered in selecting which one to use. Choosing the best one requires evaluating the options—from yield to glycosylation, to proper folding, to economics of scale-up.

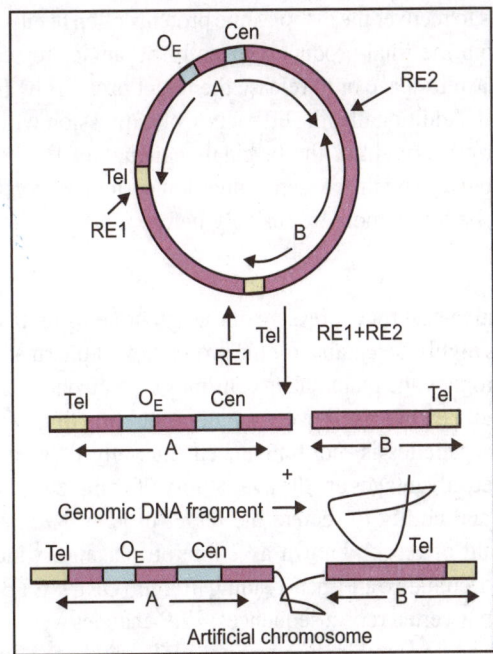

Fig. 5.2. Design of an artificial chromosome. RE1 and RE2, Restriction enzymes cleavage sequences; O_E, Eukaryotic origin of replication; Cen, Respective centromeric sequence; Tel, Respective telomeric sequence; A and B, Fragments generated by cleavage of the vector by RE1 and RE2. Cleavage of the vector by a mixture of RE1 and RE2 generates fragments A and B and another fragment which is discarded. A and B fragments have Tel sequences at one end. Larger fragments of targeted genomic DNA to be cloned can be bracketed by ligation with fragments A and B as shown. Since the construct has centromeric and telomeric sequences, it can replicate as a chromosome in the appropriate eukaryote.

Bacterial system

E. coli is by far the most widely employed host, provided post-translational modifications of the product are not essential. Its popularity is due to the vast body of knowledge about its genetics, physiology and complete genomic sequence which greatly facilitates gene cloning and cultivation. High growth rates combined with the ability to express high levels of heterologous proteins, i.e. strains producing up to 30 per cent of their total protein as the expressed gene product, result in high volumetric productivity. Furthermore, *E. coli* can grow rapidly to high densities in simple and inexpensive media. Strains used for recombinant production have been genetically manipulated so that they are generally regarded as safe for large-scale fermentation. Purification has been greatly simplified by producing recombinant fusion proteins which can be affinity-purified, e.g. glutathione-S-transferase and maltose-binding fusion proteins. However, expression in bacteria does have some serious disadvantages. It poses significant problems in post-translational modifications of proteins. Common bacterial expression systems such as *E. coli* have no capacity to glycosylate proteins in either N- or O-linked conformation. Although other bacterial strains such as *Neisseria meningirulls* have recently been shown to O-glycosylate some of their endogenous proteins, the trisaccharide added is different from O-linked sugars found in eukaryotes. Protein expressed in large amounts often precipitates into insoluble aggregates called inclusion bodies, from which it can only be recovered in an active form by solubilisation in denaturing agents followed by careful renaturation. Lysis to recover the cytoplasmic proteins often results in the release of endotoxins, which must be removed from the final product. Currently, strategies to secrete the target proteins by translocation into the periplasmic space or to release the target proteins by linking to existing excretory systems are being developed. Additionally, the efficiency of expression will also depend on differences of codon utilisation by bacteria. At times the original sequence of the heterologous gene has to be modified to reflect the codon usage by the chosen expression system. *E. coli* has toxic cell wall pyrogens and hence products need to be tested more extensively before use.

Yeast

Yeast is the favoured alternative host for expression of foreign proteins for research, industrial or medical use. As a food organism, it is highly acceptable for the production of pharmaceutical proteins. In contrast, *E. coli* has toxic cell wall pyrogens and mammalian cells may contain oncogenic or viral DNA. Compared to mammalian cells, yeast can be grown relatively rapidly (doubling time 90 min.) on simple media and to high cell density and its genetics is more advanced than any other eukaryote, so that it can be manipulated as readily. Added advantages are the availability of complete genomic sequence, the nuclear stable high copy plasmids and ability to secrete the target protein. *Saccharomyces* strains have high copy stably-inherited plasmid of 6.3 kb known as 2-micron plasmid, which codes for 4 genes *FLP*, *REP1*, *REP2* and *D*. It also contains an open reading frame (ORF), STB locus (required in *cis* for stabilisation) and two 599 bp inverted repeat sequences. *FLP* encodes a site-specific recombinase which promotes flipping about the *FLP* recombination targets (FRT) within the inverted repeats, so that cells contain two forms of 2-micron plasmids, A and B. The simple 2-micron shuttle vectors contain the 2-micron ORI-STB, a yeast selectable marker and bacterial plasmid sequence (*ori* and selection markers) and are used in host strains which supply *REP1* and *REP2* proteins.

These lower eukaryotic systems are able to glycosylate the target proteins, but it has been shown that both N- and O-linked oligosaccharide structures are however, significantly different from their mammalian counterparts. Hypermannosylation (addition of a large number of mannose residues to the core oligosaccharide) is a common feature in yeast, hindering proper folding and therefore the activity of the protein. At the moment yeast provides a good compromise between bacteria on one side and mammalian cell lines on the other.

Insect

The baculoviruses have emerged as a popular system for overproducing recombinant proteins in eukaryotic cells. Several factors have contributed to their popularity. Being eukaryotes, they use many of the protein modifications, processing, and transport systems present in higher eukaryotic cells. They use a helper-independent virus that can be propagated to high titers in insect cells adapted for growth in suspension cultures, making it possible to obtain large amounts of recombinant proteins with relative ease. Expressed proteins are usually expressed in the proper cellular compartment, i.e. membrane proteins are usually localised to the membrane, nuclear proteins to the nucleus and secreted proteins secreted into the medium. Majority of the overproduced proteins remain soluble in insect cells. Viral genome is large (130 kb) and thus can accommodate large fragments of foreign DNA. Baculoviruses are noninfectious to vertebrates and their promoters have been shown to be inactive in mammalian cells, which gives them a possible advantage over other systems when expressing oncogenes or potentially toxic proteins. Also the process development time is short. Expression using baculoviral vectors also has some limitations. Since baculoviruses infect invertebrates, it is possible that the processing of proteins produced by vertebrates is different and this seems to be the case for some post-translational modifications, e.g. internal proteolytic cleavages at arginine- or lysine-rich sequences are highly inefficient. The glycosylation capability is generally limited to producing only high mannose type and not processed to complex type oligosaccharides containing fucose, galactose and sialic acid.

Mammalian cells

Ideally, proteins requiring mammalian post-translational modifications should be expressed in mammalian cells. If product authenticity is absolutely essential for clinical efficacy, then despite the many shortcomings, a mammalian host is the only choice, as it offers the greatest degree of product fidelity. It should, however, be noted that oligosaccharide processing is species- and cell type-dependent among mammalian cells. Differences in glycosylation pattern are reported in rodent cell lines and human tissues. Even the use of human cell line is not perfect, since the transformation event required in most cases to produce a stable cell line may itself result in altered glycosylation profiles. Also mammalian expression techniques are time consuming and much more difficult to perform on a large scale. Complex nutrient requirement and low product concentration have meant that the end product must be highly value-added for this approach to be commercially viable.

Dictyostelium discoideum

Recently, the cellular slime mould *Dictyostelium discoideum* has been developed as an alternative eukaryotic system for expressing recombinant proteins. Circular plasmids are common in prokaryotes, but only a few eukaryotes have been identified and studied for having circular nuclear plasmids and *Dictyostelium* is one of them. The cellular slime moulds have families of similar plasmids which are found in the nuclei of different species. They are organised differently from the yeast 2-micron like plasmids. *Dictyostelium* plasmids are packaged in a nucleosomal structure similar to the chromatin organisation of higher eukaryotes. The best characterised family is that of the Ddp2-like plasmids. These plasmids are small (4.4–5.8 kb), encode ORF and contain an inverted repeat. The product of ORF is required in *trans* for plasmid maintenance, while an approximately 600 bp fragment, presumably containing the origin of replication is required in *cis*. The second best characterised plasmid family is Ddp1, found in wild type isolates like NC4 and V12. Ddp1 is a 13.7 kb plasmid which is present at an estimated copy number of 50–100 per cell and encodes at least 5 growth-specific and 5 development-specific transcripts. Although Ddp1 is larger and highly transcribed than the plasmids of the Ddp2-like family, none of the known transcripts seems to be essential for its replication. However, while approximately 1.2 kb region appeared to carry all the elements necessary for extra chromosomal replication, in the absence of selection, this fragment is quickly lost from the sub-population. In addition, deletion of plasmid sequences outside the region results in reduction of plasmid copy number. Therefore at least some of the Ddp1-encoded genes are required for the long-term maintenance of the plasmid at its normal copy number.

The development of reliable transformation systems for *D. discoideum* has provided the possibility of expressing heterologous genes in this microbe. *Dictyostelium* is a simple eukaryotic micro-organism with a haploid genome of 5×10^7 bp and a life-cycle that alternates between single-celled and multicellular stages. They grow to a high cell density without the serum factors or special aeration needed by animal cell cultures. There is no cell wall and the high copy number plasmid vectors allow the expression of protein in cell-associated, membrane-attached or secreted form under the control of regulatable promoters. The cells of *Dictyostelium* can carry out both O- as well as N-glycosylation. The major advantages of this system include a very simple and cheap growth medium and the potential for large-scale production of proteins.

Factors Affecting Intracellular Expression

Having the target DNA in an appropriate vector in the expression system of choice is the first step in optimising production of the heterologous proteins. Within a given system the transcription and translation processes leading to the heterologous protein production are a complex set of reactions. Each process is carried out and controlled by several enzymes/factors. In recent years we have learnt that the following few key steps or reactions are critical in determining the ultimate outcome.

Initiation of transcription

Gene expression is most frequently regulated at the level of transcription and it is generally assumed that the steady-state mRNA level is a primary determinant of the final yield of a foreign protein. The mRNA level is determined both by the rate of initiation and the rate of turnover. In most cases the yield of a foreign protein expressed using a host promoter has been much lower than the yield of the homologous protein, using the same promoter (~50 per cent). Many factors could account for these differences, e.g. downstream activating sequences (DAS) and upstream activating sequences (UAS). If DAS are characterised, it may be possible to incorporate them into upstream promoter fragments, in order to create more efficient expression vectors.

Alternatively, if DAS prove to be strongly position-dependent, they could be placed within an intron which could be excised prior to translation. If neither of these options works, then maximal transcription will only be possible using fusion proteins.

RNA elongation

The elongation of transcripts is not thought normally to affect the overall rate of transcription, but the yield of full length transcripts could be affected by fortuitous sequences in foreign genes which cause pausing or termination. These could either act in the same way as natural host terminator or else by a different mechanism, e.g. in yeast, though not widely recognised, this problem could be a very common reason for low yields or complete failure of expression of foreign genes. At present the only solution is to increase the AT/GC of the offending section of genes by chemical synthesis.

RNA stability

There is evidence that subtle changes in mRNA sequence affect the stability of mRNA, with low mRNA stability being a primary factor in poor yields of foreign proteins. Where mRNA instability is diagnosed as a problem, overall yield might be improved by: (i) using a more powerful promoter, (ii) using a promoter with more rapid induction kinetics or (iii) chemically synthesising the gene with altered codons or deleting the 3′ untranslated region in the hope that the instability determinant will be removed. Degradation of mRNA is also more pronounced under adverse growth conditions.

Gene dosage

Since the target gene is often incorporated into a plasmid vector system, gene dosage is dependent on plasmid copy number. As can be expected, an increase in copy number results in concomitantly higher recombinant protein productivity, but not indefinitely. Plasmid copy number is affected by plasmid and host genetics and also by cultivation conditions such as growth rates, media and temperature.

Initiation of translation

Translational efficiency is a function of either translational initiation or elongation rate. Translational efficiency is controlled primarily by the rate of initiation. Initiation in eukaryotes is thought to follow a scanning mechanism, whereby the 40 S ribosomal subunit plus co-factors bind the 5′ cap of the mRNA and then migrate down the untranslated leader scanning for the first AUG codon. Any part of this process, which is affected by the structure of the leader and the AUG content, could limit the initiation rate. AUG is recognised efficiently as initiation codon only when it is in the right context and optimal content is found to be GCC(A or G)CCAUGG.

The purines (A or G) three bases before AUG and G immediately following it are found to be the most important, influencing translation to the tune of 10-fold. The following factors have also been found to be important for prokaryotes: (i) the ribosome-binding nucleotide sequence or Shine–Dalgarno (S–D) sequence, (ii) the distance between the initiation codon and S–D, and (iii) the secondary structure of mRNA.

Translational elongation

Translational elongation does not effect the yield or quality of polypeptide normally, but it can become limiting with very high mRNA levels. Codon usage is considered a potential factor affecting product yield. Despite the degeneracy of the genetic code, a non-random codon usage is found in most organisms. The codon usage of most genes reflects the nucleotide composition of the genome; highly-expressed genes show a strong bias towards a subset of codons. This major codon bias, which can vary greatly between organisms, is thought to be a growth optimisation strategy such that only a subset of tRNAs and aminoacyl-tRNA synthetases are needed at high concentration for efficient translation of highly-expressed genes at fast growth rates. Rare codons, for which the cognate tRNA is less abundant, are translated at a slower rate, but this will not normally affect the level of product from an mRNA, since initiation is usually rate-limiting. A ribosome finishing translation of one mRNA molecule is most likely to initiate translation of a different mRNA species, unless the original species comprises a large proportion of the total mRNA.

Thus, the overall rate of translation of an mRNA is not usually affected by a slower elongation rate unless ribosomes become limiting, which would affect all transcripts in the cell. In contrast to the normal situation, there is evidence that codon usage may affect both the yield and quality of a protein when a gene is transcribed to very high levels. With very high levels of mRNA containing rare codons, aminoacyl-tRNAs may become limiting, increasing the probability of mistranslation, which is the incorporation of an amino acid which does not correspond to the codon being translated, and possibly causing ribosomes to drop off. Thus the codon content of a foreign gene may influence the yield of protein where the mRNA is produced at very high levels. This may more likely occur on growth in minimal medium, when the cell produces a wide variety of biosynthetic enzymes encoded by genes containing rare codons.

The effect on product quality has been difficult to measure, but requires further attention since it has further implications for therapeutic proteins. Proteins containing amino acid mis-incorporation are difficult to separate and may affect the activity and antigenicity of the product. Since small genes are now frequently synthesised chemically, they may be easily and perhaps profitably engineered to contain optimal codons for high-level expression. mRNA secondary structure, in addition to codon usage may affect translational elongation.

Polypeptide folding

During or following translation, the polypeptide must fold so as to adopt its functionally-active conformation. Since many denatured proteins can be refolded *in vitro*, it appears that the information for correct folding is contained in the primary polypeptide structure. However, folding comprises rate-limiting steps during which some molecules may aggregate, particularly at high rates of synthesis and at higher temperatures. There is evidence that certain heat shock proteins act as molecular chaperones in preventing the formation and accumulation of unfolded aggregates, while accelerating the folding reactions. Due to the intrinsic nature of polypeptide folding and low specificity of chaperones, it is very unlikely that foreign cytosolic proteins will accumulate in non-native conformations, but when fragments of proteins or fusion proteins are expressed, normal folding domains may be perturbed, resulting in an insoluble product. Insoluble proteins can often be renatured *in vitro*, though the techniques for this can be complex and unpredictable. In contrast to intracellular proteins, naturally secreted proteins encounter an abnormal environment in the cytoplasm; disulphide bond formation is not favoured and glycosylation cannot occur. In *E. coli*, foreign proteins are frequently insoluble, but low temperature has been found to increase solubility in some cases. This may be due to a decreased translation rate or to the fact that hydrophobic interactions, such as those occurring in aggregates, become less favourable. A dramatic increase in the yield of active, soluble protein is observed on reducing the rate of induction.

Post-translational processing

Prokaryotic expression systems are generally useful for producing heterologous proteins from cloned eukaryotic cDNA. In some cases however, eukaryotic proteins that have been synthesised in bacteria are either unstable or lack biological activity. The inability of prokaryotic organisms to produce authentic versions of proteins is for the most part due to the absence of appropriate mechanisms for generating certain post-translational modifications. In eukaryotes there are a number of modifications that may occur at the post-translational stage, after protein synthesis is complete.

Amino-terminal modifications of polypeptides: These are the most common processing events and occur on most cytosolic proteins. Two types of events normally occur – removal of the N-terminal Met residue, catalysed by Met aminopeptidase (MAP) and acetylation of the N-terminal residue, catalysed by N-acetyltransferase (NAT). Both enzymes are associated with ribosomes and act on nascent polypeptide. In most cases the structure of the N-terminus should not affect the biological activity of a protein, but there may be exceptions, e.g. the response of haemoglobin to physiological modifiers involves the N-terminus and correct folding of alpha and beta globins is therefore advantageous. Similarly N-acetylation of melanocyte-stimulating hormone is required for full biological activity.

Disulphide bond formation: In eukaryotes, formation of disulphide bond (*cys-s-s-cys*) occurs in the lumen of RER and is mediated by an enzyme called disulphide isomerase. Disulphide bond is confined to secretory proteins and exoplasmic membrane proteins. This is important in stabilisation of tertiary structure. An improperly folded protein is unstable and lacks activity.

Proteolytic cleavage of a precursor form: This is required in some cases. Selected segments of amino acid sequences are removed to yield a functional protein.

Glycosylation: This is the most extensive of all the post-translational modifications and has important function in secretion, antigenicity and clearance of glycoproteins. Oligosaccharides can attach to proteins in three ways: (i) via an N-glycosidic bond to the R-group of an *Asn*-residue within the consensus sequence *Asn-X-Ser/Thr* (N-glycosylation). All mature N-linked glycan structures have a common core of Man.GlcNAc, which can form part of simple oligomannose structures or be extensively modified by other residues such as fucose, galactose and sialic acid. Hybrid structures also exist where one or more arms of the glycan are modified and the remaining arms contain only mannose, (ii) via an O-glycosidic bond to the R group of the Ser or Thr (O-glycosylation). O-linked glycosylation is extensive in structural proteins such as proteoglycans. Small glycan structures can also be O-linked to the side chain of hydroxylysine or hydroxyproline, (iii) carbohydrates are also components of the glycophosphotidylinositol anchor used to secure some proteins to the cell membrane. The presence of these consensus sequences by no means guarantees their glycosylation. They show varying degrees of occupancy with oligosaccharides (macroheterogeneity) depending on their position within the protein and its conformation, the host cell type used for expression and its physiological status. These three factors also determine the extent of variation in the type of sugar residues found within each oligosaccharide (microheterogeneity). Glycosylation is both organism- and cell type-specific and therefore expression of a protein in a heterologous system will almost certainly result in a product with different modification from the native protein. This may affect the function and immunogenicity of the protein.

Modification of amino acid within proteins: Modifications of this type include phosphorylation, acetylation, sulphation, acylation (carboxylation, myristylation and palmitylation). Of these modifications, prokaryotic host cells are least likely to carry out either proper glycosylation or additions to specific amino acids within the heterologous protein. Moreover, no single eukaryotic host cell system is capable of performing all the possible post-translational modifications for every potential heterologous protein. Therefore, if a particular protein requires a specific set of modifications, then it may be necessary to examine different eukaryotic expression systems to find the one that can produce a biologically authentic product.

Stability of intracellular proteins

So far processes affecting the rate of synthesis of proteins have been considered, but the ultimate yield is equally affected by the rate of degradation. Yields might logically be improved by the following measures: (i) fusion to a stable protein, (ii) secretion to segregate the product from intracellular proteases, (iii) using a more rapidly induced promoter, (iv) using additional protease inhibitors to minimise degradation during extraction, (v) inducing at lower temperature, and (vi) harvesting cells in the exponential growth phase.

Stability of plasmid

Plasmid instability is a major problem in continuous and large-scale fermentation, since these cultures go through many generations. The resulting effects are lower productivity and increased production cost, because of the build-up of non-productive plasmid-free cells. Plasmid instability is categorised as segregational instability and structural instability. Segregational instability is the loss of plasmid from one of the daughter cells during division because of defective partitioning. Structural instability is attributed to deletions, insertions and rearrangements in the plasmid structure, resulting in the loss of the desired gene function. Plasmid stability is influenced by the vector and host genotypes; the same plasmid in different hosts exhibits different degrees of stability and vice versa. The origin and size of foreign DNA have been observed to affect the plasmid stability. Plasmid stability is also a function of physiological parameters that affect the growth rate of the host cell, which include pH, temperature, aeration rate, medium components and heterologous protein accumulation. Mathematically structured and unstructured kinetic models of plasmid stability have been developed which are ultimately useful for the design of recombinant processes.

SACCHAROMYCES CEREVISIAE

Saccharomyces cerevisiae is a species of budding yeast. It is perhaps the most useful yeast owing to its use since ancient times in baking and brewing. It is believed that it was originally isolated from the skins of grapes (one can see the yeast as a component of the thin white film on the skins of some dark-coloured fruits such as plums; it exists among the waxes of the cuticle). It is one of the most intensively studied eukaryotic model organisms in molecular and cell biology, much like *Escherichia coli* as the model prokaryote. It is the micro-organism behind the most common type of fermentation. *S. cerevisiae* cells are round to ovoid, 5–10 micrometers in diameter. It reproduces by a division process known as budding. Many proteins important in human biology were first discovered by studying their homologs in yeast; these proteins include cell cycle proteins, signalling proteins, and protein-processing enzymes. The petite mutation in *S. cerevisiae* is of particular interest. Antibodies against *S. cerevisiae* are found in 60–70 per cent of patients with Crohn's disease and 10–15 per cent of patients with ulcerative colitis.

Biology

Life cycle

There are two forms in which yeast cells can survive and grow: haploid and diploid. The haploid cells undergo a simple life cycle of mitosis and growth, and under conditions of high stress will generally simply die. The diploid cells (the preferential 'form' of yeast) similarly undergo a simple life cycle of mitosis and growth, but under conditions of stress can undergo sporulation, entering meiosis and producing a variety of haploid spores, which can proceed on to mate.

Nutritional requirements

All strains of *S. cerevisiae* can grow aerobically on glucose, maltose, and trehalose and fail to grow on lactose and cellobiose. However, growth on other sugars is variable. It was shown that galactose and fructose were two of the best fermenting sugars. The ability of yeasts to use different sugars can differ depending on whether they are grown aerobically or anaerobically. Some strains cannot grow anaerobically on sucrose and trehalose. All strains can utilise ammonia and urea as the sole nitrogen source, but cannot utilise nitrate since they lack the ability to reduce them to ammonium ions. They can also utilise most amino acids, small peptides and nitrogen bases as a nitrogen source. Histidine, glycine, cystine and lysine are, however, not readily utilised. *S. cerevisiae* does not excrete proteases so extracellular protein cannot be metabolised. Yeasts also have a requirement for phosphorus, which is assimilated as a dihydrogen phosphate ion, and sulphur, which can be assimilated as a sulphate ion or as organic sulphur compounds like the amino acids methionine and cysteine. Some metals like magnesium, iron, calcium, zinc also are required for good growth of the yeast.

Mating

Yeast has two mating types, **a** and α (alpha), which show primitive aspects of sex differentiation, and are hence of great interest. For more information on the biological importance of these two cell types, where they come from (from a molecular biology point of view), and details of the process of mating type switching, see mating of yeast.

Cell cycle

Growth in yeast is synchronised with the growth of the bud, which reaches the size of the mature cell by the time it separates from the parent cell. In rapidly growing yeast cultures, all the cells can be seen to have buds since bud formation occupies the whole cell cycle. Both mother and daughter cell can initiate bud formation before cell separation has occurred. In yeast cultures which are growing more slowly, cells lacking buds can be seen and bud formation only occupies a part of the cell cycle. The cell cycle in yeast normally consists of the following stages—G1, S, G2 and M—which are the normal stages of mitosis.

Yeast in Biological Research

A model organism

When researchers look for an organism to use in their studies, they look for several traits. Among these are size, generation time, accessibility, manipulation, genetics, conservation of mechanisms, and potential economic benefit. The yeast species *S. pombe* and *S. cerevisiae* are both well studied; these two species diverged approximately 300 to 600 million years before present, and are significant tools in the study of DNA damage and repair mechanisms. The alpha-factor of *S. cerevisiae*, has been compared to the liphophilic peptide created by the fungus *Tremella mesenterica*. *S. cerevisiae* has developed as a model organism because it scores favourably on a number of these criteria.

1. As a single-celled organism *S. cerevisiae* is small with a short generation time (doubling time 1.5–2 hours at 30°C) and can be easily cultured. These are all positive characteristics in that they allow for the swift production and maintenance of multiple specimen lines at low cost.
2. *S. cerevisiae* can be transformed allowing for either the addition of new genes or deletion through homologous recombination. Furthermore, the ability to grow *S. cerevisiae* as a haploid simplifies the creation of gene knockouts strains.
3. As a eukaryote, *S. cerevisiae* shares the complex internal cell structure of plants and animals without the high percentage of non-coding DNA that can confound research in higher eukaryotes.
4. *S. cerevisiae* research is a strong economic driver, at least initially, as a result of its established use in industry.

Genome sequencing

S. cerevisiae was the first eukaryotic genome that was completely sequenced. The genome sequence was released in the public domain on April 24, 1996. Since then, regular updates have been maintained at the *Saccharomyces* genome database (SGD). This database is a highly annotated and cross-referenced database for yeast researchers. Another important *S. cerevisiae* database is maintained by the Munich Information Center for Protein Sequences (MIPS). The genome is composed of about 12,156,677 base pairs and 6275 genes, compactly organised on 16 chromosomes. Only about 5800 of these are believed to be true functional genes. It is estimated that yeast shares about 23 per cent of its genome with that of humans .

Other tools in yeast research

The availability of the *S. cerevisiae* genome sequence and the complete set of deletion mutants has further enhanced the power of *S. cerevisiae* as a model for understanding the regulation of eukaryotic cells. A project underway to analyse the genetic interactions of all double deletion mutants through synthetic genetic array analysis will take this research one step further. Approaches have been developed by yeast scientists which can be applied in many different fields of biological and medicinal science. These include yeast two-hybrid for studying protein interactions and tetrad analysis.

Yeast in Commercial Applications

Top-fermenting yeast

Saccharomyces cerevisiae is sometimes called a top-fermenting or top cropping yeast, so called because during the fermentation process its hydrophobic surface causes the flocs to adhere to CO_2 and rise to the top of the fermentation vessel. It is one of the major types of yeast used in the brewing of ale, along with *Saccharomyces pastorianus* which is used in the brewing of lager. Top-fermenting yeasts are fermented at higher temperatures than lager yeasts and the resulting ales have a different flavour than the same beverage fermented with a lager yeast. 'Fruity esters' may be formed if the ale yeast undergoes temperatures near 21°C (70° F), or if the fermentation temperature of the beverage fluctuates during the process. Lager yeast normally ferments at a temperature of approximately 5°C (40°F), where ale yeast becomes dormant. Lager yeast can be fermented at a higher temperature normally used for ale yeast, and this application is often used in a beer style known as 'steam beer'.

Uses in aquaria

Owing to the high cost of commercial CO_2 cylinder systems, CO_2 injection by yeast is one of the most popular DIY approaches followed by aquaculturists for providing CO_2 to underwater aquatic plants. The yeast culture is generally maintained in plastic bottles and typical systems provide one bubble every 3–7 seconds. Various approaches have been devised to allow proper absorption of the gas into the water.

PRODUCTION OF HETEROLOGOUS PROTEINS USING *S. CEREVISIAE* EXPRESSION SYSTEM

Recombinant DNA expression constitutes a major approach in gene function studies that naturally complement genetic and genomic research. Well-regulated expression systems provide an invaluable tool for investigating the cellular roles of novel genes either in their original cellular environment or in specialised host organisms. These systems can be utilised to observe the biological effects of the controlled expression (or lack of it) of a given DNA sequence. Very often they also provide the means to produce and purify a desired gene product, opening the way to a comprehensive analysis and manufacture of proteins of biotechnological interest.

Traditionally, the expression and purification of heterologous proteins is accomplished using prokaryotic systems such as *Escherichia coli* or *Bacillus subtilis*. However, when the expression of eukaryotic proteins is desired, bacterial systems often fail because of a limited capacity to perform multi-step post-translational modifications such as protein *N*-glycosylation, phosphorylation and acetylation. Moreover, the production of bacterial toxins and their derivatives is highly desirable; however, attempts at heterologous expression using the traditional *E. coli* expression system are often problematic due to the formation of inclusion bodies that severely limit the final yields of a biologically active product.

Unicellular eukaryotes such as the yeasts *Saccharomyces cerevisiae*, *Pichia pastoris*, *Hansenula polymorpha*, *Kluyveromyces lactis* and *Schizosaccharomyces pombe* have become important systems in biotechnology for heterologous protein expression for both academic and industrial purposes. Yeasts combine the ability to grow on a simple medium at a very high cell density and secrete heterologous proteins. Moreover, they perform many of eukaryotic post-transductional modifications such as protein folding, proteolytic processing, disulphide bond formation and glycosylation.

S. cerevisiae has been widely employed as a host organism for expression of heterologous proteins, using regulated systems able to provide an accurate control of gene expression in the functional analysis, and the timely recombinant protein synthesis during fermentative production. For this purpose, yeast-derived promoters are used: *MET3* negatively regulated by the amino acid methionine, *PHO5* negatively regulated by inorganic phosphate, *CUP1* activated by Cu^{2+} ions, both *GAL1* and *GAL10* activated by galactose while repressed by glucose.

In the present work, the expression of hybrid proteins consisting of Abeta40 peptide fused to bacterial thioredoxin (*trx*) or pyrroloquinoline quinone (PQQ)-dependent glucose dehydrogenase (GDH) was analysed in yeast *S. cerevisiae*. An aggregated form of β-amyloid peptide (Abeta), both 40 and 42 amino acid long peptides, is the principal component of amyloid in the core of plaques, which is characteristic of Alzheimer's disease. Thioredoxin, a product of the *E. coli trxA* gene, is 12 kDa protein acting as antioxidant by facilitating the reduction of other proteins by cysteine thiol-disulphide exchange. The PQQ-dependent dimeric glucose dehydrogenase from *Acinetobacter calcoaceticus* oxidises a wide range of mono- and disaccharides to the corresponding lactones and is able to donate electrons to various artificial electron acceptors; also, it is a potential biocatalyst for an accurate monitoring of glucose in blood samples. An attractive feature of Abeta peptide to form the β-sheet fibrils was on the target in creating novel hybrid proteins able to form self-assembled nanostructures. The selection of the fused-partner is based on a possible practical application of hybrids in various areas such as biotechnology, molecular electronics, medicine, etc. The cloning, expression and purification of *trx*-ab and GDH-ab hybrid proteins have been previously performed using prokaryotic cells but have never been studied in a eukaryotic system. Given that the origin of the individual partners of the fused derivatives is both prokaryotic and eukaryotic, the expression peculiarities of these hybrids in eukaryotic organisms have a certain value to be studied.

Materials and Methods

The yeast expression plasmid pBK containing the *S. cerevisiae* K2 preprotoxin gene under the control of the inducible CYC-GAL1 promoter, as well as *URA3* and *leu2*-d auxotrophic markers and bacterial plasmids pET3a-abeta40, pET3a-abetacys2,39 bearing the double *cys* mutant of Abeta40 and pTAbEcoI containing a GDH-abeta sequence were used for constructing the recombinant plasmids pBK-*trx*-ab, pBK-*trx*-abcys2,39 and pBKGDH-ab, respectively. General procedures for the construction and analysis of recombinant DNAs were performed as described by Sambrook. All restriction enzymes (*Sma*I, *Bam*HI, *Pst*I), T4 DNA ligase, bacterial alkaline phosphatase, the Klenow fragment, Pfu DNA polymerase and DNA size marker (GeneRulerTM DNA Ladder mix) were obtained from Fermentas (Lithuania) and used according to the manufacturer's recommendations. For expression of the hybrid proteins, *S. cerevisiae* strains 3PMR-1 (*MATα ura3-52*); 21PMR (*MATα leu2 ura3-52*) and α'1 (*MATα leu2*) were used. Media for the propagation of *S. cerevisiae* yeast as well as standard genetic techniques were described in Ausubel. The *E. coli* strain DH5α (*F⁻(φ80dΔ(lacZ)M15) recA1 endA1 gyrA96 thi1 hsdR17 ($r_k^- m_k^+$) supE44 relA1 deoRΔ(lacZYA-argF) U169*) was used for plasmid isolation and maintenance.

Transformation of *S. cerevisiae* strains was performed using the LiAc/PEG method, and the transformants were selected by complementation of *URA3* or *LEU2* auxotrophy followed by isolation of a plasmid of interest and PCR analysis. The transformation of *E. coli* was carried out using the calcium chloride method. Protein production was analysed after cultivation of clones under appropriate conditions. Yeast cells were harvested by centrifugation (3000 g) at 4°C for 10 min., the biomass was (1 g) resuspended in 2 ml of A buffer (for *trx*-ab: 50 mM *tris*-HCl, pH 8.5, 100 mM NaCl, 10 per cent glycerol; for GDH-ab: 50 mM *tris*-HCl, pH 8.5, 10 per cent glycerol) and grinded using liquid nitrogen. The cell extract was cleared by centrifugation (11000 g) at 4°C for 15 min. Purification of the fused *trx-ab* protein was performed by metalochelate separation on a HiTrap HP column. GDH-*ab* was purified by an ion-exchange chromatography on a CM-cellulose column according to the manufacturer's instruction (GE healthcare). The concentration and purity of proteins were estimated from 15 per cent SDS-PAGE data after visualisation using Coomassie Brilliant Blue.

Results and discussion

The principal advantages of *S. cerevisiae* yeast in expressing recombinant proteins were used to study the expression peculiarities of the fused bacterial thioredoxin or glucose dehydrogenase genes with the Abeta peptide sequence. Basing on *S. cerevisiae* expression system pBK prepared by using *Sma*I and *Bam*HI restriction endonucleases, the recombinant plasmids pBK-*trx-ab* and pBK-trx-abcys2,39 were obtained by inserting 580 bp DNA fragments of *trx-ab* and *trx-abcys2,39* amplified by PCR (templates: pET3a-abeta40 and pET3a-abetacys2,39 and oligonucleotide primers: 4036F and 4612R) (Table 5.1), digested with *Xba*I restriction endonuclease and blunted with the Klenow enzyme with a subsequent *Bam*HI restriction [Fig. 5.3(a)]. The *GDH-ab* fragment was PCR-amplified using pTAbEcoI plasmid as a template (primers: 3021F and 3021R) (Table 5.1) for the construction of pBK-GDH-ab. The fragment was digested with *Bam*HI and *Pst*I and inserted into the pBK vector linearised by the same enzymes [Fig. 5.3(b)]. It is important to note that in all these constructs the expression of fused genes is regulated by a galactose-inducible CYC-GAL1 promoter.

The newly created heterologous expression plasmids were introduced into *S. cerevisiae* 3PMR-1 *ura*3-52, 21PMR *ura*3-52 *leu*2 and α'1 *leu*2 strains, and the transformants were selected for uracil or leucine auxotrophy. The screening of transformants by leucine marker was found to lead to an internal plasmids instability and the formation of different phenotypic groups depending on the morphology of the colonies. This effect had been observed previously and depended on the defective leucine gene *leu*2-d action. Additionally, we have found that the presence of *Abeta* sequence in combination with *leu*2-d decreases the efficiency of transformation, and yeast colonies appear only after 10–14 days in the case of selection for leucine auxotrophy, in contrast to 3–5 days for a regular transformation. We have determined that the stability of the new constructs, monitored by maintaining the *URA*+ or *LEU*+ phenotype, reaches 90–96 per cent, while the stability by Abeta is only approximately 50 per cent. The data were confirmed by PCR analysis. It is possible that the toxicity of Abeta peptide influences the yeast survival. In order to analyse the accuracy of the fused sequence, the recombinant plasmids were maintained in yeast, isolated and verified by PCR analysis. The primer pairs EclNcoF/SnaBR and 3021F/3021R were used for the analysis of the *trx-ab* and *GDH-ab* genes containing plasmids, respectivelly (Table 5.1).

Table 5.1. Sequences of oligonucleotide primers.

Name	Sequence (5' to 3')
4036F	CACAACGGTTTCCCTCTAGA
4612R	TCCTTTCGGGCTTTGTTAGC
3021F	GCATGGATCCAAATGAATAAACATTTATTG
3021R	GCATCTGCAGCACTTCACAGGTCAAGC
EclNcoF	CGCCATGGAGCTCGACGCTGAATTCCGTCACG
SnaBR	GCCGGATCCTCTACGTAAACAACACCACCAACCATC

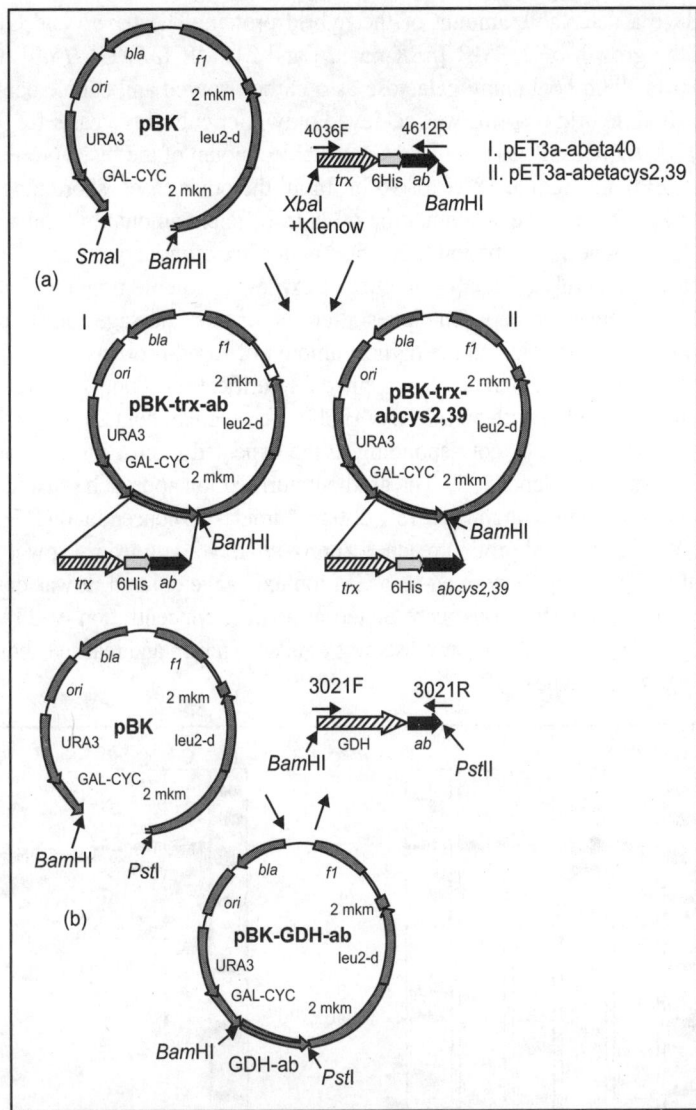

Fig. 5.3. Construction scheme of plasmids pBK-trx-ab, pBK-trx-abcys2,39 (a) and pBK-GDH-ab (b). *URA3, leu2-d* – genetic markers; 2 mkm – sequence originated from 2 μ plasmid of *S. cerevisiae; bla* – gene for β-lactamase; ori – pMB1 replication origin; GALCYC1 – galactose inducible promoter; *trx* – thioredoxin gene; 6His – hexahistidine linker; *ab* – Abeta polypeptide sequence; *abcys2,39* – Abeta with cysteine in 2 and 39 positions; *GDH-ab* – glucose dehydrogenase gene fused with Abeta; *Sma*I, *Bam*HI, *Pst*I – restriction endonuclease sites.

In the next step of this work, we investigated the growth conditions of persisting yeast transformants in order to achieve the maximal production of the hybrid proteins. Cultures were grown in liquid YEPD (2 per cent glucose), YEPG (3 per cent galactose) or minimal media supplemented with galactose or glucose by changing induction time and cultivation temperature. We have found that only the 21PMR strain bearing the recombinant constructs of interest possesses a satisfactory transformation efficiency and is able to produce a detectable amount of the hybrid protein. The *trx-ab* and GDH-ab proteins accumulate during the growth of 21PMR [*pBK-trx-ab*] and 21PMR [*pBKGDH-ab*] transformants at 18°C in the minimal medium containing galactose as a carbon source and supplemented with uracil. The highest level of both hybrid proteins was achieved only after culturing yeasts for 96 hr. However, the clone 21PMR [*pBK-trx-abcys2,39*] produced a detectable amount of the fused protein *trx-abcys2,39* after the growth in YEPG medium at 18°C for 96 hr. In all the other cases, shortening the cultivation time (24 hr, 48 hr or 72 hr) led to the accumulation of an insufficient amount of biomass or the protein started to degrade after a too long incubation (120 hr). An increase of induction temperature from 18° to 23°C or more resulted in a barely detectable amount of expressed soluble proteins. The differences in the expression level were observed between clones after two or more passages on solid media. Only a freshly-transformed yeast culture yielded the highest amount of fused proteins.

Single-step Ni-chelating chromatography was applied for purification of both *trx-ab* and *trx-abcys2,39* proteins. The proteins were eluted with 50 mM *tris*-HCl buffer, pH 8.5, containing 500 mM imidazole. A protein band migrating at 20 kDa, corresponding to the expected size of *trx-ab*, was detected after SDS electrophoresis [Fig. 5.4(a), lanes 1, 3]. The gradient purification approach showed that the protein of interest could be eluted from the column at a 150–200 mM imidazole concentration [Fig. 5.4(a), lane 2]. The maximal yield of the expressed protein reached approximately 20 μg from 1 g wet weight of yeast cells. Purification of GDH-ab was performed on a CM ion-exchange column. It was demonstrated that 45 kDa hybrid protein-enriched fractions were eluted at a NaCl concentration of 250–300 mM. The level of the heterologous protein expressed in yeasts was similar to *trx-ab* and reached about 25–30 μg/1 g wet yeast culture [Fig. 5.4(b), lanes 1, 2].

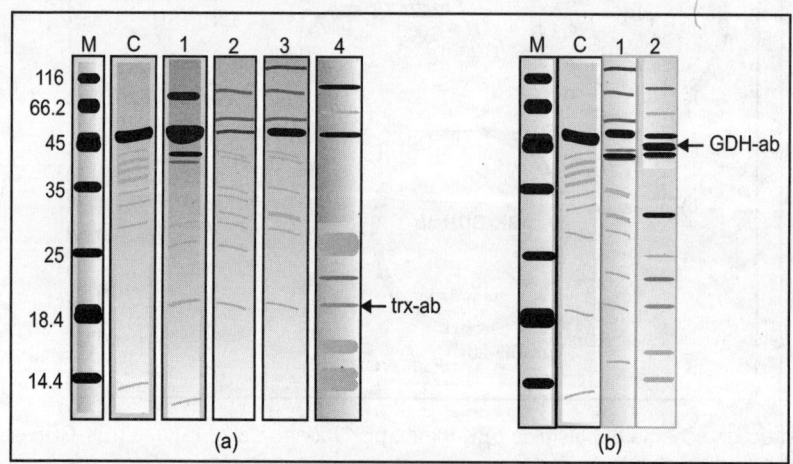

Fig. 5.4. SDS-PAGE electrophoresis of hybrid proteins. (a) Coomassie Brilliant blue-stained gel of *trx-ab* and *-trx-abcys2,39* fused proteins purified on a chelating column. Lane M – unstained protein molecular weight marker (UAB Fermentas), masses are shown in kDa; lane C – proteins of the untransformed 21PMR yeast strain purified on Ni-column; lane 1 – a single-step sample purification; His-tagged *trx-ab* eluted using 500 mM imidazole; lane 2 – gradient purification of *trx-ab* sample, elution at 250 mM imidazole; lane 3 – a single-step purification of *trx-abcys2,39*; lane 4 – a single-step purification of *trx-ab* in presence of 6 M urea (b). Coomassie Brilliant blue-stained gel of GDH-ab fused protein purified on CM column. Lane M – protein molecular weight marker; lane C – proteins of the untransformed 21PMR yeast strain purified on CM-column; lanes 1, 2 – purification of GDH-ab by ion-exchange chromatography; samples eluted at 250 mM and 300 mM NaCl, respectively).

Interestingly, using both metalochelate separation and ion-exchange chromatography, an approximately 52 kDa protein (high density band on SDS-PAGE) was observed [Fig. 5.4(a), lanes 1, 3; Fig. 5.4(b), lanes 1, 2]. Purification of the hybrid protein showed an interaction between *trx-ab* (or GDH-*ab*) and the 'leading' protein which can be distorted in the presence of 6 M urea [Fig. 5.42(a), lane 4]. In this case, only the His-tagged *trx-ab* binds to the Ni-column. It is possible that the interaction partner might be involved in the regulation of transport, folding and/or processing of the hybrid proteins (in a particular case of an Abeta peptide-bearing construct) and requires additional experiments to be proven. Thus, the expression and purification of both *trx-ab* and GDH-*ab* proteins have been successfully performed using yeast *S. cerevisiae*. The highest production output of the hybrid proteins was achieved by growing the yeast strains 21PMR [*pBKtrx-ab*] and 21PMR [*pBK-GDH-ab*] under inducing conditions of 18°C for 96 hr. The yield from 1 g of the yeast culture reached about 20–25 µg of the target proteins.

YEAST EXPRESSION PLATFORM

Yeasts can be used to produce proteins and sugars. Yeasts differ in productivity and with respect to their capabilities to secrete, to process and to modify proteins. The different 'platforms' of types of yeast make them better suited for different cooking and industrial applications.

Use of Organics in Creating Medicine and Products

Since the onset of gene technology, a plethora of bacterial micro-organisms, fungi and mammalian cells have been developed for the production of foreign proteins. These proteins are used in medicine and industry to create products such as pharmaceuticals like hepatitis B vaccines or insulin. Common organic 'platforms' for the development of medicine and products include the bacterium *E. coli*, and several yeasts and mammalian cells, most of them derived from Chinese hamster cells. In general a system used for production has to meet several criteria: it should be able grow rapidly in large fermenters, it should produce proteins in an efficient way, it should be safe and, in case of pharmaceuticals, it should produce and modify the products to be as similar to 'human' as possible.

Yeasts Include a Great Diversity of Organisms

In general, fungi are excellent hosts for the production of recombinant proteins. They offer a desired ease of genetic manipulation and rapid growth to high cell densities on inexpensive media. As eukaryotes, they are able to perform protein modifications like glycosylation (addition of sugars), thus producing even complex foreign proteins that are identical or very similar to native products from plant or mammalian sources. The first yeast expression platform was based on the commonly known baker's yeast *Saccharomyces cerevisiae*. However the baker's yeast is only one of more than 800 different yeasts with different characteristics and capabilities. For instance some of them grow on a wide range of carbon sources and are not restricted to glucose, as it is the case with baker's yeast. Several of them are also applied to genetic engineering and to the production of foreign proteins. The selection is given below:

Arxula adeninivorans (Blastobotrys adeninivorans)

Arxula adeninivorans is a dimorphic yeast (it grows as a budding yeast like the baker's yeast up to a temperature of 42°C, above this threshold it grows in a filamentous form) with unusual biochemical characteristics. It can grow on a wide range of substrates and can assimilate nitrate. It has successfully been applied to the generation of strains that can produce natural plastics or the development of a biosensor for estrogens in environmental samples.

Candida boidinii

Candida boidinii is a methylotrophic yeast (it can grow on methanol). Like other methylotrophic species such as *Hansenula polymorpha* and *Pichia pastoris*, it provides an excellent platform for the production of foreign proteins. Yields in a multigram range of a secreted foreign protein have been reported.

Hansenula polymorpha (Pichia angusta)

Hansenula polymorpha is another methylotrophic yeast. It can furthermore grow on a wide range of other substrates; it is thermo-tolerant and can assimilate nitrate (see also *Kluyveromyces lactis*). It has been applied to the production of hepatitis B vaccines, insulin and interferon alpha-2a for the treatment of hepatitis C, furthermore to a range of technical enzymes.

Kluyveromyces lactis

Kluyveromyces lactis is a yeast regularly applied to the production of kefir. It can grow on several sugars, most importantly on lactose which is present in milk and whey. It has successfully been applied among others to the production of chymosin (an enzyme that is usually present in the stomach of calves) for the production of cheese. Production takes place in fermenters on a 40,000 L scale.

Pichia pastoris

Pichia pastoris is a methylotrophic yeast (see *Candida boidinii* and *Hansenula polymorpha*). It provides an efficient platform for the production of foreign proteins. Platform elements are available as a kit and it is worldwide used in academia for the production of proteins. Strains have been engineered that can produce complex human N-glycan (yeast glycans are similar but not identical to those found in humans).

Saccharomyces cerevisiae

Saccharomyces cerevisiae is the traditional baker's yeast known to all readers for its use in brewing and baking and for the production of alcohol. Often the collective term 'yeast' is used for this single species. As protein factory it has successfully been applied to the production of technical enzymes and of pharmaceuticals like insulin and hepatitis B vaccines.

Yarrowia lipolytica

Yarrowia lipolytica is a dimorphic yeast that can grow on a wide range of substrates. It has a high potential for industrial applications but there are no recombinant products commercially available yet.

Do the Various Yeasts Perform in an Identical Way?

The answer is 'no'. They differ in productivity and with respect to their capabilities to secrete, to process and to modify proteins in particular examples. First we explain how a yeast becomes a producer of foreign proteins. Suitable yeast strains are transformed by a vector, a so-called plasmid that contains all necessary genetic elements for recognition of a transformed strain and the genetic advice for the production of a protein. The elements are summarised in the following:

1. A selection marker, required to select a transformed strain from an untransformed background—this can be done if for instance such an element enables a deficient strain to grow under culturing conditions void of a certain indispensable compound like a particular amino acid that cannot be produced by the deficient strain.

2. Certain elements to propagate and to target the foreign DNA to the chromosome of the yeast (ARS and/or rDNA sequence).

3. A segment responsible for the production of the desired protein compound a so-called expression cassette. Such a cassette is made up by a sequence of regulatory elements, a promoter that controls, how much and under which circumstances a following gene sequence is transcribed and as a consequence how much protein is eventually made. This means that the segment following the promoter is variable depending on the desired product—it could be for instance a sequence determining the amino acids for insulin, for hepatitis B vaccine or for IFN alpha-2a. The expression cassette is terminated by a following terminator sequence that provides a proper stop of the transcription. The promoter elements of the *H. polymorpha* system are derived from genes that are highly expressed. Some of them are not only very strong, but can also be regulated by certain addition of carbon sources like sugar, methanol or glycerol. However, most of them can only be recognised by a single yeast species.

However, since the yeasts differ in their characteristics to produce a certain protein it cannot be excluded at the beginning of a development that a selected yeast will not be able to produce the desired compound at all.

This in turn can lead to costly time-consuming failures. It is therefore advisable to assess several yeast platforms in parallel for their capabilities to produce such a compound. Therefore, a plasmid system was developed that can be targeted in functional form to all yeast in parallel. The basic design of this vector system, designated CoMed, is shown in the Fig. 5.5. It is composed in modular way of element for selection, a 'universal' targeting sequence that is present in all yeasts (the rDNA) and it contains within the expression cassette a promoter that is active in all yeasts (Fig. 5.5).

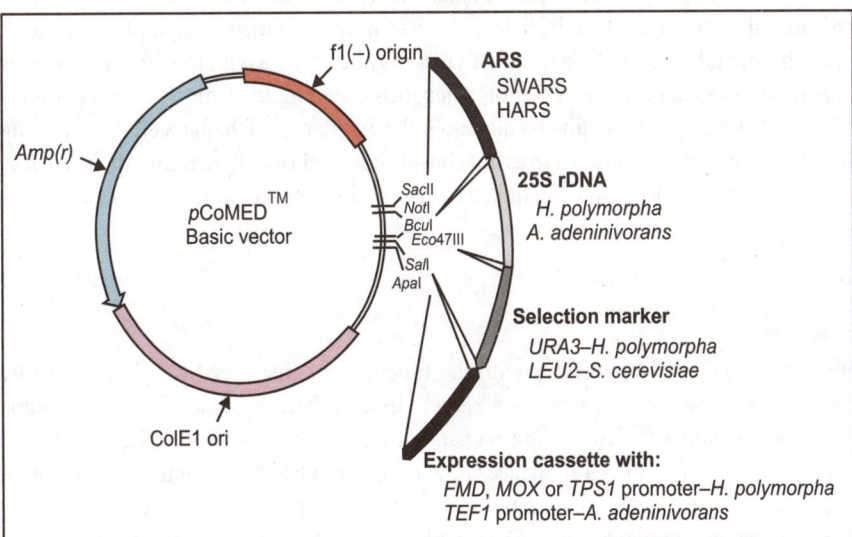

Fig. 5.5. Design and functionality of CoMed vector system. The CoMed basic vector contains all *E. coli* elements for propagation in the *E. coli* system and a MCS (multiple cloning ste) for integration of ARS, rDNA, selection marker and expression cassette modules. For this purpose, ARS fragments are flanked by *Sac*II and *Bcu*I restriction sites, rDNA regions by *Bcu*I and *Eco*47III restriction sites, selection markers by *Eco*47III and *Sal*I restriction sites and promoter elements by *Sal*I and *Apa*I restriction sites.

Hepatitis B

Hepatitis B is an infectious illness caused by hepatitis B virus (HBV) which infects the liver of hominoidae, including humans, and causes an inflammation called hepatitis. Originally known as 'serum hepatitis', the disease has caused epidemics in parts of Asia and Africa, and it is endemic in China. About a third of the world's population, more than 2 billion people, have been infected with the hepatitis B virus. This includes 350 million chronic carriers of the virus. Transmission of hepatitis B virus results from exposure to infectious blood or body fluids.

The acute illness causes liver inflammation, vomiting, jaundice and—rarely—death. Chronic hepatitis B may eventually cause liver cirrhosis and liver cancer—a fatal disease with very poor response to current chemotherapy. The infection is preventable by vaccination. Hepatitis B virus is an hepadnavirus—*hepa* from *hepatotrophic* and *dna* because it is a DNA virus—and it has a circular genome composed of partially double-stranded DNA.

The viruses replicate through an RNA intermediate form by reverse transcription, and in this respect they are similar to retroviruses. Although replication takes place in the liver, the virus spreads to the blood where virus-specific proteins and their corresponding antibodies are found in infected people. Blood tests for these proteins and antibodies are used to diagnose the infection.

Signs and symptoms

Acute infection with hepatitis B virus is associated with acute viral hepatitis—an illness that begins with general ill-health, loss of appetite, nausea, vomiting, body aches, mild fever, dark urine, and then progresses to development of jaundice. It has been noted that itchy skin has been an indication as a possible symptom of all hepatitis virus types. The illness lasts for a few weeks and then gradually improves in most affected people. A few patients may have more severe liver disease (fulminant hepatic failure), and may die as a result of it. The infection may be entirely asymptomatic and may go unrecognised. Chronic infection with hepatitis B virus may be either asymptomatic or may be associated with a chronic inflammation of the liver (chronic hepatitis), leading to cirrhosis over a period of several years. This type of infection dramatically increases the incidence of hepatocellular carcinoma (liver cancer). Chronic carriers are encouraged to avoid consuming alcohol as it increases their risk for cirrhosis and liver cancer. Hepatitis B virus has been linked to the development of Membranous glomerulonephritis (MGN).

Mechanisms

Pathogenesis

The hepatitis B virus primarily interferes with the functions of the liver by replicating in liver cells, known as hepatocytes. The receptor is not yet known, though there is evidence that the receptor in the closely related duck hepatitis B virus is carboxypeptidase D. HBV virions (DANE particle) bind to the host cell via the preS domain of the viral surface antigen and are subsequently internalised by endocytosis. PreS and IgA receptors are accused of this interaction. HBV-preS specific receptors are primarily expressed on hepatocytes; however, viral DNA and proteins have also been detected in extrahepatic sites, suggesting that cellular receptors for HBV may also exist on extrahepatic cells.

During HBV infection, the host immune response causes both hepatocellular damage and viral clearance. Although the innate immune response does not play a significant role in these processes, the adaptive immune response, particularly virus-specific cytotoxic T lymphocytes (CTLs), contributes to most of the liver injury associated with HBV infection. By killing infected cells and by producing antiviral cytokines capable of purging HBV from viable hepatocytes, CTLs eliminate the virus. Although liver damage is initiated and mediated by the CTLs, antigen-nonspecific inflammatory cells can worsen CTL-induced immunopathology, and platelets activated at the site of infection may facilitate the accumulation of CTLs in the liver.

Transmission

Transmission of hepatitis B virus results from exposure to infectious blood or body fluids containing blood. Possible forms of transmission include unprotected sexual contact, blood transfusions, reuse of contaminated needles and syringes, and vertical transmission from mother to child during childbirth. Without intervention, a mother who is positive for HBsAg confers a 20 per cent risk of passing the infection to her offspring at the time of birth. This risk is as high as 90 per cent if the mother is also positive for HBeAg. HBV can be transmitted between family members within households, possibly by contact of nonintact skin or mucous membrane with secretions or saliva containing HBV. However, at least 30 per cent of reported hepatitis B among adults cannot be associated with an identifiable risk factor.

Virology

Structure

Hepatitis B virus (HBV) is a member of the Hepadnavirus family. The virus particle, (virion) consists of an outer lipid envelope and an icosahedral nucleocapsid core composed of protein. The nucleocapsid encloses the viral DNA and a DNA polymerase that has reverse transcriptase activity. The outer envelope contains embedded proteins which are involved in viral binding of, and entry into, susceptible cells. The virus is one of the smallest enveloped animal viruses, with a virion diameter of 42 nm, but pleomorphic forms exist, including filamentous and spherical bodies lacking a core. These particles are not infectious and are composed of the lipid and protein that forms part of the surface of the virion, which is called the surface antigen (HBsAg), and is produced in excess during the life cycle of the virus (Fig. 5.6).

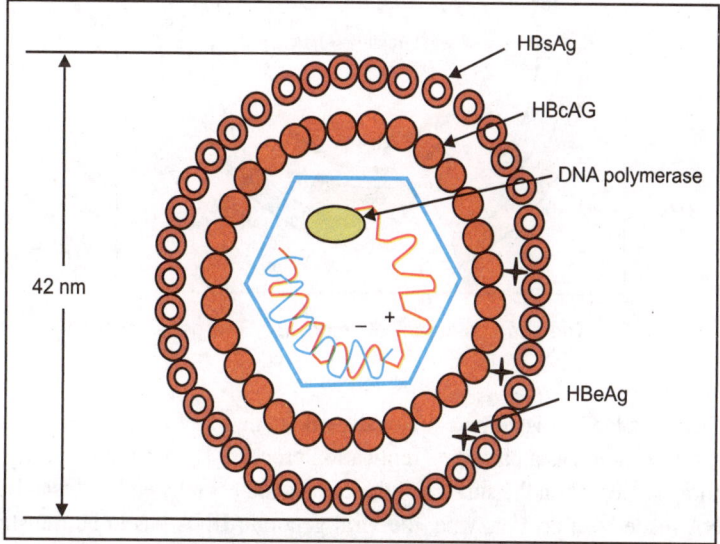

Fig. 5.6. A simplified drawing of the HBV particle and surface antigen.

Genome

The genome of HBV is made of circular DNA, but it is unusual because the DNA is not fully double-stranded. One end of the full length strand is linked to the viral DNA polymerase.

The genome is 3020–3320 nucleotides long (for the full-length strand) and 1700–2800 nucleotides long (for the short length-strand). The negative-sense, (non-coding), is complementary to the viral mRNA. The viral DNA is found in the nucleus soon after infection of the cell. The partially double-stranded DNA is rendered fully double-stranded by completion of the (+) sense strand and removal of a protein molecule from the (−) sense strand and a short sequence of RNA from the (+) sense strand. Non-coding bases are removed from the ends of the (−) sense strand and the ends are rejoined. There are four known genes encoded by the genome, called C, X, P, and S. The core protein is coded for by gene C (HBcAg), and its start codon is preceded by an upstream in-frame AUG start codon from which the pre-core protein is produced. HBeAg is produced by proteolytic processing of the pre-core protein. The DNA polymerase is encoded by gene P. Gene S is the gene that codes for the surface antigen (HBsAg). The HBsAg gene is one long open reading frame but contains three in frame 'start' (ATG) codons that divide the gene into three sections, pre-S1, pre-S2, and S. Because of the multiple start codons, polypeptides of three different sizes called large, middle, and small (pre-S1 + pre-S2 + S, pre-S2 + S, or S) are produced. The function of the protein coded for by gene X is not fully understood but it is associated with the development of liver cancer. It stimulates genes that promote cell growth and inactivates growth regulating molecules (Fig. 5.7).

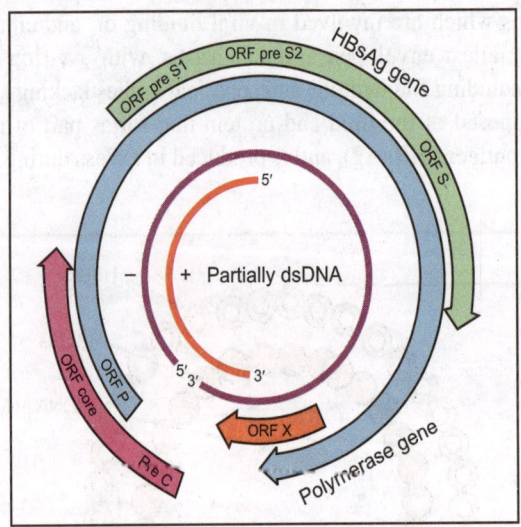

Fig. 5.7. The genome organisation of HBV. The genes overlap.

Replication

The life cycle of hepatitis B virus is complex. Hepatitis B is one of a few known non-retroviral viruses which use reverse transcription as a part of its replication process. The virus gains entry into the cell by binding to an unknown receptor on the surface of the cell and enters it by endocytosis. Because the virus multiplies via RNA made by a host enzyme, the viral genomic DNA has to be transferred to the cell nucleus by host proteins called chaperones. The partially double stranded viral DNA is then made fully double stranded and transformed into covalently closed circular DNA (cccDNA) that serves as a template for transcription of four viral mRNAs. The largest mRNA, (which is longer than the viral genome), is used to make the new copies of the genome and to make the capsid core protein and the viral DNA polymerase. These four viral transcripts undergo additional processing and go on to form progeny virions which are released from the cell or returned to the nucleus and recycled to produce even more copies. The long mRNA is then transported back to the cytoplasm where the virion P protein synthesises DNA via its reverse transcriptase activity.

Serotypes and genotypes

The virus is divided into four major serotypes (*adr*, *adw*, *ayr*, *ayw*) based on antigenic epitopes presented on its envelope proteins, and into eight genotypes (A-H) according to overall nucleotide sequence variation of the genome. The genotypes have a distinct geographical distribution and are used in tracing the evolution and transmission of the virus. Differences between genotypes affect the disease severity, course and likelihood of complications, and response to treatment and possibly vaccination.

Genotypes differ by at least 8 per cent of their sequence and were first reported in 1988 when six were initially described (A-F). Two further types have since been described (G and H). Most genotypes are now divided into subgenotypes with distinct properties.

Genotype A is most commonly found in the Americas, Africa, India and Western Europe. Genotype B is most commonly found in Asia and the United States. Genotype B1 dominates in Japan, B2 in China and Vietnam while B3 confined to Indonesia. B4 is confined to Vietnam. All these strains specify the serotype *ayw1*. B5 is most common in the Philippines. Genotype C is most common in Asia and the United States. Subgenotype C1 is common in Japan, Korea and China. C2 is common in China, South-East Asia and Bangladesh and C3 in Oceania. All these strains specify the serotype adrq. C4 specifying *ayw3* is found in Aborigines from Australia. Genotype D is most commonly found in Southern Europe, India and the United States and has been divided into 8 subtypes (D1-D8). In Turkey genotype D is also the most common type. A pattern of defined geographical distribution is less evident with D1-D4 where these subgenotypes are widely spread within Europe, Africa and Asia. This may be due to their divergence having occurred before than of genotypes B and C. D4 appears to be the oldest split and is still the dominating subgenotype of D in Oceania. Type E is most commonly found in West and Southern Africa. Type F is most commonly found in Central and South America and has been divided into two subgroups (F1 and F2). Genotype G has an insertion of 36 nucleotides in the core gene and is found in France and the United States. Type H is most commonly found in Central and South America and California in United States. Africa has five genotypes (A-E). Of these the predominant genotypes are A in Kenya, B and D in Egypt, D in Tunisia, A-D in South Africa and E in Nigeria. Genotype H is probably split off from genotype F within the New World.

Diagnosis

The tests, called assays, for detection of hepatitis B virus infection involve serum or blood tests that detect either viral antigens (proteins produced by the virus) or antibodies produced by the host. Interpretation of these assays is complex.

The hepatitis B surface antigen (*HBsAg*) is most frequently used to screen for the presence of this infection. It is the first detectable viral antigen to appear during infection. However, early in an infection, this antigen may not be present and it may be undetectable later in the infection as it is being cleared by the host. The infectious virion contains an inner 'core particle' enclosing viral genome. The icosahedral core particle is made of 180 or 240 copies of core protein, alternatively known as hepatitis B core antigen, or *HBcAg*. During this 'window' in which the host remains infected but is successfully clearing the virus, *IgM* antibodies to the hepatitis B core antigen (*anti-HBc IgM*) may be the only serological evidence of disease (Fig. 5.8).

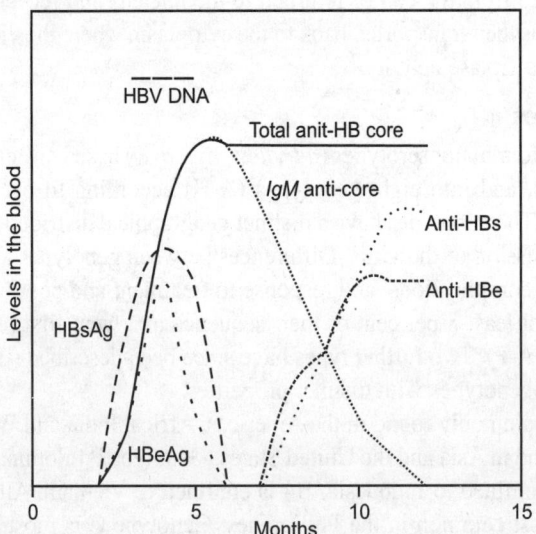

Fig. 5.8. Hepatitis B viral antigens and antibodies detectable in the blood following acute infection.

Shortly after the appearance of the HBsAg, another antigen named as the hepatitis B e antigen (*HBeAg*) will appear. Traditionally, the presence of HBeAg in a host's serum is associated with much higher rates of viral replication and enhanced infectivity; however, variants of the hepatitis B virus do not produce the 'e' antigen, so this rule does not always hold true. During the natural course of an infection, the HBeAg may be cleared, and antibodies to the 'e' antigen (*anti-HBe*) will arise immediately afterwards. This conversion is usually associated with a dramatic decline in viral replication (Fig. 5.9).

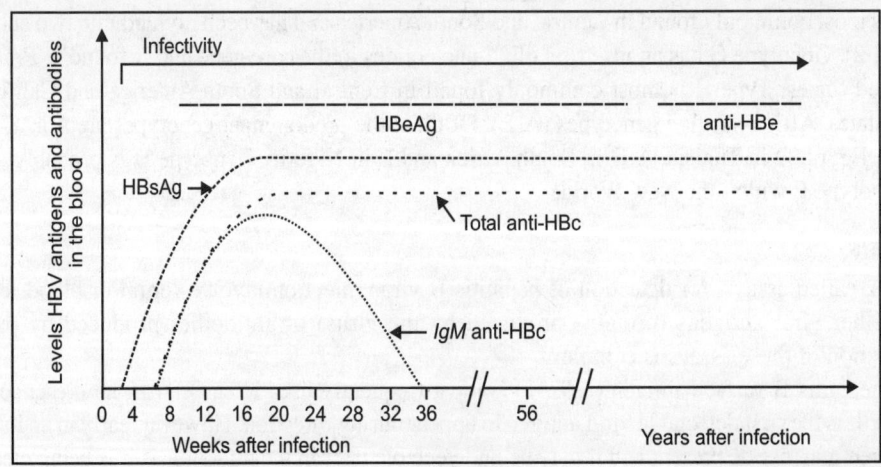

Fig. 5.9. Hepatitis B viral antigens and antibodies detectable in the blood of a chronically infected person.

If the host is able to clear the infection, eventually the HBsAg will become undetectable and will be followed by *IgG* antibodies to the hepatitis B surface antigen and core antigen, (*anti-HBs* and *anti HBc IgG*). The time between the removal of the HBsAg and the appearance of anti-HBs is called the window period. A person negative for HBsAg but positive for anti-HBs has either cleared an infection or has been vaccinated previously. Individuals who remain HBsAg positive for at least six months are considered to be hepatitis B carriers. Carriers of the virus may have chronic hepatitis B, which would be reflected by elevated serum alanine aminotransferase levels and inflammation of the liver, as revealed by biopsy. Carriers who have seroconverted to HBeAg negative status, particularly those who acquired the infection as adults, have very little viral multiplication and hence may be at little risk of long-term complications or of transmitting infection to others.

PCR tests have been developed to detect and measure the amount of HBV DNA, called the viral load, in clinical specimens. These tests are used to assess a person's infection status and to monitor treatment. Individuals with high viral loads, characteristically have ground glass hepatocytes on biopsy.

Prevention

Several vaccines have been developed by Maurice Hilleman for the prevention of hepatitis B virus infection. These rely on the use of one of the viral envelope proteins (hepatitis B surface antigen or HBsAg). The vaccine was originally prepared from plasma obtained from patients who had long-standing hepatitis B virus infection. However, currently, it is made using a synthetic recombinant DNA technology that does not contain blood products. You cannot catch hepatitis B from this vaccine.

Following vaccination, hepatitis B surface antigen may be detected in serum for several days; this is known as vaccine antigenaemia. The vaccine is administered in either two-, three-, or four-dose schedules into infants and adults, which provides protection for 85–90 per cent of individuals. Protection has been observed to last 12 years in individuals who show adequate initial response to the primary course of vaccinations, and that immunity is predicted to last at least 25 years. Unlike hepatitis A, hepatitis B does not generally spread through water and food. Instead, it is transmitted through body fluids; prevention is thus the avoidance of such transmission: unprotected sexual contact, blood transfusions, reuse of contaminated needles and syringes, and vertical transmission during child birth. Infants may be vaccinated at birth. Shi showed that besides the WHO recommended joint immunoprophylaxis starting from the newborn, multiple injections of small doses of hepatitis B immune globulin (*HBIg*, 200–400 IU per month), or oral lamivudine (100 mg per day) in HBV carrier mothers with a high degree of infectiousness ($>10^6$ copies/ml) in late pregnancy (the last three months of pregnancy), effectively and safely prevent HBV intrauterine transmission, which provide new insight into prevention of HBV at the earliest stage.

Treatment

Acute hepatitis B infection does not usually require treatment because most adults clear the infection spontaneously. Early antiviral treatment may only be required in fewer than 1 per cent of patients, whose infection takes a very aggressive course (fulminant hepatitis) or who are immunocompromised. On the other hand, treatment of chronic infection may be necessary to reduce the risk of cirrhosis and liver cancer. Chronically infected individuals with persistently elevated serum alanine aminotransferase, a marker of liver damage, and HBV DNA levels are candidates for therapy.

Although none of the available drugs can clear the infection, they can stop the virus from replicating, thus minimising liver damage. Currently, there are seven medications licensed for treatment of hepatitis B infection in the United States. These include antiviral drugs lamivudine (Epivir), adefovir (Hepsera), tenofovir (Viread), telbivudine (Tyzeka) and entecavir (Baraclude) and the two immune system modulators interferon alpha-2a and PEGylated interferon alpha-2a (Pegasys). The use of interferon, which requires injections daily or thrice weekly, has been supplanted by long-acting PEGylated interferon, which is injected only once weekly. However, some individuals are much more likely to respond than others and this might be because of the genotype of the infecting virus or the patient's heredity. The treatment reduces viral replication in the liver, thereby reducing the viral load (the amount of virus particles as measured in the blood).

Infants born to mothers known to carry hepatitis B can be treated with antibodies to the hepatitis B virus (HBIg). When given with the vaccine within twelve hours of birth, the risk of acquiring hepatitis B is reduced 90 per cent. This treatment allows a mother to safely breastfeed her child. Response to treatment differs between the genotypes. Interferon treatment may produce an e antigen seroconversion rate of 37 per cent in genotype A but only a 6 per cent seroconversion in type D. Genotype B has similar seroconversion rates to type A while type C seroconverts only in 15 per cent of cases. Sustained 'e' antigen loss after treatment is ~45 per cent in types A and B but only 25–30 per cent in types C and D.

Prognosis

Hepatitis B virus infection may either be acute (self-limiting) or chronic (long-standing). Persons with self-limiting infection clear the infection spontaneously within weeks to months.

Children are less likely than adults to clear the infection. More than 95 per cent of people who become infected as adults or older children will stage a full recovery and develop protective immunity to the virus. However, this drops to 30 per cent for younger children, and only 5 per cent of newborns that acquire the infection from their mother at birth will clear the infection. This population has a 40 per cent lifetime risk of death from cirrhosis or hepatocellular carcinoma. Of those infected between the age of one to six, 70 per cent will clear the infection.

Hepatitis D (HDV) can only occur with a concomitant hepatitis B infection, because HDV uses the HBV surface antigen to form a capsid. Co-infection with hepatitis D increases the risk of liver cirrhosis and liver cancer. *Polyarteritis nodosa* is more common in people with hepatitis B infection.

Reactivation

Hepatitis B virus DNA persists in the body after infection and in some people the disease recurs. Although rare, reactivation is seen most often in people with impaired immunity. HBV goes through cycles of replication and non-replication. Approximately 50 per cent of patients experience acute reactivation. Male patients with baseline ALT of 200 UL/L are three times more likely to develop a reactivation than patients with lower levels. Patients who undergo chemotherapy are at risk for HBV reactivation. The current view is that immunosuppressive drugs favour increased HBV replication while inhibiting cytotoxic T cell function in the liver.

Hepatitis B Virus

Hepatitis B virus, abbreviated HBV, is a species of the genus *Orthohepadnavirus*, which is likewise a part of the *Hepadnaviridae* family of viruses. This virus causes the disease hepatitis B. In addition to causing Hepatitis B, infection with HBV can lead to cirrhosis and hepatocellular carcinoma. It has also been suggested that it may increase the risk of pancreatic cancer.

Classification

The Hepatitis B virus is classified as the type species of the Orthohepadnavirus, which contains three other species: the *Ground squirrel hepatitis virus*, *Woodchuck hepatitis virus*, and the *Woolly monkey hepatitis B virus*. The genus is classified as part of the Hepadnaviridae family, which contains two other genera, the Avihepadnavirus and a second which has yet to be assigned. This family of viruses have not been assigned to a viral order. Viruses similar to Hepatitis B have been found in all the Old World great apes (orangutan, gibbons, gorillas and chimpanzees) and from a New World woolly monkey suggesting an ancient origin for this virus in primates.

The virus is divided into four major serotypes (*adr*, *adw*, *ayr*, *ayw*) based on antigenic epitopes present on its envelope proteins, and into eight genotypes (A-H) according to overall nucleotide sequence variation of the genome. The genotypes have a distinct geographical distribution and are used in tracing the evolution and transmission of the virus. Differences between genotypes affect the disease severity, course and likelihood of complications, and response to treatment and possibly vaccination.

Morphology

Components

It consists of: (i) HBsAg, (ii) HBcAg (HBeAg is a splice variant), (iii) Hepatitis B virus DNA polymerase, (v) HBx: The function of this is not yet well known. Hepatitis D virus requires HBV envelope particles to become virulent.

Genotypes

There are eight known genotypes labelled A through H. A possible new 'I' genotype has been described, but acceptance of this notation is not universal. Different genotypes may respond to treatment in different ways. The genotypes differ by at least 8 per cent of the sequence and have distinct geographical distributions and this has been associated with anthropological history. Type F which diverges from the other genomes by 14 per cent is the most divergent type known. Type A is prevalent in Europe, Africa and South-east Asia, including the Philippines. Type B and C are predominant in Asia; type D is common in the Mediterranean area, the Middle East and India; type E is localised in sub-Saharan Africa; type F (or H) is restricted to Central and South America. Type G has been found in France and Germany. Genotypes A, D and F are predominant in Brazil and all genotypes occur in the United States with frequencies dependent on ethnicity. The E and F strains appear to have originated in aboriginal populations of Africa and the New World, respectively. Within genotypes 24 subtypes have been described which differ by 4–8 per cent of the genome.

Life cycle

The life cycle of Hepatitis B virus is complex. Hepatitis B is one of a few known non-retroviral viruses which use reverse transcription as a part of its replication process.

Attachment: The virus gains entry into the cell by binding to a receptor on the surface of the cell and enters it by endocytosis. The cell surface receptor has yet to be identified however it is suspected to be a member of the ovalbumin family of serine protease inhibitors.

Penetration: The virus membrane then fuses with the host cell's membrane releasing the mRNA and core proteins into the cytoplasm.

Uncoating: Because the virus multiplies via RNA made by a host enzyme, the viral genomic DNA has to be transferred to the cell nucleus by host proteins called chaperones. The core proteins dissociate from the partially double stranded viral DNA is then made fully double stranded and transformed into covalently closed circular DNA (cccDNA) that serves as a template for transcription of four viral mRNAs.

Replication: The largest mRNA, (which is longer than the viral genome), is used to make the new copies of the genome and to make the capsid core protein and the viral DNA polymerase.

Assembly: These four viral transcripts undergo additional processing and go on to form progeny virions which are released from the cell or returned to the nucleus and recycled to produce even more copies.

Release: The long mRNA is then transported back to the cytoplasm where the virion P protein synthesises DNA via its reverse transcriptase activity.

INSECT CELL CULTURE

The utilisation of insect cell culture for heterologous protein expression has steadily increased over the last several decades. It has become a common expression system for both basic research and large-scale commercial applications. Currently, some of the common uses of insect cell expression include the research driven gene expression for protein crystallography-small molecule interaction, and FDA regulated GMP protein production. These regulated applications can include subunit vaccine production as well as the *in vitro* diagnostic and *in vivo* therapeutic markets. A key factor to the popularity of insect cell expression is the ability of insect cells to produce relatively large quantities of post-translationally modified eukaryotic proteins in a relatively short period of time. Most insect cell-produced proteins have been expressed by employing the baculovirus expression vector system (BEVS); however, other technologies that make stable transfected insect cells are gaining in popularity.

Many types of viruses infect insects, with the most common belonging to the family *baculoviridae*. The most popular invertebrate expression vector system is based on the Autographa Californica nuclear polyhedrosis virus (AcNPV), an insect baculovirus isolated from the Alfalfa looper that replicates in the nucleus of over 30 lepidopteran insect cell lines. The baculovirus expression vector system has been used to express genes derived from viruses, fungi, bacteria, plants, and animals. In this system, foreign genes placed under the control of the strong polyhedrin promoter of the AcNPV are usually expressed at high levels in cultured lepidopteran insect cells.

Baculovirus constitute one of the largest known groups of viruses, and they are capable of infecting over 500 species of insects, and more recently, these viruses have shown the ability to make ideal vectors for a variety of mammalian cell lines. The most widely used lepidopteran cells for BEVS are the Sf9 and Sf21 cell lines isolated from ovarian tissue of the fall army worm, *Spodoptera frugiperda*, and the high five cell line, designated BTI-Tn-5B1-4, originally established from the *Trichoplusia ni* embryonic tissue. Sf9 cells are a sub-clone of the Sf21 cells and were selected for their faster growth rate and higher cell densities than the Sf21 cells. *Spodoptera frugiperda* cells, either Sf9 or Sf21 are preferred for virus expansion. Sf21 cells can compare favourably, in terms of heterologous protein expression, to both High Fives and the Sf9 cell lines in certain situations.

The BEVS technology, developed by Max Summers, Gale Smith and colleagues at Texas A&M University, has unique biological advantages over bacterial, yeast or mammalian protein expression systems. A major advantage is the quick turnaround time for the expression of recombinant proteins that show biological activity, antigenicity, and immunogenicity similar to authentic natural proteins. Also, the vectors are not dependent on helper viruses nor are they pathogenic for vertebrates or plants. The replication cycle is biphasic, with gene expression occurring as a cascade of sequentially and temporally regulated events. During these events two different forms of the virus are synthesised: extracellular (or budded) virus particles (ECV) for cell to cell infection within the insect and viruses contained in occlusion bodies (OV) for spread to a new host insect.

Polyhedrin is the major viral-encoded structural protein that comprises the crystalline matrix of the occlusion body that protects the virus from environmental factors that would otherwise inactivate the ECV. Upon entry into the nucleus of a susceptible cell, the virus is uncoated and transcripts of many early genes are synthesised. DNA replication begins at around 6 hours post-infection, and expression of many of the early genes is repressed as the late genes become activated. Between 10 and 48 hours post-infection, extracellular viruses bud from the plasma membrane and spread the infection. Viral occlusions are detected by 18 hours post-infection and continue to accumulate for 4 to 5 days until the infected cells lyse.

Insect Cell Expression System

Insect cells are a higher eukaryotic system than yeast and are able to carry out more complex post-translational modifications than the other two systems. They also have the best machinery for the folding of mammalian proteins and, therefore, give you the best chance of obtaining soluble protein when you want to express a protein of mammalian origin. The most commonly used vector system for recombinant protein expression in insect is *baculovirus*, although baculoviral also can be used for gene transfer and expression in mammalian cells.

Advantages

Baculovirus-assisted insect cell expression is optimal for glycosylated protein expression in a cost-effective manner. There are many advantages to using baculovirus for heterologous gene expression. Heterologous cDNA is expressed well. Proper transcriptional processing of genes with introns occurs but is expressed less efficiently. As with other eukaryotic expression systems, baculovirus expression of heterologous genes permits folding, post-translational modification and oligomerisation in manners that are often identical to those that occur in mammalian cells. The insect cytoplasmic environment allows proper folding and S-S bond formation, unlike the reducing environment of the *E. coli* cytoplasm. Post-translational processing identical to that of mammalian cells has been reported for many proteins. These include proper proteolysis, N- and O-glycosylation, acylation, amidation, carboxymethylation, phosphorylation, and prenylation. Proteins may be secreted from cells or targeted to different subcellular locations. Single polypeptide, dimeric and trimeric proteins have been expressed in baculoviruses. Finally, expression of heterologous proteins is under the control of the strong polyhedrin promoter, allowing levels of expression of up to 30 per cent of the total cell protein.

The benefits of protein expression with baculovirus can be summarised as:
1. Eukaryotic post-translational modification.
2. Proper protein folding and function.
3. High expression levels.
4. Easy scale up with high-density suspension culture.
5. Safety

Baculoviruses infect primarily insects with a narrow host range. *Autographa californica*, the most commonly used baculovirus for protein expression, infects only two lepidopteran (moth) families in nature. Although these viruses may enter other cells types (perhaps by phagocytosis), they are not infectious in them. For example, nucleocapsid proteins are not removed in most human cells. In human hepatic cell lines that do remove these proteins, the virus fails to replicate and express proteins due to the absence of insect transcription factors. Thus, working with baculoviruses is considered safe for humans and contamination of mammalian cell lines in shared biosafety hoods is not a problem.

Recombinant DNA guidelines recommend a BL1 biosafety level for most baculovirus expression experiments.

Disadvantages

Despite these potential advantages, particular patterns of post-translational processing and expression must be empirically determined for each construct. Differences in proteins expressed by mammalian and baculovirus infected insect cells have been described and overcome in some cases. For example, inefficient secretion from insect cells may be circumvented by the addition of insect secretion signals (e.g. honeybee melittin sequence). Improperly folded proteins and proteins that occur as intracellular aggregates may be due to expression late in the infection cycle. In such cases, harvesting cells at earlier times after infection may help. Low levels of expression can often be increased with optimisation of time of expression and multiplicity of infection. The complete analysis of carbohydrate structures has been reported for a limited number of glycoproteins. Potential N-linked glycosylation sites are often either fully glycosylated or not glycosylated at all, as opposed to expression of various glycoforms that may occur in mammalian cells. Species-specific or tissue-specific modifications are unlikely to occur.

Insect cell culture

SF-9, SF-21, and High-Five insect cells are commonly used for baculovirus expression. SF-9 and SF-21 are ovarian cell lines from *Spodoptera frugiperda*. They are grown in Grace's (or a similar) media supplemented with 10 per cent fetal calf serum, lactalbumin, and yeastolate. High-Five cells are egg cells from *Trichoplusia ni*. These cells are less expensive to maintain since they may be grown without fetal calf serum. They reportedly express higher levels of recombinant proteins, although we have found these differences to be minimal.

All three cells lines may be grown at room temperature (optimum = 25°–27°C), and do not require CO_2 incubators. Their doubling time is 18–24 hours.

Outline process of expression

Given the variations of proteins to be expressed, no single protocol will satisfy every need. An outline for baculovirus expression is given below. One should plan 1–2 months to accomplish these goals:

1. Ligate the gene of interest to a bacterial transfer vector. The inserts are typically flanked by portions of viral genes to permit homologous recombination with replication defective, linear, viral DNA. Vectors or inserts may include sequences for protein targeting and purification. Verify direction of the inserts relative to the polyhedrin promoter and purify plasmids for transfections into insect cells.

2. Co-transfect insect cells with the recombinant transfer vector and a linearised viral vector. Electroporation, lipid, and calcium phosphate-mediated transformations work well. Replicative viruses are formed after intracellular homologous recombination between the ends of the viral molecules and portions of the transfer vector that flank the gene of interest. These recombination events insert your gene into the virus and complement defective viral gene(s) to permit viral replication. In some vectors, this may also generate production of marker proteins such as beta-galactosidase. Nonrecombinant viruses are kept to a minimum with this system.

3. Harvest the transfected cell supernatants.

4. Infect insect cells with dilutions of this supernatant to isolate single virus plaques. Identification of viral plaques can be difficult without the presence of a marker gene product such as beta-galactosidase.

5. Infect additional insect cells with viruses from these plaques to amplify the quantity and titer of viral stocks. Protein expression in these cells may be examined in Western blots.

6. Optimise the level of protein expression (MOI, time course of infection) and test for activity in an appropriate bioassay.

Development of vector and host

Baculoviral vector system and insect host cell lines are continually being developed. Several new systems for more robust and convenient application of baculovirus-based protein expression in insect cells have been invented and made available to researchers which are given below:

1. Transient expression system using non-viral vector system.
2. Multiple plasmid vector system for high-level expression of transgene in insect cells.
3. Novel insect cell lines with 'humanised glycosylation function' for better glycosylation of expressed recombinant protein.

RECOMBINANT BACULOVIRUSES

Recombinant baculoviruses are widely used to express heterologous genes in cultured insect cells and insect larvae. For large-scale applications, the baculovirus expression vector system (BEVS) is particularly advantageous. Specialised media, transfection reagents, and vectors have been developed in response to recent advances in insect cell culture and molecular biology methods.

The following are important choices in designing a system for recombinant protein production:

1. Selecting the expression vector, including the style or type of promoter, that provides best results with the recombinant gene product being expressed.
2. Evaluating insect cell lines, growth media (serum-supplemented or serum-free), and feeding/infection strategies that allow for optimal rAcNPV and/or product expression.
3. Choosing a scalable process of cell culture and deciding on other factors affecting downstream processing.

Overview of Baculovirology

Baculoviruses are the most prominent viruses known to affect the insect population. They are double-stranded, circular, supercoiled DNA molecules in a rod-shaped capsid. More than 500 baculovirus isolates (based on hosts of origin) have been identified, most of which originated in arthropods, particularly insects of the order *Lepidoptera*. Two of the most common isolates used in foreign gene expression are Autographa californica multiple nuclear polyhedrosis virus (AcMNPV) and Bombyx mori (silkworm) nuclear polyhedrosis virus (BmNPV).

Wild-type baculoviruses exhibit both lytic and occluded life cycles that develop independently throughout the three phases of virus replication. The following are characteristics of the three phases:

1. Early phase: In this phase (also known as the virus synthesis phase), the virus prepares the infected cell for viral DNA replication. Steps include attachment, penetration, uncoating, early viral gene expression, and shut off of host gene expression. Actual initial viral synthesis occurs 0.5 to 6 h after infection.
2. Late phase: In this phase (also known as the viral structural phase), late genes that code for replication of viral DNA and assembly of virus are expressed. Between 6 and 12 hr after infection, the cell starts to produce extracellular virus (EV), also called non-occluded virus (NOV) or budded virus (BV). The EV contains the plasma membrane envelope and glycoprotein (gp)64

necessary for virus entry by endocytosis. Peak release of extracellular virus occurs 18 to 36 hr after infection.

3. Very late phase: In this phase (also known as the viral occlusion protein phase), the polyhedrin and p10 genes are expressed, occluded virus (OV)—also called occlusion bodies (OB) or polyhedral inclusion bodies (PIBs)—are formed, and cell lysis begins. Between 24 and 96 hr after infection, the cell starts to produce OV, which contains nuclear membrane envelopes and the viral polypeptides gp41 and gp74. Multiple virions are produced and surrounded by a crystalline polyhedra matrix. The virus particles produced in the nucleus are embedded within the polyhedrin gene product and a carbohydrate-rich calyx.

Infection

Figure 5.10 summarises how baculoviruses infect cells and are transmitted *in vivo* vertically and horizontally. During the lytic cycle, enveloped and budded virions are generated. These virions promote horizontal transmission of the infection throughout the tissue in an *in vivo* infection of a worm larvae, or throughout the cell culture in an *in vitro* over-expression system. *In vitro*, this cycle is exploited to both generate virus stocks and establish a fully developed infection from subsaturating primary virus inocula. During the occluded cycle, virions packaged in the PIBs are generated. *In vivo*, these virions promote vertical transmission of the virus from insect host to insect host. *In vitro*, a polyhedrin gene modified to express a recombinant gene product in place of the PIBs is used. Biochemically, the essential difference between the lytic and occluded cycles is the induction of polyhedrin production at the beginning of the very late phase.

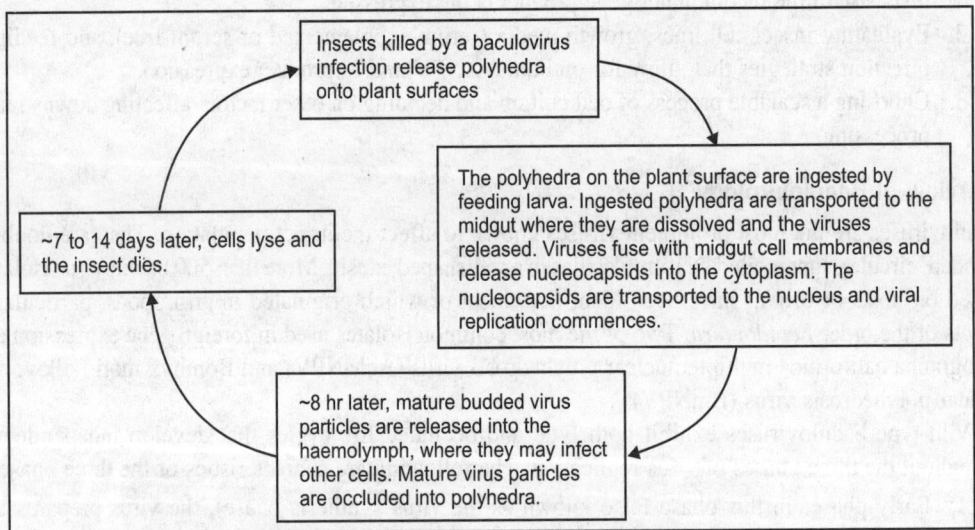

Fig. 5.10. *In vivo* baculovirus infection and replication.

We need to be able to distinguish between the initiation of virus production and budding, at approximately 8 to 10 hr post-infection, and the initiation of protein expression under control of the polyhedrin promoter, at approximately 20 to 24 hr. By doing so, you will be able to efficiently produce high-titer baculovirus stocks and high-quality recombinant product (i.e. product that is non-degraded and free of cell debris).

Vertical transmission

After the OV is ingested by insect larvae, the crystalline polyhedrin matrix is degraded in the alkaline midgut of the insect. Embedded virions are released and fuse to microvillar epithelial cells. Infected cells release EV from the basement membrane side of the midgut cell into the haemolymph system.

Horizontal transmission

EV enters the insect haemocoel and immediately spreads throughout the insect's open circulatory system, infecting many cell types. Within 10 viral generations, the insect dies and the OV, produced during the very late stage of infection, is released into the environment.

Baculoviruses as Expression Vectors

The major difference between the naturally occurring *in vivo* infection and the recombinant *in vitro* infection is that the naturally occurring polyhedrin gene within the wild-type baculovirus genome is replaced with a recombinant gene or cDNA. These genes are commonly under the control of polyhedrin and p10 promoters. In the late phase of infection, the virions are assembled and budded recombinant virions are released. However, during the very late phase of infection, the inserted heterologous genes are placed under the transcriptional control of the strong AcNPV polyhedrin promoter. Thus, recombinant product is expressed in place of the naturally occurring polyhedrin protein. Usually, the recombinant proteins are processed, modified, and targeted to the appropriate cellular locations.

Cytopathogenesis

As the recombinant infection advances, several morphological changes take place within the cells. The timing of the infection cycle and the changes in cell morphology vary with the insect cell line and strain of baculovirus used. The metabolic condition of the culture and growth medium used also can affect the timing of baculovirus infection. The following morphological changes are typical of monolayer Sf9 cells infected with recombinant AcNPV.

1. Early phase: Infection begins with the adsorptive endocytosis of one or more competent virions by a cell in a high metabolic state (peak replication rate). The nucleocapsids pass through the cytoplasm to the nucleus. When the virions enter the nucleus, they release the contents of the capsid. Within 30 min. of infection, viral RNA is detectable. Within the first 6 hr of infection, the cellular structure changes, normal cellular functions decline precipitously, and early-phase proteins become evident.

2. Late phase: Within 6 to 24 hr after infection, an infected cell ceases many normal functions, stops dividing, and is logarithmically increasing production of viral genome and budded virus. The virogenic stroma (an electron-dense nuclear structure) becomes well developed. Infected cells increase in diameter and have enlarged nuclei. The cells may demonstrate reduced refractivity under phase contrast microscopy. Infected cultures stop growing.

3. Very late phase: Within 20 to 36 hr after infection, cells cease production of budded virus and begin the assembly, production, and expression of recombinant gene product. In monolayer cultures, areas of infection display decreased density as cells die and lyse. Likewise, in suspension cultures, cell densities begin to decrease. Infected cells continue to be increased in diameter and have enlarged nuclei. The cytoplasm may contain vacuoles, and the nuclei may demonstrate granularity. As the infected cells die, plaques develop in immobilised cultures. The plaques can be identified under a microscope as regions of decreased cell density, or by eye as regions of differential refractivity.

Advantages of BEVS Technology

Since 1983, when BEVS technology was introduced, the baculovirus system has become one of the most versatile and powerful eukaryotic vector systems for recombinant protein expression. More than 600 recombinant genes have been expressed in baculoviruses to date. Since 1985, when the first protein (IL-2) was produced in large scale from a recombinant baculovirus, use of BEVS has increased dramatically. Baculoviruses offer the following advantages over other expression vector systems.

1. Safety: Baculoviruses are essentially nonpathogenic to mammals and plants. They have a restricted host range, which often is limited to specific invertebrate species. Because the insect cell lines are not transformed by pathogenic or infectious viruses, they can be cared for under minimal containment conditions. Helper cell lines or helper viruses are not required because the baculovirus genome contains all the genetic information.

2. Ease of scale up: Baculoviruses have been reproducibly scaled up for the large-scale production of biologically active recombinant products.

3. High levels of recombinant gene expression: In many cases, the recombinant proteins are soluble and easily recovered from infected cells late in infection when host protein synthesis is diminished.

4. Accuracy: Baculoviruses can be propagated in insect hosts which post-translationally modify peptides in a manner similar to that of mammalian cells.

5. Use of cell lines ideal for suspension culture: AcNPV is usually propagated in cell lines derived from the fall armyworm Spodoptera frugiperda or from the cabbage looper Trichoplusia ni. Cell lines are available that grow well in suspension cultures, allowing the production of recombinant proteins in large-scale bioreactors.

Generating a Recombinant Virus by Homologous Recombination

Using homologous recombination to generate a recombinant baculovirus is outlined in Fig. 5.11. The most common baculovirus used for gene expression is AcMNPV. AcMNPV has a large (130-kb), circular, double-stranded DNA genome. The gene of interest is cloned into a transfer vector containing a baculovirus promoter flanked by baculovirus DNA derived from a nonessential locus—in this case, the polyhedrin gene. The gene of interest is inserted into the genome of the parent virus (such as AcMNPV) by homologous recombination after transfection into insect cells. Typically, 0.1 to 1 per cent of the resulting progeny are recombinant. The recombinants are identified by altered plaque morphology. For a vector with the polyhedrin promoter, as in this example, the cells in which the nuclei do not contain occluded virus, contain recombinant DNA. Detection of the desired occlusion-minus plaque phenotype against the background of greater than 99 per cent wild-type parental viruses is difficult.

A higher percentage of recombinant progeny virus (nearly 30 per cent higher) results when the parent virus is linearised at one or more unique sites located near the target site for insertion of the foreign gene into the baculovirus genome. To obtain an even higher proportion of recombinants (80 per cent or more), linearised viral DNA that is missing an essential portion of the baculovirus genome downstream from the polyhedrin gene can be used. These approaches can take more than a month to purify plaques, amplify the virus, and confirm the desired recombinants.

Generating a Recombinant Virus by Site-Specific Transposition

A faster approach for generating a recombinant baculovirus uses site-specific transposition with Tn7 to insert foreign genes into bacmid DNA propagated in E. coli. The gene of interest is cloned into a pFASTBAC™ vector, and the recombinant plasmid is transformed into DH10BAC™ competent cells which contain the bacmid with a mini-*att*Tn7 target site and the helper plasmid.

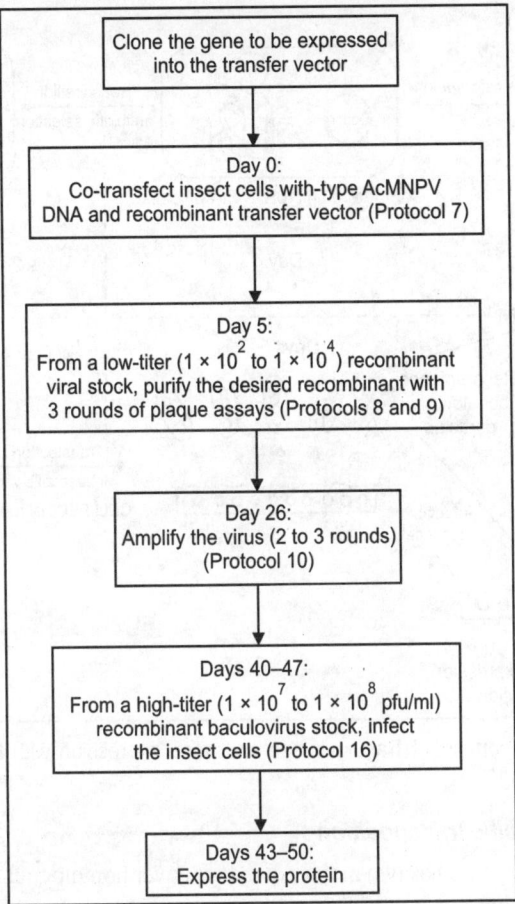

Fig. 5.11. Generating a recombinant baculovirus by homologous recombination.

The mini-Tn7 element on the pFASTBAC plasmid can transpose to the mini-*att*Tn7 target site on the bacmid in the presence of transposition proteins provided by the helper plasmid. Colonies containing recombinant bacmids are identified by antibiotic selection and blue/white screening, since the transposition results in disruption of the *lacZa* gene. High molecular weight mini-prep DNA is prepared from selected *E. coli* clones containing the recombinant bacmid, and this DNA is then used to transfect insect cells. The steps to generate a recombinant baculovirus by site-specific transposition using the BAC-TO-BAC™ baculovirus expression system are outlined in Fig. 5.12.

A variety of pFASTBAC donor plasmids are available which share common features. The plasmid pFASTBAC 1 is used to generate viruses which will express unfused recombinant proteins. The pFASTBAC HT series of vectors are used to express polyhistidine-tagged proteins which can be rapidly purified on metal affinity resins. The pFASTBAC DUAL vector has two promoters and cloning sites, allowing expression of two genes, one from the polyhedrin promoter and one from the p10 promoter.

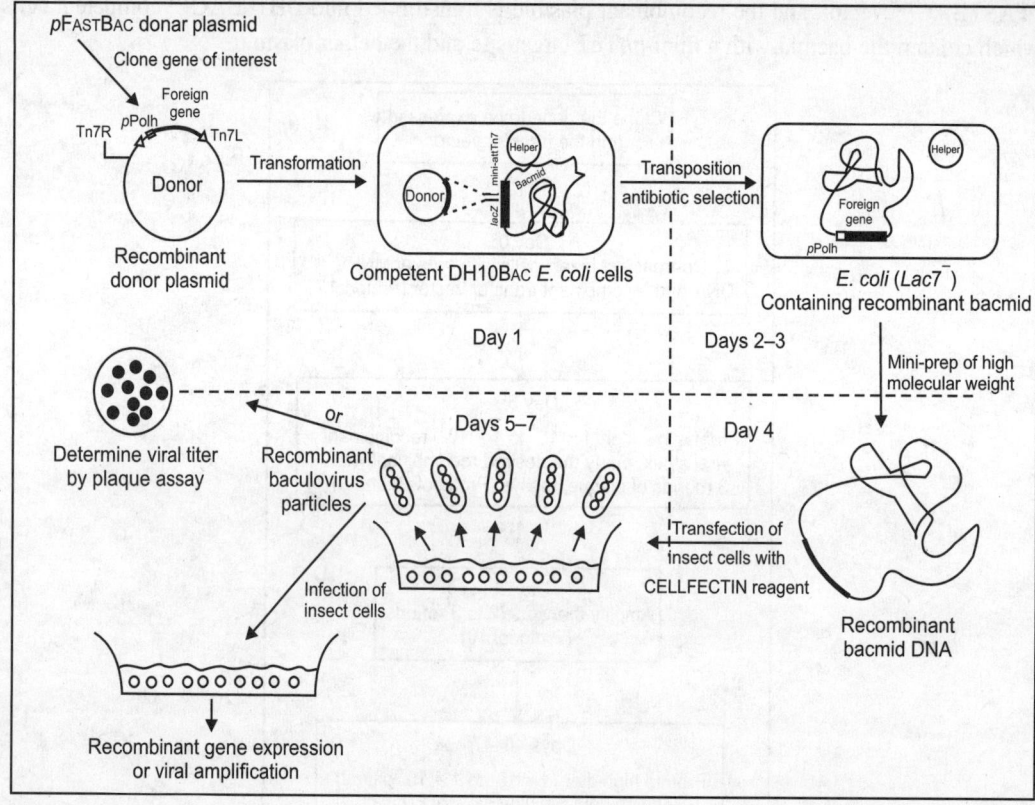

Fig. 5.12. Generation of recombinant Baculoviruses and gene expression with the BAC-TO-BAC expression system.

Advantages of site-specific transposition

Using site-specific transposition has two major advantages over homologous recombination:

1. One-step purification and amplification: Because recombinant virus DNA isolated from selected colonies is not mixed with parental, nonrecombinant virus, multiple rounds of plaque purification are not required and identification of the recombinant virus is easier. In 7 to 10 days, we will have pure recombinant virus titers of $>1 \times 10^7$ pfu/ml without any viral amplification.
2. Rapid and simultaneous isolation of multiple recombinant viruses: This feature is particularly valuable for expressing protein variants in structure/function studies.

Insect Cell Culture Techniques

Successful culture of insect cells requires a basic familiarity with insect cell physiology and general cell culture methods. The materials and methods for use with insect cell culture have evolved and contributed to the advancement of BEVS technology. The following factors have been significant:

1. Growth supplements and shear force protectants are widely used.
2. Serum-free media (SFM) have replaced serum-supplemented media, particularly for large-scale production.
3. Some insect cell lines have been optimised for use in suspension culture, especially useful for scale-up.

Cell lines

The most common cell lines used for BEVS applications are listed in Table 5.2. Of these, Sf9, a clonal isolate of the *Spodoptera frugiperda* cell line IPLB-Sf21-AE, is probably the most widely used. Sf9 was originally established from ovarian tissue of the fall armyworm. Although there is significant scientific data on the characteristics of this *Lepidopteran* cell line, it remains to be confirmed whether it is the best line for virus or recombinant protein production. Ongoing research suggests that different insect cell lines may support varying levels of expression and differential glycosylation with the same recombinant protein.

Table 5.2. Insect cell lines commonly used in BEVS applications.

Insect species	Cell line
Spodoptera frugiperda	Sf9
Spodoptera frugiperda	Sf-21
Trichoplusia ni	Tn-368
Trichoplusia ni	High-Five™ BTI-TN-5B1-4

Note: Each of these cell lines has been successfully adapted to suspension cultures.

Media and growth supplements

Commonly used insect cell culture media are listed in Table 5.3. Traditionally, Grace's supplemented (TNM-FH) medium has been the medium of choice for insect cell culture. However, other serum/haemolymph-dependent and serum-free formulations have evolved since Grace's medium was introduced.

Table 5.3. Insect cell culture media commonly used in BEVS applications.

Serum/haemolymph-dependent media	Serum-free media
Grace's supplemented (TNM-FH)	Sf-900 II SFM
IPL-41	EXPRESS-FIVE™ SFM
TC-100	
Schneider's Drosophila	

Note: Store liquid media which all contain photolabile components in the dark at 4° to 8°C.

Fetal bovine serum (FBS) has been the primary growth supplement used in insect cell culture medium. FBS has almost completely supplanted the first major supplement, insect haemolymph, which tended to melanise and deteriorate the quality of the culture medium. Of the more than 100 insect cell culture media described in the literature, a majority contain, or recommend, varying concentrations of serum as a growth supplement.

Supplementation with serum has both desirable and undesirable effects. These are summarised in Table 5.4. Serum and other undefined supplements, such as lactalbumin hydrolysate and yeastolate, provide cells with growth-promoting factors such as amino acids, peptides, and vitamins, which may not be available in defined, basal media formulations.

Before 1984, few scientific articles referenced serum-free insect cell culture media. At that time, serum-free insect culture media were used mostly to replicate insect viruses for production of viral pesticides. These early SFM formulations were not well suited for use in producing recombinant proteins.

Early formulations contained inherent flaws that limited cellular growth, suspension culture, and protein expression. For BEVS applications, these early formulations were generally poorly defined and too rich in protein.

Table 5.4. Effects of serum on cell cultures.

Desirable effects	Undesirable effects
Promotes growth	May cause excessive foaming in sparged bioreactors
Provides shear force protection	May introduce adventitious agents
Protects against proteolytic degradation and environmental toxicities	Increases cost and complexity of downstream processing
	Fluctuates in price, quality, and availability
Contributes cellular attachment factors	May demonstrate suboptimal cell growth or toxicity
	May demonstrate decreased product yields

Most commercially available serum-free insect media are essentially simple variations of IPL-41 basal medium supplemented with undefined protein hydrolysates and a lipid/surfactant emulsion. Second-generation serum-free formulations such as Sf-900 II SFM and EXPRESS-FIVE SFM are specifically designed for large-scale production of recombinant proteins. They contain optimised concentrations of amino acids, carbohydrates, vitamins, and lipids that reduce or eliminate the effect of rate-limiting nutritional restrictions or deficiencies. Both Sf-900 II SFM and EXPRESS-FIVE SFM support faster population doubling times and higher saturation cell densities than do traditional media. Thus, you can obtain both higher wild-type or recombinant baculovirus titers and increased levels or yields of recombinant protein expression by using these formulations. The optimised formulations offer the following advantages over sera:

1. Eliminate the need for costly fetal bovine and other animal sera supplements.
2. Increase cell and product yields.
3. Eliminate adventitious agents.
4. Have lot-to-lot consistency.

Environmental factors

Invertebrate cell cultures are extremely sensitive to environmental factors and conditions. The low-protein nature of most serum-free formulations often increases cellular sensitivity. To reduce problems, use materials and equipment designated for tissue culture use only, including incubators, flow hoods, autoclaves, media preparation areas, speciality gases, and bioreactors. Follow the guidelines listed here to ensure that the physical conditions of our culture optimise growth.

1. Temperature: The optimal range for growth and infection of most cultured insect cells is 25° to 30°C. Healthy serum-supplemented monolayer cultures can be stored at 2° to 8°C for periods up to 3 months.
2. pH: The pH of a growth medium affects both cellular proliferation and viral or recombinant protein production. Although many values have been reported for invertebrate cells, in most applications a pH range of 6.0 to 6.4 works well for most lepidopteran cell lines. The insect media described in this guide will maintain a pH in this range under conditions of non-CO_2 equilibration and open-capped culture systems.
3. Osmolality: The optimal osmolality of medium for use with lepidopteran cell lines is 345 to 380 mOsm/kg. To maintain reliable and consistent cellular growth patterns and minimise technical problems, maintain pH and osmolality within the ranges listed here.

4. Aeration: Invertebrate cells require sufficient transfer of dissolved oxygen by either passive or active methods for optimal cell proliferation and expression of recombinant proteins. Larger bioreactor systems using active or controlled oxygenation systems require dissolved oxygen at 10 to 50 per cent of air saturation.

5. Shear forces: Suspension culture techniques generate mechanical shear forces. Factors that contribute to the total shear stresses experienced by cells in suspension culture include the size and type of impellers within stirred vessels, the size and velocity of bubbles in airlift or sparged bioreactors, and the resulting turbulent action at the culture surface. During suspension cell culture, most insect cell lines require shear force protection. Although serum concentrations between 5 and 20 per cent in medium appear to provide some protection from shear forces, we recommend that all suspension cultures, whether serum-free or serum-supplemented, be supplemented with a shear force protectant such as PLURONIC® F-68. (If not already present in the formulation.)

IMPROVED PROTEIN PRODUCTION FROM MAMMALIAN CELLS

There is a general consensus that although non-mammalian systems can be effectively employed in the manufacture of many proteins, mammalian systems will have to be chosen for the bulk production of a large number of proteins to be used in therapeutics. The main reason being that only the latter type of system can assure the correct form of post-translational modification that many proteins require to be biologically active. In comparison to, for example, microbial systems those based on mammalian cells are extremely expensive. It is therefore evident that an intense effort is required in order to greatly improve the efficiency of mammalian cell factories such that they can become competitive with their non-mammalian counterparts. A new approach in genetic engineering is now being employed to make vast improvements in protein production using mammalian cells.

Rapid advances in disease-related research are continuously leading to the production of an increasing number of protein therapeutics and protein diagnostics. Many of these are on the market, some are currently in clinical trials whilst others are further back in company development pipelines. The market for protein therapeutics is worth some US-$ 41 billion and has been growing at a CAGR of 21 per cent over the past 5 years. More than 120 protein drugs are at present on the world market, including nine blockbuster drugs (i.e. with annual sales > US-$ 1 billion). In the field of cancer therapy 370 protein drugs are currently in company pipelines, including 47 monoclonal antibodies (mAbs). An analysis of the general market for mAbs in May 2004 showed that there were 376 preclinical-to-market products under development in 95 key companies. Opportunities for the development of 'biogenerics' are also rising, as US-$16 billion worth of protein medicines are coming off patent during the course of the next five years.

Biopharmaceutical firms are often challenged by difficulties in producing proteins in amounts large enough to allow for their proper characterisation/evaluation and for scale-up before market launch. Furthermore, a potential manufacturing shortfall and failures in achieving economically viable production yields threaten to put a brake on the rapid growth of this market. There are a number of current industrial bottlenecks which include the following: (i) failure to achieve laboratory scale production, impeding R&D success (drug lead candidates frequently falter due to an inability to produce enough quality protein for preclinical and clinical trials), (ii) commercially unviable yield levels, halting product development or hurting margins (failure to produce quality protein at yields that are economically viable is a common problem occurring in the development of novel biopharmaceuticals as well as generic protein drugs), (iii) high investment requirements in production capacity (current expectations are that the available production facilities will not suffice to meet the rapidly growing demand for the supply of protein pharmaceuticals). Within the space of a few years it is anticipated that the market supply of mAbs will represent a major challenge due to the fact that patients require long-term treatment with relatively high doses of antibody. There are forecasts suggesting that already from 2006 there will be a serious lack of production capacity for proteins derived from mammalian cell cultures. Another important factor is that of high cost: the production of 1 g mAb in CHO cells costs. It is thus quite evident that a major effort is required to vastly improve current protein production systems based on the use of mammalian cell factories.

Traditional Approaches to Improve Protein Production

Using traditional approaches, companies utilising mammalian systems to produce recombinant proteins have attempted to scale up production by strategies focusing mainly on the modulation of growth conditions (media composition and process control) or on increasing transcriptional activity of the recombinant gene within the host genome (e.g. utilisation of strong promoters/enhancers in the expression vector, amplification of gene copy number). Although leading to higher cellular levels of messenger RNA (mRNA) this in itself may not be sufficient to result in optimal protein production. An important consideration that has hitherto been poorly addressed is that of attempting to achieve the maximal efficiency of translation of the mRNA.

Genetically Engineered Cell Factories

A completely new approach is currently being developed in our laboratory where our focus is on aspects of post-transcriptional events (mRNA/protein targeting and trafficking). Genetically engineered cell factories containing selected targeting 'instructions' for the recombinant mRNA and the encoded protein of interest are generated. The move toward boosting the yield of high-quality proteins by the implementation of this unique genetic engineering technology is based on the finding that the efficiency of targeting mRNA to the endoplasmic reticulum (ER) is heavily dependent on the presence of, and correct interplay between, specific key elements (signal peptide and the 3′ untranslated region [3′ UTR]). A 'seamless' cloning methodology has been developed to insert these elements on either side of the coding region of the protein of interest, thus avoiding the use of linker sequences that may perturb the biological activity of the protein (Fig. 5.13). The protein encoded by the engineered mRNA then being efficiently directed to the cell's secretory pathway for transport out of the cell. Depending on the protein in question production has been improved by a factor of 3–50 in laboratory scale experiments.

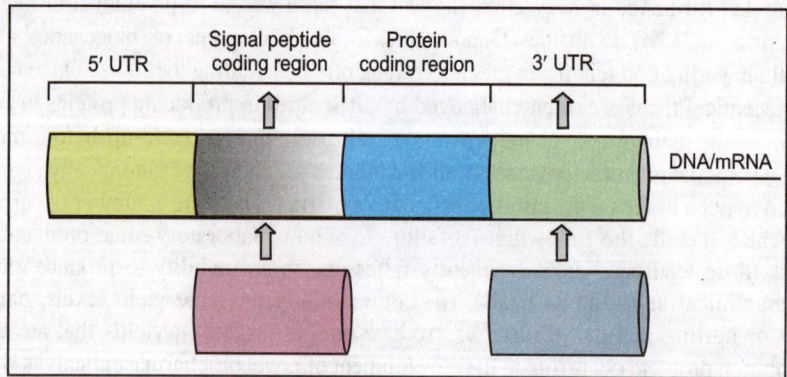

Fig. 5.13. Generation of constructs using seamless cloning for sequence element insertion/substitution.

The signal peptide is an intrinsic targeting signal located on the nascent polypeptide chain that has the property of directing the synthesis of membrane proteins and proteins destined for secretion to the ER. It has been demonstrated that different signal peptides vary greatly with respect to the efficiency by which they direct synthesis/secretion of a reporter protein in transfected CHO cells. A particular signal peptide derived from a marine organism was found to be surprisingly efficient when compared to well known signal peptides of mammalian origin (e.g. albumin, Fig. 5.14).

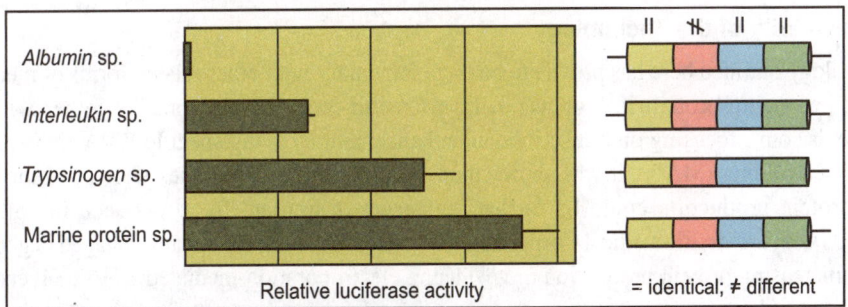

Fig. 5.14. Efficiencies of signal peptides (sp) derived from different proteins in secretion of a reporter luciferase.

Interestingly, although similar amounts of mRNA were detected when the signal peptides of the marine organism and human albumin were used (results not shown), the levels of recombinant protein differed by a factor of 50. Having previously shown that mRNA targeting to the ER is affected by the 3′ UTR, we now demonstrate that the nature of the 3′ UTR engineered into the mRNA molecule also plays an important role in enhancing the amount of the final product secreted by transfected CHO cells. Figure 5.15 exemplifies this and in addition shows that a signal peptide and 3′ UTR originating from the same gene do not necessarily form the most effective 'doublet'. Efficient doublets have been identified and it appears in principle that synthesis/secretion of any naturally secreted protein can be boosted through the cooperate action of the two components. The technology is currently being evaluated in collaboration with various pharmaceutical companies for the improved production of protein therapeutics (mAbs, erythropoietin).

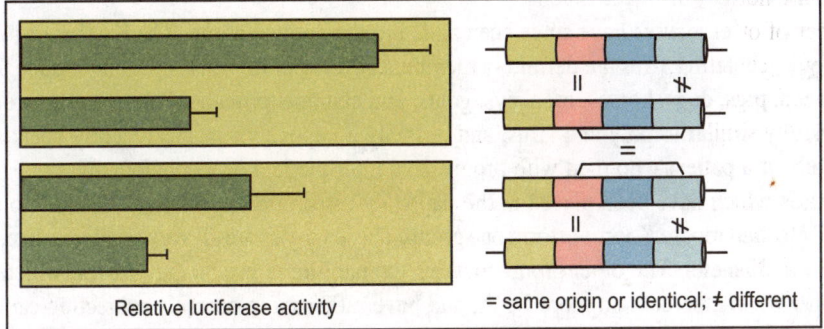

Fig. 5.15. Importance of correct choice of signal peptide/3′ UTR doublet on reporter luciferase secretion.

Production of Intracellular Proteins

The technology has another area of application, namely the production of proteins that normally reside within the cell. Intracellular proteins are commonly recovered after lysing the cell membrane to generate an extract from which the molecule in question is purified. Such proteins often represent only a minor per cent of the total cell content. It has been predicted that approximately 30,000 different proteins are produced by human cells, probably >90 per cent being synthesised for internal use. Methodology is currently being developed such that cells can be engineered to efficiently secrete large quantities of intracellular proteins of potential commercial interest (such as toxic proteins, protein targets for drug design and protein diagnostics).

Complementarity of the Technology

The technology outlined here has proven to be complementary with other related forms of methodology aiming at producing protein in high yield. In a feasibility study performed together with Selexis (www.selexis.com), focusing on transcriptional enhancement by using specific DNA elements binding to nuclear scaffolding (MAR), it was shown that when the two technologies were combined then the level of protein production could be further enhanced. A similar effect was seen in collaborative experiments with Inovio Biomedical Corporation (www.inovio.com), a company engaged in gene therapy aiming at increasing protein production *in vivo* using electroporation-mediated DNA delivery. A major increase in recombinant protein in mice serum was observed.

HUMAN PAPOVA (WART) VIRUS

The name papova virus was suggested by Melnick as a group name for the small, deoxyribonucleic acid (DNA)-containing, ether-resistant, oncogenic viruses which appeared similar in structure on electron microscopy. The viruses which he grouped together under this name were the papilloma virus of man (common wart virus), the papilloma virus of rabbits (Shope papilloma virus), the polyoma virus of mice, and the vacuolating virus of monkeys (simian virus 40 or SV40). The group name was obtained by taking the first two letters from the names of the viruses in the order in which they were discovered: papilloma, polyoma, and vacuolating.

The amount of information available on the properties of the four viruses varied, with the least being known about the human member of the group. However, they all appeared to be of similar size, to have their capsomeres arranged with cubical symmetry, to exist occasionally in a filamentous form, and to replicate in the nucleus of infected cells.

A number of other viruses have since been added to the papova group. The K virus of mice and the rabbit kidney vacuolating virus are definitely members. A number of viruses which produce papillomata in cattle, sheep, pigs, dogs, horses, monkeys, goats, and chamois probably belong to the group. A virus morphologically similar to polyoma virus, and possibly a papova virus, has recently been observed in the brain cells of a patient who died with progressive multiple leukoencephalopathy.

The viruses which have been placed in the papova virus group can be divided into two subgroups. Polyoma, SV40, and mouse K viruses form one group. These viruses are all very similar in size, measuring 40 to 45 mμ in diameter. The other group contains the papilloma-producing viruses, which are larger, 52 to 55 mμ in diameter, contain more DNA, and have rather more coarsely projecting capsomeres.

The question of virus nomenclature is at present under consideration in an attempt to obtain international agreement, and a provisional committee has recommended the term papillomaviridae as a family name for the viruses presently included in the papova virus group. This change of nomenclature seems to have few advantages, and it appears useful for the present to retain the name papova virus group, especially as it has established itself in the literature.

Types of Warts

Warts or papillomata of several different clinical or morphological types are caused by the human papova virus. However, they all have the same basic pathological features, and consist of a localised hyperplasia of epithelial cells with a sharply defined boundary. It is probable that warts of all the various clinical types are caused by the same virus, the clinical manifestation being determined by the location of the lesion. In the normal epidermis, cell division is limited to the basal layer of cells, but in a wart mitotic figures are seen in the cells situated several layers higher up. The basal cell layer is intact, with thickening of the cell layers above it. There is elongation and broadening of the interpapillary processes, with characteristic long thin papillae containing blood vessels extending high into the wart. These vessels cause bleeding points when the wart is trimmed, and if thrombosed may be seen as small dark spots.

The most common type of skin wart is the *verruca vulgaris*, which may be single or multiple, but is often found in groups. It forms a sharply circumscribed mass, 1 to 5 mm in diameter, projecting from the skin surface and having a hard roughened top. This type of wart may occur anywhere on the skin, but is most often seen on the hands. In children, flat warts, *verruca plana*, which are only slightly elevated above the skin surface, are commonly seen on the face, neck, and dorsum of the hands. Flat warts may also occur in adults, but are less common. They are usually multiple. The condition known as *epidermodysplasia verruciformis* appears to be a generalised eruption of flat warts and has been transmitted. Warts which project as fingerlike or threadlike structures have been given the descriptive names of digitate or filiform warts, and occur usually on the face or neck of young adults. Warts occurring on the plantar surface of the foot lie deep in the skin and do not project above the surface. They are surrounded, and may even be covered, by hyperkeratotic epithelial tissue. Plantar warts of this type are frequently seen in children and young adults. It is usually suggested that they are driven into the skin by the pressure exerted on the foot in walking; this is probably a factor, but it seems likely that, arising deep in the thick epidermis, they are to some extent imprisoned by the thick layer of keratinised cells on the surface. Warts of a similar type, situated deeply in the skin, may occur on the palms of the hands, on the pulp of the digits, or under the nails. Where the skin is moist and soft, on the external genitalia and in the perianal region, warts may become fungating masses with secondary bacterial infection producing ulceration. Warts of this exuberant, nonhorny type are called condylomata acuminata, fig warts, or venereal warts. Such warts may be contracted in various ways, and it is therefore undesirable to call them venereal warts. That they are caused by the same virus as other warts has been demonstrated by transmission experiments.

In addition to skin warts, the human papova virus is probably responsible for the multiple laryngeal warts of children and young adults and anorectal warts in adults. The multiple laryngeal warts behave very like skin warts. They are subject to spontaneous regression, but often recur after surgical removal; they seldom, if ever, become malignant. Extracts of laryngeal warts have produced skin warts on injection into normal skin. The solitary laryngeal papillomata of elderly patients which tend more frequently to become malignant may have a different etiology. Anorectal warts are histologically identical to virus-induced skin warts, and may be produced by the same virus; however, no transmission experiments have been reported. Inclusion bodies and virus particles cannot be demonstrated in all warts. They are most easily seen in the plantar type situated deep in the skin, whereas they are usually not demonstrable in the superficially placed verruca vulgaris. Lyell and Miles suggested that the former type had the clinical features of the myrmecia of Celcus, and should be called by this name, which is derived from their domed shape, similar to that of an anthill. They proposed to call the *verruca vulgaris* type banal warts because of their commonplace histology. Lyell and Miles were impressed by the fact that they never saw these two types of wart concurrently in the same patient, and that in transmission experiments the two types appeared to be distinct. However, the numbers involved in their transmission experiments were small, and two cases of myrmecia-type warts which recurred after removal were then of the banal type. The myrmecia type of wart appeared to be a more active type of lesion than the banal wart. It had usually been present for less than 1 year, whereas the banal wart had usually been present for more than 1 year. It seems likely that these two clinical types of wart represent different stages of a pathological process, or are different responses to the same infection, the type of lesion being determined by host factors. There seems little point in continuing to use the names myrmecia and banal; however, it is no doubt important to realise that the amount of virus in wart tissue may vary considerably, and the clinical type of lesion may help in selecting suitable specimens for experimental purposes. Although warts of many different types are caused by the human papova-virus, there are several wartlike lesions of the skin which have other causes. The lesions of *molluscum contagiosum* may in their early stages be confused with common warts, but are due to a virus of the pox group and are histologically distinct. The soft, slightly raised pigmented lesions often seen on the trunk and referred to as seborrheic warts (*seborrheic keratosis*, basal cell papilloma, verruca senilis) appear to be unrelated to common viral warts, but their etiology is unknown. They seldom if ever become malignant, and so must be distinguished from keratosis senilis (hyperkeratotic squamous cell papillomata), which often becomes malignant and is most frequently seen in the fifth or sixth decades of life. To summarise, there is ample evidence that both verruca vulgaris and the plantar type of wart are caused by the human papova virus. The same virus is probably also responsible for flat and filiform warts and for condylomata acuminata. The clinical type of lesion is determined by the local conditions at the site of infection and not by the virus. The comparatively rare multiple laryngeal and anorectal warts may be due to the human papova virus, but there is no direct evidence of this.

PROTEIN-BASED DRUGS

The future of pharmacy belongs to a special category of therapeutics and diagnostics referred to as protein-based drugs. To date, modern medicine has relied heavily on synthetically or chemically produced drugs to treat or prevent diseases and conditions.

However, developments in the field of molecular biology have led to an increase in our knowledge of biological systems and their interactions. For example, scientists know more about the sources of many diseases and how the human body fights diseases. They are now focussing on using the body's own tools to fight diseases by developing therapeutics that mimic the actions of the body's arsenal.

Proteins are biomolecules that are essential in determining the structure and carrying out most of the functions in living cells that make up all living organisms. They are made up of individual units called amino acids, which although similar in structure, have different characteristics. There are about 20 different amino acids in nature and these assemble in chains of varying lengths to form proteins. The order of amino acids determines the structure and function of the protein. This order is specified by genes. Proteins in living organisms are classified according to their biological roles.

These include:

1. Enzymatic: Proteins that trigger all the chemical reactions that occur in the cells of living organisms.
2. Transport: Proteins that carry other substances throughout the body or molecules across cell membranes. For instance, the protein haemoglobin carries oxygen from the lungs to other parts of the body.

3. Structural: Proteins that help in supporting functions in the body. For instance, Keratin is the protein that is important for supporting hair and other skin parts.
4. Storage: Proteins that store amino acids. For instance, casein is the protein in milk that provides a source of amino acids for baby mammals.
5. Hormonal: Proteins that coordinate bodily activities. For instance, insulin is the protein hormone secreted by the pancreas that regulates the level of sugar in the blood.
6. Receptor: Proteins that are built into the membrane of a cell and detect chemical signals released by other cells. They contribute to the cell's response to the chemical stimuli.
7. Contractile: Proteins that help in movement. For example, actin and myosin are responsible for the movement of muscles.
8. Defensive: Protect the body against diseases. For example, antibodies are proteins that protect the body against viruses and harmful bacteria.

Protein-based drugs are any substance that uses the different proteins that occur naturally in any living organism, to diagnose, prevent and treat diseases and conditions or to restore or maintain normal body functions. Humans have traditionally used animal and plant sources to obtain proteins (such as hormones and clotting factors) in order to treat different diseases and conditions. Many of these were extracted from human and animal corpses. Revolutionary discoveries in science and modern medicine propelled the large scale production of chemical drugs to be used in human health care.

However, today, advances in biotechnology have led to the increased use of living organisms and biological substances in the production of protein drugs for human health care. Specifically, the use of recombinant DNA (rDNA) technology has enabled the production of large quantities of protein drugs.

Types of Protein-Based Drugs

Cytokines: These drugs regulate the immune system. That is, they are proteins that activate the immune system cells to carry out different immune functions.

Hormones: Protein drugs that regulate functions in the body. As drugs, these proteins can be used to elevate levels of certain hormones, such as estrogen during menopause or growth deficiency. They can also be used to treat certain diseases such as diabetes, or conditions such as infertility.

Clotting factors: Proteins that regulate the clotting of blood. These drugs are used to treat blood clotting disorders such as haemophilia.

Vaccines: Proteins that stimulate the immune system to produce specific antibodies used to prevent or treat diseases.

Monoclonal antibodies: Proteins that mark a specific foreign material (such as cancer cells, disease-causing bacteria and viruses), for removal or destruction by other components of the immune system. These are also used as effective diagnostic tools for many specific genetic diseases and other conditions such as pregnancy.

The science – How do protein-based drugs work?

Protein-based drugs are developed by cloning the genes responsible for specific proteins naturally produced by the human body. The genes are cloned using vectors such as bacteria. The gene of interest is first isolated and then incorporated into the bacteria, which are multiplied in bioreactors to produce many copies of the gene. The cloned genes are then genetically engineered into micro-organisms or animals to produce the proteins. When the protein is used as a drug (for preventative or therapeutic purposes), it performs the same function as the already naturally-occurring protein in the body.

Biotechnology and protein-based drugs

Prior to advances in biotechnology such as rDNA technology, the few protein drugs available were taken directly from human and animal corpses. For instance, the human growth hormone was taken from human corpses and insulin required to treat diabetes was collected from slaughtered pigs. These drugs were available in limited supply and they were expensive, given their sources. Biotechnology has boosted the production of protein-based drugs in two significant ways:

Hybridoma cell technology

Hybridomas are the fusion of tumour cells with certain white blood cells. They replicate endlessly and can be used to produce specific protein-based drugs called monoclonal antibodies which are effective in treating cancers and other conditions.

Recombinant DNA technology

The introduction of rDNA technology or genetic engineering, has provided a large and cost-efficient source of protein-based drugs. Using genetic engineering, the gene that encodes for the required protein is transferred from one organism into another, which is capable of producing large amounts of the drug.

Genes determine what proteins do. If the gene encoding for a certain protein is known, it is possible to produce this protein. Biotechnology has enabled scientists to identify the different genes that encode for certain proteins. The human genome project has increased our knowledge of genes responsible for many diseases. The identified genes can be used to produce proteins and administer them to prevent and treat diseases.

Production of protein-based drugs through rDNA technology can be achieved through two common ways: through transgenic animals (pharming), micro-organisms such as *E. coli* bacteria or through hybridomas.

Transgenic animals for protein drug production

Transgenic Animals in health care are animals that have been genetically modified to produce a particular protein drug. The DNA gene for the desired protein is coupled with a DNA signal directing its production in the mammary glands.

The new gene functions in the mammary glands so that the protein drug is made only in the milk. The coupled DNA is injected into fertilised cow, sheep, goat or mouse embryo's. The injected embryos are implanted into surrogate mothers.

The surviving embryos are then born normally and after these have been raised to maturity and bred, they produce the protein during lactation. The protein is then harvested from the milk and formulated into a protein based drug.

To sum up the eventual objective of producing a desired protein in an economical heterologous host is influenced by a variety of factors. However, maximising production of heterologous proteins for commercial application is still an art. We have begun to understand factors influencing the eventual production. These factors, described in detail in this chapter are varied and at times poorly understood. Largely the approach remains empirical. However, our collective experience will permit us to rationalise our approach in designing heterologous production of commercially important proteins in a variety of expression systems. Subsequent to production, stabilisation and formulation of proteins will pose significant hurdles in utilising the natural biological catalysts and other proteins for therapeutic and industrial purposes.

Chapter 6

Changing Genes: Site-directed Mutagenesis and Protein Engineering

INTRODUCTION

The generation and characterisation of mutants is an essential component of any study on structure–function relationships. Knowledge of the three dimensional structure of a protein, RNA species, or DNA regulatory element (e.g. a promoter) can provide clues to the way in which they function but proof that the correct mechanism has been elucidated requires the analysis of mutants that have amino acid or nucleotide changes at key residues.

Classically, mutants are generated by treating the test organism with chemical or physical agents that modify DNA (mutagens). This method of mutagenesis has been extremely successful, as witnessed by the growth of molecular biology and functional genomics, but suffers from a number of disadvantages. First, any gene in the organism can be mutated and the frequency with which mutants occur in the gene of interest can be very low. This means that selection strategies have to be developed. Second, even when mutants with the desired phenotype are isolated, there is no guarantee that the mutation has occurred in the gene of interest. Third, prior to the development of gene-cloning and sequencing techniques, there was no way of knowing where in the gene the mutation had occurred and whether it arose by a single base change, an insertion of DNA, or a deletion.

As techniques in molecular biology have developed, so that the isolation and study of a single gene is not just possible but routine, so mutagenesis has also been refined. Instead of crudely mutagenising many cells or organisms and then analysing many thousands or millions of offspring to isolate a desired mutant, it is now possible to change specifically any given base in a cloned DNA sequence. This technique is known as site-directed mutagenesis. It has become a basic tool of gene manipulation, for it simplifies DNA manipulations that in the past required a great deal of ingenuity and hard work, e.g. the creation or elimination of cleavage sites for restriction endonucleases. The importance of site-directed mutagenesis goes beyond gene structure–function relationships for the technique enables mutant proteins with novel properties of value to be created (protein engineering). Such mutant proteins may have only minor changes but it is not uncommon for entire domains to be deleted or new domains added.

MUTAGENESIS

Mutagenesis is a process by which the genetic information of an organism is changed in a stable manner, either in nature or experimentally by the use of chemicals or radiation.

The various types of mutagenesis: (i) directed mutagenesis, (ii) insertional mutagenesis, (iii) PCR mutagenesis, (iv) signature tagged mutagenesis, (v) site-directed mutagenesis, and (vi) transposon mutagenesis.

Directed Mutagenesis

Directed mutagenesis is also known as directed mutation, is a hypothesis proposing that organisms can respond to environmental stresses through directing mutations to certain genes or areas of the genome.

The hypothesis was first proposed in 1988 by John Cairns, of Harvard University, who was studying Escherichia coli that lacked the ability to metabolize lactose. He grew these bacteria in media in which lactose was the only source of energy. In doing so, he found that the rate at which the bacteria evolved the ability to metabolise lactose was many orders of magnitude higher than would be expected if the mutations were truly random. This inspired him to propose that the mutations that had occurred had been directed at those genes involved in lactose utilisation.

Later support for this hypothesis came from Susan Rosenberg, then at the University of Alberta, who found that an enzyme involved in DNA recombinational repair, recBCD, was necessary for the directed mutagenesis observed by Cairns and colleagues in 1989.

The directed mutagenesis hypothesis was challenged in 2002, when John Roth and colleagues showed that the phenomenon was due to general hypermutability due to selected gene amplification, and was thus a 'standard Darwinian process'. Later research published in 2006 by Jeffrey D. Stumpf, Anthony R. Poteete, and Patricia L. Foster, however, concluded that amplification could not account for the adaptive mutation and that 'mutants that appear during the first few days of lactose selection are true revertants that arise in a single step'. Applications of directed mutagenesis are shown in Fig. 6.1.

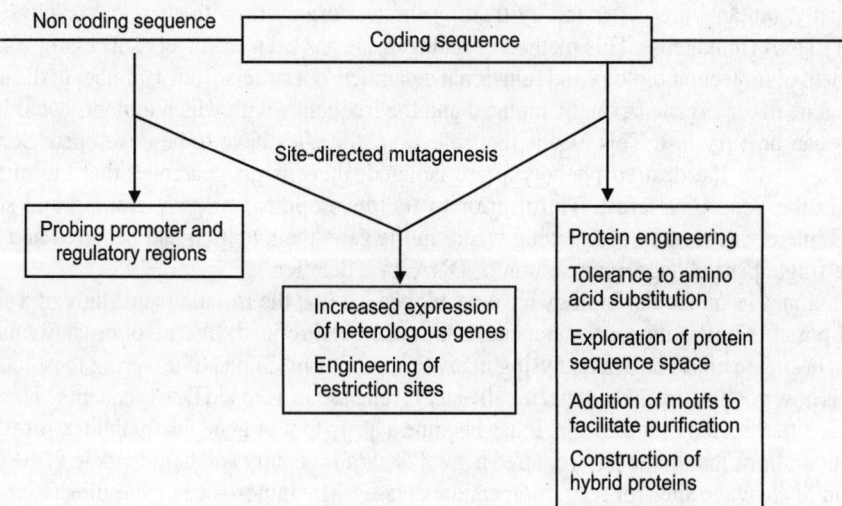

Fig. 6.1. Applications of directed mutagenesis.

Insertional Mutagenesis

Insertional mutagenesis is mutagenesis of DNA by the insertion of one or more bases. A common misconception is that the word 'Mutagenesis' derives from 'Mutation' and 'Gene'. In fact, mutagenesis refers to the Generation of Mutations. Insertional mutations can occur naturally, mediated by virus or transposon, or can be artificially created for research purposes in the lab.

Signature tagged mutagenesis: This is a technique used to study the function of genes. A transposon, such as the Drosophilla Melanogaster P-element, is allowed to integrate at random locations in the genome of the organism being studied. Mutants generated by this method are then screened for any unusual phenotypes. If such a phenotype is found then it can be assumed that the insertion has caused the gene relating to that phenotype to be inactivated. Because the sequence of the transposon is known, the gene can be identified, either by sequencing the whole genome and searching for the sequence, or using the polymerase chain reaction to amplify specifically that gene.

Virus insertional mutagenesis: As mentioned in the introduction, insertional mutagenesis refers to mutation of an organism caused by the insertion of additional DNA bases into the organism's preexisting DNA. Because many viruses (not all of them) integrate their own genome into the genome of their host cells in order to replicate, mutagenesis caused by viral infections is a fairly common occurrence. Not all integrating viruses cause insertional mutagenesis, however.

It is important to note that not all DNA insertions will lead to a noticeable mutation. In fact, most will not. However, it is a common enough occurrence in viral DNA insertions that biologists researching gene therapy will avoid using viruses that integrate their DNA in the host genome when it is not necessary to do so, opting instead for viruses that transiently express their DNA (leave their DNA free-floating within the cell, rather than integrate it into the genome of the host). For those viruses that do integrate their DNA into that of the host, the severity of any ensuing mutation depends entirely on the location within the host's genome wherein the viral DNA is inserted. If the DNA is inserted into the middle of an essential gene the effects on the cell will be drastic. Additionally, insertion into the promoter region of a gene can cause equally drastic effects. For instance, if the viral DNA is inserted into a repressor, the gene corresponding to that promoter may be over expressed - leading to an overabundance of its product and altered cellular activity. If the DNA is inserted into an enhancer region, the gene may be under-expressed-leading to relative absence of its product, which can significantly interrupt the activity of the cell.

Alteration of different genes will have varying effects on the cell. Not all mutations will significantly effect the proliferation of the cell. However, if the insertion occurs in an essential gene or a gene that is involved in cellular replication or programmed cell death, the insertion may compromise the viability of the cell or even cause the cell to replicate interminably - leading to the formation of a tumor, which may become cancerous. Below is an example of a significant change in cell activity due to insertion of a viral gene into a portion of the hosts genome that controls replication.

Virus insertional mutagenesis is only possible with a replication competent virus. The virus inserts a gene (known as a viral onocogene) normally near the cellular myc (c-myc)gene. The c-myc gene is normally turned off in the cell, however when it is turned on it is able to push the cell into the G1 phase of the cell cycle and cause the cell to begin replication which allows the viral gene to be replicated. After many replications where the viral gene stays latent tumours begin to grow. These tumours are normally derived from one mutated/transformed cell (clonal in origin). Avian leukosis virus is an example of a virus that causes a disease by insertional mutagenesis. Newly hatched chicks infected with Avian leukosis virus will begin to form tumours begin to appear in their bursa of fabricus (like the human thymus). This viral gene insertion is also known as a promoter insertion as it drives the expression of the c-myc gene. There is an example of an insertional mutagenesis event caused by a retrotransposon in the human genome where it causes Fukuyama-type muscular dystrophy.

Insertional inactivation is a technique used in recombinant DNA engineering where a plasmid is used to disable expression of a gene.

The inactivation of a gene by inserting a fragment of DNA into the middle of its coding sequence. Any future products from the inactivated gene will not work because of the extra codes added to it. pbr322 mainly having two antibiotic sites that are ampicillin and tetracyclin region.

PCR mutagenesis is simple method for generating site-directed mutagenesis. This method can generate mutations (base substitutions, insertions, and deletions) from double-stranded plasmid without the need for subcloning into M13-based bacteriophage vectors and for ssDNA rescue. The procedure involves a PCR reaction using a supercoiled plasmid vector as the template and two synthetic oligonucleotide primers containing the desired mutation with each complementary to the opposite strands of the vector. After PCR, the template (wild type) plasmid which is dam methylated in almost all *E. coli* is removed by digestion with Dpn I which is specific for methylated DNA. The new (mutant) DNA is not methylated and remains intact in the reaction. The reaction products are then transformed into competent *E. coli*, where the linear double-stranded PCR product is ligated by the host cell, and propagated by appropriate selection.

Signature-tagged mutagenesis (STM) is a genetic technique used to study gene function. Recent advances in genome sequencing have allowed us to catalogue a large variety of organisms genomes, but the function of the genes they contain is still largely unknown. Using STM, a scientist may infer what function the product of a particular gene has by disabling it and observing the effect on the organism. The original and most common use of STM is to discover which genes in a pathogen are involved in virulence in its host, so that better medical treatments can be designed.

The gene in question is inactivated by insertional mutation; a transposon is used which inserts itself into the gene sequence. When that gene is transcribed and translated into a protein, the insertion of the transposon affects the protein structure and (in theory) prevents it from functioning. In STM, mutants are created by random transposon insertion and each transposon contains a different 'tag' sequence that uniquely identifies it. If an insertional mutant bacterium exhibits a phenotype of interest, such as susceptibility to an antibiotic it was previously resistant to, then the scientist will sequence its genome and run a search (on a computer) for any of the tags used in the experiment. When a tag is located, the gene that it disrupts is also thus located (It will reside somewhere between a start and stop codon which mark the boundaries of the gene).

Scientists may use STM to discover which genes are critical to a pathogen's virulence by injecting a 'pool' of different random mutants into an animal model such as a mouse and observing which of the mutants survive and proliferate in the host. Those mutant pathogens that didn't survive in the host must have had an inactivated gene that was needed for virulence. This is hence an example of a negative selection method.

Site-directed mutagenesis, also called site-specific mutagenesis or oligonucleotide-directed mutagenesis, is a molecular biology technique in which a mutation is created at a defined site in a DNA molecule, typically a circular molecule known as a plasmid. In general, this form of mutagenesis requires that the wild type gene sequence be known.

Site-directed mutagenesis using oligonucleotides was first described in 1978. Michael Smith, its pioneer, shared the Nobel Prize in Chemistry in October 1993 with Kary B. Mullis, who invented polymerase chain reaction.

In 1987 Kunkel introduced an improvement to this technique that eliminated the need for selection of the mutants. The plasmid to be mutated is transformed into an *E. coli* strain deficient in two enzymes, UTPase and uracil deglycosidase. The UTPase deficiency prevents the breakdown of UTP, a nucleotide that normally replaces dTTP in RNA, resulting in an abundance of UTP; the uracil deglycosidase deficiency prevents the removal of UTP from newly-synthesised DNA. As the double-mutant *E. coli* replicates the transformed plasmid, its enzymatic machinery incorporates UTP, resulting in a distinguishable copy. This copy is extracted, and then incubated with the Klenow fragment, dNTPs, DNA ligase, and an oligonucleotide containing the desired mutation, which attaches by base pairing to the complementary wild type gene sequence. The ensuing reaction replicates the UTP-containing plasmid using the oligonucleotide as primer, thus incorporating the desired mutation. This forms a chimeric plasmid, with one strand unmutated and containing UTP, and the other strand mutated and containing dTTP. When this plasmid is transformed into an *E. coli* strain with normal UTPase and uracil deglycosidase, the UTP-containing strand is broken down, whereas the mutation-containing strand is replicated, forming a plasmid lacking UTP but containing the desired mutation on both strands.

The basic procedure requires the synthesis of a short DNA primer containing the desired base change. This synthetic primer has to hybridise with a single-stranded DNA containing the gene of interest. The single stranded fragment is then extended using a DNA polymerase, which copies the rest of the gene. The double stranded molecule thus obtained is then introduced into a host cell and cloned. Finally, mutants are selected for.

Cassette mutagenesis involves the cleavage by a restriction enzyme at a site in the plasmid and subsequent ligation of an oligonucleotide containing the mutation in the gene of interest to the plasmid. Usually the restriction enzyme that cuts at the plasmid and the oligonucleotide is the same, permitting sticky ends of the plasmid and insert to ligate to one another.

The same result can be accomplished using polymerase chain reaction with oligonucleotide 'primers' that contain the desired mutation. As the primers are the ends of newly-synthesised strands, by engineering a mis-match during the first cycle in binding the template DNA strand, a mutation can be introduced. Because PCR employs exponential growth, after a sufficient number of cycles the mutated fragment will be amplified sufficiently to separate from the original, unmutated plasmid by a technique such as gel electrophoresis, and reinstalled in the original context using standard recombinant molecular biology techniques.

For plasmid manipulations, this technique has largely been supplanted by a PCR-like technique where a pair of complementary mutagenic primers is used to amplify the entire plasmid. This generates a nicked, circular DNA which can undergo repair by endogenous bacterial machinery. However, this process does not amplify the DNA exponentially, but linearly. Yields are complicated by the fact that the product DNA must undergo the nick repair and is not supercoiled, resulting in reduced efficiency of bacterial transformation. Finally, the product DNA is of the same size as the plasmid. Therefore, the template DNA must be eliminated by enzymatic digestion with a restriction enzyme specific for methylated DNA. The template, which for this technique should be biosynthesised will be digested, but the mutated plasmid is preserved because it was generated *in vitro* and is therefore unmethylated.

Transposon mutagenesis, or transposition mutagenesis, is a biological process that allows genes to be transferred to a host organism's chromosome, interrupting or modifying the function of an extant gene on the chromosome and causing mutation.

Transposon mutagenesis was first studied by Barbara McClintock in the mid-20th century during her Nobel Prize-winning work with corn.

In the case of bacteria, transposition mutagenesis is usually accomplished by way of a plasmid from which a transposon is extracted and inserted into the host chromosome. This usually requires a set of enzymes including transposase to be translated.

Primer Extension (The Single-primer Method) is a Simple Method for Site-directed Mutation

The first method of site-directed mutagenesis to be developed was the single-primer method. As originally described the method involves *in vitro* DNA synthesis with a chemically synthesised oligonucleotide

(7–20 nucleotides long) that carries a base mismatch with the complementary sequence. As shown in Fig. 6.2, the method requires that the DNA to be mutated is available in single-stranded form, and cloning the gene in M13-based vectors makes this easy. However, DNA cloned in a plasmid and obtained in duplex form can also be converted to a partially single-stranded molecule that is suitable.

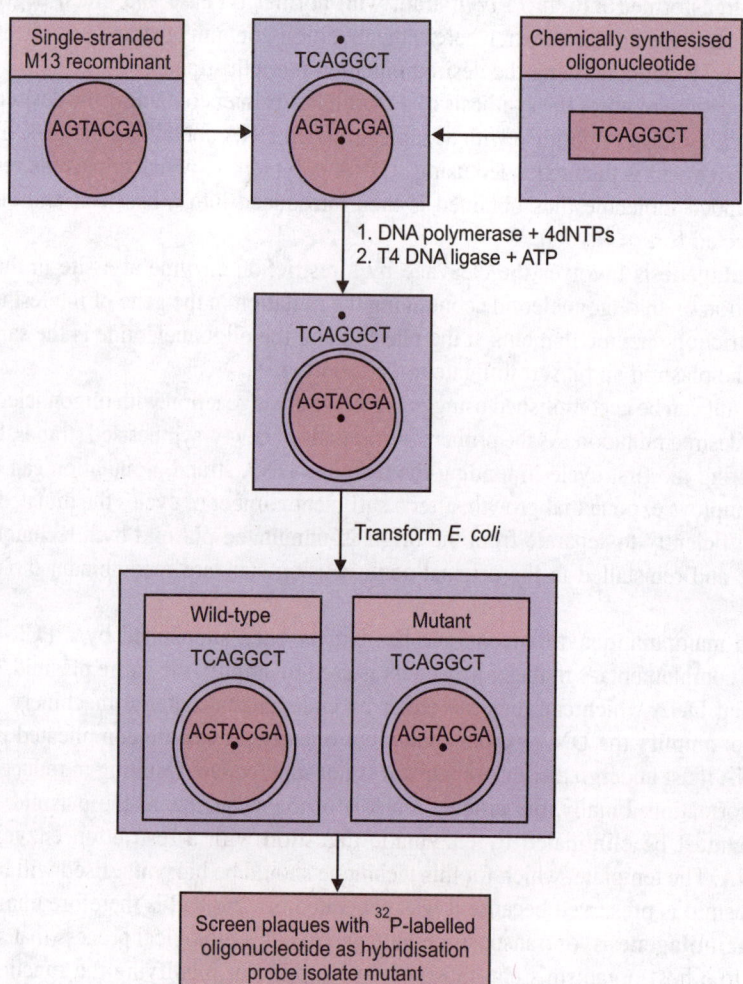

Fig. 6.2. Oligonucleotide directed mutagenesis. Asterisks indicate mismatched bases. Originally the Klenow fragment of DNA polymerase was used, but now this has been largely replaced with T7 polymerase.

The synthetic oligonucleotide primes DNA synthesis and is itself incorporated into the resulting heteroduplex molecule. After transformation of the host *E. coli*, this heteroduplex gives rise to homoduplexes whose sequences are either that of the original wild-type DNA or that containing the mutated base. The frequency with which mutated clones arise, compared with wild-type clones, may be low. In order to pick out mutants, the clones can be screened by nucleic acid hybridisation with ^{32}P-labelled oligonucleotide as probe. Under suitable conditions of stringency, i.e. temperature and cation concentration, a positive signal will be obtained only with mutant clones. This allows ready detection of the desired mutant. It is prudent to check the sequence of the mutant directly by DNA sequencing, in order to check that the procedure has not introduced other adventitious changes. This was a particular necessity with early versions of the technique which made use of *E. coli* DNA polymerase. The more recent use of the high-fidelity DNA polymerases has minimised the problem of extraneous mutations as well as shortening the time for copying the second strand. Also, these polymerases do not 'strand-displace' the oligomer, a process which would eliminate the original mutant oligonucleotide.

A variation of the procedure (Fig. 6.3) outlined above involves oligonucleotides containing inserted or deleted sequences. As long as stable hybrids are formed with single-stranded wild-type DNA, priming of *in vitro* DNA synthesis can occur, ultimately giving rise to clones corresponding to the inserted or deleted sequence.

Multiple point mutations	Insertion mutagenesis	Deletion mutagenesis
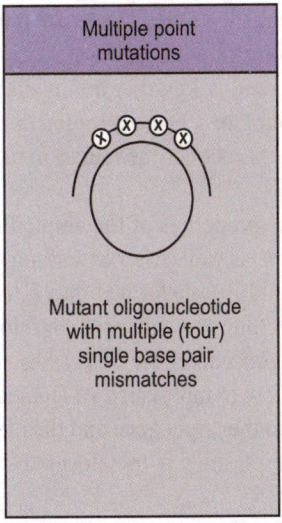	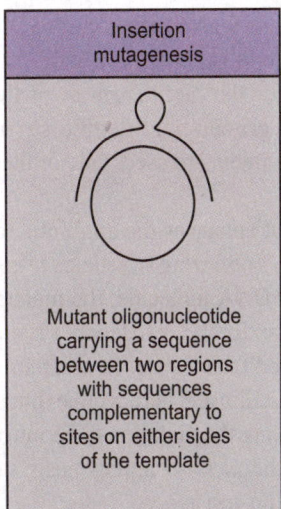	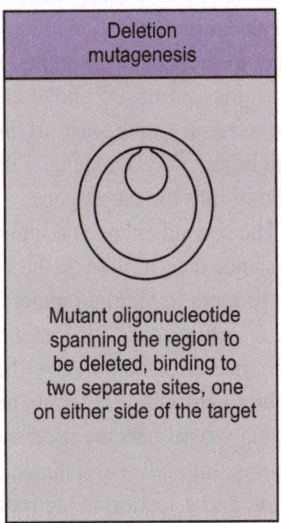
Mutant oligonucleotide with multiple (four) single base pair mismatches	Mutant oligonucleotide carrying a sequence between two regions with sequences complementary to sites on either sides of the template	Mutant oligonucleotide spanning the region to be deleted, binding to two separate sites, one on either side of the target

Fig. 6.3. Oligonucleotide directed mutagenesis used for multiple point mutation, insertion mutagenesis, and deletion mutagenesis.

Single-primer Method has a Number of Deficiencies

The efficiency with which the single-primer method yields mutants is dependent upon several factors. The double-stranded heteroduplex molecules that are generated will be contaminated both by any single-stranded non-mutant template DNA that has remained uncopied and by partially double-stranded molecules. The presence of these species considerably reduces the proportion of mutant progeny. They can be removed by sucrose gradient centrifugation or by agarose gel electrophoresis, but this is timeconsuming and inconvenient.

Following transformation and *in vivo* DNA synthesis, segregation of the two strands of the heteroduplex molecule can occur, yielding a mixed population of mutant and non-mutant progeny. Mutant progeny have to be purified away from parental molecules, and this process is complicated by the cell's mismatch repair system. In theory, the mismatch repair system should yield equal numbers of mutant and non-mutant progeny, but in practice mutants are counterselected. The major reason for this low yield of mutant progeny is that the methyldirected mismatch repair system of *E. coli* favours the repair of non-methylated DNA. In the cell, newly synthesised DNA strands that have not yet been methylated are preferentially repaired at the position of the mismatch, thereby eliminating a mutation. In a similar way, the non-methylated *in vitro*-generated mutant strand is repaired by the cell so that the majority of progeny are wild type.

The problems associated with the mismatch repair system can be overcome by using host strains carrying the *mut*L, *mut*S, or *mut*H mutations, which prevent the methyl-directed repair of mismatches. A heteroduplex molecule with one mutant and one non-mutant strand must inevitably give rise to both mutant and non-mutant progeny upon replication. It would be desirable to suppress the growth of non-mutants, and various strategies have been developed with this in mind.

Another disadvantage of all of the primer extension methods is that they require a single-stranded template. In contrast, with PCR-based mutagenesis the template can be single-stranded or double-stranded, circular or linear. In comparison with single-stranded DNAs, double-stranded DNAs are much easier to prepare. Also, gene inserts are in general more stable with double-stranded DNAs.

The issues raised above account for the fact that most of the mutagenesis kits that are available commercially make use of multiple primers and double stranded templates. For example, in the GeneEditor™ system (Fig. 6.4), two primers are used. One of these primers encodes the mutation to be inserted into the target gene.

The second encodes a mutation that enhances the antibiotic resistance properties of the ampicillin-resistance determinant on the vector by conferring resistance to ceftazidime as well. After extending the two primers to yield an intact circular DNA molecule, the mutated plasmid is transformed into *E. coli* and selection made for the enhanced antibiotic resistance. Plasmids encoding the enhanced antibiotic resistance also should carry the mutated target gene. In a variant of this procedure, the vector has two antibiotic resistance determinants (ampicillin and tetracycline) but one of these (Amp^R) carries a mutation. Again, two primers are used: one carrying the mutation to be introduced to the target gene and the other restores ampicillin resistance. After the *in vitro* mutagenesis steps, the plasmid is transformed into *E. coli* and selection made for ampicillin resistance.

Methods have been Developed that Simplify the Process of Making all Possible Amino Acid Substitutions at a Selected Site

Using site-directed mutagenesis it is possible to change two or three adjacent nucleotides so that every possible amino acid substitution is made at a site of interest. This generates a requirement for 19 different mutagenic oligonucleotides assuming only one codon will be used for each substitution. An alternative way of changing one amino acid to all the alternatives is cassette mutagenesis. This involves replacing a fragment of the gene with different fragments containing the desired codon changes. It is a simple method for which the efficiency of mutagenesis is close to 100 per cent. However, if it is desired to change the amino acids at two sites to all the possible alternatives then 400 different oligos or fragments would be required and the practicality of the method becomes questionable. One solution to this problem is to use doped oligonucleotides (Fig. 6.5).

PCR CAN BE USED FOR SITE-DIRECTED MUTAGENESIS

Early work on the development of the PCR method of DNA amplification showed its potential for mutagenesis. Single bases mismatched between the amplification primer and the template become incorporated into the template sequence as a result of amplification (Fig. 6.6).

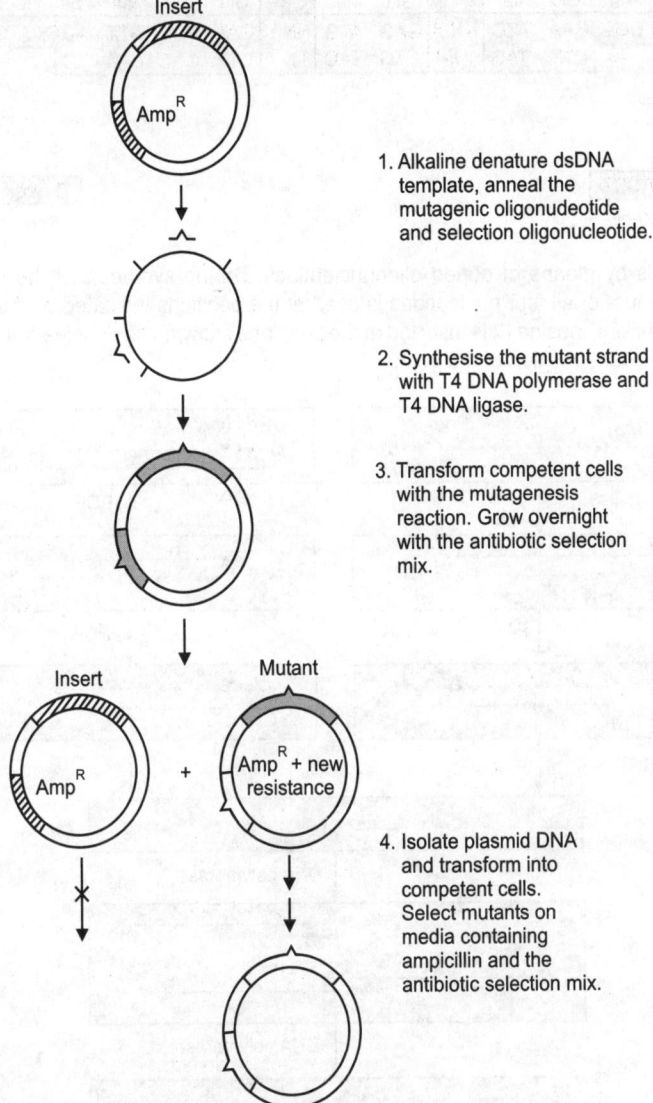

1. Alkaline denature dsDNA template, anneal the mutagenic oligonudeotide and selection oligonucleotide.

2. Synthesise the mutant strand with T4 DNA polymerase and T4 DNA ligase.

3. Transform competent cells with the mutagenesis reaction. Grow overnight with the antibiotic selection mix.

4. Isolate plasmid DNA and transform into competent cells. Select mutants on media containing ampicillin and the antibiotic selection mix.

Fig. 6.4. The GeneEditor™ system for generating a high frequency of mutations using site-directed mutagenesis.

Higuchi have described a variation of the basic method which enables a mutation in a PCR-produced DNA fragment to be introduced anywhere along its length. Two primary PCR reactions produce two overlapping DNA fragments, both bearing the same mutation in the overlap region. The overlap in sequence allows the fragments to hybridise (Fig. 6.6).

One of the two possible hybrids is extended by DNA polymerase to produce a duplex fragment. The other hybrid has recessed 5′ ends and, since it is not a substrate for the polymerase, is effectively lost from the reaction mixture. As with conventional primer-extension mutagenesis, deletions and insertions can also be created.

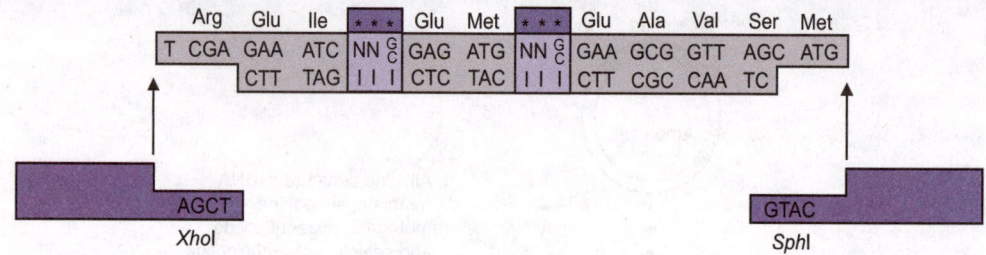

Fig. 6.5. Mutagenesis by means of doped oligonucleotides. During synthesis of the upper strand of the oligonucleotide, a mixture of all four nucleotides is used at the positions indicated by the letter N. When the lower strand is synthesised, inosine (I) is inserted at the positions shown. The double-stranded oligonucleotide is inserted into the relevant position of the vector.

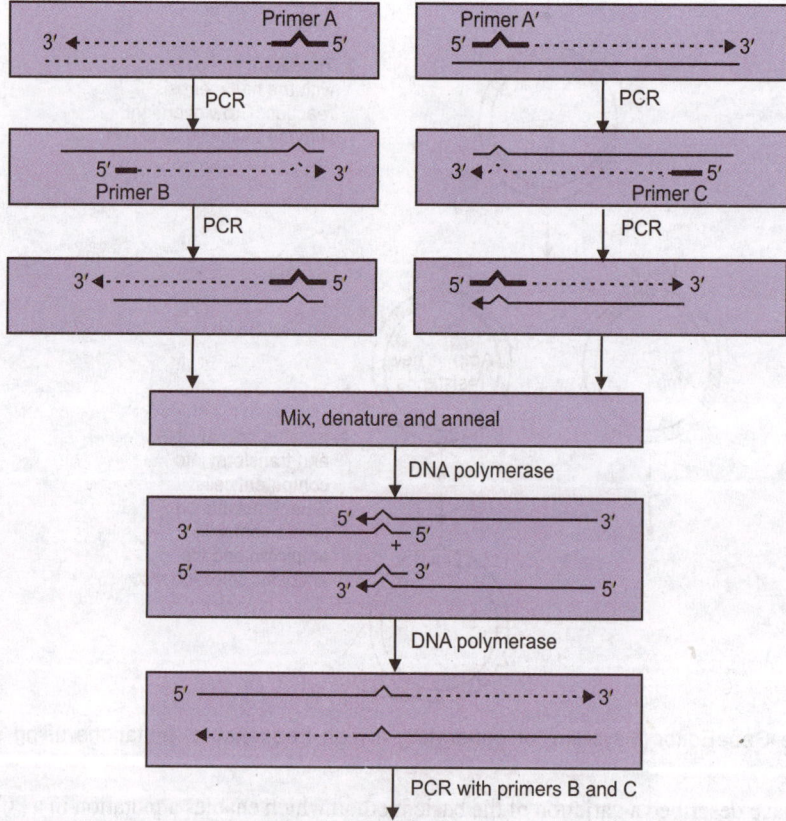

Fig. 6.6. Site-directed mutagenesis by means of the PCR. The steps shown in the top-left corner of the diagram show the basic PCR method of mutagenesis. The bottom half of the figure shows how the mutation can be moved to the middle of a DNA molecule. Primers are shown in bold and primers A and A′ are complementary.

The method of Higuchi is rather complicated in that it requires four primers and three PCRs (a pair of PCRs to amplify the overlapping segments and a third PCR to fuse the two segments). Commercial suppliers of reagents have developed simpler methods and two of these methods are described below.

Two features of PCR mutagenesis should be noted. First, the procedure is not restricted to single base changes: by selecting appropriate primers it is possible to make insertions and deletions as well. Second, Taq polymerase copies DNA with low fidelity and there is a significant risk of extraneous mutations being introduced during the amplification reaction. This problem can be minimised by using a high fidelity thermostable polymerase, and a high template concentration, and fewer than 10 cycles of amplification.

In the Exsite™ method (Fig. 6.7), both strands of the vector carrying the target gene are amplified using the PCR but one of the primers carries the desired mutation.

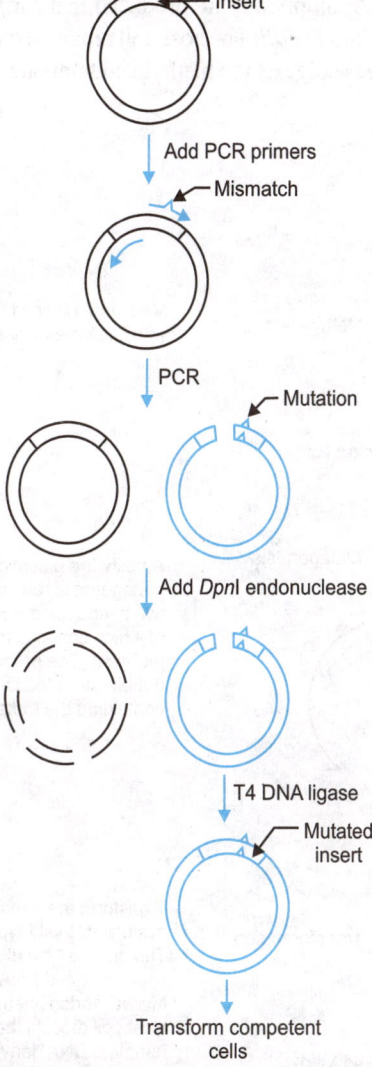

Fig. 6.7. (Left) The exsite™ method for generating mutants using the PCR. The parental plasmid (shown in blue) carrying the target gene is derived from a restriction-proficient strain of *E. coli* and so is methylated. This makes it sensitive to the *Dpn*I endonuclease and hence it can be eliminated selectively from the final PCR mixture.

This results in the production of a population of linear duplexes carrying the mutated gene that is contaminated with a low level of the original circular template DNA. If the template DNA was derived from an *E. coli* cell with an intact restriction modification system then it will be methylated and will be sensitive to restriction by the *Dpn*I endonuclease. The linear DNA produced by amplification will be resistant to *Dpn*I cleavage and after circularisation by blunt-end ligation can be recovered by transformation into *E. coli*. Any hybrid molecules consisting of a single strand of the methylated template DNA and unmethylated amplicon also will be destroyed by the endonuclease. In the GeneTailor™ method (Fig. 6.8), the target DNA is methylated *in vitro* before the mutagenesis step and overlapping primers are used. Once again, linear amplicons are produced that carry the desired mutation but in this case they are transformed directly into *E. eoli*. The host-cell repair enzymes circularise the linear mutated DNA while the *Mcr*BC endonuclease digests the methylated template DNA leaving only unmethylated, mutated product.

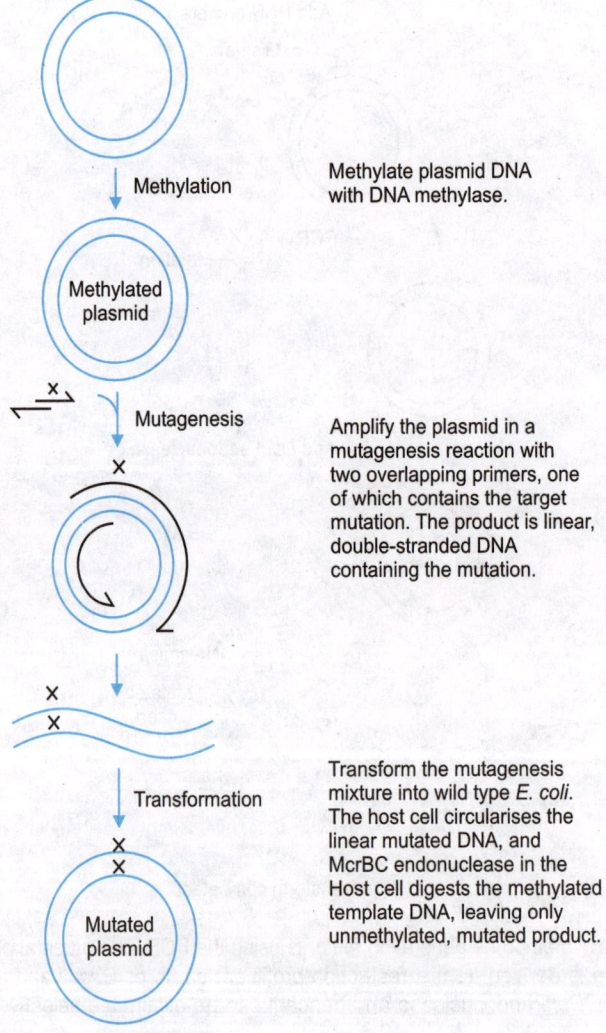

Methylate plasmid DNA with DNA methylase.

Amplify the plasmid in a mutagenesis reaction with two overlapping primers, one of which contains the target mutation. The product is linear, double-stranded DNA containing the mutation.

Transform the mutagenesis mixture into wild type *E. coli*. The host cell circularises the linear mutated DNA, and McrBC endonuclease in the Host cell digests the methylated template DNA, leaving only unmethylated, mutated product.

Fig. 6.8. The GeneTailor™ method for generating mutants using the PCR.

METHODS ARE AVAILABLE TO ENABLE MUTATIONS TO BE INTRODUCED RANDOMLY THROUGHOUT A TARGET GENE

The methods described above enable defined mutations to be introduced at defined locations within a gene and are of particular value in determining structure–activity relationships. However, if the objective of a study is to select mutants with altered and/or improved characteristics then a better approach is to mutate the gene at random and then positively select those with the desired properties. Methods for the random mutagenesis of cloned genes are described in this section and the next while selection methods are described later.

It is well known that the polymerase chain reaction is error prone and that there is a high probability of base changes in amplicons. However, even the relatively low fidelity *Taq* polymerase is too accurate to be of value in generating mutant libraries. Nevertheless, increases in error rates can be obtained in a number of ways. One of the commonest ways of achieving this is to introduce a small amount of Mn^{2+}, in place of the normal Mg^{2+}, and to include an excess of dGTP and dTTP relative to the other two nucleotide triphosphates.

With this protocol it is possible to achieve error rates of one nucleotide per kilobase. Even higher rates of mutagenesis can be achieved by using nucleoside triphosphate analogs.

The methodologies for error-prone PCR all involve either a misincorporation process in which the polymerase adds an incorrect base to the growing daughter strand or a lack of proofreading ability on the part of the polymerase. It might be expected that they generate a completely random set of mutants but in reality the mutant libraries produced are heavily biased. There are three sources of bias. First, the inherent characteristics of the DNA polymerase used mean that some types of errors are more common than others. The second source of bias arises because of the nature of the genetic code. For example, a single point mutation in a valine codon can change it to one encoding phenylalanine, leucine, isoleucine, alanine, aspartate, or glycine but two or three adjacent point mutations are required to change it to one encoding all the other amino acids. The final source of bias arises from the process of amplification. A mutant that is generated early in the amplification process will be over-represented in the final library compared to one that arises in later rounds of amplification.

Error-prone PCR protocols are effective as a means of randomly changing one amino acid into another in the final protein. However, sometimes it might be desirable to explore the effect of randomly deleting or inserting amino acids and this is possible using the random insertion/deletion (RID) process devised by Murakami. The method is based on ligating an insertion or deletion cassette at nearly random locations within the gene.

ALTERED PROTEINS CAN BE PRODUCED BY INSERTING UNUSUAL AMINO ACIDS DURING PROTEIN SYNTHESIS

All the mutation methods described above result in the replacement of one or more amino acid residues in a protein with other natural amino acids, e.g. the replacement of a phenylalanine residue with tyrosine, tryptophan, histidine, etc. The ability to incorporate unnatural amino acids into proteins *in vivo* would permit the production of large quantities of proteins with novel properties. For example, the replacement of methionine with selenomethionine facilitates the determination of the three-dimensional structure of proteins. While it is possible to 'force' bacteria to incorporate unnatural amino acids into proteins a better method is to engineer the translational apparatus.

This is achieved by generating an aminoacyl-tRNA synthetase and tRNA pair that function independently of the synthetases and tRNAs endogenous to *E. coli*.

Such a pair are said to be *orthogonal* and satisfy a number of criteria:

1. The tRNA is not a substrate for any of the endogenous *E. coli* synthetases but functions efficiently in protein translation.
2. The orthogonal synthetase efficiently aminoacylates the orthogonal tRNA whose anticodon has been modified to recognise an amber (UAG) or opal (UGA) stop codon.
3. The synthetase does not aminoacylate any of the endogenous *E. coli* tRNAs.

Archaebacteria appear to be an especially good source of orthogonal pairs for use in *E. coli*. Modifying the anticodon on the tRNA such that it recognises amber and opal codons is relatively easy. However, the synthetase also needs to be modified such that it charges the cognate tRNA with unusual amino acids more efficiently than the normal amino acid. To do this a library of synthetase mutants is generated and subjected to positive selection based on suppression of an amber codon located in a plasmidborne gene encoding chloramphenicol acetyltransferase. Using this approach the tyrosyl-tRNA synthetase of *Methanococcus jannaschii* was modified to permit the site-specific incorporation into proteins of phenylalanine and tyrosine derivatives such as *O*-allyltyrosine, *p*-acetyl-phenylalanine, and *p*-benzoyl-phenylalanine. These modified amino acids can be used as sites for chemical modification of the protein *in vitro* after purification, e.g. the attachment of fluorescent labels.

There have been two significant developments of the above technique. In the first of these, Zhang have shown that chemical modification of proteins can occur *in vivo* as well as *in vitro*. For example, *m*-acetylphenylalanine was substituted for Lys7 of the cytoplasmic domain of protein Z and for Arg200 of the outer membrane protein LamB. On addition of a membrane-permeable dye (fluorescein hydrazide) to intact cells, these modified proteins were selectively labelled. In the case of cells expressing the modified LamB derivative, labelling was possible with a range of fluorescein derivatives that are not membrane permeable. The second development is the ability to charge the orthogonal tRNA with glycosylated amino acids. For example, Zhang were able to synthesise in *E. coli* a myoglobin derivative containing β–N-acetylglucosamine (GlcNAc) at a defined position. This GlcNAc moiety was recognised by a saccharide-binding protein and could be modified by a galactosyltransferase.

PHAGE DISPLAY CAN BE USED TO FACILITATE THE SELECTION OF MUTANT PEPTIDES

In phage display, a segment of foreign DNA is inserted into either a phagemid or an infectious filamentous phage genome and expressed as a fusion product with a phage coat protein. It is a very powerful technique for selecting and engineering polypeptides with novel functions. The technique was developed first for the *E. coli* phage M13, but has since been extended to other phages such as T4 and λ.

The M13 phage particle consists of a singlestranded DNA molecule surrounded by a coat consisting of several thousand copies of the major coat protein, P8. At one end of the particle are five copies each of the two minor coat proteins P9 and P7 and at the other end five copies each of P3 and P6. In early examples of phage display, a random DNA cassette was inserted into either the P3 or the P8 gene at the junction between the signal sequence and the native peptide. *E. coli* transfected with the recombinant DNA molecules secreted phage particles that displayed on their surface the amino acids encoded by the foreign DNA. Particular phage displaying peptide motifs with, for example, antibody-binding properties were isolated by affinity chromatography (Fig. 6.9). Several rounds of affinity chromatography and phage propagation can be used to further enrich for phage with the desired binding characteristics. In this way, millions of random peptides have been screened for their ability to bind to an anti-peptide antibody or to streptavidin, and variants of human growth hormone with improved affinity and receptor specificity have been isolated.

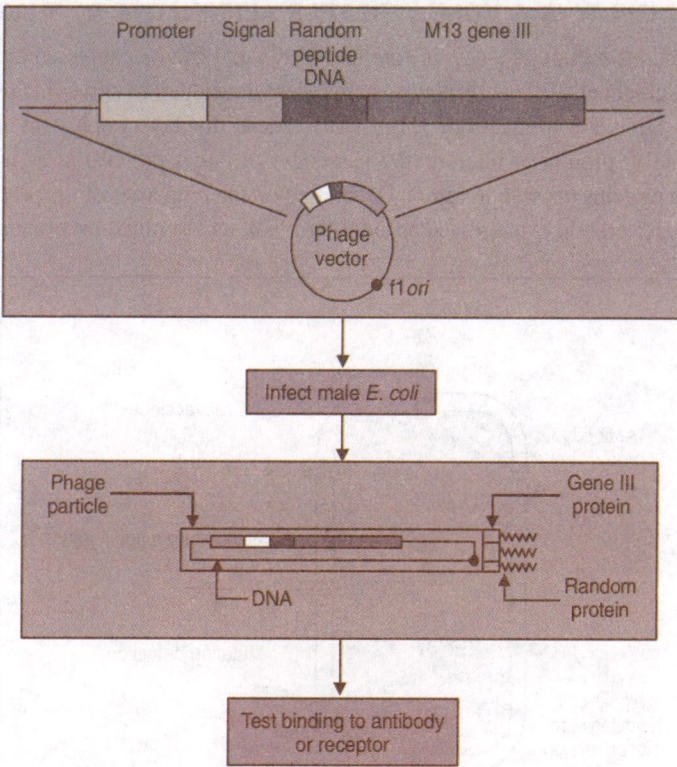

Fig. 6.9. The principle of phage display of random peptides.

One disadvantage of the original method of phage display is that polypeptide inserts greater than 10 residues compromise coat-protein function and so cannot be efficiently displayed. This problem can be solved by the use of phagemid display. In this system, the starting-point is a plasmid carrying a single copy of the P3 or P8 gene from M13 plus the M13 *ori* sequence. As before, the random DNA sequence is inserted into the P3 or P8 gene downstream from the signal peptide-cleavage site and the construct transformed into *E. coli*.

Phage particles displaying the amino acid sequences encoded by the DNA insert are obtained by superinfecting the transformed cells with helper phage. The resulting phage particles are phenotypically mixed and their surfaces are a mosaic of normal coat protein and fusion protein.

Specialised phagemid display vectors have been developed for particular purposes. For example, phagemids have been constructed that have an amber (chain-terminating) codon immediately downstream from the foreign DNA insert and upstream from the body of P3 or P8. When the recombinant phagemid is transformed into non-suppressing strains of *E. coli*, the protein encoded by the foreign DNA terminates at the amber codon and is secreted into the medium. However, if the phagemid is transformed into cells carrying an amber suppressor, the entire fusion protein is synthesised and displayed on the surface of the secreted phage particles. Other studies have shown that proteins can be displayed as fusions to the carboxy terminus of P3, P6, and P8. Although amino-terminal display formats are likely to dominate established applications, carboxyterminal display permits constructs that are unsuited to amino-terminal display.

CELL-SURFACE DISPLAY IS A MORE VERSATILE ALTERNATIVE TO PHAGE DISPLAY

As noted in the previous section, the size of foreign protein that can be expressed by phage display is rather limited. Microbial cell-surface display systems were developed to solve this problem and these systems also have far more applications (Fig. 6.10). These display systems involve expressing a heterologous peptide or protein of interest (the passenger or target protein) as a fusion protein with various cell-surface proteins (carrier proteins). Depending on the properties of the passenger and carrier proteins, the passenger protein is expressed as an N-terminal, a C-terminal or a sandwich fusion.

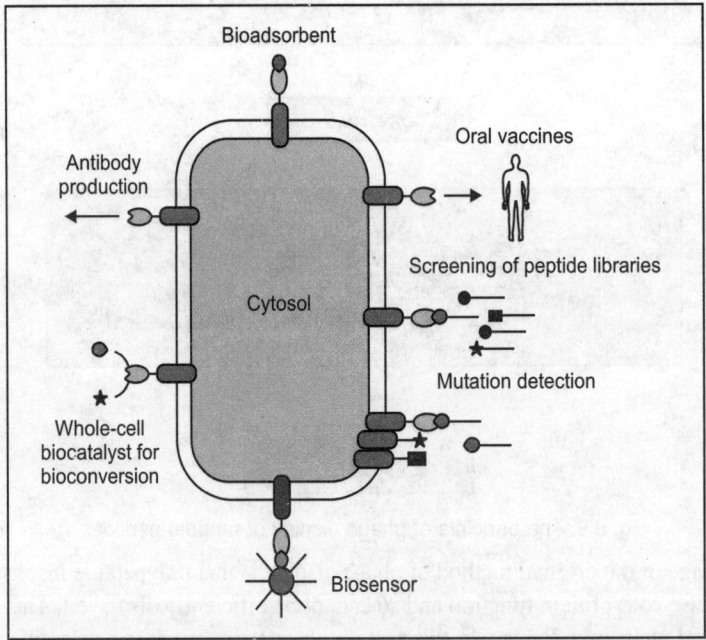

Fig. 6.10. Applications of microbial cell-surface display. Reproduced from Lee, with permission from Elsevier.

Applications of Cell-Surface Display

There are many different biotechnological and industrial applications of the cell-surface display technology. For example, key proteins from microbial pathogens can be displayed on the surface of bacteria and their ability to elicit antigen-specific responses determined as a major step towards the development of live vaccines. Proteins that bind heavy metals or specific organic pollutants can be expressed on the surface of cells and these cells can be used as specific bioadsorbents for environmental remediation. Alternatively, new enzyme activities can be expressed on the cell surface to promote environmental degradation of pollutants or for use in industrial biocatalysis. Finally, by anchoring enzymes, receptors, or other signal-sensitive components to the cell's surface new biosensors could be developed.

For a cell-surface protein to be a successful carrier it should satisfy four requirements. First, it should have an efficient signal peptide to permit the fusion protein to pass through the inner membrane. Second, it should have a strong anchoring structure to keep fusion proteins on the cell surface without detachment. Third, it should be compatible with the passenger protein such that the fusion is not unstable. Finally, it should be resistant to attack by proteases present in the periplasmic space or the growth medium. In Gram-negative bacteria such as *E. coli* many different proteins have been subjugated as carriers. Basically, these proteins fall into two classes: outer membrane proteins (e.g. the adhesin protein, peptidiglycan-associated lipoprotein, and the OmpC and TraT proteins) and protein components of appendages such as pili and flagella. Where outer membrane proteins are used as the carrier it is important to know which part of them is exposed on the outer surface of the cell since this needs to be the site of insertion of the passenger protein.

The passenger protein to be displayed is selected by the required application but its properties influence the translocation process and the effectiveness of the display procedure. For example, the formation of disulphide bridges at the periplasmic side of the outer membrane can affect the efficiency of translocation. Also, the presence of many charged or hydrophobic residues can result in inefficient secretion. Thus, if display technology is used to screen variants produced by random mutagenesis, there may be negative or positive selection for those mutants that affect the efficiency of translocation.

PROTEIN ENGINEERING

Protein engineering is the process of developing useful or valuable proteins. It is a young discipline, with much research taking place into the understanding of protein folding and recognition for protein design principles. There are two general strategies for protein engineering, rational design and directed evolution. These techniques are not mutually exclusive; researchers will often apply both. In the future, more detailed knowledge of protein structure and function, as well as advancements in high-throughput technology, may greatly expand the capabilities of protein engineering. Eventually, even unnatural amino acids may be incorporated thanks to a new method that allows the inclusion of novel amino acids in the genetic code.

One of the most exciting aspects of recombinant DNA technology is that it permits the design, development, and isolation of proteins with improved operating characteristics and even completely novel proteins (Table 6.1). The principle of the methods described so far in this chapter is that the gene is mutated, either at a discrete site or at random, and then selection made for a protein variant with the desired property. The improved variant can be subjected to further rounds of mutagenesis and selection, a process known as directed evolution.

Table 6.1. Some examples of protein engineering.

Example	Method
Increased rate and extent of biodesulphurisation of diesel by modification of dibenzothiophene mono-oxygenase	RACHITT
Generation of a subtilisin with a half-life at 65°C that is 50 times greater than wild type by recombining segments from five different subtilisin variants	StEP
Conversion of a galactosidase into a fucosidase	Shuffling
Enhanced activity of amylosucrase	Random mutagenesis plus shuffling
Generation of novel DNA polymerases from a combination of rat DNA polymerase beta and African swine fever virus DNA polymerase X	SCOPE
Generation of novel β-lactamase by recombining two genes with 40% amino acid identity and 49% nucleotide sequence identity	SISDC

The paradigm for this approach is the enzyme subtilisin. Every property of this serine protease has been altered including its rate of catalysis, substrate specificity, pH-rate profile, and stability to oxidative, thermal, and alkaline inactivation. Variants also have been produced that favour aminolysis (synthesis) over hydrolysis in aqueous solvents.

An alternative approach to directed evolution is gene shuffling. The principle of this method is that many protein variants with desirable characteristics already exist in nature and novel combinations of these variants may have even more desirable properties (Fig. 6.11). There are three sources of variants for gene shuffling. First, different polymorphisms of the gene of interest might exist naturally in a single organism or might have been created by random *in vitro* mutagenesis. Second, the same protein with the same activity may be found in other organisms but the gene and protein sequences will be different. Third, the protein of interest might belong to a protein family where the different members have different but related activities.

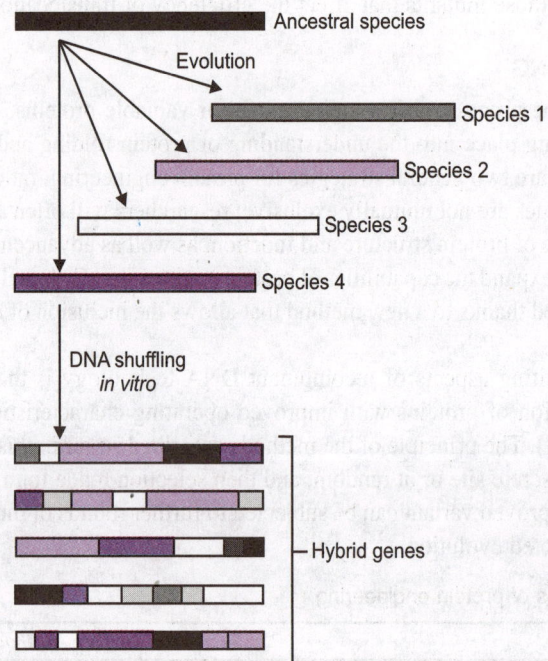

Fig. 6.11. Schematic representation of gene shuffling.

In directed evolution, random mutagenesis is applied to a protein, and a selection regime is used to pick out variants that have the desired qualities. Further rounds of mutation and selection are then applied. This method mimics natural evolution and generally produces superior results to rational design. An additional technique known as DNA shuffling mixes and matches pieces of successful variants in order to produce better results. This process mimics the recombination that occurs naturally during sexual reproduction.

The great advantage of directed evolution is that it requires no prior structural knowledge of a protein, nor is it necessary to be able to predict what effect a given mutation will have. Indeed, the results of directed evolution experiments are often surprising in that desired changes are often caused by mutations that were not expected to have that effect. The drawback is that they require high-throughput, which is not feasible for all proteins. Large amounts of recombinant DNA must be mutated and the products screened for desired qualities.

The sheer number of variants often requires expensive robotic equipment to automate the process. Furthermore, not all desired activities can be easily screened for.

Examples of engineered proteins: Using computational methods, a protein with a novel fold has been designed, known as Top7, as well as sensors for unnatural molecules. The engineering of fusion proteins has yielded rilonacept, a pharmaceutical which has secured FDA approval for the treatment of cryopyrin-associated periodic syndrome.

Rational Design of Proteins

In rational protein design, the scientist uses detailed knowledge of the structure and function of the protein to make desired changes. This generally has the advantage of being inexpensive and technically easy, since site-directed mutagenesis techniques are well-developed. However, its major drawback is that detailed structural knowledge of a protein is often unavailable, and even when it is available, it can be extremely difficult to predict the effects of various mutations.

Computational protein design algorithms seek to identify novel amino acid sequences that are low in energy when folded to the pre-specified target structure. While the sequence-conformation space that needs to be searched is large, the most challenging requirement for computational protein design is a fast, yet accurate, energy function that can distinguish optimal sequences from similar suboptimal ones.

A good example of gene shuffling is work done on subtilisin by Ness and others. They started with the genes for 26 members of the subtilisin family and created a library of chimeric proteases. When this library was screened for four distinct enzyme properties, variants were found that were significantly improved over any of the parental enzymes for each individual property. Similarly, Lehmann started with a family of mesophilic phytases whose amino acid sequence had been determined. Using these data they constructed a 'consensus' phytase sequence and found that an enzyme with this sequence was much more thermostable than any of the parent enzymes.

Different Methods of Gene Shuffling

In the original method of gene shuffling, one starts by purifying the different genes that will provide the source of variation. These genes are digested with DNase to generate the fragments that will be recombined. The fragments from the different sources are mixed together and subjected to repeated rounds of melting, annealing, and extension (Fig. 6.12). Eventually a full-length gene should be synthesised and this can be amplified by the PCR and cloned. The smaller the fragments that are produced in the initial step the greater the number of single site variations that can be incorporated in the final product. However, the smaller the fragments the greater the number of cycles needed to reassemble a complete gene.

An alternative method is the staggered extension process. This also relies on repeated cycles of melting, annealing, and extension to build the variant genes. However, in the StEP process one starts with a mixture of full-length genes, denatures them, and then primes the synthesis of complementary strands (Fig. 6.13). After a short period of primer extension, the DNA is subjected to a round of melting, annealing, and extension.

Some of the extended primers will anneal to templates with a different base sequence and on further extension will generate chimeras. The more cycles of extension, melting, and annealing the greater the variability that can be produced.

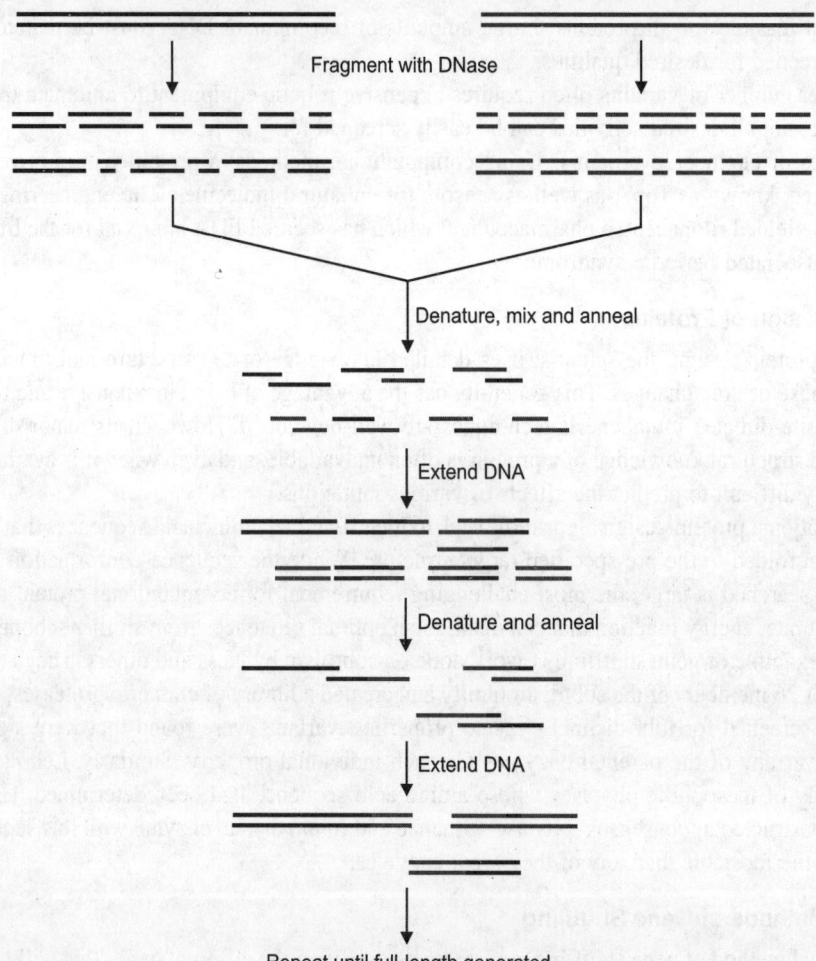

Fragment with DNase

Denature, mix and anneal

Extend DNA

Denature and anneal

Extend DNA

Repeat until full-length generated

Fig. 6.12. The original method of gene shuffling. After fragmentation of the two homologous genes, the cycles of denaturation, annealing, and extension are continued until full-length genes can be detected by gel electrophoresis.

Random chimeragenesis on transient templates (RACHITT) is conceptually similar to the original DNA-shuffling method but is designed to produce chimeras with a much larger number of crossovers. In this method the gene fragments are generated from one strand of all but one of the parental DNAs (Fig. 8.14). These fragments then are reassembled on the full-length opposite strand of the remaining parent (the transient template). The fragments are cut back to remove mismatched sections, extended, and then ligated to generate full-length genes. Finally, the template strand is destroyed to leave only the ligated gene fragments to be converted to double-stranded DNA.

Each of the methods described above has its advantages and disadvantages and all of them rely to a greater or lesser extent on the annealing of mismatched DNA sequences. Thus there is always a chance that the parental molecules will be recreated preferentially or that the degree of variation generated will not be as great as expected. However, methods for 'forcing' the generation of recombinants have been developed.

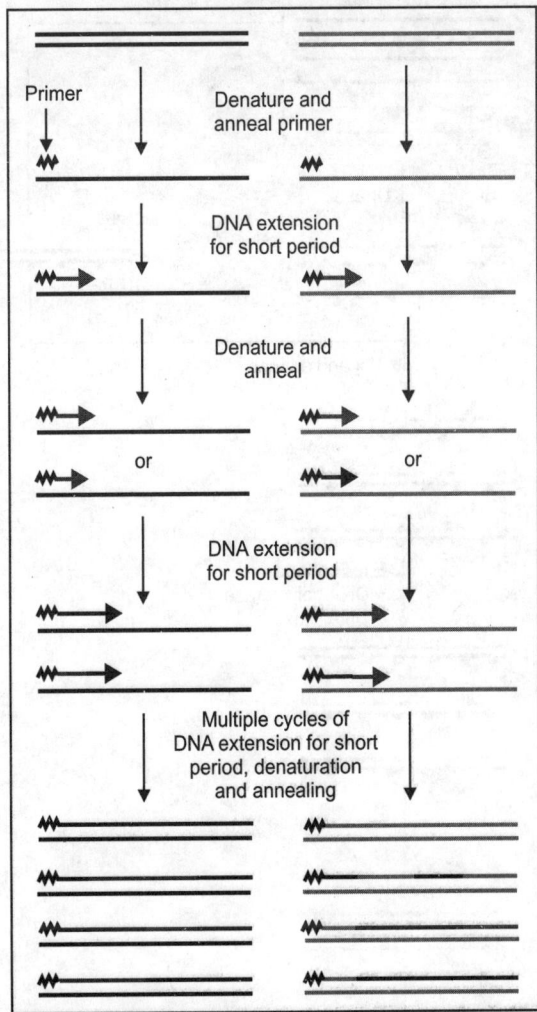

Fig. 6.13. The StEP method for generating hybrid proteins. In the example shown, a hybrid gene will be constructed from two homologous genes (shown in grey and black). Cloning of the hybrid gene will result in the production of a hybrid protein. For clarity, only one strand of each gene is shown after the initial denaturation step.

Chimeric Proteins can be Produced in the Absence of Gene Homology

The gene-shuffling methods described above have an absolute requirement for significant homology between the parental sequences. However, there may be a wish to create hybrids between proteins with functional similarities but whose sequence homology is less than 50 per cent. Achieving this requires methods for combining non-homologous sequences and the first one to be developed was ITCHY (incremental truncation for the creation of hybrid enzymes). This method is based on the direct ligation of libraries of fragments generated by the truncation of two template sequences, each template being truncated from opposite ends (Fig. 8.15). This ligation procedure removes any need for homology at the point of crossover but the downside is that the DNA fragments may be reconnected in a way that is not at all analogous to their position in the template gene.

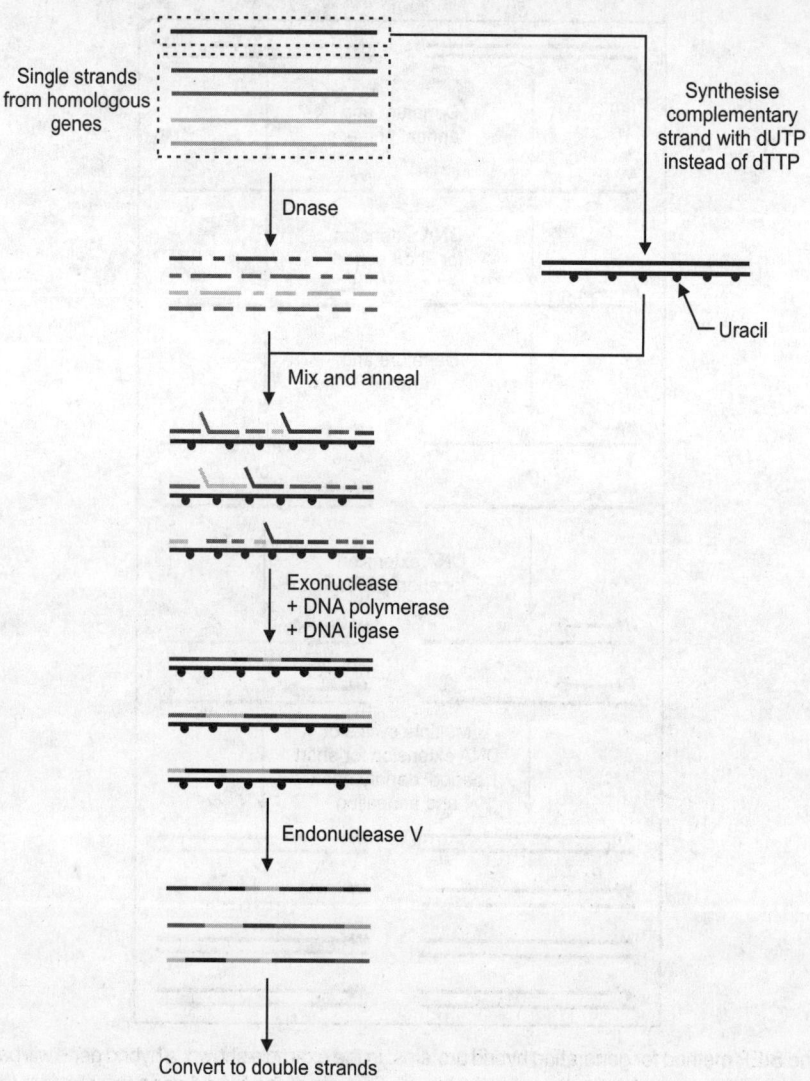

Fig. 6.14. The RACHITT method for creating hybrid proteins.

In the original ITCHY process the incremental truncation was performed using timed exonuclease digestions. In practice, these digestions are difficult to control. An improved process was developed where the initial templates are generated with phosphorothioate linkages incorporated at random along the length of the gene. Complete exonuclease digestion then generates fragments with lengths determined by the position of the nucleaseresistant phosphorothioate linkage. This method is known as thio-ITCHY and is much simpler to perform. One drawback of ITCHY libraries is that they contain only one crossover per gene. However, by combining ITCHY libraries with DNA-shuffling methods, a process known as SCRATCHY, it is possible to generate additional variation.

A major problem with methods such as ITCHY is that they generate large numbers of non-functional sequences due to mutations, insertions, and deletions. Furthermore, when one examines the three dimensional structure of proteins it is clear that they are organised into domains and motifs. Therefore, a more attractive way of generating chimeric proteins might be to recombine these domains and motifs in novel ways.

Two general methods of doing this have been developed and these are SCOPE (structure-based combinatorial protein engineering) and SISDC (sequence-independent site-directed chimeragenesis).

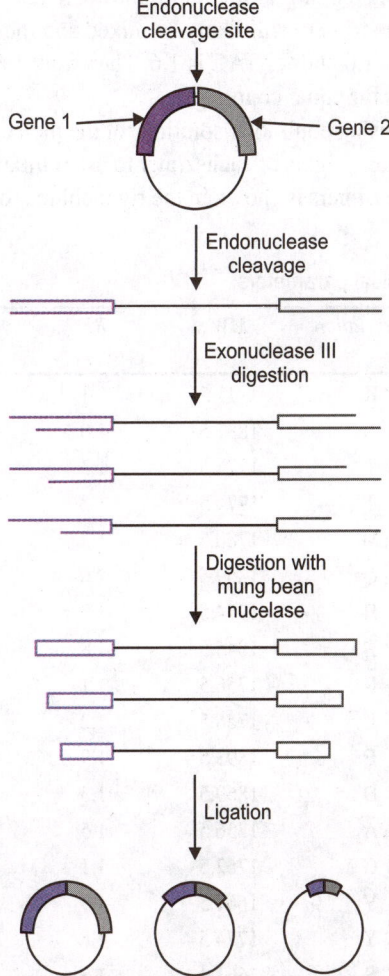

Fig. 6.15. The ITCHY method for creating hybrids of two related proteins. In the figure, the two related proteins are encoded by genes 1 (shown in purple) and 2 (shown in grey). The end result is a hybrid gene comprising the 5′ end of gene 1 and the 3′ end of gene 2.

OLIGONUCLEOTIDE-DIRECTED MUTAGENESIS

In principle, the simplest approach for oligonucleotide-directed mutagenesis would be the use of trimer phosphoramidites. Of the 64 possible combinations of codons, only 20 codons would be required to cover the 20 amino acids, although, in practice, several codons will likely be duplicated depending on the organism. Our trimers use the protection scheme described by Kayushin and others. There is a concern that the sequence of the trimers has to be verified. For example, CAT coding for histidine, has to be differentiated from TAC, coding for tyrosine. These two trimers have virtually identical lipophilicity and their identity cannot be clearly confirmed by HPLC. This problem has been solved[4] using HPLC electrospray mass spectrometric analysis of the trimers, which provides data confirming molecular weight and sequence.

In Table 6.2, the trimers, their coding amino acid and their reaction factor (RF) are listed. The reaction factor is critical since the trimers will likely be mixed and they have differing reactivity in the coupling reaction. RF for AAC is 1.0 and for TAC is 1.6. Therefore, 1.6 equivalents of TAC are needed for every 1.0 equivalent of AAC for equal coupling.

Mixtures can easily be made using equimolar solutions or the molecular weight of each trimer has to be used to generate the appropriate weights of each trimer to use if mixing by weight. An example of the preparation of a mixture of all 20 trimers is shown in the right column of Table 6.2 and completed in the footnotes.

Table 6.2. Trimer coding and physical parameters.

Trimer	Amino Acid	Abbreviation	MW	RF	MWxRF	mg/10μmol (adjusted for RF)
AAA	Lys	K	1911.5	1.1	2102.65	21.0 (11)
AAC	Asn	N	1887.5	1.0	1887.50	18.9 (10)
ACT	Thr	T	1774.5	1.3	2306.85	23.1 (13)
ATC	Ile	I	1774.5	1.2	2129.40	21.3 (12)
ATG	Met	M	1780.5	1.3	2314.65	23.1 (13)
CAG	Gln	Q	1869.5	2.0	3739.00	37.4 (20)
CAT	His	H	1774.5	1.9	3371.55	33.7 (19)
CCG	Pro	P	1845.5	1.8	3321.90	33.2 (18)
CGT	Arg	R	1756.5	1.1	1932.15	19.3 (11)
CTG	Leu	L	1756.5	1.2	2107.80	21.1 (12)
GAA	Glu	E	1893.5	1.9	3597.65	36.0 (19)
GAC	Asp	D	1869.5	1.3	2430.35	24.3 (13)
GCT	Ala	A	1756.5	1.5	2634.75	26.3 (15)
GGT	Gly	G	1762.5	1.1	1938.75	19.4 (11)
GTT	Val	V	1667.5	1.9	3168.25	31.7 (19)
TAC	Tyr	Y	1774.5	1.6	2839.20	28.4 (16)
TCT	Ser	S	1661.4	1.3	2159.82	21.6 (13)
TGC	Cys	C	1756.5	1.5	2634.75	26.3 (15)
TGG	Trp	W	1762.5	2.4	4230.00	42.3 (24)
TTC	Phe	F	1661.4	1.3	2159.82	21.6 (13)
= 530.0 mg						

All of the trimers are now available individually so that researchers can prepare custom mixtures. A mixture of all 20 trimers designed to produce equal coupling of all 20 is also available. Example of preparation of trimer mixture: Prepare 530 mg of the trimer mix, taking the amount (mg) for each trimer from the right column.

Dissolve the trimer mix in dichloromethane (highest grade possible; acid-free). Evaporate to dryness to produce a homogenous mixture of all 20 trimers.

Example of preparation of trimer mixture for the synthesiser: Dissolve 530 mg, which is equivalent to 20×10 µmoles (normalised for RF) of the trimer mix in 2.0 ml of acetonitrile-dichloromethane mixture, $1:3$ v/v to produce a 0.10 N solution of trimers, ready for use in a synthesiser.

APPROACHES TO RANDOM MUTAGENESIS

Random mutagenesis is an incredibly powerful tool for altering the properties of enzymes. Imagine, for example, you were studying a G-protein coupled receptor (GPCR) and wanted to create a temperaturesensitive version of the receptor or one that was activated by a different ligand than the wild-type. How could you do this?

Firstly, you would clone the gene encoding the receptor, then randomly introduce mutations into the gene sequence to create a 'library' containing thousands of versions of the gene. Each version (or 'variant') of the gene in the library would contain different mutations and so encode receptors with slightly altered amino acid sequences giving them slightly different enzymatic properties than the wild-type.

Next you could transform the library into a strain where the receptor would be expressed and apply a high throughput screen to pick out variants in the library that have the properties you are looking for. Using a high throughput screen for GPCR activity you could pick out the variants from the library that were temperature sensitive or were activated by different ligands.

Random Mutant Library

Creating a random mutant library that contains enough variants to give you a good chance of obtaining the altered enzyme you desire is a challenge in itself. There are many ways to create random mutant libraries, each with it's own pros and cons. Here are some of them:

1. Error-prone PCR: This approach uses a 'sloppy' version of PCR, in which the polymerase has a fairly high error rate (up to 2 per cent), to amplify the wild-type sequence. The PCR can be made error-prone in various ways including increasing the $MgCl_2$ in the reaction, adding $MnCl_2$ or using unequal concentrations of each nucleotide. Here is a good review of error prone PCR techiques and theory. After amplification, the library of mutant coding sequences must be cloned into a suitable plasmid. The drawback of this approach is that size of the library is limited by the efficiency of the cloning step. Although point mutations are the most common types of mutation in error prone PCR, deletions and frameshift mutations are also possible. There are a number of commercial error-prone PCR kits available, including those from Stratagene and Clontech.

2. Rolling circle error-prone PCR: Rolling circle error-prone PCR is a variant of error-prone PCR in which wild-type sequence is first cloned into a plasmid, then the whole plasmid is amplified under errorprone conditions. This eliminates the ligation step that limits library size in conventional error-prone PCR but of course the amplification of the whole plasmid is less efficient than amplifying the coding sequence alone.

3. Mutator strains: In this approach the wild-type sequence is cloned into a plasmid and transformed into a mutator strain, such as Stratagene's XL 1-red. XL 1-red is an *E. coli* strain whose deficiency in three of the primary DNA repair pathways (mutS, mutD and mutT) causes it to make errors during replicate of it's DNA, including the cloned plasmid. As a result each copy of the plasmid

replicated in this strain has the potential to be different from the wild-type. One advantage of mutator strains is that a wide variety of mutations can be incorporated including substitutions, deletions and frame-shifts. The drawback with this method is that the strain becomes progressively sick as it accumulates more and more mutations in it's own genome so several steps of growth, plasmid isolation, transformation and re-growth are normally required to obtain a meaningful library.

4. Temporary mutator strains: Temporary mutator strains can be built by over-expressing a mutator allele such as mutD5 (a dominant negative version of mutD) which limits the cell's ability to repair DNA lesions. By expressing mutD5 from an inducible promoter it is possible to allow the cells to cycle between mutagenic (mutD5 expression on) and normal (mutD5 expression off) periods of growth. The periods of normal growth allow the cells to recover from the mutagenesis, which allows these strains to grow for longer than conventional mutator strains.

    If a plasmid with a temperature-sensitive origin of replication is used, the mutagenic plasmid can easily be removed restore normal DNA repair, allowing the mutants to be grown up for analysis/screening. An example of the construction and use of such a strain can be found here.

5. Insertion mutagenesis: Finnzymes have a kit that uses a transposon-based system to randomly insert a 15-base pair sequence throughout a sequence of interest, be it an isolated insert or plasmid. This inserts 5 codons into the sequence, allowing any gene with an insertion to be expressed (i.e. no frame-shifts or stop codons are cause). Since the insertion is random, each copy of the sequence will have different insertions, thus creating a library.

6. Ethyl methanesulfonate (EMS): Ethyl methanesulfonate (EMS) is a chemical mutagen. EMS aklylates guanidine residues, causing them to be incorrectly copied during DNA replication. Since EMS directly chemically modifies DNA, EMS mutagenesis can be carried out either *in vivo* (i.e. whole-cell mutagenesis) or *in vitro*. An example of *in vitro* mutagenesis with EMS in which a PCR-amplified gene was subjected to reaction with EMS before being ligated into a plasmid and transformed can be found here.

7. Nitrous acid: Nitrous acid is another chemical mutagen. It acts by de-aminating adenine and cytosine residues (although other mechanisms are discussed here) causing transversion point mutations (A/T to G/C and vice versa). An example of a study using nitrosoguanidine mutagenesis can be found here.

    Note: Chemical mutagens are, of course mutagens and therefore should be handled with great care. Be especially careful with EMS as it is volatile at room temperature.

8. DNA shuffling: DNA shuffling is a very powerful method in which members of a library (i.e. copies of same gene each with different types of mutation) are randomly shuffled. This is done by randomly digesting the library with DNAsel then randomly re-joining the fragments using self-priming PCR. Shuffling can be applied to libraries produced by any of the above method and allows the effects of different combinations of mutations to be tested.

Asparagine

Asparagine (abbreviated as Asn or N; Asx or B represent either asparagine or aspartic acid) is one of the 20 most common natural amino acids on earth. It has carboxamide as the side chain's functional group. It is not an essential amino acid. Its codons are AAU and AAC.

A reaction between asparagine and reducing sugars or reactive carbonyls produces acrylamide (acrylic amide) in food when heated to sufficient temperature. These products occur in baked goods such as french fries, potato chips, and roasted coffee.

Asparagine was first isolated in 1806, under a crystalline form, by French chemists Louis Nicolas Vauquelin and Pierre Jean Robiquet (then a young assistant) from asparagus juice, in which it is abundant — hence the name they chose for that new matter—becoming the first amino acid to be isolated. The characteristic smell observed in the urine of individuals after their consumption of asparagus is attributed to various metabolic byproducts of asparagine.

A few years later, in 1809, Pierre Jean Robiquet again identified, this time from liquorice root, a substance with properties he qualified as very similar to those of asparagine, that Plisson in 1828 will confirm effectively as asparagine itself.

Structural function in proteins

Since the asparagine side chain can form hydrogen bond interactions with the peptide backbone, asparagine residues are often found near the beginning and the end of alpha-helices, and in turn motifs in beta sheets. Its role can be thought as 'capping' the hydrogen bond interactions that would otherwise be satisfied by the polypeptide backbone. Glutamines, with an extra methylene group, have more conformational entropy and thus are less useful in this regard.

Asparagine also provides key sites for N-linked glycosylation, modification of the protein chain with the addition of carbohydrate chains.

Sources

Dietary Sources

Asparagine is not an essential amino acid, which means that it can be synthesised from central metabolic pathway intermediates in humans and is not required in the diet. Asparagine is found in:

1. Animal sources: Dairy, whey, beef, poultry, eggs, fish, lactalbumin, seafood.
2. Plant sources: Asparagus, potatoes, legumes, nuts, seeds, soya, whole grains.

Biosynthesis

The precursor to asparagine is oxaloacetate. Oxaloacetate is converted to aspartate using a transaminase enzyme. The enzyme transfers the amino group from glutamate to oxaloacetate producing α-ketoglutarate and aspartate. The enzyme asparagine synthetase produces asparagine, AMP, glutamate, and pyrophosphate from aspartate, glutamine, and ATP. In the asparagine synthetase reaction, ATP is used to activate aspartate, forming β-aspartyl-AMP. Glutamine donates an ammonium group which reacts with β-aspartyl-AMP to form asparagine and free AMP (Fig. 6.16).

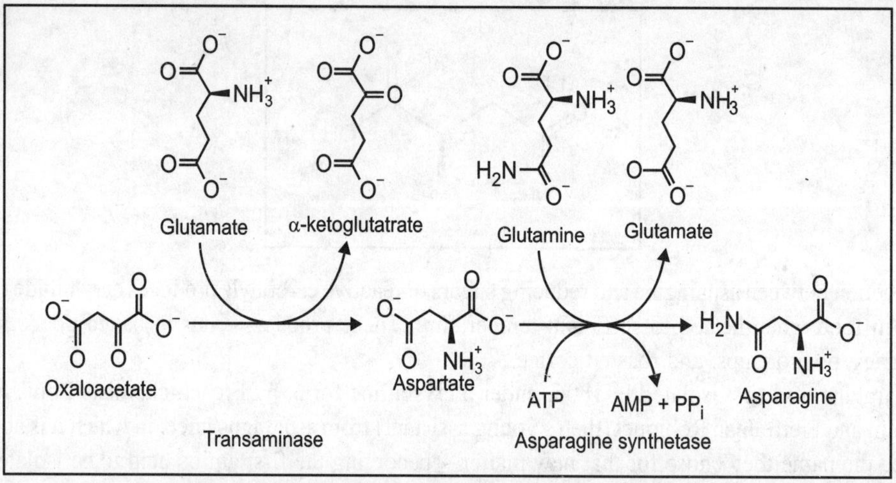

Fig. 6.16. The biosynthesis of asparagine from oxaloacetate.

Degradation

Aspartate is a glucogenic amino acid, L-asparaginase hydrolyses the amide group to form aspartate and ammonium. A transaminase converts the aspartate to oxaloacetate which can then be metabolised in the citric acid cycle or gluconeogenesis. The nervous system requires asparagine. It also plays an important role in the synthesis of ammonia.

Chapter 7

Microbial Synthesis of Commercial and Allied Products

INTRODUCTION

There is currently great interest in pharmaceutical proteins, and work in this area, from basic research to drug marketing, is expanding vigorously. The starting points of these developments are genetic engineering and biotechnology, which contribute to the discovery of new proteins and allow them to be produced on a worthwhile scale. Ever since the commercial introduction of insulin in 1923, of thyroid hormone in 1934, of factor VIII in 1948, and of calcitonin in 1970, hormones, serum proteins, and enzymes have been firmly established as therapeutic agents. Immunomodulators and various tissue proteins are in a turbulent phase of development as a new approach to the therapy of tumours. Increasingly, diagnostic aids now take the form of enzymes and monoclonal antibodies, and recently there has even been development of vaccines based on defined single proteins and oligopeptides. Of the more than 200 pharmaceutical proteins which have been investigated to date, more than half are undergoing research and development, about 100 are in clinical trials, and a dozen or so have already been marketed. The most important indications for them are cardiovascular disorders, tumours, autoimmune diseases, and infections. Genetically engineered proteins can be used as active substances, which are chemically and biologically exactly defined, for new drug products and in research to acquire new information on therapeutic use, based on the concept of therapy with endogenous proteins. Very recent developments have shown that proteins, either in their natural form or modified, are becoming of increasing importance for research into active substances.

PRODUCTION OF RECOMBINANT PHARMACEUTICAL PROTEINS IN PLANTS

Proteins are widely used in research, medicine and industry, but the extraction of proteins from their natural sources can be difficult and expensive. Also, the use of pharmaceutical proteins from natural sources can pose risks. For example, many people have contracted diseases from contaminated blood products or hormones. Other proteins, such as single-chain FV fragments (scFvs), are not found naturally. So, a simple and inexpensive system that allows the large-scale production of safe recombinant proteins would be highly desirable.

Traditional production systems that use microbial fermentation, insect and mammalian cell cultures, and transgenic animals have drawbacks in terms of cost, scalability, product safety and authenticity. Recent studies have shown that molecular farming in plants has many practical, economic and safety advantages compared with more conventional systems, and so the use of plants for large-scale protein synthesis is gaining wider acceptance.

This chapter discusses the technological basis of molecular farming in plants, with a focus on proteins that can be used for diagnostic, therapeutic and prophylactic applications. Chapter also provides a broad account of the types of pharmaceutical protein that can be produced on a commercial scale and examine the different expression systems that are being developed. The advantages and limitations of each system, with a focus on the biochemical constraints that need to be addressed for the technology to reach its full potential are also discussed.

Recombinant Proteins Expressed in Plants

Plants have provided humans with useful molecules for many centuries, but only in the past 20 years has it become possible to use plants for the production of specific heterologous proteins. The first pharmaceutically relevant protein made in plants was human growth hormone, which was expressed in transgenic tobacco in 1986. In this study, the hormone was expressed as a fusion with the *Agrobacterium* nopaline synthase enzyme. Since then, many other human proteins have been produced in an increasingly diverse range of crops. In 1989, the first antibody was expressed in tobacco, which showed that plants could assemble complex functional glycoproteins with several subunits. The structural authenticity of plant derived recombinant proteins was confirmed in 1992, when plants were used for the first time to produce an experimental vaccine: the hepatitis B virus (HBV) surface antigen. In a further report, the same group showed that the vaccine produced in tobacco plants induced the expected immune response after it had been injected into mice. More recently, the range of recombinant proteins made in plants has extended to include industrial enzymes, technical proteins that are used in research, milk proteins that are suitable nutritional supplements and new protein polymers with both medical and industrial uses. Examples of pharmaceutical proteins that have been produced in plants are listed in Table 7.1.

Table 7.1. Important pharmaceutical proteins that have been produced in plants.

Protein	Host plant system	Comments
Human biopharmaceuticals		
Growth hormone	Tobacco, sunflower	First human protein expressed in plants; initially expressed as fusion protein with *nos* gene in transgenic tobacco; later the first human protein expressed in chloroplasts, with expression levels ~7 per cent of total leaf protein
Human serum albumin	Tobacco, potato	First full size native human protein expressed in plants; low expression levels in transgenics (0.1 per cent of total soluble protein) but high levels (11 per cent of total leaf protein) in transformed chloroplasts
α-Interferon	Rice, turnip	First human pharmaceutical protein produced in rice
Erythropoietin	Tobacco	First human protein produced in tobacco suspension cells
Human-secreted alkaline phosphatase	Tobacco	Produced by secretion from roots and leaves
Aprotinin	Maize	Production of a human pharmaceutical protein in maize
Collagen	Tobacco	First production of human structural-protein polymer; correct modification achieved by co-transformation with modification enzyme
α1-Antitrypsin	Rice	First use of rice suspension cells for molecular farming

(Contd ...)

Protein	Host plant system	Comments
Recombinant antibodies		
IgG1 (phosphonate ester)	Tobacco	First antibody expressed in plants; full length serum IgG produced by crossing plants that expressed heavy and light chains
IgM (neuropeptide hapten)	Tobacco	First IgM expressed in plants and protein targeted to chloroplast for accumulation
SIgA/G (*Streptococcus mutans* adhesin)	Tobacco	First secretory antibody expressed in plants; achieved by sequential crossing of four lines carrying individual components; at present the most advanced plant-derived pharmaceutical protein
scFv-bryodin 1 immunotoxin (CD 40)	Tobacco	First pharmaceutical scFv produced in plants; first antibody produced in cell-suspension culture
IgG (HSV)	Soyabean	First pharmaceutical protein produced in soyabean
LSC (HSV)	*Chlamydomonas reinhardtii*	First example of molecular farming in algae
Recombinant subunit vaccines		
Hepatitis B virus envelope protein	Tobacco	First vaccine candidate expressed in plants; third plant-derived vaccine to reach clinical trials stage
Rabies virus glycoprotein	Tomato	First example of an 'edible vaccine' expressed in edible plant tissue
Escherichia coli heat-labile enterotoxin	Tobacco, potato	First plant vaccine to reach clinical trials stage
Norwalk virus capsid protein	Potato	Second plant vaccine to reach clinical trials stage
Diabetes autoantigen	Tobacco, potato	First plant-derived vaccine for an autoimmune disease
Cholera toxin B subunit	Tobacco, potato	First vaccine candidate expressed in chloroplasts
Cholera toxin B and A2 subunits, rotavirus enterotoxin and enterotoxigenic *E. coli* fimbrial antigen fusions	Potato	First plant-derived multivalent recombinant antigen designed for protection against several enteric diseases
Porcine transmissible gastroenteritis virus glycoprotein S	Tobacco, maize	First example of oral feeding inducing protection in an animal

HSV, herpes simplex virus; IgG, immunoglobulin G; IgM, immunoglobulin M; LSC, long single chain; *nos*, nopaline synthase; scFv, single-chain FV fragment; SIgA, secretory immunoglobulin A.

Proteins as pharmaceuticals

Many pharmaceutical proteins of mammalian origin have been synthesised in plants. These range from blood products, such as human serum albumin for which there is an annual demand of more than 500 tonnes, to cytokines and other signalling molecules that are required in much smaller amounts. Until recently, most plant-derived proteins have been produced in transgenic tobacco and extracted directly from leaves. Generally, these proteins are produced at low levels, typically less than 0.1 per cent of the total soluble protein. This low level of production probably reflects a combination of factors, with poor protein folding and stability among the most important. In the past few years, the tobacco chloroplast system has been used to express human proteins at much higher levels. Human growth hormone was produced in transplastomic tobacco leaves at levels exceeding 7 per cent of the total soluble protein and human serum albumin was produced at levels greater than 11 per cent of the total soluble protein. Higher expression levels have also been obtained in other plant species. For example, hirudin, which is expressed as a fusion to the oil-body protein oleosin, has been produced in transgenic canola at 0.3 per cent of the total seed protein.

Recombinant antibodies

Antibodies are complex glycoproteins that recognise and bind to target antigens with great specificity. This individual and specific binding activity allows antibodies to be used for a range of applications, including the diagnosis, prevention and treatment of disease.

The production of antibodies in plants represents a special challenge because the molecules must fold and assemble correctly to recognise their cognate antigens. Typical serum antibodies are tetramers of two identical heavy chains and two identical light chains; however, there are more complex forms, such as secretory antibodies, which are dimers of the typical serum antibody and include two extra polypeptide chains. Two different cell types are required to assemble such antibodies in mammals, but plants that express four different transgenes can assemble these antibodies in a single cell.

As well as full size immunoglobulins, further antibody derivatives have been expressed successfully in plants, including Fab fragments, scFvs, bispecific Fvs, diabodies, minibodies, single variable domains, antibodyfusion proteins, large single-chain antibodies and camelid heavy-chain antibodies. Unlike the proteins discussed above, antibodies have been expressed in many different plant systems and extensive comparisons have been carried out to determine optimal parameters for expression. Therefore, yields in excess of 1 per cent of the total soluble protein are routine and antibodies are set to become the first generation of plant-derived therapeutic proteins to be produced on a commercial basis. Although tobacco was used in the early studies, many antibodies are now produced in cereal seeds instead, as protein accumulation in dry seeds allows long-term storage at ambient temperatures without notable degradation or loss of activity. Antibodies have also been produced in less established plant-based expression platforms such as agroinfiltrated leaves, cell suspension cultures and virus-infected plants. A particular advantage of these systems is the short development time and rapid onset of protein production, which can be counted in weeks rather than the several months that are required to establish a production line of transgenic or transplastomic plants.

At least six types of plant-derived recombinant antibody have progressed to the preclinical testing stage, with the most advanced product now undergoing phase II clinical trials.

Recombinant subunit vaccines

Since the HBV vaccine was produced and tested, the concept of oral vaccination with raw fruit, vegetables, leaves and seeds has risen in popularity. Edible plants, rather than tobacco, are now the focus of research into HBV vaccine production in plants, and clinical trials have been carried out with the surface antigen that is expressed in potato and lettuce. Two further vaccine candidates have reached the clinical trials stage, both of which are expressed in potato: the heat-labile toxin B subunit (LT-B) of enterotoxigenic *Escherichia coli* (ETEC) and the capsid protein of Norwalk virus (NVCP). These antigens, from two important enteric pathogens, might be ideal oral-subunit vaccine candidates, as both are multimeric structures that survive in the extreme conditions of the human gut. Each protein accumulated to high levels in potato tubers and was correctly assembled into oligomers. Clinical trials with the LT-B vaccine showed that the consumption of raw potato tubers that contained 0.3–10 mg of LT-B produced high titres of mucosal and systemic antibodies.

Other proteins of medical relevance

Plants have been used to produce several other proteins with direct or indirect medical applications. These include the milk proteins β-casein and lysozyme, which could be used to improve child health, and protein polymers that could be used in surgery and tissue replacement. Early experiments with artificial polymers that were based on bovine elastin provided disappointing yields, even though mRNA levels were high, which indicated inefficient protein synthesis. More recently, it has been shown that human collagen can be produced in transgenic tobacco plants and that the protein is spontaneously processed and assembled into its typical triple-helical conformation. The original plant-derived collagen had a low thermal stability owing to the lack of hydroxyproline residues, but this was remedied by coexpressing the enzyme proline-4-hydroxylase.

A synthetic spider silk has also been expressed in transgenic plants. Genes that were modelled on the endogenous silk protein genes of the spider *Nephila clavipes* were synthesised in the laboratory and introduced into tobacco and potato. Proteins up to 100 kDa in size and with 90 per cent identity to the genuine silk protein were produced in tobacco leaves, potato leaves and potato tubers, at up to 2 per cent of the total soluble protein.

Genetic Aspects of Molecular Farming in Plants

Gene constructs

One of the main aims in molecular farming is the production of recombinant proteins at high yields. To achieve high yields, expression-construct design must optimise all stages of gene expression, from transcription to protein stability. Expression constructs are chimeric structures in which the transgene is bracketed by various regulatory elements that are known to be active in plants. For high-level transcription, the two most important elements are the promoter and the polyadenylation site, which are often derived from the 19S and 35S transcripts of the cauliflower mosaic virus (CaMV). The CaMV 35S promoter is now the most popular choice in dicotyledonous plants (dicots). It is a strong constitutive promoter that can be made even more active by duplicating the enhancer region. However, this promoter has a lower activity in monocotyledonous plants (monocots), so alternatives such as the maize ubiquitin-1 promoter are preferred. The presence of an intron in the 5′ untranslated region of the expression construct has also been shown to enhance transcription in monocots. Widely used polyadenylation sites include those from the CaMV 35S transcript, the *Agrobacterium tumefaciens nos* gene and the pea *ssu* gene.

Promoters that allow the expression of a transgene in a particular environmental, developmental or tissue-specific manner might also be useful.

For example, there are several advantages to the restriction of transgene expression to cereal seeds and potato tubers using tissue-specific promoters, such as those from the maize zein, rice glutelin, wheat glutenin and pea legumin genes. The advantages of such promoters include the increased stability of the protein and the avoidance of protein accumulation in vegetative organs, so preventing toxicity to the host plant and contact with nontarget organisms. Inducible promoter systems, which respond to external chemical and physical stimuli, might also be used to restrict transgene expression on a temporal basis.

For example, the mechanical gene activation (MeGA) system that was developed by Cramer (CropTech Corp., Virginia, United States) uses a tomato hydroxy-3-methylglutaryl CoA reductase 2 (HMGR2) promoter, which is inducible by mechanical stress. Transgene expression is activated when harvested tobacco leaves are sheared during processing, which leads to the rapid induction of protein expression, usually within 24 hours. Many other inducible promoters have been developed—for example, those that use ethanol, dexamethasone and the insecticide methoxyfenozide—and have recently been reviewed.

Transgenes from heterologous species often have a different codon bias to the host plant, which might result in pausing at disfavoured codons and truncation, misincorporation or frameshifting. Such effects can be avoided by introducing silent mutations into the coding region of the transgene by site-directed mutagenesis, which brings transgene codon usage in line with that of the host. One of the most important factors governing the yield of recombinant proteins is subcellular targeting, which affects the interlinked processes of folding, assembly and post-translational modification. Comparative experiments with recombinant antibodies have shown that the secretory pathway is a more suitable environment for folding and assembly than the cytosol, leading to higher yields. Proteins are targeted to the secretory pathway through the inclusion of an N-terminal signal peptide in the expression construct.

Although most antibodies accumulate to higher levels in the secretory pathway compared with the cytosol, there are some notable exceptions, which indicate that intrinsic features of each antibody might also influence their overall stability. The oxidising environment of the endoplasmic reticulum (ER), the lack of proteases and the abundance of molecular chaperones are important factors for correct protein folding and assembly. Also, protein glycosylation occurs only in the endomembrane system and this modification is required for the correct function of many proteins of human origin.

In the absence of further targeting information, proteins in the endomembrane system are secreted to the apoplast, where they might be retained or secreted into the environment. However, antibody yields can be increased even further if the protein is retained in the ER lumen using an H/KDEL C-terminal tetrapeptide tag, as this compartment has a stabilising influence. Yields are generally twofold to tenfold greater for ER-retention compared with secretion. Proteins that are retained in this manner are not modified in the Golgi apparatus, which means that they have high-mannose glycans but no plant-associated xylose and fucose residues. Although the measures discussed above will help to achieve high intrinsic yields, the actual amount of recombinant protein that is then obtained ultimately depends on the processing and purification methods.

Other factors that influence transgene expression

Transgene expression is influenced by several factors that cannot be controlled precisely through construct design, which lead to variable transgene expression and, in some cases, its complete inactivation. Such factors include the position of transgene integration, the structure of the transgenic locus, gene-copy number and the presence of truncated or rearranged transgene copies. Several strategies have been adopted in an attempt to minimise variation in transgene expression, including, most recently, the use of viral genes that suppress gene silencing. Preliminary studies have indicated that the co-transformation of plants with a primary transgene and a viral-silencing suppressor notably increases transgene expression level. The ability to integrate single-copy transgenes into precise locations in the plant nucleus would eliminate position effects and the problems that are associated with variable locus structure. Several laboratories are therefore investigating ways to improve the efficiency of gene targeting in plants. In practice, however, commercially developed transgenic plants undergo an enormous amount of screening to identify phenotypic, yield and agronomic variation. The screening includes identification of the site of transgene insertion, which allows a rational risk assessment to be made of the likelihood of adverse unintentional effects that result from the transformation process.

Transformation methods

Two general methods are used to generate transgenic plant lines for molecular farming: agrobacterium-mediated transformation and particle bombardment, in which DNA-coated microprojectiles are accelerated into plant tissue. Each method has advantages and disadvantages, and the choice depends on a combination of factors, including the selected host species, local expertise and intellectual property issues. Other methods, such as whisker transformation, electroporation and protoplast transformation, have not so far been used for molecular-farming applications. The soil pathogen A. *tumefaciens* provides a simple method for the transformation of most dicot species and is commonly used for molecular farming in tobacco, alfalfa, pea, tomato and potato. Monocots can also be transformed by *Agrobacterium*, but in most cases the technology has been optimised for selected model varieties. Particle bombardment shows less genotype dependence and might be the preferred transformation method for cereals, such as rice, wheat and maize, as well as soyabean and other legumes. Particle bombardment is also necessary for plastid transformation, as the *Agrobacterium* T-DNA complex is targeted to the nucleus and is therefore unsuitable for gene transfer to chloroplasts. Transformation can also be achieved using *Agrobacterium rhizogenes*, but this organism is preferred for the production of transgenic root cultures. These transformation methods generally lead to the introduction of superfluous DNA sequences into the nuclear genome. In the case of *Agrobacterium* mediated transformation, this is because inefficient processing of the T-DNA border sequences often results in the co-transfer of flanking vector sequences that might sometimes correspond to the entire plasmid. In the case of particle bombardment, superfluous DNA transfer occurs because whole plasmids are generally used to coat the microprojectiles. Superfluous DNA transfer is a regulatory problem under the strict new guidelines for the release of genetically modified organisms into the environment. Therefore, several strategies have been developed to avoid the transfer of vector sequences during transformation. Incorporation of the *barnase* gene outside the T-DNA border sequences is one approach that works during *Agrobacterium*-mediated transformation. This ensures that all plant cells that contain vector sequences linked to the T-DNA are killed, as *barnase* expression is lethal. Clean-DNA techniques, in which only the necessary transgenes but no vector backbone or superfluous marker genes are introduced into the plant, were also developed for particle bombardment, after it was shown that the microprojectiles can be coated with minimal cassettes (essentially the promoter, transgene and polyadenylation site), without compromising transformation efficiency. Furthermore, transgenic loci in clean-DNA plants are considerably simpler than those of whole-plasmid transformants, and the plants show a notable reduction in the frequency of transgene silencing.

Post-translational modification

The protein-synthesis pathway is highly conserved between plants and animals, so human transgenes that are expressed in plants yield proteins with identical amino-acid sequences to their native counterparts. However, there are some important differences in post-translational modification. One example, as discussed above, concerns the inability of transgenic plants to correctly modify human collagen unless a gene that encodes proline-4-hydroxylase is also expressed. The main difference between proteins that are produced in animals and plants, however, concerns the synthesis of glycan side chains. All eukaryotes add glycan chains to proteins as they pass through the secretory pathway, but owing to differences in the levels of different modification enzymes, the glycanchain structures vary widely across different taxa. Plant derived recombinant proteins tend to lack the terminal galactose and sialic-acid residues that are normally found in mammals, but have the carbohydrate group α(1,3)fucose, which has a (1,6) linkage in animal cells, and β(1,2)xylose, which is absent in mammals although present in invertebrates (Fig. 7.1).

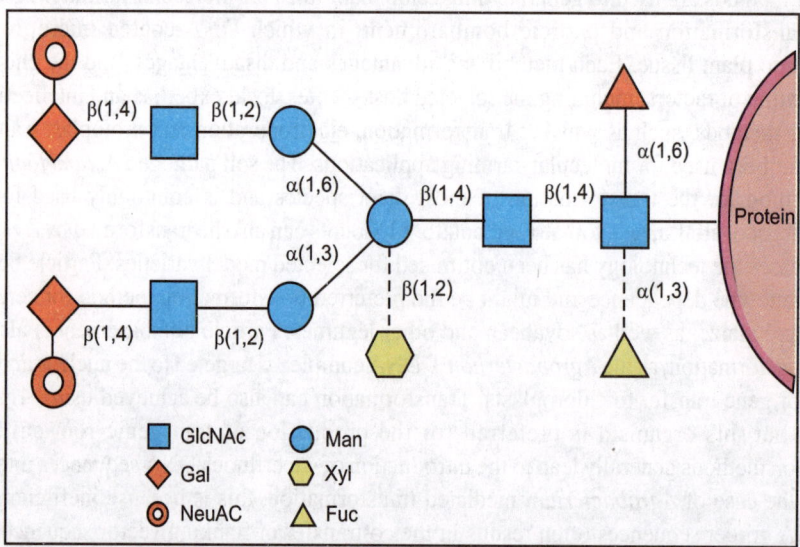

Fig. 7.1. Complex long-chain glycan structure in plants and humans. To 'humanise' the recombinant proteins that are made in plants, α(1,3) fucose and α(1,2) xylose residues must be removed (dotted lines), whereas galactose and sialic-acid residues must be added. Blue residues are common to plants and humans. Red residues are found in humans and not plants, so they need to be added. Yellow residues are found in plants but not humans and need to be removed. Fuc, fucose; Gal, galactose; GlcNAc, N-acetylglucosamine; Man, mannose; NeuAC, acetylneuraminic acid (sialic acid); Xyl, xylose.

These minor differences in glycan structure could potentially change the activity, biodistribution and longevity of recombinant proteins compared with the native forms. The possibility of plant-specific glycans inducing allergic responses in humans has been considered and the finding that human serum contains antibodies that are reactive against these residues has been interpreted as evidence that the α(1,3)fucose and β(1,2)xylose residues might lead to adverse reactions. However, carbohydrate epitopes are rarely allergenic. Moreover, the presence of antibodies in serum is not indicative of an adverse reaction. Finally, these glycan residues are also associated with every normal plant glycoprotein that is found in our diet. So, it is highly unlikely that they will be associated with adverse reactions. Indeed, studies in which mice were administered a recombinant antibody that contained plant-specific glycans showed no evidence of an antiglycan immune reaction. Nevertheless, the perceived negative effect of 'foreign' glycan structures is one of the most important issues that affect the use and acceptance of plant-derived recombinant proteins. Therefore, recent attention has focused on the development of strategies to 'humanise' the glycosylation patterns of recombinant proteins. Warner provides an overview of the biochemistry of glycanchain synthesis in different expression hosts, and lists the changes that are required to produce proteins with typical human glycan structures in plants. In the moss *Physcomitrella patens*, gene targeting has been used to disable the plant-specific fucosyltransferase and xylosyltransferase enzymes. Strategies that have been attempted in transgenic plants include the use of purified human $\beta(1,4)$-galactosyltransferase and sialyltransferase enzymes to modify plant-derived recombinant proteins *in vitro*, and the expression of human $\beta(1,4)$-galactosyltransferase in transgenic tobacco plants to produce recombinant antibodies with galactose-extended glycans. In the latter case, ~30 per cent of the recovered antibody was galactosylated. This is similar to the proportion of galactosylated antibodies that are produced by hybridoma cells. *In vivo* sialylation is unlikely to be achieved in the near future because plants seem to lack the metabolic pathway for the precursors of sialic acid, so several new enzymes would need to be introduced and coordinately expressed.

To place the issue in perspective, it should be remembered that there is natural variation in glycan structures, with many proteins having several glycosylation sites and, even in mammalian cells, a range of glycoforms. There are recognisable differences in glycan structure even when comparing native human proteins to those produced in rodent cell lines. For example, human antibodies contain only the sialic-acid residue N-acetylneuraminic acid (NANA), whereas rodents produce a mixture of NANA and N-glycosylneuraminic acid (NGNA). At this stage, it is hard to generalise about how crucial the humanised glycosylation of plant-derived pharmaceuticals is, and whether it might be more important for some classes of proteins than for others. Similarly, there are still not enough data to address whether the method of administration of recombinant proteins (oral versus injection) could make a difference in terms of the immune response that might occur.

Plant-expression Hosts

Tobacco production systems

Tobacco has an established history as a model system for molecular farming and is the most widely used species for the production of recombinant pharmaceutical proteins at the research laboratory level. The main advantages of tobacco include the mature technology for gene transfer and expression, the high biomass yield (more than 1,00,000 kg per hectare for close-cropped tobacco), the potential for rapid scale-up owing to prolific seed production, and the availability of large-scale infrastructure for processing. Although many tobacco cultivars produce high levels of toxic alkaloids, there are low-alkaloid varieties that can be used for the production of pharmaceutical proteins.

In most cases, nuclear transgenic plants have been used for production and the proteins have been extracted from leaf tissue. Targeting proteins to the secretory pathway in tobacco can result in them being exuded from the roots or leaves (rhizosecretion and phyllosecretion, respectively). Although not widely adopted so far, this strategy is potentially useful because no cropping or harvesting is necessary. The technology is under commercial development for the production of human secreted alkaline phosphatase. Perhaps surprisingly, even large molecules can be rhizosecreted from transgenic plants. For example, a monoclonal antibody was secreted into hydroponic culture medium resulting in a yield of 11.7 μg antibody per gram of dry root mass per day. Plants can reasonably be expected to survive in a hydroponic system for many months, and proteins are relatively easily purified from culture medium compared with extraction from leaves, so rhizosecretion represents an attractive option for antibody production.

As an alternative to nuclear transgenics, transplastomic plants are produced by introducing DNA into the chloroplast genome rather than the nuclear genome, a process that is generally achieved by particle bombardment. The advantages of chloroplast transformation include the high transgene-copy number (there can be several thousand chloroplasts in a photosynthetic cell) and the absence of position effects and transgene silencing. In combination, these properties can lead to astonishing levels of expression, in the best cases exceeding 25 per cent of the total soluble protein. Further advantages of chloroplast engineering include the ability to express several genes as operons and the accumulation of recombinant proteins in the chloroplast (which reduces toxicity to the host plant). As discussed above, both human growth hormone and serum albumin have been produced at high levels in tobacco chloroplasts, and each protein was found to be structurally authentic and biologically active. More recently, a tetanus toxin fragment has been expressed in tobacco chloroplasts and was shown to induce protective levels of anti-tetanus antibodies. The cholera toxin B subunit has also been expressed in chloroplasts, which shows that plastids can fold and assemble oligomeric proteins correctly. One disadvantage of the chloroplast transgenic system is that plastids do not carry out glycosylation. It is therefore unlikely that chloroplasts could be used to synthesise human glycoproteins in cases in which the glycan-chain structure is crucial for protein activity. Another limitation is that chloroplast transformation outside the solanaceae still presents a formidable technical challenge.

Recombinant proteins can also be produced in plant cell cultures. Tobacco suspension cells are generated by the continuous agitation of friable callus tissue, which results in a homogeneous suspension of single cells and small clumps. The cultures can be maintained in conventional microbial fermenters with only minor technical modifications, and various different culture modes can be used, including batch, fed-batch, perfusion and continuous fermentation. Fischer and colleagues have reported the expression of several recombinant proteins, including several antibody derivatives, in a suspension cell line that was derived from the tobacco strain BY-2. This approach is particularly advantageous when defined and sterile production conditions are required together with straightforward purification protocols. Recombinant proteins that are secreted into the culture medium are more easily purified, although proteins that are larger than 20–30 kDa tend to be retained in the apoplast and must be released by mechanical or enzymatic disruption.

Cereals and legumes

One of the disadvantages of recombinant-protein production in tobacco is the instability of the product, which means that the leaf tissue must be frozen or dried for transport, or processed at the farm. By contrast, the accumulation of recombinant antibodies in seeds allows long-term storage at ambient temperatures because the proteins amass in a stable form. Seeds have the appropriate biochemical environment for protein accumulation, and achieve this through the creation of specialised storage compartments, such as protein bodies and storage vacuoles, which are derived from the secretory pathway. Seeds are also desiccated, which reduces the exposure of stored proteins to non-enzymatic hydrolysis and protease degradation. It has been shown that antibodies that are expressed in seeds remain stable for at least three years at room temperature with no detectable loss of activity. Cereal seeds also lack the phenolic substances that are present in tobacco leaves, so increasing the efficiency of downstream processing. The main concern about the use of cereals and other established food crops for the production of pharmaceuticals relates to the potential for genes to spread into crops that are grown for food purposes, and the possibility of inadvertent contamination during seed collection and storage.

Important variables that must be considered when choosing a cereal production crop include the grain yield per hectare, the yield of recombinant protein per unit biomass, the ease of transformation and the speed of scale-up. The same single-chain variable-fragment antibody has been expressed in rice, wheat and tobacco to compare production levels in leaves and seeds. With the optimal promoter system (the enhanced CaMV35S promoter for tobacco and the ubiquitin-1 promoter for rice) it was found that rice plants showed the highest yields per unit biomass, and levels were lowest in wheat.

However, the wheat system is still under development and improved construct design will probably give rise to higher yields. Maize is now the main commercial production crop for recombinant proteins, which reflects advantages such as high biomass yield, ease of transformation and *in vitro* manipulation, and ease of scale-up. These factors, as well as intellectual property issues, prompted Prodigene to choose maize as the crop for the first commercial molecular-farming venture, which involved the production of the technical proteins avidin and β-glucuronidase. Maize is also being used for the production of recombinant antibodies and further technical/pharmaceutical enzymes, such as laccase, trypsin and aprotinin. Alfalfa and soyabean are legumes. They each produce lower amounts of leaf biomass than tobacco, but have the advantage of using atmospheric nitrogen through nitrogen fixation, thereby reducing the need for chemical inputs. Both species have been used to produce recombinant antibodies. One of the potential advantages of alfalfa is the recent finding that recombinant antibodies are produced as a single glycoform rather than the heterogeneous collection of different glycoforms that is found in other plant systems. Grain legumes are also useful production crops because of the high protein content in the seeds. For example, pea is being developed as a production system, although at present the yields that are possible with this species are low.

Fruit and vegetables

The main benefit of fruit, vegetable and leafy salad crops is that they can be consumed raw or partially processed, which makes them particularly suitable for the production of recombinant subunit vaccines, food additives and antibodies for topical passive immunotherapy. As discussed above, potatoes have been widely used for the production of plant-derived vaccines and have been administered to humans in most of the clinical trials carried out so far. The potential of potato tubers for antibody production was first shown by Artsaenko and colleagues, and recently this crop has been investigated as a possible bulk-production system for antibodies. Potatoes have also been used for the production of diagnostic antibody-fusion proteins and human milk proteins. Tomatoes, which were used to produce the first plant-derived rabies vaccine, are more palatable than potatoes and offer other advantages including high biomass yields (~68,000 kg per hectare) and the increased containment that is offered by growth in greenhouses. Lettuce is also being investigated as a production host for edible recombinant vaccines, and has been used in one series of clinical trials for a vaccine against HBV20. Bananas have been considered as hosts for the production of recombinant vaccines, as they are widely grown in the countries in which vaccines are most needed and can be consumed raw or as a puree by both adults and children.

Acceptability

Molecular farming involves the use of genetically enhanced plants to produce pharmaceuticals, and is therefore covered by a myriad of established and emerging regulations. Environmental biosafety issues, such as the potential for transgene spread and the possible toxicity of the recombinant proteins to nontarget organisms, need to be addressed on a case-by-case basis depending on the location, production host and product, taking into account measures that have been used to reduce biosafety risks. The rigorous scientific evaluation of each application for release will help in the development of effective risk-management strategies that will facilitate future decision-making processes. The main perceived risks are transgene spread by pollen dispersal, seed dispersal and horizontal gene transfer, and the effects of potentially toxic recombinant proteins on herbivores, pollinating insects and micro-organisms in the rhizosphere. There is also concern that plant material that contains recombinant proteins could inadvertently enter the food chain. Although it is apparent that pharmaceutical crops do not suffer the same acceptability problems as genetically modified food crops, risk assessment and environmental impact studies must be carried out to the same level, to ensure the highest standards of responsibility and regulatory compliance. The removal of selectable marker genes or the use of innocuous plant-derived markers for metabolic selection is required to limit the incorporation of superfluous DNA sequences. The risk of transgene spread by pollen dispersal can be addressed by several physical and genetic barrier techniques, as well as by the choice of a suitable production crop that does not outcross with wild plants near the production site.

The risk of horizontal gene transfer is thought to be extremely low. The potential for the horizontal spread of DNA from transgenic plants to bacterial populations has been considered. No such gene flow has been shown with nuclear transgenic plants, despite many attempts to create conditions in the laboratory that would simulate such an occurrence. Recently, Kay showed the horizontal transfer of an antibiotic-resistance marker from the chloroplasts of transplastomic tobacco plants to opportunistic strains of *Acinetobacter* spp. However, transfer was achieved only under idealised conditions in which the bacteria were modified to contain a sequence that was homologous to the transgene. No transfer was observed to wild-type bacteria. The potential for transfer is not surprising in light of the prokaryotic origin of plastids, but the transferred gene would need to offer a selective advantage to the recipient bacteria to persist in natural populations. All plants, both natural and transgenic, have been shown to be covered with antibiotic resistant bacteria, and these are a much more likely source of resistance genes that could jump to human pathogens. The possible negative effect of recombinant proteins on nontarget organisms can be addressed by the use of regulated promoters to restrict transgene expression to particular organs (for example, seeds) or to induce protein expression at particular times. The retrieval of proteins to the ER lumen, or the direction of proteins to other compartments such as the vacuole or chloroplast, can also improve the containment of proteins by preventing secretion to the apoplast and possible leaching into the leaf guttation fluid or the root exudates. Another strategy is to express the recombinant protein as an inactive precursor that must be proteolytically cleaved before it shows biological activity. Recently publicised incidents in which genetically enhanced crops have been inadvertently mixed with those destined for human consumption have highlighted the need for mechanisms to ensure the segregation of plants that express pharmaceuticals. Although greenhouse containment would address many of these biosafety issues, this negates the advantages of the technology in terms of low cost and large-scale production. If the main goal is to provide affordable medicines to developing countries, then these are important considerations for regulatory authorities. In any case, if food and feed crops are chosen for molecular farming, many other levels of safety can be built into the system. These include geographical isolation, differential planting seasons, the use of malesterile plants and transplastomic plants, and the use of inducible promoters, as discussed above. It would also be helpful to use identity-preserved varieties, such as white tomatoes or maize, which are easily identified by their pigmentation. Identity preservation and tracking are important parts of the regulatory procedure for the production of pharmaceuticals in transgenic plants.

ISOLATION AND USE OF cDNA CLONES

One of the more powerful approaches which has been developed over the last twenty years is the ability to make, isolate and use DNA that are complementary (cDNA) to messenger RNAs (mRNAs) that encode proteins of interest. It is also true that there are dozens of different approaches to isolating cDNAs of interest and these will be briefly discussed here. We will begin by describing how a cDNA for a known protein can be isolated using amino acid sequence information, which, historically, was the first way that a cDNA encoding for a known protein was isolated. In this first section we will also consider how cDNAs are made and how cDNA libraries are constructed.

Let us begin with three definitions:

1. Clone: Cloning refers to the isolation of a genetically homogeneous strain of any organism. Within a clone, all organisms are identical to all other organisms at a genetic level. It is possible to clone bacteria or phage or even higher plants by isolating a single cell and allowing that single cell to produce a colony, or a plaque, or an entire plant. Since most plants are derived from a single cell with a unique genotype, the act of rooting leaves to produce a collection of identical African violets is cloning.

    (a) cDNA cloning is isolating and amplifying a single, self-replicating organism that includes within its DNA, a cDNA that is of interest to the experimenter.

    (b) In some cases cDNA cloning may simply refer to the isolation of any single cDNA, since, in some circumstances, an experimentalist may be interested in any cDNA produced by a particular tissue. More frequently, the challenge of cDNA cloning is not the isolation of any cDNA but the selection of a single cDNA that is of interest to the experimentalist for a particular reason. In the same way it is possible to isolate clones that are not cDNA clones but rather are genomic clones.

    (c) Genomic clones are simply DNA derived directly from a genome. Genomic DNA would incorporate some sequences such as introns or regulatory sequences that would not be found in cDNAs.

    (d) Likewise, the isolation of a monoclonal antibody refers to the isolation of a single cell that expresses a mRNA for a unique antibody. Thus, making monoclonal antibodies an exercise in cloning.

2. Library: The second concept that is important in understanding the strategy needed to isolate a cDNA clone, a genomic clone, or even a monoclonal antibody is the idea of a library. A library is defined simply as a collection of different DNA sequences that have been incorporated into a vector.

3. Vector: A vector is simply a self-replicating organism which is usually designed for the convenience of its experimental purpose. For experimental convenience, vectors are usually derivatives of viruses (plasmids, bacteriophages, animal viruses, retroviruses). Since the essence of being able to isolate clones is the ability to replicate to make large amounts of biological material, the essence of a vector is that it must incorporate some mechanism of reproduction, (i.e. one must expand the clone to make many copies of the same organism). Thus, one would expect that vectors would incorporate an origin of DNA replication. Since vectors are an important experimental approach, a considerable amount of effort has gone into designing vectors that are particularly easy to use in an experimental sense. It would be impossible to provide even a brief description of the tricks that have been incorporated into various classes of vectors. The incorporation of selectable markers is certainly a significant experimental advantage in many cases.

Cloning Strategy

The underlying experimental approach to cloning can be divided into four parts:

1. First, it is necessary to produce or obtain a library including the sequence of interest.
2. Second, it is necessary to isolate clones that may be of interest.

3. Third, it is essential to develop a formal test to ensure that the clones that have been isolated are indeed the correct clones.

4. Fourth, it is essential to put the cDNA that has been isolated to some interesting biological use.

cDNA libraries

Let's consider the important aspects of constructing a cDNA library. A cDNA library simply contains sequences that are complementary to mRNAs. There are a number of different criteria that might be used to judge the quality of a cDNA library. A cDNA library is generally better if the size of the inserts (that is the amount of continuous cDNA in each clone) is large, ideally full-length. Ideally, no member of the library should include cDNAs derived from different mRNAs (this could be confusing). The library should be sufficiently large that it contains the cDNA of interest (or more precisely, it should have enough independently derived clones that it contains the cDNA of interest). In general this means that it should be representative of all the mRNAs present in a particular tissue. Of course, choosing a tissue that has a relatively large amount of the mRNA of interest is an important experimental choice. In general it is easier to isolate a cDNA from a library where it is represented many times than from a library where it is present rarely. Some characteristics of a library depend on the vector chosen. Vectors are frequently chosen because they allow the screening of a large number of independent members of the library with experimental ease. Some vectors are designed to express only the cDNAs, while others have been modified to express not only the cDNA but also to express it in a context so the cDNA is made into a protein or a fusion protein. Before using a cDNA library it is wise to determine if it is a good quality library.

Making cDNA

Generation of cDNAs can also be done by a wide variety of processes, but, in virtually all cases, cDNA is generated by the enzyme reverse transcriptase (RT) which has the ability to use the information in an RNA to generate a complementary DNA. Thus, reverse transcriptase is a RNA-dependent DNA polymerase. Like all DNA polymerases it cannot initiate synthesis *de novo* but depends on the presence of a primer. Since many mRNAs have a poly-A tail at the 3′ end, oligo-dT is frequently used to prime DNA synthesis (it is also possible, and frequently essential, to generate cDNAs by using either random primers or primers designed to amplify a specific mRNA). Once the initial cDNA has been generated it is generally necessary to produce a second strand of DNA. Again, there are many strategies for doing this, but a convenient mechanism involves exposure of the DNA/RNA hybrid to a combination of RNAase-H and DNA polymerase. RNAase-H has the ability to cause single-stranded nicks in the RNA, and DNA polymerase can then use these single-stranded nicks to initiate 'second strand' DNA synthesis. This two-step procedure has been optimised to maximise fidelity and length of cDNAs.

Incorporating cDNA into the vector

The next challenge is to incorporate this collection of cDNAs into a vector so that it can be manipulated. One of the most convenient ways of doing this is to attempt to manipulate the cDNAs so that each one has a unique restriction site at those ends. To do this, the cDNAs are frequently methylated with a specific methyl transferase that incorporates a methyl group into particular restriction site to protect them from the restriction enzyme that will be used later. Any 3′ or 5′ extensions must be then either eliminated by nuclease treatment or filled in with polymerase. This produces a 'blunt ended' molecule in which the 3′ and 5′ bases are in 'register'. It is then possible to ligate a synthetic oligonucleotide to the ends of this cDNA . Blunt end ligation is generally a low efficiency process; but, by using a high concentration of these synthetic oligonucleotides, it is possible to drive the reaction to near completion. These synthetic oligonucleotides can either be 'linkers' (which are synthesised to have one blunt end and one end that have an 'overhang' (i.e. region of single stranded DNA) that is complementary to that produced by restriction enzymes or they can be 'adapters' (which are a double-stranded DNA molecule that can be treated with a nuclease to produce the appropriate overhang).

The value of producing an overhang is that it will facilitate the introduction of the cDNA into a vector. The vector can also be prepared by treating it with the same nuclease, or a nuclease that produces the same restriction site, to produce a single-stranded region that is complementary to the single-stranded region in the cDNA. Mixing the cDNA of interest with the vector in the presence of ligase allows incorporation of the cDNA into the vector. One of the experimental difficulties in doing this is that the vector itself will have a high tendency to re-ligate to form a vector without any cDNA insert. This is frequently minimised by treating the vector with the phosphatase to remove the terminal phosphates. These phosphates are required for ligase to act, so this strategy prevents this unwanted side reaction.

The choice of the vector used also has an important impact on experimental outcome. Initially, plasmids were chosen as vectors and were modified to include markers that could be used to determine whether a plasmid had been introduced into a bacterial cell or whether there was a cDNA insert in the cloning site. More recently, derivatives of bacteria phage lambda has been made that can be effective vectors for cDNA cloning. The advantage of bacteria phage lambda is that it is possible to isolate more independent clones from a given amount of mRNA/cDNA and to screen a higher number of clones using hybridisation techniques. The extent of understanding of lambda and lambda genetics has made it possible to isolate lambda derivatives where some nonessential genes have been removed making it possible to carry inserts of up to 11 kb of cDNA, which is a convenient size and sufficient for the isolation of most cDNAs. The lambda genome is a linear molecule when it is packaged into the bacteriophage and the cDNA can be incorporated into the central region of the DNA. The lambda 'arms' (the more distal parts of the DNA) encode all the essential information for replication of lambda in an infectious cycle. The cloning site in lambda -gt10 was chosen to interrupt genes that are essential for lambda to undergo lysogeny. If the lambda arms re-ligate in the absence of an insert, and an appropriate host is chosen (*hfl*, for high frequency of lysogeny), then these particles will not form plaques. Thus only particles carrying an insert will form plaques. The remarkable power of bacteriophage lambda as a vector is that once the cDNA has been ligated into the lambda arms, the DNA can then be incorporated into a phage particle *in vitro*. Extracts prepared from cells that have all the necessary proteins for the assembly of lambda can then be mixed with the library DNA and ATP and particles will be assembled. These particles can then be used to infect *E. coli* and each individual plaque is an independent clonal population which represents a single cDNA species. This ability can be used both to amplify the cDNA library (which is somewhat dangerous because repeated amplification can lead to a loss of some cDNA sequences) and for the screening of the cDNA library to isolate the cDNA of interest.

Screening

A lambda-gt10 library can be conveniently screened by plating it at relatively high concentrations on a bacterial lawn of *E. coli*. High density screening allows the experimentalist to screen between 1,00,000 and 10,00,000 independent plaques on a single plate and makes it theoretically possible to screen for a cDNA that is present only at one copy per cell in a particular tissue. Screening is done by a 'replica plating' procedure. After the phage infect *E. coli* and form individual plaques, a perfect spatial representation of the infected plaque can be produced by placing a piece of nitrocellulose on top of the lawn of *E. coli*. Nitrocellulose binds DNA with great avidity and so some of the DNA of each plaque can be transferred to nitrocellulose paper or even several different nitrocellulose papers, each nitrocellulose sheet should have a representation of the original pattern of infected cells on a 'petri dish'. The DNA from the library can then be cross-linked to the filter and extraneous protein can be washed off. The plaques of interest can then be screened using a hybridisation assay.

This takes us to the question of how a library can be screened to isolate candidates for the cDNA of interest. One of the most straight forward ways to do this is to take advantage of DNA hybridisation. If one can design an oligonucleotide that is complementary to the mRNA of interest this can be used to screen the library. Such an oligonucleotide probe can be designed by sequence information from the amino acid sequence of a known protein. In the 50s and 60s biochemical methods were developed to produce amino acid sequence of overlapping fragments of known purified proteins. Our task is much simpler. It is now necessary only to know the amino acid sequence of a couple of regions of the protein. To do this, a purified protein is generally digested either with proteases or biochemical method to produce a series of peptides. Unlike proteins, which must be treated with care to ensure that they retain their native conformation, peptides can be treated as bio-organic molecules. They can be fractionated by fairly standard procedures using HPLC (high pressure liquid chromatography) which is capable of resolving individual peptides. If a series of individual peptides can be resolved, the sequence of those peptides can be determined, or at least partially determined, by Edmund degradation. This series of reaction cleaves individual amino acids one at a time from a peptide and the resultant amino acid derivatives can be identified.

This procedure can produce sequence information on a series of peptides. To do this intelligently it is essential that each of the peptides is derived from a single protein molecule, and the criterion for insuring that this is likely to be the case were discussed in the section on protein purification. Edmund degradation works via removing single amino acids from the N-terminal end and can in some cases be applied to an intact protein, however, generally the N-terminal amino group is chemically modified so this approach usually fails.

Designing a probe

A probe is an oligonucleotide that is designed to be complementary to the mRNA of interest so that it can be used to screen a library. Of course, any mRNA produces a unique polypeptide when it is translated; but the reverse is not true. Because the triplet code is degenerate, there are many mRNA sequences that might produce the same amino acid sequences. Because of this the design of an oligonucleotide probe is not straight forward, but a clever experimentalist can make good choices in designing a probe. There are basically two strategies that can be used. Either the experimentalist can choose to design a relatively short oligonucleotide that hopefully will have a high degree of homology to the mRNA of interest or the experimentalist can choose to design a longer probe that is more likely to have some regions that are not complementary to the mRNA of interest but hopefully will have at least some sequences that can form a stable duplex. In many cases it makes sense to make a mixture of different probes, which are homologous, but have different bases in positions where it is not possible to make a good prediction of which one should be present. This is called degeneracy. A probe can frequently be 64 or 128 fold degenerate; but too much degeneracy reduces the specific activity of a probe and increases the chance of hybridisation with the 'wrong' cDNA. The choice of which strategy depends on the amino acid sequences that are available.

There are a number of other factors that should also be taken into consideration. In many organisms, there is a preference for the use of particular triplets over the use of other triplets (codon utilisation). Designing a probe that has homology to a known mRNA is generally not recommended since this may lead to the cloning of the wrong cDNA. Testing of any probe for its correspondence to known sequences in the data base is, thus, essential. Using amino acids or amino acid combinations that have fewer potential triplet coding sequences or lower degree of degeneration (i.e. potential sequences) is of great importance. If multiple related probes are possible, it is often sensible to screen with a degenerate oligonucleotide. Once a probe or a series of probes are designed they can be synthesised chemically and labelled to high specific activity with ^{32}P. The oligonucleotide probes can then be incubated with the nitrocellulose filters to allow hybridisation. Conditions are chosen to try to maximise the specificity of the hybridisation, but allow for some potential mismatch. Most importantly, conditions should be chosen so that hybridisation which is nonspecific or occurs only with high degree of mismatch is not allowed. Thus, filters are washed to remove unlabelled or non-specifically bound oligonucleotides. The filters can then be autoradiographed to identify the regions of the filter corresponding to a, hopefully, specific signal. Since the filter is a replicate of the original plate, the experimentalist can then return to this plate and isolate the original plaque or group of plaques responsible for the signal. The plaques can then be re-plated on fresh *E. coli* (remember each plaque contains phage that can infected and replicate in *E. coli*), and the process is repeated to eventually isolate a single plaque that is responsible for the signal (i.e. Plaque purify it).

Test for specificity

While the isolation of a plaque that gives a strong signal is clearly an exciting step, it is only the first step. The next question must be asked: is the isolated cDNA really the one of interest? It could certainly be a cDNA for a related protein or a completely unrelated protein that just happened to have a sequence that would hybridise to the probe that was chosen. Thus, it is essential to develop some criteria that the right cDNA has been isolated or eliminated from contention. There are a number of criteria that will fulfil this need. The simplest advantage of sequence information that can be obtained from the isolated cDNA. In contrast to proteins where getting sequence information is experimentally difficult, it is relatively straight forward to get sequence information from DNA. The cDNA can be subcloned into a convenient vector and sequence information can be obtained. If the sequence of the cDNA that has been isolated also encodes the sequence of some of the peptides that had been sequenced but not used to design a probe, this is certainly persuasive evidence that the correct cDNA has been isolated. It would be hard to argue that the wrong cDNA had been isolated if sequence of several independent peptides were all predicted by a cDNA.

Frequently, there are also elements of the structure of the predicted protein that can be used to help confirm the correctness of the cloning procedure. During the characterisation of the protein, it is frequently known that the protein for example may be a membrane protein in which case one might predict the existence of transmembrane sequences. Some proteins are known to be phosphoproteins which suggest the presence of either serines or threonines in particular context that will allow kinase to phosphorylate them. Likewise, some proteins are glycosylated and the presence of amino acid sequences that are associated with glycosylation will also support the correctness of the cloning approach. Again, it must be emphasised that all of these are simply criteria that the correct cDNA has been isolated. These must be used by the experimentalist to develop a convincing case, but none are absolutely foolproof. In some cases, the pattern of expression of a protein (a tissue-specific manner) or a change in mRNA in organisms that carry a particular mutation that is known to influence the activity of the protein of interest can be a powerful criterion that will allow the experimentalist to make a persuasive case that the correct cDNA has been isolated. One of the most convincing approaches is to determine if the protein encoded by the isolated DNA has the biological activity of interest, but it sometimes takes time to do this experiment.

Getting full length cDNAs

In some cases, indeed in most cases, the cDNA that is isolated will not be full-length, i.e. it will correspond only to parts of mRNA but not the entire sequence. In this case it is necessary to re-screen the library, generally using the cDNA that already has been isolated to identify either a full-length cDNA or a series of partial cDNAs that would encompass the entire cDNA of interest. This brings up the interesting question of how an experimentalist knows whether a full-length cDNA has indeed been isolated. Consideration of basic molecular biology can provide a number of clues in this question. The molecular weight of a mRNA can be estimated by northern analysis and this can be compared to the size of the cDNA that has been isolated. Of it is possible that several mRNAs may be generated from a single gene by alternative splicing and this should be remembered. A mRNA should include both a coding region which has a long open-reading frame as well as non-coding sequences (frequently called UTRs, for untranslated regions) at both the 3′ and 5′ ends. An open reading frame is simply an uninterrupted series of triplets that does not contain stop codons. Such a coding sequence should predict a protein of an appropriate molecular weight which can often be compared to the molecular weight of the known protein. Upstream of the translation start site are frequently, but not always, found stop codons. The 3′ end of the message frequently has a poly-A tail. There is almost always special interest in clearly identifying the 5′ end of the mRNA. This sequence is often most difficult to obtain from a cDNA library since it requires effective reverse transcriptase to the extreme end of the mRNA. Often it is necessary to return to a cDNA library repeatedly or use specialised approaches to isolate an authentic 5′ end. Often, the best way to identify sequences at the 5′ end of a cDNA is to use RACE, which is a PCR based technique to amplify DNA sequences near either the 5′ or the 3′ end of a DNA. The authenticity of a particular 5′ end can be confirmed by doing 'primer extension' experiments. In this technique, reverse transcriptase is used to extend an oligonucleotide primer which has been designed to hybridise near the predicted 5′ end of a mRNA. The extension of such a primer should produce a polymer of a specific and predicted size.

Other Methods of Isolating cDNAs

The choice of how to isolate cDNAs depends on the interest of the investigator and the tools that are available. Design of an oligonucleotide probe has been used effectively in many cases but there are many other additional approaches that can be used. A few of them will be listed and described in this section.

Cloning from expression libraries

In many cases a vector can be designed so that the cDNA will be expressed, frequently as a fusion protein. In this case the cDNA has been incorporated into a vector in a position where it is within a coding sequence of another protein. The vector also incorporates promoter sequences that allows the protein to be expressed (both transcribed and translated). When such a vector is used to make a library it is called an expression library. Expression libraries have the advantage and disadvantage that the protein is present. In some cases this may mean that there may be selective pressure against the expression a cDNA of interest, but in many cases this expression allows for a novel screening approaches. The most straight forward of these is the use of antibodies to screen a library.

Screening with an antibody is quite similar to screening with an oligonucleotide probe, but in this case an antibody to the protein is the reagent that is available. This antibody can be generated experimentally, but it can also be available because of interesting autoimmune response in an animal model or in a human population. For example, some cancer patients develop an autoimmune disease that leads to neuronal degeneration. The antisera from these patients can then be used to isolate a gene which produces a protein that is recognised by this antibody. The antibody can be added to nitrocellulose filters under conditions where it binds specifically and the antibody can be then detected by a secondary antibody that is either labelled with an isotope or covalently attached to an enzyme like horse radish peroxidase that can be detected using standard enzymatic reactions.

If a cDNA is thought to encode a soluble factor that has a known biological effect, and if that effect can be easily assayed, then the assay could be a way to screen the library, although it may be difficult to screen a large number of independent isolates.

Complementation

Some genes can be isolated by a classic genetic complementation approach. If there is a method to select for the expression of a particular gene then this selection can be used to isolate a cDNA that encodes for that gene. For example it is relatively straight forward to select either for or against the presence of the enzyme HGPRTase (hypoxanthine guanine phospho ribosol transferase) in *E. coli* or in eukaryotic cells. If HGPRTase-deficient *E. coli* can be isolated and then transformed with an expression vector, those cells expressing the appropriate activity would become HGPRTase+. Since it is possible to select for such colonies, this would be an easy way to isolate a cDNA for HGPRTase from any organism. Complementation has been used to isolate many types of cDNAs including some that regulate complex phenomenon like the cell cycle or membrane trafficking. The power of this approach is that it provides such strong evidence for specific *in vivo* function. Of course, it is essential to independently establish that the correct clone has been isolated.

Expression on the cell surface with antibody screening

Cell surface receptors are special interest in biology and they can sometimes be isolated using an expression strategy. Cell surface molecules on lymphocytes for example have been identified by the isolation of specific monoclonal antibodies. Likewise, the ligand for many receptors has been isolated before the nature of the receptor is established. In both cases a cDNA for the cell surface molecule when expressed, will lead to the presence of a binding site on the cell surface. This binding site can be used to screen a library either by a method analogous to the antibody screening mentioned above or by using the ligand or antibody as an affinity reagent to 'pan' for cells that express the binding site.

Functional cloning of receptors

One of the more interesting classes of cell surface molecules are molecules that encode ionic channels. Because of the tremendous power and sensitivity of the electrophysiology (electrophysiologists can even measure the function of a single molecule), the presence of one or a few mRNA molecules in a single cell can produce enough ion channels to be detected relatively easily using an electrophysiological approach. Injection of mRNAs in frog oocytes can lead to the appearance of particular ion channels that can be detected either because of their responsiveness to electrical signals or the presence of extracellular ligands. This approach provided a straight forward assay for the cell-surface receptor for glutamic acid (glutamate), which is the most common neurotransmitter receptor in the central nervous system. This type of approach can either rely on expression vectors that can produce the mRNA of interest or it can rely on a negative criterion. Co-injection of cDNAs can squelch a signal by hybridising specifically with the mRNA. Of course the difficulty with any of these approaches is that it becomes more difficult to screen a large number of mRNAs. This problem has been successfully conquered by using strategies involving 'sib (for sibling) selection'. In this strategy, thousands of independent clones are screened at once, and, once a signal is identified in any one pool, the pool itself can then be subdivided until an individual clone can be isolated.

Homology screening

One of the most productive, although perhaps less creative approaches to isolating cDNAs is homology screening. Once an interesting gene has been isolated from one species, it is relatively straight forward to use a low stringency hybridisation strategy to isolate cDNAs from another species. Likewise, additional family members from the same species can frequently be identified. The power of this approach should not be underestimated. Interesting mutants are frequently obtained in Drosophila by using genetic screens and identifying the existence of corresponding genes in humans can be tremendously important. Likewise, because of the large population of humans in the careful monitoring of their medical care, human genetic diseases are proving an abundant source of interesting genes and eventually interesting cDNAs. Determining the existence of such cDNAs in model systems can then be extremely valuable. Good examples of this come from the field of apoptosis.

Some of the original genes like the ICE protease were originally identified in studies of *C. elegans* and subsequently human homologs of this genes were isolated. Likewise, the human oncogene, *bcl*2, was initially isolated by genetic studies which led to the isolation of the cDNA and subsequently homologs were identified in model systems.

PCR-based screens

PCR-based screening is also a method to isolate novel cDNAs. After two or more members of a family have been isolated, regions of homology can be identified. These regions of homology are conserved within the family, PCR primers can be designed and used to amplify reverse transcriptase products of mRNAs in an appropriate tissue. The molecular weight of known members of the family can be predicted and novel mRNAs may give rise to novel amplification products. These amplification products in turn can be used to screen cDNA libraries. In some cases even a single region of conserved structure may be sufficient to isolate novel genes using the following strategy. Reverse transcriptase can be used to extend a primer which has been made to a conserved sequence. Such products of course could be heterogeneous because different reverse transcriptase molecules would extend to different degrees. However, some restriction enzymes are capable of cleaving single stranded DNA and treatment of such a product with an enzyme of this type would produce a fragment of a unique size. Such a fragment can then be homopolymer tailed (i.e. a sequence of Cs can be added to the end of the molecule) using terminal transferase.

This sequence of Cs can then be used as a site to anchor an oligonucleotide primer containing a stretch of Gs. If this primer is extended the resulting product will be suitable for PCR amplification between the two primers that were used in its creation.

Plus/minus screening and differential display

Another useful approach to isolating cDNAs of interest relies not on knowledge of their primary structure, but rather on assumptions about their expression. Both plus/minus screening and differential display rely on strategies that seek to isolate cDNAs that are expressed in one situation but not another. For example, growth factors like NGF or PDGF and hormones like estrogen are known to induce the expression of novel genes. Thus, a population of cells that are cultured or grown in the presence and absence of such an experimental manipulation (e.g. +/–NGF, +/–estrogen, +/–retinoic acid) should express some genes in common, but have some distinct mRNAs. Likewise, tissues at different developmental stages may have expression patterns that are of special interest. Tissues that are related but distinct may also express interesting subset of genes. There are presumably interesting genes that are expressed in cerebellum, but not basal ganglia; or in T cells, but not B cells. An isolation of those genes may give a clue to the function of those tissues or the way gene expression is regulated.

1. In plus/minus screening, mRNA is isolated from two populations of cells and reverse transcribed to produce a population of cDNAs. Aliquots of these cDNAs can then be converted to probe by random hexamer priming and used to screen duplicate lifts from a library (i.e. two nitrocellulose filters produced from the same plate of plaques or cells. Any plaque or colony that hybridises duplicate lifts from a library to one probe but not the other is a potential candidate for interest, and differential expression can be tested by northern analysis or a related approach.

2. Differential display is a simple modification of PCR amplification. In this approach, mRNA is reverse transcribed using a series of primers. Frequently primers are chosen to have a random set of oligonucleotide and an oligo-dT section that would hybridise to a poly-A tail. mRNAs that are homologous to the randomly chosen sequence should be reverse transcribed, producing a single-stranded cDNA. The addition of another primer, again, randomly chosen will allow amplification of a subset of the reverse transcribed cDNAs. Depending on the distance between the two primers, fragments of varying molecular weights will be obtained. By doing this procedure with mRNA that has been isolated from two different cell populations, the pattern of expression between the two cell types or cell states can be determined. Again, an amplified product that is thought to be unique to a particular cell type, can then be used a probe to screen a library or test expression by northern analysis. Both of these methods have been used to isolate large number of interesting genes using only their expression pattern.

Two hybrid screening

One of the more active approaches to isolating cDNA are the two-hybrid screens. These screens are named because they take advantage of a specific protein–protein interaction that occurs between two proteins each of which is itself a hybrid protein. The entire assay relies on the ability of one part of each of the hybrid protein to form a specific interaction that is reasonably stable under physiological conditions with the other. A number of variations of this approach have been developed, but they all rely on the same feature.

1. In the most straight forward version a test cell which expresses an easily assayed gene, like beta-galactosidase, under the control of a well characterised promoter is produced. The promoter is chosen so that it has a low basal activity in the absence of stimulation from a specific regulatory element.

2. The same cell is then transfected with an expression vector for a hybrid protein. One part of the hybrid protein is derived from a transcription factor which is designed to recognise the DNA

regulatory element. Binding to the site, however, is not sufficient to induce gene expression; rather, a specific mechanism to activate transcription is required. A second part of this hybrid protein includes a sequence isolated from a particular gene of interest. This protein can be derived from another transcription factor, from a structural protein, or from an intracellular signalling protein. The only requirement is that the hybrid itself is not sufficient to activate expression of the reporter gene.

3. This cell system is then transfected with an expression library that also expresses a collection of fused protein. In this case the fusion protein consists of two part. One part of the fusion protein is coded by the collection of the cDNA libraries that the experimentalist hopes may encode a protein which will interact with target in the hybrid protein already expressed in the cell. The second part of this fusion protein is an activator of transcription, frequently the activating region of VP16, a potent transcription factor. If a cell is transfected with a hybrid protein that does not recognise the hybrid protein already present in the cell (the bate) nothing should happen.

4. In the rare case where VP16 is expressed as a hybrid with the protein that interacts with the hybrid already present in the cell, this should result in activation of beta-galactosidase. Thus, the screen serves as an initial assay for protein-protein interaction and is structured in such a way that a large number of members of a cDNA library can be quickly screened and selected for testing for specific interaction. Of course, there are always the possibility that activation can occur by a nonspecific mechanism, but this possibility can be tested for without too much difficulty.

Screening by databases

The rapid accumulation of sequence information and genetic data often allows scientists to bypass the steps required to isolate cDNAs. For example, if partial protein sequence or partial cDNA sequence is available, searching data bases may result in identifying candidate clones that can be ordered and tested to determine if they are the 'right' clone. Databases include the sequence of entire genomes as well as short sequences from cDNAs that serve to tag individual clones (ESTs, or expressed sequence tags).

Thus, each of these methods of screening a cDNA library provides a specific screen or assay for cDNAs that may be of interest. Just as it is true that when purifying a protein, one is likely to get what one assays for, in screening a cDNA library one is likely to get what one screens for. Determining whether the cDNA that has been isolated is indeed the one that is of most interest to the experimentalist requires additional tests.

In the absence of understanding of what those tests should be, it will makes little sense to do initial screenings. Likewise, careful consideration of what are the best screens for a specific purpose is likely to result in a more fruitful search with a higher percentage of successes.

INTERFERONS

Interferons are proteins produced by a cell infected by a virus, and provide protection to other healthy cells from viruses. Interferon was discovered in 1957 when Issacs and Lindenmann observed that virus-free fluid obtained from cultured cells infected with virus protected other cells from virus infection. They called the substance present in these fluids, which interfered with virus infection, interferon. There are three major types of interferons: (i) interferon-α (INF-α; produced by leucocytes or white blood cells), (ii) interferon-β (INF-β; produced by fibroblasts), and (iii) interferon-γ (INF-γ; produced by stimulated T-lymphocyte cells, hence also called immune interferon.

The mechanism of protection by interferons appears to be as follows. When interferon reacts with the interferon receptors of a cell the cell enters in a state called interferon-induced antiviral state. In this state, a rapid degradation of mRNA occurs if the cell is infected by any virus. Interferon induces in cells the production of 2,5-adenosine polymerase. When such a cell is infected by a virus, the 2,5-A polymerase is activated to produce 2,5 adenosine (2,5-A), which in turn activates preexisting but inactive molecules of ribonuclease-L.

Activated ribonuclease-L degrades all mRNA (of host as well as virus origin) present in the cell bringing the protein synthesis to a halt in such cells. This interferes with multiplication of the virus so that virus infection is either stopped or sufficiently slowed down to allow the production of adequate antibodies against the invading virus. The protection due to interferons is nonspecific in that interferon induced by anyone virus will provide protection against all viruses. It is possible that interferons modify ribosomes so that they no longer translate viral mRNAs, although they are fully capable of translating mRNAs of the host origin.

Interferons enhance the cytotoxic activity of natural killer cells (NK cells), which are a type of lymphocytes identifiable as large granular lymphocytes (LGL), NK cells are cytotoxic to some types of tumour cells.

Interferons are known to inhibit growth of some types of tumours; most of these tumours are also responsive to chemotherapy. Interferons, therefore, have been employed in treatment of the responsive tumours despite their prohibitive cost.

Interferons are produced from human leucocytes isolated from donor blood and cultured *in vitro*, and from mouse fibroblast cultures. The production scheme, in simple terms, is as follows. Large scale (1000 l to 10,000 l) cell cultures are infected with Sendai virus, and incubated for 24 hr after which the supernatant (clear fluid) is collected, centrifuged, and used for interferon isolation. The amount of interferon recovered is relatively small (1 g interferon of low purity from leucocytes separated from blood of about 90,000 donors), and the normal leucocytes are difficult to culture preventing scaling up from relatively small inocula. These contributed to the enormous price of the product.

GROWTH FACTORS

Growth factors belong to the group of proteins called cytokines; they can alter cell production, organogenesis, and disease susceptibility in animals. The effect produced by a growth factor will mainly depend on the presence of other growth factors, the target cells and their receptors on target cells. The nomenclature of cytokines is confusing and terms like interleukins, growth factors, colony stimulating factors, etc. are used often for a single protein. The term interleukin is the preferred one and new leucocyte products are designated by this name followed by a number, e.g. interleukin-13. The various growth factors can be grouped into the following families: (i) insulin like growth factors (IGF, e.g. IGF-I and IGF-II), (ii) nerve growth factors (NGF), (iii) epidermal growth factors (EGF), (iv) transforming growth factor β (TGF-β), (v) platelet-derived growth factors (PDGF), (vi) fibroblast growth factors (FGFs), (vii) hepatocyte growth factors (HGF), and (viii) haemopoietic growth factors (at least 16 cytokines; affect production and function of blood cells).

Many of the growth factors have been approved for treatment of human diseases. Erythropoietin (EPO) is used on a considerable scale for the treatment of anemia. Interleukin-2 in conjunction with LAK cells are being used for cancer therapy. Similarly, granulocyte macrophage colony stimulating factor and gramulocyto-colony stimulating factor are used to accelerate neutrophil recovery after chemotherapy or bone marrow transplantation. EPO is also used to stimulate red blood cell production in kidney dialysis or cancer patients. Several other growth factors have been/are likely to be approved for similar and other applications.

Human Growth Hormone (HGH)

Human growth hormone is safe when taken under the supervision of a reputed medical practitioner in cases of HGH deficiency. It is used by many today to build muscle and increase stamina without medical consultation. This could lead to a series of serious side effects.

Human growth hormone (HGH) is a naturally occurring hormone in a healthy human body. HGH is produced by the pituitary gland situated deep inside the brain, just behind the eyes. It is responsible for proper growth and development in all humans. Normal growth in children is dependent on the proper secretion of HGH and once adulthood is reached it plays an important role in metabolism.

It is a well-known fact that HGH is responsible for a person growing taller, but there are other areas where HGH helps in human development. HGH is proven to reverse muscle wasting in persons suffering from AIDS. It is claimed (not yet proven) that HGH supplements slow down the ageing process making one live longer.

HGH is today made of advent genetic engineering which is a complex procedure. A few decades ago HGH was made by removing the pituitary gland from dead bodies and processing it. The processed hormones were injected into HGH deficient persons.

HGH today need not be given by your doctor as an injection. They are available as pills and nasal sprays. HGH is helpful for children with HGH deficiency. This deficiency keeps their growth stunted. HGH supplements help them grow normally. This treatment will not be of any use to a stunted child who has got a normal secretion of HGH, but is stunted due to some other reason. Many athletes have taken to using HGH for its claimed muscle building and stamina increasing properties.

The use of HGH has increased of late since advertisers make you believe that HGH is the magic potion that can cure a vast variety of ailments. Many fall for these false and unproved claims and take HGH without any medical consultation. It is very possible that such people will suffer from some side effects, not benefiting at all.

OPTIMISING GENES FOR PROTEIN EXPRESSION

A vast number of different nucleic acid sequences can all be translated by the genetic code into the same amino acid sequence. These sequences are not all equally useful however; the exact sequence chosen can have profound effects on the expression of the encoded protein. Despite the importance of protein-coding sequences, there has been little systematic study to identify parameters that affect expression. This is probably because protein expression has largely been tackled on an adhoc basis in many independent projects: once a sequence has been obtained that yields adequate expression for that project, there is little incentive to continue work on the problem. Synthetic biology may now provide the impetus to transform protein expression folklore into design principles, so that DNA sequences may easily be designed to express any protein in any system.

At the heart of biotechnology is our ability to cause a cell to produce a protein it would not normally make. These proteins may be useful in themselves, for example as therapeutics or industrial catalysts. They may enable a cell to produce new compounds or to interact with other cells in a novel way. Whether a protein is a modified version of proteins that are naturally produced by the intended expression host or comes from another kingdom, its sequence must be encoded in a gene that the host cell recognises as instructions to produce appropriate amounts of the specified amino acid sequence.

One aspect of the design process that needs more attention, however, is the treatment of coding sequences. As in biotechnology, these are at the centre of synthetic biology: it is proteins that will catalyse the reactions in a novel metabolic pathway or be the signal transducers or the new biomaterials. There is an implicit assumption that, because we know the genetic code, it will be straightforward to choose a DNA sequence to encode any protein.

But we need to think about more than the sequences that will ensure enough mRNA and an adequate rate of translational initiation: the codon choices themselves must not limit expression under the anticipated conditions of use.

ENDONUCLEASE

Endonucleases are enzymes that cleave the phosphodiester bond within a polynucleotide chain, in contrast to exonucleases, which cleave phosphodiester bonds at the end of a polynucleotide chain. Restriction endonucleases (restriction enzymes) cleave DNA at specific sites, and are divided into three categories, Type I, Type II, and Type III, according to their mechanism of action. These enzymes are often used in genetic engineering to make recombinant DNA for introduction into bacterial, plant, or animal cells.

Restriction Endonucleases

Endonucleases are enzymes that produce internal cuts, called cleavage, in DNA molecules. Many endonucleases cleave DNA molecules at random sites. But a class of endonucleases cleaves DNA only within or near those sites which have specific base sequences; such endonucleases are known as restriction endonucleases, and the sites recognised by them are called recognition sequences or recognition sites. The recognition sequences are different and specific for the different restriction endonucleases' or restriction enzymes.

Restriction enzymes were discovered due to and named after the phenomenon of host restriction of bacterial phages. When a phase (say λ C) DNA released from one bacterial strain (Say, *E. coli* strain C; such a λ phage is designated as λ C) is used, to infect another strain (say, *E. coli* strain K) the efficiency of phage growth on the latter (strain K) is only a very small-fraction of the efficiency on the former (strain C). Some phages that survive grow normally on the second strain, and are now referred to as λ K; these phage particles infect strain K with the same efficiency as λ C does on strain C. Thus multiplying a phage on one bacterial strain seems to restrict the growth of that phage to the strain concerned. This restriction on phage host range is due to the presence of restriction enzymes in the host cells which recognise and cleave foreign DNA introduced in the cell. The DNA of a cell is protected from its own endonucleases by methylation (usually of A and C) within their recognition sites. Thus DNA molecules having the same methylation pattern as that of a bacterial cell itself will be recognised as own DNA, while those lacking this will be regarded as foreign DNA.

Restriction endonucleases are indispensable for DNA cloning and sequencing. They serve as the tools for cutting DNA molecules at predetermined sites, which is the basic requirement for gene cloning or recombinant DNA technology.

SMALL BIOLOGICAL MOLECULES

With recombinant DNA technology, it is possible to modify metabolic pathways of organisms either by introducing new genes or by altering existing ones. The goal is to create an organism with a novel enzymatic activity that can convert an existing substrate into a commercial compound that with current technology can only be produced by a combination of chemical treatments and ferementation steps.

L-Ascorbic Acid

Vitamin C (Fig. 7.2) or L-ascorbic acid or L-ascorbate is an essential nutrient for humans and certain other animal species, in which it functions as a vitamin. In living organisms, ascorbate is an anti-oxidant, since it protects the body against oxidative stress. It is also a cofactor in at least eight enzymatic reactions, including several collagen synthesis reactions that cause the most severe symptoms of scurvy when they are dysfunctional. In animals, these reactions are especially important in wound-healing and in preventing bleeding from capillaries.

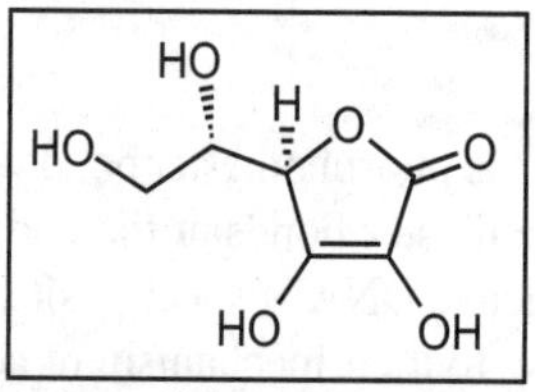

Fig. 7.2. Vitamin C or L-ascorbic structure.

Ascorbate (an ion of ascorbic acid) is required for a range of essential metabolic reactions in all animals and plants. It is made internally by almost all organisms; notable mammalian group exceptions are most or all of the order chiroptera (bats), and one of the two major primate suborders, the *Anthropoidea* (*Haplorrhini*) (tarsiers, monkeys and apes, including human beings). Ascorbic acid is also not synthesised by guinea pigs, capybaras, and some species of birds and fish. All species that do not synthesise ascorbate require it in the diet. Deficiency in this vitamin causes the disease scurvy in humans. It is also widely used as a food additive.

Biological significance

Vitamin C is purely the L-enantiomer of ascorbate; the opposite D-enantiomer has no physiological significance. Both forms are mirror images of the same molecular structure. When L-ascorbate, which is a strong reducing agent, carries out its reducing function, it is converted to its oxidised form, L-dehydroascorbate. L-dehydroascorbate can then be reduced back to the active L-ascorbate form in the body by enzymes and glutathione.

During this process semidehydroascorbic acid radical is formed. Ascorbate free radical reacts poorly with oxygen, and thus, will not create a superoxide. Instead two semidehydroascorbate radicals will react and form one ascorbate and one dehydroascorbate. With the help of glutathione, dehydroxyascorbate is converted back to ascorbate. The presence of glutathione is crucial since it spares ascorbate and improves antioxidant capacity of blood. Without it dehydroxyascorbate could not convert back to ascorbate.

L-Ascorbate is a weak sugar acid structurally related to glucose that naturally occurs attached either to a hydrogen ion, forming ascorbic acid, or to a metal ion, forming a mineral ascorbate.

Biosynthesis

The vast majority of animals and plants are able to synthesise their own vitamin C, through a sequence of four enzyme-driven steps, which convert glucose to vitamin C. The glucose needed to produce ascorbate in the liver (in mammals and perching birds) is extracted from glycogen; ascorbate synthesis is a glycogenolysis-dependent process. In reptiles and birds the biosynthesis is carried out in the kidneys.

Among the animals that have lost the ability to synthesise vitamin C are simians and tarsiers which together make up one of two major primate suborders, the anthropoidea, also called haplorrhini. This group includes humans. The other more primitive primates (strepsirrhini) retained the ability to make vitamin C, so this loss probably occurred in a common ancestor of the haplorrhini. Synthetic ability has been lost in a number of species (perhaps all species) in the small rodent family Caviidae that includes guinea pigs and capybaras, but lost in other rodents (rats and mice do not need vitamin C, for example). A number of species of passerine birds also lost the ability, but not all of them, and those that have lost it are not clearly related; there is some evidence that the ability was lost separately a number of times in birds. All tested families of bats, including major insect and fruit-eating bat families have lost the ability to make vitamin C, and this loss may derive from a common bat ancestor, as a single mutation.

These animals all lack the L-gulonolactone oxidase (GULO) enzyme, which is required in the last step of vitamin C synthesis, because they have a defective form of the gene for the enzyme (Pseudogene ΨGULO). Some of these species (including humans) are able to make do with the lower levels available from their diets by recycling oxidised vitamin C.

An adult goat, a typical example of a vitamin C-producing animal, will manufacture more than 13 g of vitamin C per day in normal health and the biosynthesis will increase 'manyfold under stress'. Trauma or injury has also been demonstrated to use up large quantities of vitamin C in humans. Some micro-organisms such as the yeast *Saccharomyces cerevisiae* have been shown to be able to synthesise vitamin C from simple sugars.

MICROBIAL BIOSYNTHESIS OF INDIGO

Indigo is considered to be the oldest dye. It was generally extracted from various species of plants initially. However, by the end of nineteenth century the commercial synthetic indigo almost completely replaced indigo production from the natural source. More recently, research work has been undertaken to find a way to replace the chemical synthesis of indigo by using bacterial systems.

The dye indigo is found in mammalian urine. P450 enzymes are found throughout nature from archbacteria to humans and can catalyse the monoxygenation of a diverse range of chemicals. It is generally believed that tryptophan is degraded by intestinal bacteria to indole. Some research workers considered the hypothesis that indole might be hydroxylated by P450 enzymes and finally carried out oxidation and dimerisation to form indigo spontaneously.

Human cytochrome P450 enzymes expressed in *Escherichia coli* can oxidise indole to indigo. The wild P450 BM3 enzyme from *Bacillus megaterium* catalyses subterminal hydroxylation of saturated long-chain fatty acids. However, P450 BM3 enzyme with novel function of converting indole into indigo has been obtained by directed evolution.

But most P450 enzymes act supported by one or more redox partners. NAD(P)H serves as the electron donor. However, use of whole cell system containing the P450 BM3 monooxygenase can ensure the regeneration of the cofactor NAD(P)H during the bioconversion. But free cells can be used only once in biocatalysis. To ensure reuse of the cells and reduce the cost, immobilisation technique is necessary to be applied. The encapsulation of biocatalysts in calcium alginate capsule is a widespread technique. It can enclose the biocatalysts in an aqueous solution inside a semipermeable membrane capsule. This technique has all the advantages of immobilisation in calcium alginate gels: biocompatibility, simplicity, and low cost. Moreover, the main advantage of this technique is that it has a specific liquid core which enables substrate and biocatalyst contact easily. This technique has been applied to immobilise microbial cells, such as *Lactobacillus rhamnosus* and *Lactobacillus casei*.

Indigo and indigoid pigments are widely used in the industry of textile, food, and medicine. Now people pay more and more attention to developing environment-friendly methods for indigo production, especially to microbial biosynthesis of indigo. Numbers of micro-organisms involved in the biosynthesis of indigo have been isolated and characterised, and monooxygenase and dioxygenase have been identified responsible for catalysing indigo biosynthesis. Some genes encoding for these enzymes have been cloned and used to construct 'engineering bacteria'. With this kind of bacteria, more efficient fermentation systems for indigo production have been exploited. In the meantime, biotransformation of the indigo produced by micro-organisms is under investigation. These progresses will bring us a greener method of indigo and indigo-like pigments production. New route of bacterial production of indigo: Cells of *Escherichia coli* K–12 containing a cloned fragment of *Pseudomonas putida* TOL plasmid pWW0 produce the dye indigo. Analysis of the cloned fragment and Tn1000 transposon insertion mutagenesis has identified the *xyl*A gene as being responsible for this phenotype. The xylA gene specifies xylene oxidase, a relaxed specificity enzyme that hydroxylates or monooxygenates toluene and xylenes and their corresponding alcohols. Indole, which is formed from tryptophan by tryptophanase in *E. coli*, was shown to be a precursor in the reaction sequence leading to indigo formation. These results suggest a novel route for bacterial production of indigo via hydroxylation of indole.

AMINO ACID PRODUCTION

The amino acid business is a multi-billion dollar enterprise. All twenty amino acids are sold, albeit each in greatly different quantities (Table 7.2).

Table 7.2. Processes for different amino acids and their uses.

Amino acid	Process	Uses
L-Glutamate	Fermentation	Flavour enhancer
D,L-Methionine	Chemical	Food , Feed pharmaceutical
L-Lysine HCL	Fermentation	Feed supplement
Glycine	Chemical	Pharmaceutical, soya sauce
L-Phenylalanine	Fermentation, synthesis	Aspartame
L-Aspartic acid	Enzymatic	Aspartame, pharmaceutical
L-Threonine	Fermentation	Feed supplement
L-Cysteine	Extraction, enzymatic	Pharmaceutical
D,L-Alanine	Chemical	Flavour, sweetener
L-Glutamine	Fermentation	Pharmaceuticals
L-Arginine	Fermentation	Flavour, pharmaceuticals
L-Tryptophan	Fermentation, enzymatic	Feed supplementation, phamaceutical
L-Valine	Fermentation	Pharmaceuticals
L-Leucine	Fermentation, extraction	Pharmaceuticals
L-Alanine	Enzymatic	Pharmaceutical
L-Isoleucine	Fermentation	Pharmaceuticals
L-Histidine	Fermentation	Pharmaceuticals
L-Proline	Fermentation	Pharmaceuticals
L-Serine	Fermentation	Pharmaceuticals
L-Tyrosine	Extraction	Pharmaceuticals

Amino acids are used as animal feed additives (lysine, methionine, threonine), flavour enhancers (monosodium glutamic, serine, aspartic acid) and as speciality nutrients in the medical field. Glutamic acid, lysine and methionine account for the majority, by weight, of amino acids sold. Glutamic acid and lysine are made by fermentation; methionine is made by chemical synthesis. The major producers of amino acids are based in Japan, the US, South Korea, China and Europe. Many microbe-based industries have their origins in traditions that go back hundreds or thousands of years. The amino acid industry has its roots in food preparation practices in Japan. Seaweeds had been used for centuries there and in other Asian countries as a flavouring ingredient. In 1908, Kikunae Ikeda of Tokyo Imperial University isolated the flavour enhancing principle from the seaweed *konbu* (also spelled *kombu, Laminaria japonica;* related to kelp) as crystals of monosodium glutamate (MSG).

Adding MSG to meat, vegetables and just about any other type of prepared food makes it savoury, a property referred to as *umami*. Soon after Ikeda's discovery, and recognising the market potential of MSG, Ajinomoto Co. in Japan began extracting MSG from acid-hydrolysed wheat gluten or defatted soyabean and selling it as a flavour enhancer.

Monosodium Glutamate (MSG)

Glutamate is the most abundant free amino acid in bacterial cytoplasm. Nevertheless, in order to be useful, glutamate producers must do two things well: they must overproduce glutamate in excess of their normal metabolic needs, and they must excrete it into culture broth. The precise mechanism by which *C. glutamicum* does these things is still not completely understood despite over forty years of study. Some physiological traits, however, are clearly involved. These include biotin auxotrophy of producing strains, a marked decrease in α-ketoglutarate dehydrogenase activity during production, and a predilection for exporting glutamate, perhaps via a specific transporter.

Many of the original glutamate-excreting strains were biotin auxotrophs, and growing in biotin deficient medium was found to 'trigger' glutamate production. Biotin is a cofactor (a vitamin) used by enzymes that carboxylate substrates. One such enzyme is acetyl-CoA carboxylase that converts Acetyl-CoA + CO_2 to malonyl-CoA in the first step of fatty acid biosynthesis. Biotin auxotrophs growing in biotin deficient medium were proposed to have altered membranes due to suboptimal fatty acid biosynthesis. Supporting the notion of altered permeability is the observation that growth at higher temperatures, or including detergents or cell-wall biosynthesis inhibitors like penicillin in the growth medium can also trigger excretion. Reduced levels of α-ketoglurate dehydrogenase during production may also be linked to membrane integrity. In corynebacteria, the enzyme has three activities on two peptides: the α-kg dehydrogenase + dihydrolipoamide S-succinyltransferase peptide and the dihydrolipoamide dehydrogenase peptide. The latter is shared with pyruvate dehydrogenase and is likely to be membrane bound and thus prone to being affected by trigger factors that alter membrane composition.

Since α-ketoglurate dehydrogenase catalyses a step in the TCA cycle, the cycle is largely incomplete during glutamate production, a circumstance requiring that pools of oxaloacetate be filled, as carbon is lost through glutamate. Anaplerotic enzymes replace OAA; these enzymes include pyruvate carboxylase (Rxn. 1), malic enzyme (Rxn. 2), PEP carboxylase (Rxn. 3) and glyoxylate pathway enzymes.

1. Pyruvate + CO_2 + ATP $\longleftrightarrow$ oxaloacetate + ADP + P_i
2. Pyruvate + CO_2 + NADPH $\longleftrightarrow$ malate + $NADP^+$ + H^+
3. Phosphoenol pyruvate + CO_2 $\longleftrightarrow$ oxaloacetate + P_i

The actual contribution of each anaplerotic enzyme or pathway depends on the growth conditions, production phase and a host of interacting metabolic signals. However, mutants lacking pyruvate carboxylase produce as much glutamate as wild type suggesting that PEP carboxylase is the major anaplerotic enzyme when growing on sugars. When growing on acetate or fatty acids, the glyoxylate pathway assumes a major role in filling OAA pools, although acetate is not normally used in the industrial process.

For many years, increased membrane permeability was thought to promote glutamate excretion. Recently, however, export via a specific efflux transporter has been proposed as a mechanism for avoiding exceptionally high levels of intracellular glutamate. Such an exporter has been proposed by analogy with the *Lys*E transporter that is responsible for lysine and arigine export in *C. glutamicum*. Other factors contributing to glutamate overproduction include metabolic flux alterations based on cell growth limitations. The following chain of events seems likely: A triggering mechanism (biotin depletion, high temperature, cell membrane alterations by detergents, oleic acid or antibiotics) results in a decrease or repression of α-kg dehydrogenase. The result is a redistribution of metabolites at the branch point in the TCA cycle leading from α-kg to succinyl-CoA or glutamate. The increase in glutamate levels, beyond that needed for cell growth, stimulates glutamate efflux as the cell attempts to maintain the proper level of intracellular glutamate. The result is the excretion of glutamate from the cell.

ANTIBIOTIC BIOSYNTHETIC PATHWAYS

Antibiotics of industrial, agricultural and medicinal significance like erythromycin, avermectin and validamycin are produced in vast amounts every year. Great efforts are constantly being made for the screening of natural compounds and for strain improvement by traditional means, but a rapid growth in research on diverse antibiotic biosynthetic pathways and metabolic engineering for new drug discovery has only started to emerge over the last decade or so. This section deals with the identification and characterisation of a series of gene clusters of diverse antibiotic groups and various biological activities, followed by the elucidation of their biosynthetic pathways and extensive effort for the generation of novel antibiotic derivatives by modern biotechnology related to metabolic engineering and combinatorial biosynthesis.

MOLECULAR CLONING OF THE WHOLE BIOSYNTHETIC PATHWAY OF A *STREPTOMYCES* ANTIBIOTIC AND ITS EXPRESSION IN A HETEROLOGOUS HOST

The application of molecular cloning to antibiotic-producing micro-organisms should lead to enhanced antibiotic productivity and to the biosynthesis of novel antibiotics by *in vitro* interspecific recombination. To allow such approaches, the genes for antibiotic synthesis must be isolated, analysed and perhaps modified. Certain *Streptomyces* species produce nearly two-thirds of the known natural antibiotics; the recent development of cloning systems in the genus makes it possible to isolate and analyse *Streptomyces* genes. However, antibiotics are metabolites which require sets of several enzymes for their synthesis and attempts to isolate the corresponding genes have so far yielded clones carrying either individual genes of the set, or only incomplete gene sets. Not only can the cloned DNA 'complement' all available classes of actinorhodin non-producing mutants of *S.coelicolor* but, on introduction into a different host, *Streptomyces parvulas*, it directs the synthesis of the antibiotic. The tendency for the genes for antibiotic synthesis to be clustered together on the chromosomes of *Streptomyces* species and the availability of plasmid vectors which can carry stable inserts of DNA larger than 30 kilobase pairs (kb) and which can be introduced efficiently into *Streptomyces* protoplasts, suggest that the experiments described have general significance for this area of biotechnology. Antibiotics—cloning of biosynthetic pathways: Biosynthetic pathways leading to antibiotics have often been found to be clustered, and new organisational forms of multifunctional enzymes have been discovered. Such polyenzymes accomplish the synthesis of complex metabolites such as peptides or polyketides by a sequence of enzymatic reactions. So, reactions leading to the tripeptide precursor of beta-lactam antibiotics, ACV, or to the cycloundecapeptide cyclosporine have been fused into single polypeptide chain synthetases, respectively. In certain isofunctional sites restricted similarities have been detected.

BIOPOLYMERS

Biopolymers can be produced through a variety of mechanisms. They can be derived from microbial systems, extracted from higher organisms such as plants, or synthesised chemically from basic biological building blocks. A wide range of emerging applications rely on all three of these production techniques. Biopolymers are being developed for use as medical materials, packaging, cosmetics, food additives, clothing fabrics, water treatment chemicals, industrial plastics, absorbents, biosensors, and even data storage elements. Table 7.3 provides a partial list of the biopolymers now in use.

Table 7.3. A Snapshot of the biopolymer family.

Polyesters	Polysaccharides (plant/algal)
Polyhydroxyalka noates	Starch (amylose/amylopectin)
Polylactic acid	Cellulose
Proteins	Agar
Silks	Alginate
Collagen/gelatine	Carrageenan
Elastin	Pectin
Resilin	Konjac
Adhesives	Various gums (e.g. guar)
Polyamino acids	Polysaccharides (animal)
Soya, zein, wheat gluten, casein	Chitin/chitosan
Serum albumin	Hyaluronic acid
Polysaccharides (bacterial)	Lipids/surfactants
Xanthan	Acetoglycerides, waxes, surfactants
Dextran	Emulsan
Gellan	Polyphenols
Levan	Lignin
Curd Ian	Tannin
Polygalactosamine	Humic acid
Cellulose (bacterial)	Speciality polymers
Polysaccharides (fungal)	Shellac
Pullulan	Poly-gamma-glutamic acid
Elsinan	Natural rubber
Yeast glucans	Synthetic polymers from natural fats and oils (e.g. nylon from castor oil)

Xanthan

Xanthan gum, a complex copolymer produced by a bacterium, was one of the first commercially successful bacterial polysaccharides to be produced by fermentation. The xanthan polymer building blocks or 'repeat units' contain five different sugar groups (Fig. 7.3). The xanthan-producing bacterium, *Xanthomonas campestris*, is one of the frost bacterial polysaccharide production systems targeted for genetic engineering. Under certain conditions, genetic modification of *Xanthomonas* by using recombinant DNA technology has increased the rate of xanthan production by more than 50 per cent. In the future, recombinant DNA technology may enable entirely new xanthan biosynthetic pathways to be created in host organisms.

Xanthan gum is produced by large-scale fermentation of *X. campestris* using a number of different feedstocks including molasses and corn syrup. The gum is extruded from the bacteria during the polymerisation process and can be recovered by alcohol precipitation following removal of the bacterial cells. For some applications such as enhanced oil recovery, the crude culture broth can be used directly following sterilisation.

Probably the most significant technical problem in the production of xanthan is the fact that as the polymer is produced, the fermentation medium becomes increasingly viscous. This increases the energy required for the mixing process that feeds oxygen to the bacterial cells.

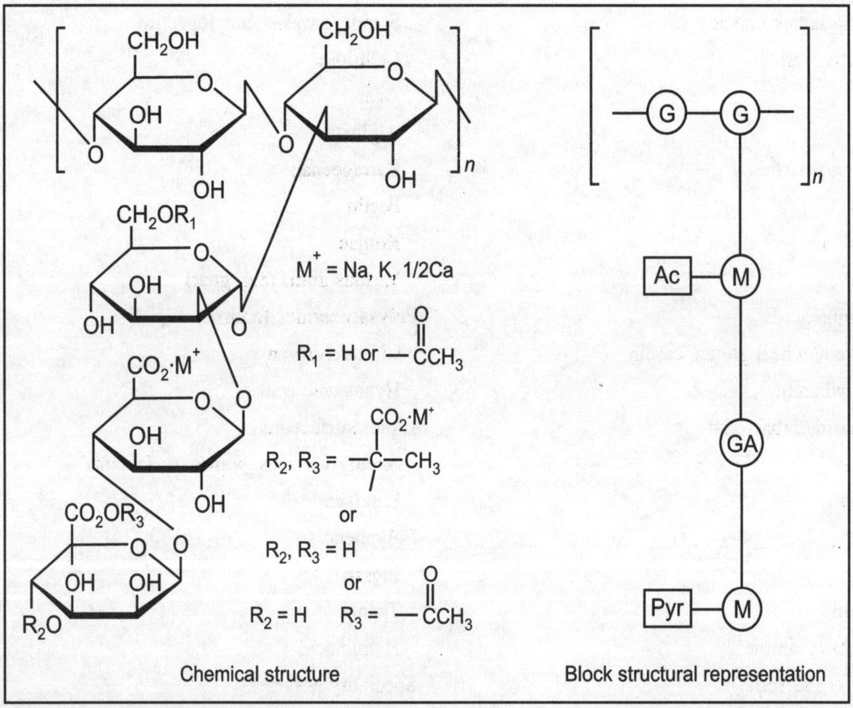

Fig. 7.3. The structure of xanthan gum. The Xanthan gum repeat unit is made of 5 sugar groups: two glucose (G) groups, two mannose (M) groups, and one gluouronic acid (GA) unit. Pyruvate (Pyr) and acetyl (Ac) units are also present in the mannose structures. The degree of pyruvate and acetate substitution varies with the specific fermentation conditions. The charged pyruvate molecule alters xanthan's electrical properties, while the acetate serves to stabilise the conformation or spatial arrangement of xanthan.

Dextrans

Dextran is the generic name of a large family of microbial polysaccharides that are assembled or polymerised outside the cell by enzymes called dextran sucrases. This class of polysaccharides is composed of building blocks (monomers) of the simple sugar glucose and is stored as fuel in yeasts and bacteria. Dextrans are produced by fermentation or enzymatic conversion of the feedstock sucrose, a product of the sugar beet and sugarcane industries. Most commercial dextran production uses the micro-organism *Leuconstoc mesenteroides*. Dextran can be synthesised by using either large-scale industrial fermentors or enzymatic filtration methods. The latter approach is generally favoured since it results in an enhanced dextran yield and a uniform product quality, which allows the product to be readily purified. Both of these production methods permit system conditions to be adjusted so as to control the molecular weight range of the products. This feature is an integral requirement for polysaccharide biosynthesis.

Pullulan

Pullulan is a water-soluble polysaccharide produced outside the cell by several species of yeast, most notably *Aureobasidium pullulans*. *Pullulan* is a linear polymer made up of monomers that contain three glucose sugars linked together (Fig. 7.4). For more than a decade, a Japanese firm, Hayashibara Biochemical Laboratories, has used a simple fermentation process to produce pullulan. A number of feedstocks are used for this process, including waste streams containing simple sugars. Pullulan can be chemically modified to produce a polymer that is either less soluble or completely insoluble in water. The thermal and ionic (electrical) properties of pullulans can also be altered.

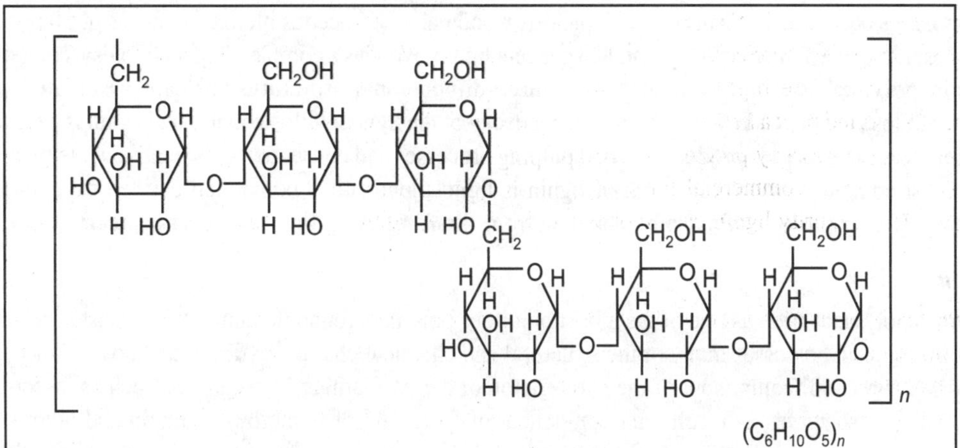

Fig. 7.4. The structure of pullulan. Pullulan is made up of glucose sugars linked together in groups of three. The three member repeat units are connected together in a branched fashion.

Selected Polymers of Plants and Higher Organisms

Starch

Starch is the principal carbohydrate storage product of higher plants. The term starch actually refers to a class of materials with a wide range of structures and properties. Starch polymers can be extracted from corn, potatoes, rice, barley, sorghum, and wheat. The principal source of starch for industrial and food purposes is corn. Starches are mixtures of two glucan polymers, amylose and amylopectin. These polymers are accumulated in plants as insoluble energy storage granules, with each granule containing a mixture of the two polymers. Plant breeding techniques have been used to produce new strains with altered ratios of amylose to amylopectin (e.g. waxy corn contains only 0.8 per cent amylose compared with natural corn, which contains 28 per cent amylose, and amylomaize can contain up to 80 per cent amylose). The ability to manipulate the ratio of amylose to amylopectin by strain development has drastically reduced the economic costs associated with physical separation of the two polymers. This is important because amylose and amylopectin have different properties and applications.

Plant cellulose

As mentioned previously, cellulose is one of the most abundant constituents of biological matter. It is the principal component of plant cell walls. Among the plant cellulose, cotton fibre is the most pure, containing around 90 per cent cellulose. Wood, on the other hand, consists of about 50 per cent cellulose. Cellulose serves as an important material feedstock for many industries. By adding various functional groups to the basic glucose building blocks of cellulose, a range of useful derivatives (cellulosics) can be created.

Lignin

Lignin is a polymer found in woody and herbaceous plants. Its principal function is to provide structural support in plant cell walls. Lignin consists of phenylpropane building blocks and belongs to the polyphenol family of polymers. Along with cellulose and hemicellulose, lignin is one of the three chemically distinct components occurring in plant tissue. Typically, woody and herbaceous biomass consists of 50 per cent cellulose, 25 per cent hemicellulose, and 25 per cent lignin. Wood is a complex lingocelluolosic composite. Lignin polymers are highly amorphous, three-dimensional structures that are associated with hemicellulose and play a key role in preventing decay of the lignocellulosic material. Lignin is generated in great quantities as a by-product of wood pulping processes and consequently is relatively inexpensive. The most common commercial form of lignin is lignosulphonate, a compound derived from sulphite pulping. Higher purity lignin can be obtained from 'kraft' pulping, but this process is more costly.

Chitin

Chitin, a polysaccharide, is one of the most ubiquitous polymers found in nature. It is almost as common as cellulose, and possesses many of the structural and chemical characteristics of cellulose. Chitin is an important structural component of the exoskeleton of a great number of organisms such as insects and shellfish. It also serves as a cell wall component of fungi and of numerous plankton and other small organisms in the ocean. Because of the different biological requirements of these various species, chitin is an extremely versatile natural polymer. Chitin and its most important derivative, chitosan, have a number of useful physical and chemical properties, including high strength, biodegradability, and nontoxicity. Currently, the principal source of chitin is shellfish waste, but given the seasonal fluctuation of shellfish harvests, genetically engineered microbial systems might be used to provide a stable supply of high-grade chitin compounds.

Hyaluronic acid

Hyaluronic acid (HA) is a natural product that is found throughout vertebrate tissue. It also occurs as an extracellular polysaccharide in a variety of bacteria. HA plays an important physiological role in many organisms. Research indicates that HA aids tissue formation and repair, provides a protective matrix for reproductive cells, serves as a regulator in the lymphatic system, and acts as a lubricating fluid in joints. Currently, most of the HA used for research and commercial purposes is extracted from rooster combs. In the future, it is likely that this biopolymer will be produced from fermentation broths of *Streptococcus* and other bacteria. Hyduronic acid is a long, unbranched polysaccharide chain, composed of repeating twin sugar units. Because of the high density of negative charges along the polymer chain, HA is very hydrophilic (has a strong affinity for water) and adopts highly extended, random-coil conformations. This structure occupies a large volume relative to its mass and forms gels even at very low concentrations. It is extremely flexible and has a high viscosity.

Chapter 8

Molecular Diagnostics and Antibodies

INTRODUCTION

The range of diagnostic tools available to the clinician has been steadily expanding since the advent of modern medicine. We are, however, at the threshold of seeing an exponential rise in this area, akin to the rapid developments in the field of digital technology that occurred over the last decade. The driving force behind the rapid expansion of the diagnostic market can be attributed to developments in biomolecular and genomic technologies.

The popular press regularly provides tantalising stories of how all disease diagnosis and therapy will soon become tailored to an individual's genetic makeup (often referred to as personalised medicine). Although the emerging field of pharmacogenomics (targeted drug therapy by taking account of an individual's genetic makeup) is expected to make rapid progress in the years ahead, there have been some setbacks and disappointments. Gene therapy is one of the more notable areas where the early enthusiasm has been tempered by difficulties in obtaining successful outcomes. Similarly, the discovery of the *brca* gene family and its putative link to breast cancer was followed by the realisation that genetic testing may not be highly predictive, especially for the Indian genetic makeup.

Molecular diagnostics has, however, been extremely successful in the area of infectious diseases where viral and bacterial genotyping has made rapid progress. Similarly, cancer diagnostics through mutational analysis and gene expression profiling, though still at an embryonic stage, is likely to be the next major breakthrough area in clinical practice. Although clinicians require a large range and high efficacy of tests to undertake correct diagnosis, laboratory testing currently accounts for only 1 per cent of total health costs worldwide, according to the World health organisation.

The current *in vitro* diagnostic segment is composed of various well-established tests that clinicians have come to depend on, including clinical chemistry, immunoassay, and others. Indeed, infectious disease and blood screening tests together are responsible for over 70 per cent of all diagnostic tests. The united states provides the major driving force, accounting for more that 50 per cent of sales. In this context, the overall market share of molecular diagnostics currently holds a modest position.

Although molecular diagnostics currently occupies a modest position in comparison to other segments, it is also clear that in many respects this is where the future is, as evidenced by its growth rate. Although estimates vary depending on the reporting methodology, there is general consensus that the current growth rate is in excess of 25 per cent. These estimates do not take into account many cutting-edge tests that are making their way into the marketplace, the so-called esoteric tests. This segment is increasing at a rapid rate for two reasons. First, a number of innovative companies are introducing early-stage, often fledgling new technologies, into clinical labs. And second, the rapid development of automated systems and point-of-care platforms is adding to the throughput of molecular testing. Together, these factors augur well for the future growth of molecular diagnostics with the accompanying prospect of greater affordability down the road.

The emergence of ultra high-end tests is in general accompanied by consumer concerns of high cost. The initial introduction of such tests therefore must often be targeted to the economic sector that can afford such tests. In this regard, there are three demographic factors that provide for an encouraging outlook in terms of market prospects. First, the economic boom has led to a striking increase in purchasing power among the middle-to upper-tier economic groups. Thus, although esoteric testing and disease-screening programs are largely at an embryonic stage compared to the West, the shift in economics and attitude provides for a more encouraging outlook in terms of the success of such efforts in the future.

The second encouraging demographic factor also relates to the economic boom. The arrival of multinational corporations in large numbers to the Indian scene has been accompanied by a similar growth in indigenous corporate entities, especially those catering to information technology (IT), business process outsourcing (BPO), and other related sectors. As a result, a new corporate mentality is emerging in India, one in which employee health issues, especially those of managers and executives, are of increasing importance. A parallel development has been the progressive expansion of health insurance programs that cover curative, diagnostic, and health screening programs. The continuing rapid expansion of the all over the world economy suggests that this trend will only accelerate, and with it, state-of-the-art diagnostic technologies should have a bright future in this marketplace.

Given the above demographic facts and trends, the future market potential for molecular diagnostics is widely believed to be extremely positive in terms of sales growth. These overall trends have made the manufacturers and distributors of premium-priced products and services very bullish on the Indian market. The benefit to the overall medical community in the world is that once market penetration has been achieved, the combined factors of financial return from investment coupled with advancing technology are likely to lead to cost reduction, allowing greater economic segments of the Indian society to afford these tests.

IMMUNOLOGY

Immunology is a broad branch of biomedical science that covers the study of all aspects of the immune system in all organisms. It deals with the physiological functioning of the immune system in states of both health and disease; malfunctions of the immune system in immunological disorders (autoimmune diseases, hypersensitivities, immune deficiency, transplant rejection); the physical, chemical and physiological characteristics of the components of the immune system *in vitro*, *in situ*, and *in vivo*. Immunology has applications in several disciplines of science, and as such is further divided.

Even before the concept of immunity was developed, numerous early physicians characterised organs that would later prove to be part of the immune system. The key primary lymphoid organs of the immune system are like thymus and bone marrow, and secondary lymphatic tissues such as spleen, tonsils, lymph vessels, lymph nodes, adenoids, and skin. When health conditions warrant, immune system organs including the thymus, spleen, portions of bone marrow, lymph nodes and secondary lymphatic tissues can be surgically excised for examination while patients are still alive.

Many components of the immune system are actually cellular in nature and not associated with any specific organ but rather are embedded or circulating in various tissues located throughout the body.

Classical Immunology

Classical immunology ties in with the fields of epidemiology and medicine. It studies the relationship between the body systems, pathogens, and immunity.

Clinical Immunology

Clinical immunology is the study of diseases caused by disorders of the immune system (failure, aberrant action, and malignant growth of the cellular elements of the system). It also involves diseases of other systems, where immune reactions play a part in the pathology and clinical features.

Immunotherapy: The use of immune system components to treat a disease or disorder is known as immunotherapy. Immunotherapy is most commonly used in the context of the treatment of cancers together with chemotherapy (drugs) and radiotherapy (radiation). However, immunotherapy is also often used in the immunosuppressed (such as HIV patients) and people suffering from other immune deficiencies or autoimmune diseases.

Diagnostic immunology: Diagnostic immunology is a collective term for a variety of diagnostic techniques that rely on the specificity of the bond between antibodies and antigens. Diagnostic immunology is well-suited for the detection of even the smallest of amounts of (bio)chemical substances. Antibodies specific for a desired antigen can be conjugated with a radiolabel, fluorescent label, or colour-forming enzyme and are used as a 'probe' to detect it.

The specificity of the bond between antibody and antigen has made it an excellent tool in the detection of substances in a variety of diagnostic techniques. Antibodies specific for a desired antigen can be conjugated with a radiolabel, fluorescent label, or colour-forming enzyme and are used as a 'probe' to detect it. However, the similarity between some antigens can lead to false positives and other errors in such tests by antibodies cross-reacting with antigens that aren't exact matches.

Immunoassay: An immunoassay is a biochemical test that measures the presence or concentration of a substance in solutions that frequently contain a complex mixture of substances. Analytes in biological liquids such as serum or urine are frequently assayed using immunoassay methods. Such assays are based on the unique ability of an antibody to bind with high specificity to one or a very limited group of molecules. A molecule that binds to an antibody is called an antigen. Immunoassays can be carried out for either member of an antigen/antibody pair.

ENZYME-LINKED IMMUNOSORBENT ASSAY (ELISA)

Enzyme-linked immunosorbent assay (ELISA), also known as an enzyme immunoassay (EIA), is a biochemical technique used mainly in immunology to detect the presence of an antibody or an antigen in a sample. The ELISA has been used as a diagnostic tool in medicine and plant pathology, as well as a quality control check in various industries. In simple terms, in ELISA, an unknown amount of antigen is affixed to a surface, and then a specific antibody is applied over the surface so that it can bind to the antigen. This antibody is linked to an enzyme, and in the final step a substance is added that the enzyme can convert to some detectable signal. Thus in the case of fluorescence ELISA, when light of the appropriate wavelength is shone upon the sample, any antigen/antibody complexes will fluoresce so that the amount of antigen in the sample can be inferred through the magnitude of the fluorescence.

Performing an ELISA involves at least one antibody with specificity for a particular antigen. The sample with an unknown amount of antigen is immobilised on a solid support (usually a polystyrene microtiter plate) either non-specifically (via adsorption to the surface) or specifically (via capture by another antibody specific to the same antigen, in a 'sandwich' ELISA). After the antigen is immobilised the detection antibody is added, forming a complex with the antigen. The detection antibody can be covalently linked to an enzyme, or can itself be detected by a secondary antibody which is linked to an enzyme through bioconjugation. Between each step the plate is typically washed with a mild detergent solution to remove any proteins or antibodies that are not specifically bound. After the final wash step the plate is developed by adding an enzymatic substrate to produce a visible signal, which indicates the quantity of antigen in the sample.

Traditional ELISA typically involves chromogenic reporters and substrates which produce some kind of observable colour change to indicate the presence of antigen or analyte. Newer ELISA-like techniques utilise fluorogenic, electrochemiluminescent, and real-time PCR reporters to create quantifiable signals. These new reporters can have various advantages including higher sensitivities and multiplexing. Technically, newer assays of this type are not strictly ELISAs as they are not 'enzyme-linked' but are instead linked to some non-enzymatic reporter. However, given that the general principles in these assays are largely similar, they are often grouped in the same category as ELISAs.

Applications of ELISA

Because the ELISA can be performed to evaluate either the presence of antigen or the presence of antibody in a sample, it is a useful tool for determining serum antibody concentrations (such as with the HIV test or West Nile Virus). It has also found applications in the food industry in detecting potential food allergens such as milk, peanuts, walnuts, almonds, and eggs. ELISA can also be used in toxicology as a rapid presumptive screen for certain classes of drugs (Fig. 8.1).

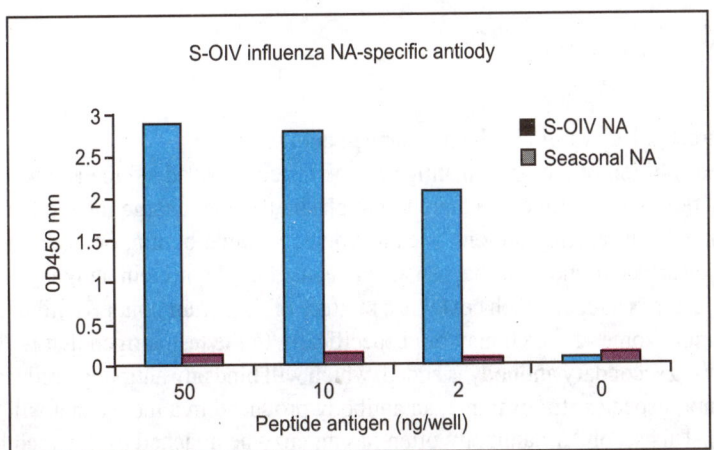

Fig. 8.1. ELISA results using S-OIV A neuraminidase antibody at 1 µg/ml to probe the immunogenic and the corresponding seasonal influenza A neuraminidase peptides at 50, 10, 2 and 0 ng/ml.

The ELISA was the first screening test widely used for HIV because of its high sensitivity. In an ELISA, a person's serum is diluted 400-fold and applied to a plate to which HIV antigens are attached. If antibodies to HIV are present in the serum, they may bind to these HIV antigens. The plate is then washed to remove all other components of the serum. A specially prepared 'secondary antibody' — an antibody that binds to other antibodies — is then applied to the plate, followed by another wash. This secondary antibody is chemically linked in advance to an enzyme. Thus, the plate will contain enzyme in proportion to the amount of secondary antibody bound to the plate. A substrate for the enzyme is applied, and catalysis by the enzyme leads to a change in colour or fluorescence. ELISA results are reported as a number; the most controversial aspect of this test is determining the 'cut-off' point between a positive and negative result.

A cut-off point may be determined by comparing it with a known standard. If an ELISA test is used for drug screening at workplace, a cut-off concentration, 50 ng/ml, for example, is established, and a sample will be prepared which contains the standard concentration of analyte. Unknowns that generate a signal that is stronger than the known sample are 'positive'. Those that generate weaker signal are 'negative.' ELISA can also be used to determine the level of antibodies in faecal content specifically the direct method.

Before the development of the EIA/ELISA, the only option for conducting an immunoassay was radioimmunoassay, a technique using radioactively-labelled antigens or antibodies. In radioimmunoassay, the radioactivity provides the signal which indicates whether a specific antigen or antibody is present in the sample.

Because radioactivity poses a potential health threat, a safer alternative was sought. A suitable alternative to radioimmunoassay would substitute a non-radioactive signal in place of the radioactive signal. When enzymes (such as peroxidase) react with appropriate substrates (such as ABTS or 3, 3', 5, 5'-Tetramethylbenzidine), this causes a change in colour, which is used as a signal. However, the signal has to be associated with the presence of antibody or antigen, which is why the enzyme has to be linked to an appropriate antibody. This linking process was independently developed by Stratis Avrameas and G. B. Pierce. Since it is necessary to remove any unbound antibody or antigen by washing, the antibody or antigen has to be fixed to the surface of the container, i.e. the *immunosorbent* has to be prepared.

Types of ELISA

Indirect ELISA

The steps of 'indirect' ELISA follows the mechanism below:
1. A buffered solution of the protein antigen to be tested for is added to each well of a microtiter plate, where it is given time to adhere to the plastic through charge interactions.
2. A solution of non-reacting protein, such as bovine serum albumin, or casein is added to block any plastic surface in the well that remains uncoated by the protein antigen.
3. Then the serum is added, which contains a mixture of the serum donor's antibodies, of unknown concentration, some of which may bind specifically to the test antigen that is coating the well.
4. Afterwards, a secondary antibody is added, which will bind any antibody produced by a member of the donor's species (for example, an antibody produced in a mouse that will bind any rabbit antibody). This secondary antibody often has an enzyme attached to it, which has a negligible effect on the binding properties of the antibody.
5. A substrate for this enzyme is then added. Often, this substrate changes colour upon reaction with the enzyme. The colour change shows that secondary antibody has bound to primary antibody, which strongly implies that the donor has had an immune reaction to the test antigen. This can be helpful in a clinical setting, and in R & D.
6. The higher the concentration of the primary antibody that was present in the serum, the stronger the colour change. Often a spectrometer is used to give quantitative values for colour strength.

The enzyme acts as an amplifier; even if only few enzyme-linked antibodies remain bound, the enzyme molecules will produce many signal molecules. Within common-sense limitations the enzyme can go on producing colour indefinitely, but the more primary antibody is present in the donor serum, the more secondary antibody + enzyme will bind, and the faster colour will develop. A major disadvantage of the indirect ELISA is that the method of antigen immobilisation is non-specific; when serum is used as the source of test antigen, all proteins in the sample may stick to the microtiter plate well, so small concentrations of analyte in serum must compete with other serum proteins when binding to the well surface. The sandwich or direct ELISA provides a solution to this problem, by using a 'capture' antibody specific for the test antigen to pull it out of the serum's molecular mixture.

ELISA may be run in a qualitative or quantitative format. Qualitative results provide a simple positive or negative result (yes or no) for a sample. The cutoff between positive and negative is determined by the analyst and may be statistical. Two or three times the standard deviation (error inherent in a test) is often used to distinguish positive from negative samples. In quantitative ELISA, the optical density (OD) of the sample is compared to a standard curve, which is typically a serial dilution of a known-concentration solution of the target molecule. For example if your test sample returns an OD of 1.0, the point on your standard curve that gave OD = 1.0 must be of the same analyte concentration as your sample.

Sandwich ELISA

A less-common variant of this technique, called 'sandwich' ELISA, is used to detect sample antigen. The steps are as follows:
1. Prepare a surface to which a known quantity of capture antibody is bound.
2. Block any non specific binding sites on the surface.
3. Apply the antigen-containing sample to the plate.
4. Wash the plate, so that unbound antigen is removed.
5. Apply enzyme linked primary antibodies as detection antibodies which also bind specifically to the antigen.
6. Wash the plate, so that the unbound antibody-enzyme conjugates are removed.
7. Apply a chemical which is converted by the enzyme into a colour or fluorescent or electrochemical signal.
8. Measure the absorbency or fluorescence or electrochemical signal (e.g. current) of the plate wells to determine the presence and quantity of antigen.

The Fig. 8.2 includes the use of a secondary antibody conjugated to an enzyme, though technically this is not necessary if the primary antibody is conjugated to an enzyme. However, use of a secondary-antibody conjugate avoids the expensive process of creating enzyme-linked antibodies for every antigen one might want to detect. By using an enzyme-linked antibody that binds the Fc region of other antibodies, this same enzyme-linked antibody can be used in a variety of situations. Without the first layer of 'capture' antibody, any proteins in the sample (including serum proteins) may competitively adsorb to the plate surface, lowering the quantity of antigen immobilised. Use of the purified specific antibody to attach the antigen to the plastic eliminates a need to purify the antigen from complicated mixtures before the measurement, simplifying the assay, and increasing the specificity and the sensitivity of the assay. A descriptive animation of the application of sandwich ELISA to home pregnancy testing can be found here.

Competitive ELISA

A third use of ELISA is through competitive binding. The steps for this ELISA are somewhat different than the first two examples:
1. Unlabelled antibody is incubated in the presence of its antigen.
2. These bound antibody/antigen complexes are then added to an antigen coated well.

3. The plate is washed, so that unbound antibody is removed. (The more antigen in the sample, the less antibody will be able to bind to the antigen in the well, hence 'competition.')
4. The secondary antibody, specific to the primary antibody is added. This second antibody is coupled to the enzyme.
5. A substrate is added, and remaining enzymes elicit a chromogenic or fluorescent signal.

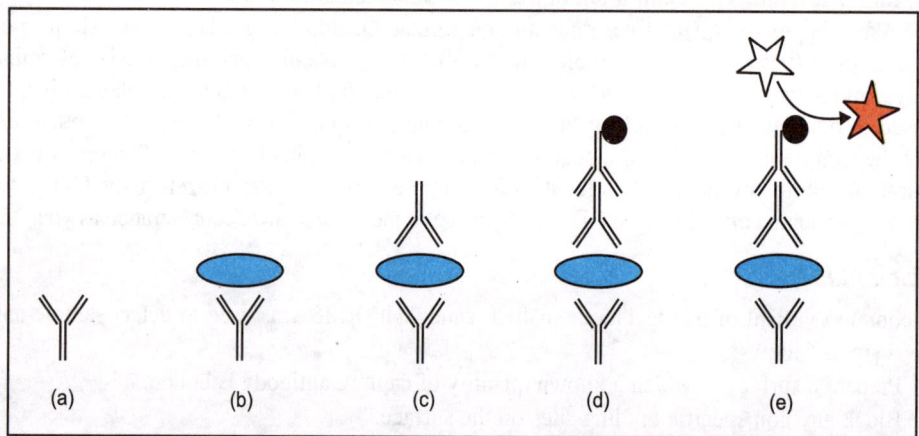

Fig. 8.2. A sandwich ELISA. (a) Plate is coated with a capture antibody, (b) sample is added, and any antigen present binds to capture antibody, (c) detecting antibody is added, and binds to antigen, (d) enzyme-linked secondary antibody is added, and binds to detecting antibody, (e) substrate is added, and is converted by enzyme to detectable form.

For competitive ELISA, the higher the sample antigen concentration, the weaker the eventual signal. The major advantage of a competitive ELISA is the ability to use crude or impure samples and still selectively bind any antigen that may be present.

(Note that some competitive ELISA kits include enzyme-linked antigen rather than enzyme-linked antibody. The labelled antigen competes for primary antibody binding sites with your sample antigen (unlabelled). The more antigen in the sample, the less labelled antigen is retained in the well and the weaker the signal). Commonly the antigen is not first positioned in the well.

Reverse ELISA

A new technique uses a solid phase made up of an immunosorbent polystyrene rod with 4–12 protruding ogives. The entire device is immersed in a test tube containing the collected sample and the following steps (washing, incubation in conjugate and incubation in chromogenous) are carried out by dipping the ogives in microwells of standard microplates pre-filled with reagents.

The advantages of this technique are as follows:

1. The ogives can each be sensitised to a different reagent, allowing the simultaneous detection of different antibodies and different antigens for multi-target assays.
2. The sample volume can be increased to improve the test sensitivity in clinical (saliva, urine), food (bulk milk, pooled eggs) and environmental (water) samples.
3. One ogive is left unsensitised to measure the non-specific reactions of the sample.
4. The use of laboratory supplies for dispensing sample aliquots, washing solution and reagents in microwells is not required, facilitating ready-to-use lab-kits and on-site kits.

STRUCTURE AND FUNCTION OF ANTIBODY

Antibodies (also known as immunoglobulins, abbreviated Ig) are gamma globulin proteins that are found in blood or other bodily fluids of vertebrates, and are used by the immune system to identify and neutralise foreign objects, such as bacteria and viruses. They are typically made of basic structural units—each with two large heavy chains and two small light chains—to form, for example, monomers with one unit, dimers with two units or pentamers with five units. Antibodies are produced by a kind of white blood cell called a plasma cell. There are several different types of antibody heavy chains, and several different kinds of antibodies, which are grouped into different isotypes based on which heavy chain they possess. Five different antibody isotypes are known in mammals, which perform different roles, and help direct the appropriate immune response for each different type of foreign object they encounter (Fig. 8.3).

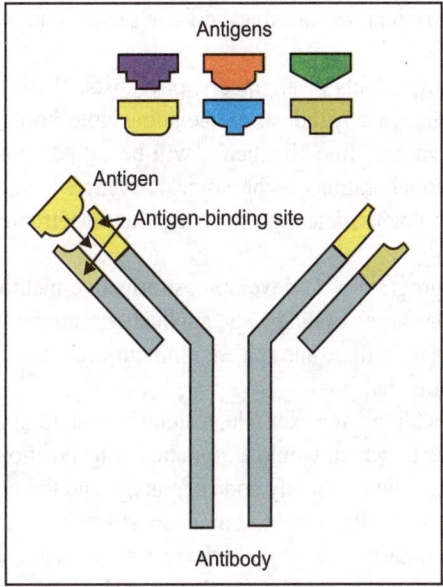

Fig. 8.3. Each antibody binds to a specific antigen; an interaction similar to a lock and key.

Though the general structure of all antibodies is very similar, a small region at the tip of the protein is extremely variable, allowing millions of antibodies with slightly different tip structures, or antigen binding sites, to exist. This region is known as the hypervariable region. Each of these variants can bind to a different target, known as an antigen. This huge diversity of antibodies allows the immune system to recognise an equally wide variety of antigens. The unique part of the antigen recognised by an antibody is called the epitope. These epitopes bind with their antibody in a highly specific interaction, called induced fit, that allows antibodies to identify and bind only their unique antigen in the midst of the millions of different molecules that make up an organism. Recognition of an antigen by an antibody tags it for attack by other parts of the immune system. Antibodies can also neutralise targets directly by, for example, binding to a part of a pathogen that it needs to cause an infection.

The large and diverse population of antibodies is generated by random combinations of a set of gene segments that encode different antigen binding sites (or paratopes), followed by random mutations in this area of the antibody gene, which create further diversity. Antibody genes also re-organise in a process called class switching that changes the base of the heavy chain to another, creating a different isotype of the antibody that retains the antigen specific variable region. This allows a single antibody to be used by several different parts of the immune system. Production of antibodies is the main function of the humoral immune system.

TOOLS FOR DNA DIAGNOSTICS

The tools for DNA diagnostics focused program will develop low-cost automated systems that can be used to obtain DNA sequence information efficiently and accurately and that will provide the basis for a broad spectrum of economical products and applications. These systems will be integrated and miniaturised, provide high-throughput, and be easily integrated in parallel processes. This program will build upon the strong molecular biology and instrumentation base that is evolving to serve the research market, but it will take a non-traditional, collaborative approach by bringing together the talents of industrial cooperators from different sectors that will each contribute specialised expertise toward a common goal.

The program will require the talents of engineers, physicists, chemists, mathematicians, computer scientists, and molecular biologists. Many industries, including biotechnology, microelectronics, software, instrumentation, pharmaceutical, and fine chemicals, will be called upon to participate in this critical national effort. Through these collaborations, technological advances in microchemistry, micromachining, microfluidics, separation technologies, detection systems, microelectronics, and information technology will be efficiently integrated.

The technical goal of the program is to develop cost-effective methods to determine, analyse, and store DNA sequences for a wide variety of diagnostic applications, ranging from health care to agriculture to the environment. These systems will be automated, miniaturised whenever possible, high-throughput, accurate, low-cost, and user-friendly.

In medical diagnostic applications, for example, a suitable system might begin with the injection of a biological sample into a cassette, which would automatically be positioned in a reader. All the steps of the analysis would be performed automatically and accurately, and the results displayed on a computer screen and immediately transferred to the patient's computerised record. For environmental or agricultural uses, readily transportable, miniaturised, hand-held devices are envisioned. Sequencing instruments for studying the effects of environmental mutagens require a very high degree of sensitivity since the goals will include searching for rare genetic changes in cell populations.

The business goal of the program is to support the development of a new and very large, potential market for DNA-diagnostic systems. Recent advances in DNA technology have set the stage for development of systems that will have a wide variety of commercial applications. Successful accomplishment of these goals would create new opportunities in many fields, including health care, agriculture, veterinary medicine, environmental monitoring, and personal identification.

The program should enable industry to deliver DNA diagnostics to a variety of industrial sectors at 1/10 to 1/100 the current price. It should also enable the industry to reduce the cost of DNA sequencing and make DNA sequencing apparatus available at significantly less than the current cost.

DNA is the universal code for all biological organisms. The availability of technology which provides cost-efficient, sequence-based analysis of that code will affect virtually all industries that currently rely upon or service biological organisms. Therefore, this program will not only provide for cost savings in existing markets such as diagnostics, drug discovery, forensics, and infectious-agent identification, but will allow for the creation and expansion of new markets and applications.

In the long term, DNA sequence/diagnostic analysis technologies are likely to yield increased activity and greater efficiencies in such areas as: (i) health care, (ii) forensics and personnel identification, (iii) biomedical research, including pure and applied biology, (iv) environmental monitoring, (v) toxicology, (vi) drug discovery and design, (vii) biomass diversity, assessment, maintenance, (viii) bioremediation, (ix) infectious agent monitoring, (x) quality control in the food industry, (xi) industrial processing, including the monitoring of biological processes, and (xii) animal husbandry and agriculture, including assessing and maintaining diversity, improving yield, monitoring disease resistance, assessing nutritional value, and targeting biocontrol.

Together with the information that will be forthcoming from the Human genome project and other genome efforts, this technology can aid in increasing the use and decreasing the cost of DNA diagnostics for preventive screening, symptomatic and presymptomatic testing; create a market for cost-effective therapeutic monitoring of patients; and create a market for monitoring of endogenous gene expression to aid in informed diagnosis, the combination of which should yield more individually-tailored rational therapy regimens.

DNA diagnostic tests for agriculture could supplant the presently used methodologies to identify plants with special characteristics such as hardiness, diseases resistance, etc. The use of these tests will become widespread if the cost of analysis is significantly reduced. In a similar way, use of this technology will become widespread in animal genetics, plant and animal design, husbandry and the treatment of disease. Market penetration will very much depend on the costs of these tests. For example, a reduction of the costs to ten dollars per test will lead to a use of these in the control of the germ lines in artificial insemination of cattle. Furthermore, the reduction of the costs of doing DNA analysis will widen the market for these instruments and diagnostics. Chemical process technologies will be affected by this program. It is expected that inexpensive DNA diagnostics will be used to monitor bioprocessing for the production of specialty and commodity chemicals. At present, there exist no apparent barriers to the commercialisation of the resulting products from research applications.

Other applications related to health care and the agribusiness are likely to require approval by the Food and Drug Administration as well as more thorough optimisation of conditions, definition of standards, and evaluation of error rates. These issues should be addressed in applications for awards. There is precedent for the use of biological or DNA-based technologies for most of the applications listed above and therefore, the potential to achieve commercialisation has been demonstrated, although optimisation of the process for individual cases will still need to occur.

Technical scope of program: The following discussion addresses some of the technical areas eligible for proposals in the tools for DNA diagnostics program together with some examples.

At present, there exist three approaches to DNA analysis that appear to be the most promising for automated DNA diagnostics applications: serial sequence analysis, hybridisation analysis, and amplification-based analysis. Previous government investments in basic research, including the Human Genome Project, have supported the acquisition of preliminary data to demonstrate the proof of principle of these approaches. However, these programs, including the Human Genome Project, will not support the development of these techniques for use in diagnostic applications.

The utility of DNA diagnostics already is apparent, even with only a small proportion of the human genome sequenced. The application of DNA diagnostics will greatly expand as more of the human genome is sequenced. The use of any of the three approaches listed for diagnostic applications will require miniaturisation, parallelisation, and automation of current technology. Independent of the approach, improvements will need to be made in the areas of sample preparation, assay technology, detection systems, integration, and data management and analysis. Specific improvements in each of these areas will depend upon the specific approach and the ultimate diagnostic application of the technology. Beyond this, however, many of the technological improvements that are required are sufficiently basic and enabling that the improvements will benefit industries and markets beyond DNA diagnostics.

In the areas of sample preparation and assay, it is clear that miniaturisation is key. To reduce the size of samples by a factor of 10 or greater, barriers in microfluidics, micromachining, robotics, microchemistry, nucleic acid chemistry, and surface chemistry must be overcome. To implement miniaturised protocols accurately and efficiently, substantial automation of the process will be required. In the development of miniaturised systems, it is essential that the system can be adapted for high levels of parallelisation.

Miniaturisation

Miniaturisation poses significant technological risks. Currently, there exists no universally accepted precedent for the handling, replication, amplification, or cloning of DNA in nanoliter volumes. Due to the size and charge of the DNA molecule, and the relative instability of many of the enzymes involved in the sample preparation processes, nanoliter and less volumes may pose substantial challenges. In addition, interactions of the biological molecules with the surfaces of the reaction chambers must be minimised. For some methodologies, it is not clear what the optimal sample will be, so substantial improvement in DNA fragmentation technologies or DNA cloning vectors may be required for the ultimate efficient application to diagnostics. Improvements in any of these areas are likely to be of value to other non-DNA based diagnostic applications such as antibody screening protocols and enzyme-based diagnostics, because miniaturised robotic or micro-electro mechanical systems developed for DNA could be modified to be used for these purposes.

Assay

Assay capabilities improvements for DNA diagnostics are likely to be somewhat dependent upon the specific approach. For instance, in serial sequence DNA analysis application of capillary gel electrophoresis, ultrathin gels, and microchannel arrays to the separation step will increase the speed and parallelisation of DNA analysis by a least one order of magnitude. New efforts that are being undertaken to apply microfabrication and micro-electro mechanical systems technology to the separation step could afford an increase in the speed of two to three orders of magnitude. All of these approaches require the development of improved separation matrices. In addition, improved capillary fabrication or microfabrication will be required and fluid handling and surface chemistry issues addressed.

Assay capabilities for hybridisation-based DNA analysis also will require overcoming a variety of technical barriers. Improved technologies for the production of low cost oligonucleotide arrays will need to be developed. This requires new approaches to oligonucleotide synthesis, improved surface chemistry for oligonucleotide attachment, and microfabrication improvements utilising many substrates including silicon, glass and polymers. Optimisation of the biochemistry involved in the actual hybridisation is also required and may be specific for the detection format. Automation to allow for the processing of many parallel units is also be required.

For amplification-based DNA analysis, there are two possibilities for the assay step, one of which includes a separation step similar to that used for serial sequence analysis, and therefore would require overcoming similar technical barriers to those listed above. An alternative assay would involve enzymatic detection similar to current antibody assays, which could possibly allow for future 'dip stick' formats for particular diagnostic applications. This assay would require the development of biochemistry for the attachment of appropriate enzymatic substrates to DNA and optimisation of surface chemistry to promote specific sample binding and prevent anomalous sample binding. As with other approaches, automation to allow for the processing of many parallel units will be required.

Detection

The detection step of each of the three DNA analysis approaches will require both improved reporter groups and improved detector technology. With the proposed miniaturisation described above, detection will have to be increasingly more sensitive. In addition, new detection technologies could allow for increased multiplicity of samples per unit of the assay step. A limited number of fluorescent, energy transfer, or infrared dyes constitute the most commonly used current reporter groups. Additional dyes are being sought, but other reporters such as electrophores and heavy metals are also being developed. Improved chemistry for the production of these reporters and the attachment of the reporters to DNA will be required. The sensitivity of the appropriate detectors for each of these reporters will have to be increased. The development of more sensitive charge coupled device (CCD) arrays and photodiode arrays may also be required. Some approaches to detection that do not rely on reporter groups include measurement of changes in impedance following hybridisation and measurement of electron conduction along double stranded DNA. Optimisation of such to allow parallelisation and high throughput approaches requires development of improved micromachining and microelectronic capabilities.

Data Processing

With the expected improvement in diagnostic capability, better systems will need to be made available to handle the increased information output. This will include better data management tools, and better analysis software. It is likely that individual software packages will be required for each type of application to make the systems user friendly. In addition, improvements in systems integration will be necessary for all applications, such that the interface between components of the individual systems is transparent to the user.

Integration

The ultimate challenge of all the areas described above is to integrate the steps outlined from sample preparation to analysis in an economic way so that DNA analysis can be performed substantially quicker for orders of magnitude less cost than existing tests for simpler monogenic diseases. This involves thoughtful integration in the preliminary design of the methodology to be developed.

Proposals are welcome in all of these areas as well as any other approaches that address the fundamental technical issues described here. This program will not accept proposals which differ in content and focus from the scope discussed above. Proposed projects should focus on developing enabling technologies; the ATP will not fund product development. Examples of proposals that will not be accepted include studies to design, develop or target drugs, agrochemicals, herbicides, etc. based on genomic information, studies involving gene discovery and the de novo sequencing of any DNA fragment or genome. Proposals that are primarily directed towards the development of lasers are also not included since laser development is already being supported in various ATP projects and programs.

The strong industry commitment to a program in the area of improved technologies for sequenced-based DNA analysis is clear from the number and quality of white paper submissions (this area was the subject of more white-paper proposals than any other biotechnology-related topic.) and to the quality of the proposals submitted to the competitions. The development of improved technologies for sequenced-based DNA analysis involves a diverse group of both large and small industries with varied expertise and interests in areas including, but not limited to, biological sample preparation and molecular biology; microfabrication; surface chemistry; separation sciences; nucleic acid chemistry; instrumentation development and engineering; detection technologies, in particular various forms of excitable wavelength spectroscopy; and information handling, data analysis, and systems integration. White papers defining programs related to this area were received from a broad spectrum of companies, including representatives of the pharmaceutical industry, drug development companies, molecular biologicals suppliers, instrumentation development firms, and software developers, as well as others. In addition, the contributors of white papers in this area were broadly distributed in size, ranging from large corporations to small start-up companies.

The real opportunity and enthusiasm for industry involvement in this area is also reflected by the significant level of industry participation in meetings of the scientific community related to this area such as the international genome gequencing and analysis conferences, as well as the appearance of national meetings directed toward industries interested in this area, such as 'The Human Genome Project: Commercial Implications', 'Genetic Screening and Diagnosis of Human Disease', 'BioChips' and 'Nanotechnology'. But perhaps the most persuasive testimony to industry interest in this area is the number of start-up companies which have formed in response to the opportunities in this area.

There is a strong industry commitment to the development of DNA technologies for sequencing, diagnostics, and the development of drug and gene therapies. Large and small companies are involved in these activities. Several companies are involved in the development of the concepts and technology necessary for oligonucleotide array hybridisation, capillary electrophoresis, and mass spectrometry. Laser development is being pursued by several companies for the development of cheaper, more efficient, solid-state lasers. Micromanufacturing technologies are being pursued for the manufacture of chips, capillaries and detector arrays.

Hybridisation Probe

In molecular biology, a hybridisation probe is a fragment of DNA or RNA of variable length (usually 100–1000 bases long), which is used in DNA or RNA samples to detect the presence of nucleotide sequences (the DNA target) that are complementary to the sequence in the probe. The probe thereby hybridises to single-stranded nucleic acid (DNA or RNA) whose base sequence allows probe-target base pairing due to complementarity between the probe and target. The labelled probe is first denatured (by heating or under alkaline conditions such as exposure to sodium hydroxide) into single DNA strands and then hybridised to the target DNA (Southern blotting) or RNA (northern blotting) immobilised on a membrane or *in situ*.

To detect hybridisation of the probe to its target sequence, the probe is tagged (or labelled) with a molecular marker of either radioactive or (more recently) fluorescent molecules; commonly used markers are ^{32}P (a radioactive isotope of phosphorus incorporated into the phosphodiester bond in the probe DNA) or Digoxigenin, which is non-radioactive antibody-based marker. DNA sequences or RNA transcripts that have moderate to high sequence similarity to the probe are then detected by visualising the hybridised probe via autoradiography or other imaging techniques. Normally, either X-ray pictures are taken of the filter, or the filter is placed under UV light. Detection of sequences with moderate or high similarity depends on how stringent the hybridisation conditions were applied—high stringency, such as high hybridisation temperature and low salt in hybridisation buffers, permits only hybridisation between nucleic acid sequences that are highly similar, whereas low stringency, such as lower temperature and high salt, allows hybridisation when the sequences are less similar. Hybridisation probes used in DNA microarrays refer to DNA covalently attached to an inert surface, such as coated glass slides or gene chips, and to which a mobile cDNA target is hybridised.

Depending on the method the probe may be synthesised using phosphoramidite method or generated and labelled by PCR amplification or cloning (older methods). In order to increase the *in vivo* stability of the probe RNA is not used, instead RNA analogues may be used, in particular morpholino. Molecular DNA- or RNA-based probes are now routinely used in screening gene libraries, detecting nucleotide sequences with blotting methods, and in other gene technologies like microarrays.

In forensic science, hybridisation probes are used, for example, for detection of short tandem repeats (microsatellite) regions and in RFLP methods, all of which are widely used as part of DNA profiling analysis.

Diagnosis of Malaria

Diagnosis of malaria involves identification of malaria parasite or its antigens/products in the blood of the patient. Although this seems simple, the efficacy of the diagnosis is subject to many factors. The different forms of the four malaria species; the different stages of erythrocytic schizogony; the endemicity of different species; the population movements; the inter-relation between the levels of transmission, immunity, parasitemia, and the symptoms; the problems of recurrent malaria, drug resistance, persisting viable or non-viable parasitemia, and sequestration of the parasites in the deeper tissues; and the use of chemoprophylaxis or even presumptive treatment on the basis of clinical diagnosis can all have a bearing on the identification and interpretation of malaria parasitemia on a diagnostic test. The diagnosis of malaria is confirmed by blood tests and can be divided into microscopic and non-microscopic tests.

DIAGNOSIS OF GENETIC DISEASES BY DNA TECHNOLOGY

During the last twenty years the recombinant DNA technology has developed very powerful and sensitive techniques, which are listed in Table 8.1, useful in the study and for the identification of the molecular defects of human inherited diseases.

Table 8.1. Recombinant DNA technology.

Restriction	
Endonucleases	Vectors
Cloning	Oligonucleotides
Libraries	PCR (b)
Electrophoresis	Sequencing
Blotting	Probes
Mapping	DGGE (c)
PFGE (a)	SSCP (d)
Chemical Cleavage	RNAseA mismatch analysis

(a) Pulse field gel electrophoresis.
(b) Polymerase chain reaction.
(c) Denaturing gradient gel electrophoresis.
(d) Single strand conformational polymorphism.

DNA technology has allowed an enormous increase of basic knowledge on inherited diseases and has had great effect on biodiagnostics; in general it has increased the knowledge on the human genome. The development of DNA based diagnostic tests for genetic disorders is still in progress. It will take time for experimental validation and for standardisation of protocols. However their transferibility to the clinical field will depend on other factors, like the simplicity of procedures, the speed of execution and the cost of the analysis. Since 1973, 75 human genes have been mapped. Table 8.2 shows all the genes mapped in the 1st edition of 'Human gene mappingt'. Every year, during the Human gene mapping conference, the DNA Committee has three primary responsibilities: (i) summarising information on cloned and mapped human genes, (ii) summarising information on polymorphisms detected by using molecular techniques, and (iii) the development of a nomenclature appropriate for loci identified by anonymous DNA probes and assignment of symbols to those loci. Since 1983, these data have been collected also on Database to facilitate and to speed up the access. There are also others Database with the list of papers on cloned sequences both for genes and for anonimous sequences. The number and chromosome distribution of cloned sequences and polymorphisms are shown in Fig. 8.4 and Table 8.3.

Table 8.2. Summary of human gene map. New haven HGM 1–1973.

Chromosome	Mendelian markers	In vitro markers
1	Iqh+, Cae, Fy, AOD Amy1, Amy2, EL1, Rh	PGM1, PGD, PPH, UGPP, FH, GuK, Pep-Cl, RN5S, AK-2
2	Acpl, MNSs	IDH-1, MDH-1, GallPT, If1, Hb
3		No assignment
4 or 5		Hb, ade+B, Es-Act
5		If2, Hex B
6		Me-1, IPO-B, PGM3, HLA
7		MPI, PKIII, HexA
8		No assignment
9		No assignment
10		GOT-1, HK
11		LDH-A, Es-A1, AL AcP2
12		LDH-B, Pep-B, TPI Gly+A, CS
13		RNr
14		RNr, NP
15		RNr
16	αHp	APRT
17		TK
18		Pep-A
19		GPI
20		ADA
21	Ag	RNr, IPO-A, AVP
22		RNr
X	mp, rp, rs, oa, Xg, ich, cbD, cbP, sp, md, mdc, HemA, HemB, Xm, MPS 2	PGK, αGal, HPRT, G6PD, TATr

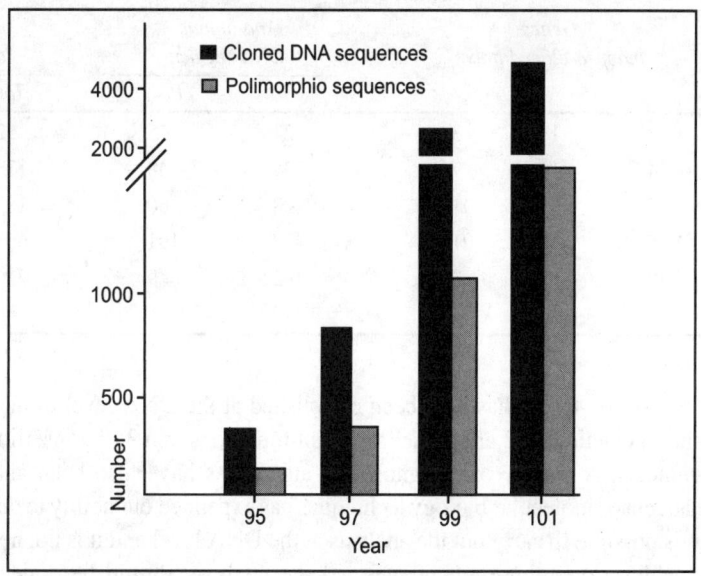

Fig. 8.4. Cumulative annual number of cloned sequences and polymorphisms.

Table 8.3. Chromosome distribution of cloned human DNA (HGM 10).

Chrom	Genes mapped cloned poly*			Anonimous DNA segment		All cloned DNA	
				Tot	Poly*	Tot	Poly*
1	181	98	33	97	88	278	121
2	103	62	26	65	53	168	79
3	63	40	17	184	46	247	63
4	71	45	28	157	96	228	124
5	66	32	9	103	86	169	95
6	98	61	28	76	42	174	70
7	104	41	21	417	155	521	176
8	56	30	14	72	36	128	50
9	58	25	9	44	33	102	42
10	55	30	13	87	65	142	78
11	133	68	37	404	67	537	104
12	86	50	15	37	31	123	46
13	27	17	8	61	42	88	50
14	50	33	25	33	23	83	48
15	48	25	8	71	38	119	46
16	55	32	9	255	98	310	107
17	83	57	21	217	112	300	133
18	22	14	6	28	22	50	28
19	75	35	15	53	33 ·	128	48

(Contd...)

Chrom	Genes mapped cloned poly*			Anonimous DNA segment		All cloned DNA	
				Tot	Poly*	Tot	Poly*
20	28	17	3	24	15	52	18
21	34	16	7	144	48	178	55
22	55	31	11	108	60	163	71
X	17 5	44	21	478	191	663	212
Y	14	8	2	192	9	216	11
XY				10	6		6

* polymorphism.

The nature of the genetic lesion has now been established at the DNA level in many diseases: the majority, 58, are due to deletions, 52 are caused by point mutations and 34 by insertions, duplications and gene rearrangements. A variety of chromosomal alterations have also been analysed and well characterised. The advent of molecular biology techniques has expanded our ability to diagnose inherited diseases. In fact , it is possible to carry out the analysis at the DNA level and it is not necessary to know the gene product, which gives three advantages: (i) the analysis should be done for example on limphocytes and not only on the disease target cells, (ii) it allows carrier detection, and (iii) it allows the molecular defect characterisation.

PCR-OLIGONUCLEOTIDE LIGATION ASSAY FROM DRIED BLOOD SPOTS

PCR followed by oligonucleotide ligation assay (PCR-OLA) is a molecular method that can be used for the detection of nucleotide sequence variants. During the past 10 years it has been used successfully for numerous diagnostic applications. PCR-OLA is based on the enzymatic ligation of two oligonucleotides that anneal next to each other onto the PCR-amplified target DNA. Even a single-nucleotide mismatch between the oligonucleotides and the template precludes the ligation. Automated PCR-OLA on a microplate format in combination with ELISA detection technology is a powerful method for testing numerous samples. One bottleneck for the effective use of PCR-OLA in population screening programs has been the time-consuming and tedious preparation of DNA samples that is necessary to eliminate PCR inhibitors. Dried blood spot (DBS) specimens on filter blotters are widely used for collection, storage, and shipping of blood samples in screening programs for newborns, and they have been used for genotypic confirmation of positive screening tests. PCR inhibitors can be eliminated from DBS specimens by eluting the spots, by fixing the spots to the disk with methanol, or by extracting DNA from the disk. To increase the throughput of PCR-OLA, we treated DBS specimens with methanol and used the methanol-fixed samples for the PCR-OLA analysis of the major mutation (AGU$_{Fin}$), which is responsible for Finnish-type aspartylglycosaminuria (AGU). The methanol treatment tested on DBS specimens collected on five different types of glass fiber or filter paper blotters. The results show that PCR-OLA from methanol-treated DBSs enables rapid and reliable detection of genetic variances.

On collecting EDTA blood samples from 115 Finnish individuals with unknown genotype and 20 carriers of AGU$_{Fin}$, making these anonymous after collection. The genotype of the AGU$_{Fin}$ carriers was confirmed by restriction fragment length polymorphism. DBS specimens were prepared by dropping 10–20 μL of fresh or previously frozen (–20°C) blood onto Merckoquant® blank strips (Merck), GF/C glass microfiber filters (Whatman), BFC 180 specimen collection paper (Whatman), Schleicher and

Schuell (S&S) filter paper no. 2992, or S & S filter paper no. 903. The membranes were air-dried for 2 hr, followed by application of one drop of methanol (~50 μL) to the DBS area. The methanol was allowed to evaporate in a fume hood for 1 hr, and the membranes were stored desiccated at room temperature until analysis. In addition, for each membrane type, 10 DBS specimens that had not been treated with methanol were analysed by PCR-OLA as controls.

A disk 1.5 mm in diameter, representing ~0.5–1 μL of whole blood, was punched out of the membrane with a handheld punch and placed directly into a PCR tube. The punch was first rinsed in 2 mol/L HCl and then in distilled water after each sample to prevent cross-contamination between specimens. A 429-bp segment of the glycosylasparaginase gene containing the AGU_{Fin} mutation site was amplified using primers 5′-TGTAGCTCACTTAAGATG-3′ and 5′-CCAGTAGCTCTCCATGCT-3′ in a final volume of 30 μL. Amplification reactions contained 10 mmol/L Tris-HCl (pH 8.3), 50 mmol/L KCl, 1.5 mmol/L $MgCl_2$, 6 μmol of each dNTP, 7.5 pmol of primers, and 0.24 U of DynaZyme DNA polymerase (Finnzymes). The cycling program in a PTC-100 Thermal Cycler (MJ Research) consisted of a first cycle of 96°C for 10 min, 84°C for the time needed to add DNA polymerase, 51°C for 45 s, and 72°C for 1 min, followed by 30 cycles of 1 min at 94°C, 45 s at 51°C, and 1 min at 72°C, with a final extension for 9 min at 72°C. The oligonucleotide ligation assay for the detection of the AGU_{Fin} mutation was performed as described by Delahunty. The absorbance readings of the mutant and the wild-type (WT) ELISA reactions after a constant colour development time of 15 min were measured at 510 nm with a Tecan Spectrafluor spectrophotometer. The ratio of the absorbance of the WT allele-specific reaction to the mutant allele-specific reaction was calculated to determine the genotype of the sample. A homozygote for the WT allele was identified by a ratio >5, and a homozygote for the mutant allele was identified by a ratio <0.2. The ratio of the two absorbances for a heterozygous individual was close to 1. In each PCR-OLA series, we used one negative control in which no DBS was added, and as a positive control we used DNA from a known carrier of the AGU_{Fin} mutation. For confirmation of the genotype obtained in PCR-OLA analysis of the DBS specimens, DNA from each EDTA blood sample was isolated with a Split Second® DNA Preparation kit (Roche), and 0.5 μL of the DNA preparation was used for PCR amplification as described above. PCR-OLA has been shown to accurately detect both the WT genotype and the heterozygous AGU_{Fin} genotype.

When PCR amplification of the AGU_{Fin} mutation site was applied to untreated DBS specimens collected on various membranes, the PCR mixtures became deep brown because of the elution of heme and its degradation products from the filter blotters, and the OLA reaction was successful for only 30 of 50 of these samples. In the other 20 samples, no amplified target DNA was detected after PCR in ethidium bromide-stained agarose gel electrophoresis, indicating that a failure in the PCR step was the cause for unsuccessful OLA assays. When the corresponding DBS specimens were amplified after the methanol treatment, the reaction mixtures were colourless and clear after PCR, and OLA was successfully accomplished for every specimen, verifying the importance of the methanol treatment of the blotters. We also found that prolongation of the denaturation step at 96°C to 10 min before addition of DNA polymerase improved the PCR amplification of the target DNA. The PCR procedure was optimised for DBS disks of 1.5 mm in diameter in a reaction volume of 30 μL. The amplification of the target DNA was often lower when disks with 2 mm in diameter were used in the same conditions, and disks larger than 2 mm did not properly fit into the V-bottomed PCR tubes or plates. On testing the applicability of five different filter blotters for collection of blood for PCR-OLA by genotyping 115 Finnish blood samples with unknown AGU_{Fin} genotype and 20 blood samples from known carriers of the AGU_{Fin} mutation. PCR-OLA was successful after the methanol treatment on each DBS collected on various filter blotters (Table 8.4).

Table 8.4. Absorbances of the WT and AGU$_{Fin}$ mutant PCR-OLA reactions and absorbance ratios of the WT to the mutant reactions.

Sample	WT genotype[1]				Heterozygous genotype[1]			
	n[2]	WT reaction, A_{cin}	Mutant reaction, A_{cin}	Ratio of absorbances	n[2]	Wt reaction, A_{cin}	Mutant reaction, A_{cin}	Ratio of absorbances
Filter blotter								
Merckoquant blank strips	64	0.918 (2.380) ≥3.0	0.062 (0.078) 0.136	11.8 (27.6) 37.6	11	1.363 (≥3.0) ≥3.0	1.675 (≥3.0) ≥3.0	0.8 (1.0) 1.4
GF/C glass microfiber filters	10	0.820 (1.522) 2.689	0.081 (0.116) 0.159	7.1 (13.3) 29.5	10	1.656 (≥3.0) ≥3.0	1.310 (≥3.0) ≥3.0	1.0 (1.0) 1.3
BFC 180	10	≥3.0[3]	0.078 (0.096) 0.121	24.8 (30.0) 38.5	10	0.509 (2.443) ≥3.0	0.495 (2.297) ≥3.0	1.0 (1.0) 1.1
S&S filter paper no. 2992	20	0.714 (2.350) 2.705	0.052 (0.109) 0.166	5.3 (19.8) 45.3	20	0.512 (≥3.0) ≥3.0	0.480 (≥3.0) ≥3.0	0.9 (1.0) 1.8
S&S filter paper no 903	10	1.185 (2.779) 2.929	0.067 (0.085) 0.107	15.8 (29.7) 41.5	10	0.626 (2.550) ≥3.0	0.542 (2.522) ≥3.0	1.0 (1.0) 1.2
Split second DNA	114	1.173 (2.636) ≥3.0	0.055 (0.071) 0.187	7.4 (30.9) 49.1	21	1.511 (≥3.0) ≥3.0	1.001 (≥3.0) ≥3.0	0.9 (1.0) 2.4

[1] Absorbances and absorbance ratios are given as 2.5th (50th) 97.5th percentiles.
[2] Number of samples analyses.
[3] absorbance ≥3.0 in all samples.

The constant colour development time of 15 min in the ELISA led to absorbance readings higher than the measuring range of the spectrophotometer in many samples. These absorbances are marked as ≥ 0 3.0 in Table 8.4. In 114 of 115 samples collected on five different membranes (Table 8.4), the absorbance ratio of the WT reaction to the mutant reaction was 5.3 – 45.3 (median, 26.0), indicating the normal genotype. In 1 of the 115 samples, the ratio was 0.8, which was in the same range as in DBS prepared from frozen blood of known carriers of AGU_{Fin} mutation (range, 0.8–1.8; median, 1.0; n = 60; Table 8.6), indicating a carrier phenotype. All of the genotyping results of PCR-OLA from DBS were verified with PCR-OLA from Split second DNA samples, and they were in full conformity.

The 2.5th, 50th, and 97.5th percentile absorbances for the WT and the mutant PCR-OLA reaction, and the absorbance ratio of the WT and the mutant reactions for DBS specimens collected on five different filter blotters and for Split Second DNA samples are shown in Table 8.4. With each filter blotter type that was studied, the absorbance ratio of the WT reaction to the mutant reaction in normal samples was significantly higher (Mann–Whitney U-test, P <0.001) than the corresponding ratio in samples with the heterozygous genotype. Although the absorbances were lower for the DBS than for the Split Second DNA samples, the genotype was determined correctly in each DBS sample. DBS specimens prepared from blood samples that had been stored frozen at $-20°C$ for several years were also analysed successfully by PCR-OLA. The results show that all of the five tested blotters can be used for reliable DNA diagnostics by PCR-OLA according to the present procedure. The membrane type seemed to affect the assay to some extent because a slight variation in absorbance readings was seen (Table 8.4). However, this variation did not prevent the interpretation of the genotype in any of the samples.

Thus that this novel methodology can easily be adapted to various PCR-OLA applications for research or diagnostic purposes. The use of DBS specimens in the detection of nucleotide sequence variations by PCR-OLA simplifies the collection, storage, and shipment of blood samples. Rapid handling of DBS specimens would be facilitated by use of an automated punching equipment, which is already commercially available. The simplified sample preparation reduces risk of human error and increases the usefulness of PCR-OLA, e.g. for use in large-scale population screening programs.

MUTANT SELECTION

Large scale mutant selection programes begin when favourable reports of clinical trials are obtained. In the early stages, selection of spontaneous mutants may be helpful, but induced mutations are the most common sources of improvements. Mutations occurring without any specific treatment are called spontaneous mutation, while those resulting due to a treatment with certain agents are known as induced mutations, such agents are referred to as *mutagens*. Either physical and chemical mutagens can be employed. Usually, the frequency of mutants with desirable phenotype is quite low; hence the major bottleneck is the identification and isolation of such cells from among the large number of non-mutant/undesirable mutant cells.

Many mutations (a sudden and heritable change in the traits of an organism) bring about marked changes in a biochemical character of practical interest; these are called major mutations. Some major mutations can be useful in strain improvement. For example, the original strain of *Streptomyces griseus* produced small amounts of streptomycin and large amounts of mannosidostreptomycin which has low antibiotic activity. A major mutant isolated from this strain produced negligible amounts of mannosidostreptomycin and much larger quantities of streptomycin. Similarly, a mutant strain (S-604) of *Streptomyces aureofaciens* produces 6-demethyl tetracycline in place of tetracycline; this demethylated form of tetracycline is the major commercial form of tetracycline.

In contrast, most improvements in biochemical production have been due to the stepwise accumulation of so called *minor genes*. These genes lead to small increases (or decreases) in the antibiotic or other biochemical production, and selection may be expected to result in a 10–15 per cent increase in yield The selected strains are usually subjected to successive cycles of mutagenesis and selection, and after several cycles large increases is yields are likely to be obtained. Application of mutagens to induce mutations is called *mutagenesis*. In some cases, improvements have been obtained even without the use of mutagens. *Mutants* of *Penicillium chrysogenum* were selected for increased penicillin production; each cycle of selection was preceded by mutagen (chemical) treatment and resulted in only small changes in penicillin yield. But after several (about dozen) cycles of selection, a strain. (E 15–1) was obtained that yielded 55 per cent more penicillin than the original strain (Fleming Strain).

Selective isolation of mutants: A majority of desirable mutants, especially the 'minor gene' mutants showing increased production, are isolated by screening a large number of clones surviving the mutagen treatment; this is called secondary screening, but this approach requires a large amount of work. Therefore, efforts have increasingly focussed on developing techniques for the isolation of particular classes of mutants which are likely to be overproducers (Table 8.5).

Table 8.5. A summary of different approaches in utilisation of mutation and genetic recombination for strain improvement.

Approach	Chief feature	Example/remark
Mutant Selection: Types		The main approach to strain improvement; produces new alleles of existing genes.
Spontaneous mutations	Occurs without any treatment with a mutagen	Used in the initial stages of strain improvement; also for maintenance of improved strains.
Induced mutations	Induced by chemical (mainly) or physical mutagens	Mutagenesis followed by selection; several cycles employed.
Major mutations	Affect the pattern of metabolite production	Production of 6-demethyl tetracycline in place of tetracycline by *S. griseus*.
Minor mutations	Affect the rate of metabolite production	Small gains in each cycle of selection; substantial improvement after several cycles
Mutant Selection: Strategies		
Auxotrophic mutants	Defective biosynthesis of a biochemical	Enhanced production of an amino acid, e.g. *phe⁻* mutants accumulate tyrosine.
Analogue-resistant mutants	Feed-back insensitive enzymes	Overproduction of metabolites, e.g. amino acids by *C. glutamicus*
Revertants of nonproducing mutants		Some mutants are high producers, e.g. chlortetracycline by *S. viridifaciens*
Revertants of auxotrophic mutants		Some are high produces, e.g. chlortetracycline by *S. viridifaciens*
Resistance to the antibiotic produced by the organism itself		Increased production, e.g. chlortetracyline by *S. aureofaciens*
Recombination		Produces new combinations of existing alleles

(Contd...)

Approach	Chief feature	Example/remark
Sexual reproduction	Conjugation; fusion of gametes	Some bacteria and Actinomycetes.; fungi and yeast.
Heterokaryosis	Nuclear fusion followed by mitotic recombination and mitotic reduction	Fungi
Protoplast fusion	Protoplasts produced by lytic enzymes; fusion by PEG, recombinant recovery	Bacteria, Actinomycetes, fungi; quite successful.

Some of the strategies are briefly summarised below; the selection for these classes of mutants is simple, easy and effective.

1. Isolation of auxotrophic mutants is the basis for commercial amino acid production in Japan from the bacterium *Corynebacterium glutamicus*. An *auxotrophic mutant* has a defect in one of its biosynthetic pathways so that it requires a specific biochemical for normal growth and development. For example, *phe⁻* mutants require phenylalanine for growth; such mutants of *C glutamicus* accumulate tyrosine. Similarly, *tyr⁻* mutants accumulate phenylalanine, while *phe⁻* + *tyr⁻* mutants accumulate tryptophan.

2. Many anologue-resistant mutants have feed-back insensitive enzymes of the biosynthetic pathway the analogue of whose product was used for selection of such cells. In feed-back inhibition, activity of all enzyme is inhibited by the end-product of the biosynthetic pathway in which the enzyme participates, For example, when *tyr⁻* mutants of *C. glutamicus* were selected for resistance to 50 mg/l *p*-fluorophenylalanine (analogue of phenylalanine), there was a nearly 7-fold increase in phenylalanine accumulation over that of the *tyr⁻* mutant.

3. Sometimes revertants from non producing mutants of a strain are high producers, e.g. one such reversion mutant of *Streptomyces viridifaciens* showed over 6-fold increase in chlortetracycline production over the original strain from which the nonproducing mutant was obtained. When a mutant mutates back to its original phenotype it is called reversion, and the mutant is known as revertant, e.g. nonproducer mutant mutating to back producer.

4. Reversion mutants of appropriate auxotrophs may often be high producers, e.g. in case of *S. viridifaciens* reversion mutants of an auxotrophic mutant requiring homocysteine showed 28 per cent more chlortetracycline yield than the original strain.

5. In some cases, selection for resistance to the antibiotic produced by the organism itself may lead to increased yields. For example, *Streptomyces aureofaciens* mutants selected for resistance to 200–400 mg/l chlortetracycline showed a four-fold increase in the production of this antibiotic.

6. Sometimes, mutants with altered cell membrane permeability show high production of some metabolites. A mutant *E. coli* strain has defective lysine transport; it actively excretes L-lysine into the medium to 5-times as high concentration as that within its cells.

7. Mutants have been selected to produce altered metabolites, especially in case of aminogycoside antibiotics. For example, *Pseudomonas aureofaciens* produces the antibiotic pyrrolnitrin; a mutant of this fungus yields 4'-fluoropyrrolnitrin.

The above and many other approaches for selection of mutants can be most profitably used when the biosynthetic pathway for the concerned product is known, as are the precursors and the regulatory mechanisms. Mutant selection has been the most successful approach for strain improvement, but major advances are being made in the expostulation of other strategies, i.e. recombination and recombinant DNA technology.

Chapter 9

Vaccines and Therapeutic Agents

INTRODUCTION

A number of diseases are caused by micro-organisms. For many bacterial diseases, and some fungal diseases, there are antibiotics, produced by other micro-organisms. There are also chemical agents produced by higher plants that can control microbial pathogens. But there are very few means of fighting viral diseases. Even when there are therapeutic agents to control several microbial diseases, in course of time the pathogen acquires resistance, making the therapeutic agent ineffective. In this eternal race between the pathogen and the pathologist, the pathogens seem to be always a step ahead. Against this background, production of vaccines against the microbial pathogens, and more particularly the pathogenic viruses, in order to immunise the susceptible populations, is a safe and more certain recourse. More importantly, the immunological approach is both preventive and curative, while other means are only curative. Advances in immunology and biotechnology have made it now possible to produce immunological agents to afford protection from diseases to large numbers of people. This area is immunotechnology, an arm of biotechnology.

VACCINES

A vaccine is an agent, sourced from the pathogen, and is deliberately introduced into the mammalian system in order to impart a 'memory' of the pathogen or its pathogenic component. The memory is imparted on the first contact of the vaccine with the mammalian immune system. Vaccine usually contains the modified pathogenic organism or a protein or a low molecular weight non-protein compound (hapten) conjugated with the protein, obtained from the pathogen.

Vaccines contain antigens (that elicit the production of antibodies), or immunogens (that trigger the cellular component of immune response). In the event of an encounter with the corresponding antibodies, only the antigens can bind with the antibodies, and form an antigen-antibody complex that neutralises the harmful effects of the antigens or the organisms that produce them.

Since vaccines employ a part of the chemical machinery of the organisms themselves, pathogens cannot easily acquire resistance to vaccines, as they do for antibiotics and chemical therapeutic agents.

Vaccination/Immunisation

The process of the deliberate introduction of a vaccine into the organism is vaccination, for which the term inoculation is also often used. Since vaccination immunises the organism, the process is also called immunisation.

When an organism is vaccinated, the immune system is readied to show an immune response by way producing antibodies against the pathogen, in the event of a second encounter with the pathogen, basing on the memory imparted by the vaccine used for the first encounter.

Immunotherapy

Immunotherapy differs from vaccination in that in the former antibodies isolated from an immunised organism (polyclonal or monoclonal immunoglobulin antibodies or cytokines) is used to cure the patient. Immunotherapy becomes essential when there is no time to prepare the patient through vaccination or when the patient is physically and/or physiologically not competent to respond to vaccination.

Composition of Vaccines

Vaccines are suspensions, in saline or buffered saline, of weakened pathogenic organisms or their fractions or the proteins they secrete, which have the potential to cause a disease. A virulent organism cannot be used as a vaccine.

Adjuvants

Antigens often need to be coupled with an adjuvant, which is a compound that holds the antigen and releases it slowly over a longer period of time. The most commonly used immunological adjuvant in experimental systems is Freund's Complete Adjuvant (FCA), which contains mineral oil and heat killed mycobacteria. The bacteria are intended to heighten immunological response, but may produce hypersensitivity in many patients. The mineral oil also may prove to be harmful. Hence FCA is not normally used in human immunisation schedules. Aluminium hydroxide is human safe but is a poor adjuvant. Some plant saponins are now projected as efficient and human safe adjuvants. There are some effective and safe synthetic adjuvants, but their composition is a trade secret.

Various types of vaccines

1. Inactivated vaccines: The pathogen is killed using heat or formalin, as for example, typhoid or Salk poliomyelitis vaccines.
2. Attenuated vaccines: The pathogen is weakened (attenuated) by ageing or altering growth conditions, but is alive, as in the case of measles, mumps and rubella vaccines. There is some risk of the concerned virus becoming virulent.
3. Avirulent organisms: A non-pathogenic strain of a pathogenic organism is used as a vaccine, as in *Bacillus* Calmette Guerin (BCG) vaccine against *Mycobacterium tuberculosis,* the tuberculosis bacterium.
4. Toxoids: The toxin from the pathogen is used as an antigen to produce the vaccine. The severity of the toxicity of the antigen is reduced by treating it with aluminium salts while preparing the 'toxoid', as in the case of diphtheria and tetanus.
   In the case of allergy, the allergenic proteins from pollen and other allergenic material are isolated and used to immunise the patient.
5. Acellular vaccines: Only the antigenic component of the organism is used instead of the whole organism, as in haemophilus influenza B vaccine.
6. Subunit vaccines: Genetic engineering techniques have now made it possible to use as a vaccine only a part of an organism that is adequate to stimulate the immune response. An appropriate segment of genetic material is isolated from the pathogens and introduced into bacteria or yeasts,

to transcribe and translate the inserted foreign DNA. The product is used as a vaccine, as in the case of Hepatitis B vaccine. These vaccines cannot cause the disease even in patients whose immunological system is impaired (immunocompromised) patients.

7. DNA vaccines: Described as the third vaccine revolution, DNA vaccines are an offshoot of gene therapy. Selected segments of DNA, when introduced into the patients system synthesise and deliver proteins that are needed to replace the defective enzyme system or tag a cell for destruction. Viruses or lipid vehicles are used to deliver the DNA into the cells. This recent technology is being tried to produce vaccines against HIV, by a direct injection of plasmid borne DNA.

Herd Immunity

Use of vaccines to prevent disease in communities is herd immunity, which affords protection by decreasing the number of susceptible people in a community, with time. This basically constitutes mass immunisation. Polio vaccination programmes now target an enormous number of children throughout the world, to eradicate polio, as was done for smallpox earlier.

Booster Doses

The effectiveness of certain vaccines is life long as for example of smallpox, measles, mumps and rubella. Attenuated vaccines normally afford life long immunity. But in the case of certain others, the effectiveness is short lived and the immune system needs to be re-educated through periodical booster doses. The vaccine is administered one or more times, with appropriate time gaps, after the initial vaccination, to boost to the immune system to produce adequate quantities of antibodies against the intended pathogen.

Toxoid vaccines require a booster every ten years or so. Booster doses are also needed in case of inactivated or acellular vaccines, which are very safe, as they cannot cause the disease.

Multiple Vaccines

While most vaccines contain antigens of a single pathogen, there is a practice of multiple vaccines, which combine antigens of more than one pathogen. For example, diphtheria, tetanus and pertussis are administered together as DTP vaccination.

Vaccine Administration

Vaccines are administered, as injections (DTP), or dermally (smallpox, anthrax), or orally (polio) or as a nasal spray (influenza virus).

Edible Vaccines

Now transgenic plants are being developed through genetic engineering techniques, where the vaccine is synthesised in the edible part of a food plant (edible vaccines). Transgenic bananas, melons, and tomatoes are choice candidates for carrying edible subunit vaccines, as for example against rabies. The obvious advantage is the ease of transportation and storage of the vaccine bearing material and administration without technical support.

Conventional vaccination programmes in many countries are seriously handicapped due to a lack of equipment for storage and transport of the vaccines and the shortage of paramedical staff to administer the vaccines.

Safety of Vaccines

By and large vaccination programmes have proven to be reasonably safe for the human populations. However, at certain times complications may arise mostly due to an incorrect handling of the vaccines and/or vaccination or due to individual metabolic deficiencies. In spite of all that is adverse in vaccination, immunisation is one of the most efficient means of disease prevention, particularly in large sections of the human population. In the case of HIV and epidemic diseases and even cancer, immunisation is probably the only hope.

BIOTECHNOLOGICAL APPROACHES TO VACCINE PRODUCTION

At present, the majority of veterinary vaccines are produced by conventional methods similar to those implemented by Jenner or Pasteur. These include live, attenuated vaccines and killed or inactivated vaccines. Both of these types of vaccines have proven to be effective particularly in reducing the clinical manifestation following exposure to virulent filed strains of the pathogens.

One of the important impediments in the case of live vaccines is to ensure that the organism is attenuated sufficiently not to cause the disease, but still replicate to a sufficient level to induce an appropriate immune response. However, only a limited number of viral disease can be prevented by live attenuated viral vaccines state and most DNA-containing viruses have the potential to establish persistent (or latent) infection. New viral strains may arise by recombination of the vaccine virus with other viral strains in animal populations; pregnant animals or their offspring may be adversely affected by the vaccine strain. Certain apparently avirulent viral strains can revert to virulence, either by host induced proteolysis or surface proteins of the phenotype, as in the activation of the HN and F0 proteins of influenza virus or by mutations in the genotype, as in the reversion of attenuated oral Sabin poliovirus vaccine. Similarly the so called inactivated foot and mouth disease (FMD) viral vaccines are found to be infectious far frequently. For example, at least 44 per cent of the outbreaks of FMD in Europe from 1968 to 1981 were caused by incompletely inactivated vaccines or due to escape of virus from vaccine manufacturing facilities (FAQ 1981). Similarly, outbreaks of FMD in three South American countries in 1979 and 1980 were caused by three different vaccines that contained infectious virus. In addition, conventional whole agent vaccines, particularly crude preparations, have been implicated in post vaccinal pyrogenic and allergic reactions, abortions, Guillain-Barre neurological syndromes and adverse sequelae.

Conventional killed or inactivated viral vaccines also have potential risks, for example, incompletely or improperly killed batches of virus could result in contamination of the vaccines with active wild, type virus or with contaminating virus in the vaccine. Therefore, elaborate safety testing is a crucial and costly part of the production process. Improvements in conventional biochemistry, recombinant DNA technology, peptide synthesis, molecular genetics and protein purification had laid the foundation for the development of new vaccines which should be more efficacious, cost effective and which have fewer side effects.

Animal vaccines must be cheap, easy to administer and effective. To produce a vaccine, genetic engineers move genes around in the infectious organisms to separate the pathogenic factors (components that cause the disease) from the antigens (components that stimulate an immune response).

Five strategies are currently being applied to the generation of new types of vaccines:

1. Recombinant DNA cloning of immunogenic surface protein.
2. Chemical synthesis of polypeptide vaccines.
3. Construction of recombinant vaccines having guest genes for foreign surface proteins.

4. Genetic engineering of non pathogenic mutant agents.
5. Production of monoclonal epitopes of the surface proteins of infectious agents.
6. Nucleic acid vaccines.

One approach is to remove virulent genes from the infectious organisms. Scours is a disease caused by *E. coli* that affects newborn calves and piglets. The resulting diarrhoea and severe dehydration can cause heavy mortality. Disease, causing strains of the bacteria produce one protein which allows the bacteria to adhere to the gut of the young animals and another which governs the water loss. If the gene for the water loss protein is removed, scours can be prevented. The organism sticks to the gut without causing diarrhoea and acts as a vaccine, stimulating an immune response against the adhering protein. The vaccine is often given to pregnant animals which pass immunity to their offspring.

Recently, recombinant DNA technology has helped to develop new generation vaccines, which are cheaper, safer and more effective. Some vaccines are made not by disarming the pathogen, but by transforming the genes coding for the antigens of pathogen into those coding for harmless characteristics. This method has been used to produce rabies vaccine. The gene for the surface glycoprotein of the rabies virus is inserted into the DNA of another virus vaccinia. Vaccinia virus causes cowpox, but is relatively harmless to dogs. It acts as a vector, transporting the piece of rabies virus RNA into a vaccinated individual and subsequently producing rabies antibodies. This stimulates a protective immune response against rabies.

Subunit vaccines are produced by genetic engineering. They are purified single proteins from the surface of a pathogen which can be produced cheaply in fermenters. The great advantage of subunit vaccines is that they contain no live, potentially infectious organisms. The synthetic vaccines are advantageous because the immune system of the animal is challenged with only one antigen, thereby omitting other components of the virion that might adversely affect the immune response. The major drawback with subunit/peptide vaccines is that the antigenic mass cannot be greater than the amount injected. There is no amplification of the antigen. The conventional vaccine for FMD (killed vaccine) was responsible for nearly half of the outbreaks of the disease in Europe between 1968 and 1981, because it contained a low percentage of live organisms. It may now be replaced by a subunit vaccine.

Many important antigens are proteins and can be made in harmless organisms through genetic engineering. Genetic engineering also provides a way to produce vaccines even if the infectious organisms cannot be grown in animals or in artificial cultures. Genetic engineers have taken a gene that codes for a surface protein (hepatitis B surface antigen) and inserted it into *E. coli* or into yeast. When the proteins are produced by gene expression in new hosts, it is easy to purify the whole protein to obtain a genetically engineered vaccine. Only small regions of the proteins called epitopes are bound by antibodies.

Immunity of flu lasts for a year or so, not because the vaccines are no good, but because the virus keeps changing its protein coat. Scientists have investigated several strains of the flu virus, looking for regions that do not vary and were exposed sufficiently to stimulate an immune reaction. They found a peptide of 18 amino acids which they knew, from the protein structure studies, was located in an exposed part of a viral protein called haemagglutinin. This region was short enough to be produced chemically in a peptide synthesiser. Joining this synthetic peptide to a carrier protein provides a vaccine that protected mice from several different strains of the influenza virus.

Protein and peptide preparations are dead vaccines. Live vaccines can also be produced by genetic engineering. If genes from other organisms are inserted into the DNA of vaccinia, the virus used as a vaccine will produce the corresponding proteins as it grows inside human cells. Experimental vaccines to protect animals against infection from rabies, herpes, hepatitis B and influenza have been produced in this way. Up to 25 genes can be inserted into vaccinia DNA and there are plans to produce multiple vaccines to confer immunity to several diseases simultaneously. Anti-idiotype antibodies have been produced against very many antigens and are being used as an antigen. One of the biggest advantages of this is that the virulent inactivated microbe need not be used, instead anti-idiotypic antibodies could be used for development of immune response. Anti-idiotypic antibody mimics the structure of the original antigen. Anti-idiotypic MAbs have also been evaluated as immunogen.

TYPES OF VACCINE

Whole virus vaccines, either live or killed, constitute the vast majority of vaccines in use at present. However, recent advances in molecular biology had provided alternative methods for producing vaccines. Listed below are the possibilities:
1. Live whole virus vaccines.
2. Killed whole virus vaccines.
3. Subunit vaccines: purified or recombinant viral antigen.
4. Recombinant virus vaccines.
5. Anti-idiotype antibodies.
6. DNA vaccines.

Live Vaccines

Live virus vaccines are prepared from attenuated strains that are almost or completely devoid of pathogenicity but are capable of inducing a protective immune response. They multiply in the human host and provide continuous antigenic stimulation over a period of time. Primary vaccine failures are uncommon and are usually the result of inadequate storage or administration. Another possibility is interference by related viruses as is suspected in the case of oral polio vaccine in developing countries. Several methods have been used to attenuate viruses for vaccine production.

Use of a related virus from another animal—the earliest example was the use of cowpox to prevent smallpox. The origin of the vaccinia viruses used for production is uncertain.

Administration of pathogenic or partially attenuated virus by an unnatural route—the virulence of the virus is often reduced when administered by an unnatural route.

Passage of the virus in an 'unnatural host' or host cell—the major vaccines used in man and animals have all been derived this way. After repeated passages, the virus is administered to the natural host. The initial passages are made in healthy animals or in primary cell cultures. There are several examples of this approach: the 17D strain of yellow fever was developed by passage in mice and then in chick embryos. Polioviruses were passaged in monkey kidney cells and measles in chick embryo fibroblasts. Human diploid cells are now widely used such as the WI-38 and MRC-5. The molecular basis for host range mutation is now beginning to be understood.

Development of temperature sensitive mutants—this method may be used in conjunction with the above method.

Inactivated Whole Virus Vaccines

These were the easiest preparations to use. The preparation was simply inactivated. The outer virion coat should be left intact but the replicative function should be destroyed. To be effective, non-replicating virus vaccines must contain much more antigen than live vaccines that are able to replicate in the host. Preparation of killed vaccines may take the route of heat or chemicals.

The chemicals used include formaldehyde or beta- propiolactone. The traditional agent for inactivation of the virus is formalin. Excessive treatment can destroy immunogenicity whereas insufficient treatment can leave infectious virus capable of causing disease. Soon after the introduction of inactivated polio vaccine, there was an outbreak of paralytic poliomyelitis in the USA use to the distribution of inadequately inactivated polio vaccine.

This incident led to a review of the formalin inactivation procedure and other inactivating agents are now available, such as Beta-propiolactone. Another problem was that SV40 was occasionally found as a contaminant and there were fears of the potential oncogenic nature of the virus.

Live vs dead vaccines

Live vs dead vaccines shown in Table 9.1.

Table 9.1. Live vs dead vaccines.

Feature	Live	Dead
Dose	Low	High
No. of doses	Single	Multiple
Need for adjuvant	No	Yes
Duration of immunity	Many years	Less
Antibody response	IgG,	IgA IgG
CMI	Good	Poor
Reversion to virulence	Possible	Not possible

Because live vaccines replicate inside host cells, bits of virus antigen are presented to the cell surface and recognised by cytotoxic cells

Potential safety problems

Live vaccines

1. Underattenuation.
2. Mutation leading to reversion to virulence.
3. Preparation instability.
4. Contaminating viruses in cultured cells.
5. Heat liability.
6. Should not be given to immunocompromised or pregnant patients.

Killed vaccines

1. Incomplete inactivation.
2. Increased risk of allergic reactions due to large amounts of antigen involved.

Present problems with vaccine development include:

1. Failure to grow large amounts of organisms in laboratory.
2. Crude antigen preparations often give poor protection, e.g. key antigen not identified, ignorance of the nature of the protective or the protective immune response.
3. Live vaccines of certain viruses can: (i) induce reactivation, and (ii) be oncogenic in nature.

Subunit Vaccines

Originally, non-replicating vaccines were derived from crude preparations of virus from animal tissues. As the technology for growing viruses to high titres in cell cultures advanced, it became practicable to purify virus and viral antigens. It is now possible to identify the peptide sites encompassing the major antigenic sites of viral antigens, from which highly purified subunit vaccines can be produced. Increasing purification may lead to loss of immunogenicity, and this may necessitate coupling to an immunogenic carrier protein or adjuvant, such as an aluminium salt. Examples of purified subunit vaccines include the HA vaccines for influenza A and B, and HBsAg derived from the plasma of carriers.

Steps in subunit vaccine production

Steps in subunit vaccine production are:
1. Identify protective proteins or epitopes on the proteins. Once this is done, an individual can either produce a subunit vaccine by rDNA technology or by synthetic peptide technology.
2. Identify gene coding for the protein.
3. Clone the gene coding for the specific protein and express it in a suitable expression system.
4. Purify the protective protein to homogeneity using bovine herpes virus-1. BHV-1 has four glycoproteins—GVPI, GVPII, GVPIII and GVPIV.
5. Immunosorbent columns with monoclonal antibodies are prepared and used for purification of large quantities of the BHV-I glycoproteins. These glycoproteins are then mixed with the adjuvant avidine and used to immunise animals against BHV-I virus.

The host organism used for expression of immunogenic proteins to be used as vaccines may be a genetically engineered micro-organism.

Hepatitis B virus-core protein is planted in *E. coli*, yeast, *Bacillus*, etc. AIDS viral coat protein is engineered in vaccinia virus; foot-and-mouth disease (FMD) core protein is planted in *E. coli*. Malarial parasites and syphilis organism which are difficult to be grown has been planted in *E. coli*.

Myrin and others have developed a more effective and less toxic cholera vaccine. It gives immunity equivalent to infection with natural bacterium. It was genetically altered Vibrio cholerae cells of E1T/ Incaba strain. Side effects like diarrhea can be eliminated by scaling the dose.

Malarial vaccine from Hoffmann La Roche of Switzerland is on the horizon. Surface antigen in sporozoite stage has been identified and isolated to give protection. Antigens and concerned genes from organisms in other parts of parasitic life cycle are under search, for the preparation of a multiple vaccine, which may give a broader spectrum protection against malaria.

DNA of spirochaete (*Treponema pallidum*, the causative agent of syphilis) has been isolated from infected rabbit testicles and is cloned in *E. coli* using vector coliphage. This has enabled development of a more specific diagnostic screening test for syphilis and manufacturing of an effective vaccine.

Need for such vaccine is due to the difficulty of extraction and purification of antigen by conventional techniques, on the one hand, and *Treponema pallidum* becoming resistant to antibiotics in current use and therefore, difficulty faced in the treatment on the other.

Foot-and-mouth disease (FMD), a highly contagious disease in cattle, sheep and swine worldwide, is caused by the virus with a single-stranded RNA. German scientists have successfully cloned double-stranded DNA copies of viral RNA into plasmid pBR 322 and grown in *E. coli*. It was found that more than 100 molecules of viral proteins were synthesised per bacterial ell with a positive serological test.

FMD virus is having a capsid with 60 copies of polypeptides GVP I, GVP II, GVP III and GVP IV. Treatment with trypsin results in the cleavage of VP I and considerable decrease in infectivity and loss of immunising activity. Synthesis of VP I protein precursor is being attempted to give long-lasting immunity. Rabies is a zoonosis endemic in animals and humans countries of Africa, South America and Asia and increasing Europe.

Virus propagation is difficult, so the cost of vaccine production is high. The virus has to be propagated in human cells. Rabies virus-protein-encoding gene is now cloned in *E. coli*, thus producing cheaper vaccine will be possible. Hepatitis B virus-antigen-producing gene can be clone in *E. coli* to produce antigen and the vaccine. But with *E. coli*, complications can be there due to the risk of contamination by endotoxins.

Recombinant Viral Proteins

Virus proteins have been expressed in bacteria, yeast, mammalian cells, and viruses. *E. coli* cells were first to be used for this purpose but the expressed proteins were not glycosylated, which was a major drawback since many of the immunogenic proteins of viruses such as the envelope glycoproteins, were glycosylated. Nevertheless, in many instances, it was demonstrated that the non-glycosylated protein backbone was just as immunogenic. Recombinant hepatitis B vaccine is the only recombinant vaccine licensed at present.

An alternative application of recombinant DNA technology is the production of hybrid virus vaccines. The best known example is vaccinia; the DNA sequence coding for the foreign gene is inserted into the plasmid vector along with a vaccinia virus promoter and vaccinia thymidine kinase sequences. The resultant recombination vector is then introduced into cells infected with vaccinia virus to generate a virus that expresses the foreign gene. The recombinant virus vaccine can then multiply in infected cells and produce the antigens of a wide range of viruses. The genes of several viruses can be inserted, so the potential exists for producing polyvalent live vaccines. HBsAg, rabies, HSV and other viruses have been expressed in vaccinia.

Hybrid virus vaccines are stable and stimulate both cellular and humoral immunity. They are relatively cheap and simple to produce. Being live vaccines, smaller quantities are required for immunisation. As yet, there are no accepted laboratory markers of attenuation or virulence of vaccinia virus for man. Alterations in the genome of vaccinia virus during the selection of recombinant may alter the virulence of the virus. The use of vaccinia also carries the risk of adverse reactions associated with the vaccine and the virus may spread to susceptible contacts. At present, efforts are being made to attenuate vaccinia virus further and the possibility of using other recombinant vectors is being explored, such as attenuated poliovirus and adenovirus.

Recombinant vaccines used by humans

Besides Gardisal cervical cancer vaccine, one of the only other few recombinant vaccines currently used in humans is the Hepatitis B Virus (HBV) vaccine, which contains a surface protein from the hepatitis virus. This protein is produced by recombinant yeast cells and then purified for injection. The HBV vaccine is much safer to use than a weakened form of the actual virus, which, if it reverts back to its original form, could cause liver cancer or hepatitis.

Another recombinant vaccine that has been successfully trialled for human use is the recombinant influenza vaccine, although it has not yet been produced on a commercial basis. Feder, 2009, in fact argues that the US should have had batches of this recombinant vaccine prepared in advance during the swine flu (H1N1) outbreak in 2009, as it is fast to produce and obviates the reliance on vaccines from overseas. Recombinant influenza vaccines are composed of haemagglutinin, a protein present in various strains of the influenza virus. This protein is expressed by recombinant cell cultures and later purified to produce the vaccine.

Recombinant vaccines for animal use

Several commercially used recombinant vaccines used on animals employ a vector based delivery system. These include the VRG vaccine, which protects animals against rabies, and the Purevax recombinant feline leukaemia vaccine. As mentioned above, the VRG vaccine consists of a recombinant *Vaccinia* virus that carries the gene for a rabies glycoprotein. The virus has been modified in several ways, one of which involves the removal of the thymidine kinase gene, making it safer to administer than in its original form. Studies have in fact shown it has not caused any side effects in over 10 avian species and 35 mammalian species.

The Purevax leukaemia vaccine contains a harmless recombinant canarypox virus that incorporates the FeLV gene. This gene produces a protein identical to that produced by the FeLV (feline leukaemia) virus, with the result that the cat's immune response is triggered without the danger of the actual virus being introduced. The canarypox virus is also used as a vector in dog and ferret vaccines.

Live Recombinant Vaccines

An approach holding considerable promise employs a live vector for the delivery of immunogen encoding gene into the vaccinated individuals. The vectors are, vaccinia viruses, adenoviruses, *E. coli*, *Salmonella typhimurium*, etc.

The concerned gene is introduced into the genome of selected viral/bacterial vector, which is suitably attenuated, and the live micro-organism is used for vaccination. Of the various vectors studied, vaccinia virus appears to be the most promising.

Vaccinia virus (VV) is a close relative of the variola virus causing small pox and was used as the vaccine to generate protection against small pox. Generally, antigen encoding genes are inserted within its thymidine kinase (TK) locus, which makes the virus TK- and attenuates its pathogenicity. Further attenuation of VV can be achieved by integration, in its genome, of lymphokine genes like interferon gamma (IFN-γ) or interleukin-2 (IL-2). A large number of genes encoding antigenic proteins have been integrated into the VV genome, which was then used for vaccination.

Recently, a highly effective vaccine against rinderpest virus has been developed by inserting the viral genes Hand F in the VV genes TK and HA. Cattle immunised with the recombinant VV vaccine were completely protected even when they were challenged by a more than 1000 times the normally lethal inoculum. A VV expressing rabies virus glycoprotein (G protein) is widely used vaccine.

Recombinant VV

Recombinant VV is not transmitted from vaccinated to contact animals and induces both humoral and cellular immune responses. But (i) individuals previously immunised or exposed to infection by VV may respond poorly to recombinant VV vaccines. In addition (ii) children and adults with congenital or acquired immunodeficiency may run the risk of severe infections; this could be resolved by incorporating into the VV genome the gene IL-2 or IFN-γ. DNA vaccines offer the following advantages:

1. Purification and preparation of DNA for vaccines is easier, cheaper and more rapid.
2. They are safer and more specific because of high purity.
3. They elicit a more potent immune response than purified protein vaccines.

Future of recombinant vaccines

Further research is likely to increase the availability and effectiveness of recombinant vaccines, resulting in safer preparations that are tailor made to specific diseases in both animals and humans. Vaccines against noninfectious diseases such as diabetes and for protection against parasitic organisms in animals may also become a possibility. Methods of delivery will also undergo improvement, especially in relation to orally introduced treatments.

Synthetic Peptides

The development of synthetic peptides that might be useful as vaccines depends on the identification of immunogenic sites. Several methods have been used. The best known example is foot and mouth disease, where protection was achieved by immunising animals with a linear sequence of 20 amino acids. Synthetic peptide vaccines would have many advantages. Their antigens are precisely defined and free from unnecessary components which may be associated with side effects. They are stable and relatively cheap to manufacture. Furthermore, less quality assurance is required. Changes due to natural variation of the virus can be readily accommodated, which would be a great advantage for unstable viruses such as influenza.

Synthetic peptides do not readily stimulate T cells. It was generally assumed that, because of their small size, peptides would behave like haptens and would therefore require coupling to a protein carrier which is recognised by T-cells. It is now known that synthetic peptides can be highly immunogenic in their free form provided they contain, in addition to the B cell epitope, T-cell epitopes recognised by T-helper cells. Such T-cell epitopes can be provided by carrier protein molecules, foreign antigens, or within the synthetic peptide molecule itself.

Synthetic peptides are not applicable to all viruses. This approach did not work in the case of polioviruses because the important antigenic sites were made up of 2 or more different viral capsid proteins so that it was in a concise 3-D conformation.

Advantages of defined viral antigens or peptides

1. Production and quality control simpler.
2. No NA or other viral or external proteins, therefore less toxic.
3. Safer in cases where viruses are oncogenic or establish a persistent infection.
4. Feasible even if virus cannot be cultivated.

Disadvantages

1. May be less immunogenic than conventional inactivated whole-virus vaccines.
2. Requires adjuvant.
3. Requires primary course of injections followed by boosters.
4. Fails to elicit CMI.

Anti-idiotype Antibodies

The ability of anti-idiotype antibodies to mimic foreign antigens has led to their development as vaccines to induce immunity against viruses, bacteria and protozoa in experimental animals. Anti-idiotypes have many potential uses as viral vaccines, particularly when the antigen is difficult to grow or hazardous. They have been used to induce immunity against a wide range of viruses, including HBV, rabies, Newcastle disease virus and FeLV, reoviruses and polioviruses.

DNA Vaccines

Recently, encouraging results were reported for DNA vaccines whereby DNA coding for the foreign antigen is directly injected into the animal so that the foreign antigen is directly produced by the host cells. In theory these vaccines would be extremely safe and devoid of side effects since the foreign antigens would be directly produced by the host animal. In addition, DNA is relatively inexpensive and easier to produce than conventional vaccines and thus this technology may one day increase the availability of vaccines to developing countries. Moreover, the time for development is relatively short which may enable timely immunisation against emerging infectious diseases. In addition, DNA vaccines can theoretically result in more long-term production of an antigenic protein when introduced into a relatively nondividing tissue, such as muscle.

Indeed some observers have already dubbed the new technology the 'third revolution' in vaccine development—on par with Pasteur's ground-breaking work with whole organisms and the development of subunit vaccines. The first clinical trials using injections of DNA to stimulate an immune response against a foreign protein began for HIV in 1995. Four other clinical trials using DNA vaccines against influenza, herpes simplex virus, T-cell lymphoma, and an additional trial for HIV were started in 1996.

The technique that is being tested in humans involves the direct injection of plasmids—loops of DNA that contain genes for proteins produced by the organism being targeted for immunity. Once injected into the host's muscle tissue, the DNA is taken up by host cells, which then start expressing the foreign protein. The protein serves as an antigen that stimulate an immune responses and protective immunological memory. Enthusiasm for DNA vaccination in humans is tempered by the fact that delivery of the DNA to cells is still not optimal, particularly in larger animals. Another concern is the possibility, which exists with all gene therapy, that the vaccine's DNA will be integrated into host chromosomes and will turn on oncogenes or turn off tumour suppressor genes. Another potential downside is that extended immunostimulation by the foreign antigen could in theory provoke chronic inflammation or autoantibody production

Presentation of immunogenic proteins and peptides

Proteins separated from virus particles are generally much less immunogenic than the intact particles. This difference in activity is usually attributed to the change in configuration of a protein when it is released from the structural requirements of the virus particle. Many attempts have been made to enhance the immunogenic activity of separated proteins.

Adjuvants

Used to potentiate the immune response:

1. Functions to localise and slowly release antigen at or near the site of administration.
2. Functions to activate APCs to achieve effective antigen processing or presentation.

Materials that have been used include:

1. Aluminium salts.
2. Mineral oils.
3. Mycobacterial products, e.g. Freud's adjuvants.

Immunostimulating complexes (ISCOMS)

1. An alternative vaccine vehicle.
2. The antigen is presented in an accessible, multimeric, physically well defined complex.

3. Composed of adjuvant (Quil A) and antigen held in a cage like structure.
4. Adjuvant is held to the antigen by lipids.
5. Can stimulate CMI.
6. Mean diameter 35 nm.

In the most successful procedure, a mixture of the plant glycoside saponin, cholesterol and phosphatidylcholine provides a vehicle for presentation of several copies of the protein on a cage-like structure. Such a multimeric presentation mimics the natural situation of antigens on micro-organisms. These immunostimulating complexes have activities equivalent to those of the virus particles from which the proteins are derived, thus holding out great promise for the presentation of genetically engineered proteins.

Similar considerations apply to the presentation of peptides. It has been shown that by building the peptide into a framework of lysine residues so that 8 copies instead of 1 copy are present, the immune response induced was of a much greater magnitude. A novel approach involves the presentation of the peptide in a polymeric form combined with T cell epitopes. The sequence coding for the foot and mouth disease virus peptide was expressed as part of a fusion protein with the gene coding for the Hepatitis B core protein. The hybrid protein, which forms spherical particles 22 nm in diameter, elicited levels of neutralising antibodies against foot and mouth disease virus that were at least a hundred times greater than those produced by the monomeric peptide.

Immunisation and Herd immunity

The following questions should be asked when a vaccination policy against a particular virus is being developed.

1. What proportion of the population should be immunised to achieve eradication.
2. What is the best age to immunise?
3. How is this affected by birth rates and other factors?
4. How does immunisation affect the age distribution of susceptible individuals, particularly those in age-classes most at risk of serious disease?
5. How significant are genetic, social, or spatial heterogeneities in susceptibility to infection?
6. How does this affect herd immunity?

A basic concept is that of the basic rate of the infection R_0. for most viral infections, R_0 is the average number of secondary cases produced by a primary case in a wholly susceptible population. Clearly, an infection cannot maintain itself or spread if R_0 is less than 1. R_0 can be estimated from as B/(A–D); B = life expectancy, A = average age at which infection is acquired, D = the characteristic duration of maternal antibodies.

The larger the value of R_0, the harder it is to eradicate the infection from the community in question. A rough estimate of the level of immunisation coverage required can be estimated in the following manner: eradication will be achieved if the proportion immunised exceeds a critical value pinc = $1-1/R_0$. Thus the larger the R_0, the higher the coverage is required to eliminate the infection. Thus the global eradication of measles, with its R_0 of 10 to 20 or more, is almost sure to be more difficult to eradicate than smallpox, with its estimated R_0 of 2 to 4. Another example is rubella and measles immunisation in the US. Rubella (A = 9 years) has an R_0 roughly half that of measles (A = 5 years) and indeed rubella has been effectively eradicated in the US while the incidence of measles have declined more slowly.

Why do we not require 100 per cent coverage to eradicate an infection? Immunisation has both a direct and indirect effect. The susceptible host population is reduced by mass immunisation so that the transmission of infection has become correspondingly less efficient and eventually, the infection will be unable to maintain itself.

	Average age of infection	Epidemic period	R_0	Critical coverage
Measles	4–5	2	15–17	92–95
Pertussis	4–5	3–4	15–17	92–95
Mumps	6–7	3	10–12	90–92
Rubella	9–10	3–5	7–8	85–87
Diptheria	11–14	4–6	5–6	80–85
Polio	12–15	3–5	5–6	80–85

Other Type of Vaccines

Attenuated vaccine

An attenuated vaccine is a vaccine created by reducing the virulence of a pathogen, but still keeping it viable (or live). Attenuation takes a living agent and alters it so that it becomes harmless or less virulent. These vaccines contrast to those produced by 'killing' the virus (inactivated vaccine).

An attenuated vaccine is a vaccine which uses live pathogenic material for the purposes of inducing immunity. The strength of the pathogen is weakened or attenuated during the processing of the vaccine to make it less likely to cause disease. A number of vaccines including typhoid, tuberculosis, polio, measles, mumps, and rubella vaccines may be offered in attenuated form.

Attenuation is usually accomplished by culturing the pathogen in a foreign host such as a tissue culture, a live animal, or an egg, with chicken eggs being especially popular. The cultured pathogen is introduced in low amounts to a patient, often through inhalation, where it multiplies in the body. Exposed to the pathogen in the form of an attenuated vaccine, the immune system responds and develops antibodies so that when someone encounters a full strength version, the body will be able to fight it off.

The idea behind an attenuated vaccine is that it is strong enough to cause immunity, but too weak to cause disease. However, the use of such vaccines has sometimes been linked with disease in some patients.

In some cases this appears to be because a batch of vaccines was not handled properly, while in others, the patient reacted poorly, or the virus mutated inside the body to become virulent. This is why attenuated vaccines are viewed as more risky than killed or inactivated vaccines, in which the pathogen is killed before being introduced into the body so that it cannot make someone sick.

Given that attenuated vaccines can sometimes cause disease, one might be reasonably led to wonder why they are used at all when inactive vaccines are available and would presumably be much safer. One of the key reasons to use an attenuated vaccine is that they are more effective, with some vaccinations not even available in killed form.

Live vaccines also stimulate a greater immune system response, lead to the development of more antibodies, and confer longer-lasting immunities. Additionally, they are less costly to produce than killed vaccines, making them appealing for rapid mass-vaccination efforts.

When someone is vaccinated with an attenuated vaccine, it is not uncommon to develop some minor symptoms of illness such as fever, fatigue, or sluggishness as the body's immune system reacts. A doctor can discuss common side effects of specific vaccines with patients and their families, and a doctor can also talk about more serious side effects which could occur. As a general rule, the personal and social benefit of vaccination is believed to outweigh the risks, but there are some specific circumstances in which it may be dangerous for someone to be vaccinated, making it critical to give a complete history to a doctor or nurse before receiving a vaccination or booster.

MMR vaccine

The MMR vaccine is an immunisation shot against measles, mumps and rubella (also called German measles). It was first developed by Maurice Hilleman while at Merck in the late 1960s.

The vaccine is a mixture of three live attenuated viruses, administered via injection. The shot is generally administered to children around the age of one year, with a second dose before starting school (i.e. age 4/5). The second dose is not a booster; it is a dose to produce immunity in the small number of persons (2–5 per cent) who fail to develop measles immunity after the first dose.

MMRV vaccine

The MMRV vaccine, a combined measles, mumps, rubella and varicella vaccine, has been proposed as a replacement for the MMR vaccine to simplify administration of the vaccines. Preliminary data indicate a rate of fever-induced seizure of 9 per 10,000 vaccinations with MMRV, as opposed to 4 per 10,000 for separate MMR and varicella injections; US health officials therefore do not express a preference for use of MMRV vaccine over separate injections.

Pneumococcal conjugate vaccine

Pneumococcal conjugate vaccine (PCV) is a vaccine used to protect infants and young children against disease caused by the bacterium *Streptococcus pneumoniae* (pneumococcus). There are currently two PCV vaccines available on the global market: Prevnar (called Prevenar in some countries) and Synflorix.

Prevnar is a heptavalent vaccine, meaning that it contains the cell membrane sugars of seven serotypes of pneumococcus, conjugated with Diphtheria proteins.

Pneumococcal polysaccharide vaccine

Pneumococcal polysaccharide vaccine (PPSV), is a vaccine used to prevent *Streptococcus pneumoniae* (pneumococcus) infections such as pneumonia and septicaemia. PNEUMOVAX 23, manufactured by Merck, is the currently licensed PPSV. PPSV is not the same vaccination as the pneumococcal conjugate vaccine (PCV) that is routinely administered to infants in the US, Canada, and the UK.

Risks: Approximately half of people who receive PPSV experience pain and soreness at the vaccination site. Less than 1 per cent develop a fever and/or muscle aches.

Polio vaccine

Two polio vaccines are used throughout the world to combat poliomyelitis (or polio). It consists of an injected dose of inactivated (dead) poliovirus.

In the generic sense, vaccination works by priming the immune system with an 'immunogen'. Stimulating immune response, via use of an infectious agent, is known as immunisation. The development of immunity to polio efficiently blocks person-to-person transmission of wild poliovirus, thereby protecting both individual vaccine recipients and the wider community.

Oral vaccine: Oral polio vaccine (OPV) is a live-attenuated vaccine, produced by the passage of the virus through non-human cells at a sub-physiological temperature, which produces spontaneous mutations in the viral genome.

Rotavirus vaccine

A rotavirus vaccine protects children from rotaviruses, which are the leading cause of severe diarrhea among infants and young children. The rotavirus vaccine program aims to reduce child morbidity and mortality from diarrhoeal disease by accelerating the availability of rotavirus vaccines in developing countries.

Smallpox vaccine

The smallpox vaccine was the first successful vaccine to be developed. The process of vaccination was discovered by Edward Jenner in 1796, who acted upon his observation that milkmaids who caught the cowpox virus did not catch smallpox. Prior to widespread vaccination, mortality rates in individuals with smallpox were high—up to 35 per cent in some cases.

Post-eradication vaccination

The vaccine consists of the virus which causes the related, yet far milder, cowpox disease; this virus is appropriately named vaccinia, from the Latin *vacca* which means cow. This vaccine has functional viruses in it which improves its effectiveness but, unfortunately, causes serious complications for people with impaired immune systems (for example chemotherapy and AIDS patients, and people with eczema) and is not yet considered safe for pregnant women. A woman planning on conceiving within one month should not receive the smallpox immunisation until after the pregnancy.

In the event of an outbreak the woman should delay pregnancy if possible. A small, yet significant, percentage of healthy individuals also suffer adverse side-effects which, in rare cases, include permanent neurological damage.

HIV protection

Recent studies suggest that the smallpox vaccine provides some level of defense against HIV. Both the smallpox and HIV virus exploit a receptor called CCR5, which is expressed in white blood cells as the result of smallpox vaccination.

Bacillus Calmette-Guérin

Bacillus Calmette-Guérin (or Bacille Calmette-Guérin, BCG) is a vaccine against tuberculosis that is prepared from a strain of the attenuated (weakened) live bovine tuberculosis bacillus, *Mycobacterium bovis*, that has lost its virulence in humans by being specially cultured in an artificial medium for years. The bacilli have retained enough strong antigenicity to become a somewhat effective vaccine for the prevention of human tuberculosis. At best, the BCG vaccine is 80 per cent effective in preventing tuberculosis for a duration of 15 years; however, its protective effect appears to vary according to geography.

Anthrax vaccines

Anthrax vaccines are vaccines against the infectious disease anthrax. Anthrax is caused by the spore-forming bacterium *Bacillus anthracis*, that most commonly occurs in wild and domestic mammals. Anthrax also occurs in humans when they are exposed to infected animals, hides, or tissue from infected animals, or when they are directly exposed to *B. anthracis*. Depending on the route of infection, anthrax disease can occur in three forms: cutaneous, inhalational, and rarely, gastrointestinal.

Cholera Vaccine

Cholera is a severe bacterial infection caused by the bacteria *Vibrio cholerae*, which primarily affects the small intestine. The main symptoms include profuse watery diarrhea and vomiting. Transmission is primarily by the acquisition of the pathogen through contaminated drinking water or infected food. The severity of the diarrhea and associated vomiting can lead to rapid dehydration and electrolyte loss, which can lead to death. Cholera is a major cause of death in the world. The study of cholera has been used as an example of early epidemiology. Study of the *V. cholerae* bacterium has also shed light on many of the mechanisms used by bacteria to infect and survive in their hosts.

DPT vaccine

DPT (also DTP and DTwP) refers to a class of combination vaccines against three infectious diseases in humans: diphtheria, pertussis (whooping cough) and tetanus. The vaccine components include diphtheria and tetanus toxoids, and killed whole cells of the organism that causes pertussis (wP).

DTaP (also DTPa and TDaP) refers to similar combination vaccines in which the pertussis component is acellular. Also available is the DT or TD vaccine, which lacks the pertussis component. In the Netherlands, the acronym DTP refers to a combination vaccine against diphtheria, tetanus, and poliomyelitis. There, pertussis is known as *kinkhoest* and DKTP refers to a combination vaccine against diphtheria, pertussis/kinkhoest, tetanus, and polio.

The usual course of childhood immunisation is five doses between 2 months and 15 years. For adults, separate combination vaccines are used that adjust the relative concentrations of their components.

Hib vaccine

Haemophilus influenzae type B vaccine (Hib vaccine or PRP vaccine) is a conjugate vaccine developed for the prevention of invasive disease caused by *Haemophilus influenzae* type B bacteria. Vaccinations against *Haemophilus influenzae* (Hib) have decreased early childhood meningitis significantly in developed countries and recently in developing countries.

Hepatitis A vaccine

The vaccine protects against the virus in more than 95 per cent of cases and provides protection from the virus for at least ten years. The vaccine contains inactivated Hepatitis A virus which stimulates active immunity against a future infection. The vaccine should be given in the muscle of the upper arm and be given in two doses for the best protection. The initial dose of the vaccine should be followed up by a booster six to twelve months later. Protection against Hepatitis A occurs two to four weeks after the initial vaccination; protection following the initial course of two or three doses is proven to last at least 10 years and is estimated to last 21 to 27 years.

Hepatitis B vaccine

Hepatitis B vaccine is a vaccine developed for the prevention of hepatitis B virus infection. The vaccine contains one of the viral envelope proteins, hepatitis B surface antigen (HBsAg). It is produced by yeast cells, into which the genetic code for HBsAg has been inserted. A course of three vaccine injections are given with the second injection at least one month after the first dose and the third injection given six months after the first dose. Afterward an immune system antibody to HBsAg is established in the bloodstream. The antibody is known as *anti-HBsAg*. This antibody and immune system memory then provide immunity to hepatitis B infection.

Recommended populations

Babies born to mothers with active hepatitis B infections are recommended to receive treatment reducing the risk of mother-to-child transmission of the hepatitis B infection. As soon as possible and within 48 hours of birth, newborns are vaccinated with hepatitis B surface antigen (HBsAg) and injected with hepatitis B immunoglobulin (HBIG).

HPV vaccine

The human papillomavirus (HPV) vaccine may prevent infection with certain serotypes of human papillomavirus associated with the development of cervical cancer, genital warts, and some less common cancers. Two HPV vaccines are currently on the market: Gardasil and Cervarix. Both vaccines protect against two of the HPV types (HPV-16 and HPV-18) that can cause cervical cancer and some other genital cancers; Gardasil also protects against two of the HPV types that cause genital warts. In addition, some commercially available vaccines have been shown to prevent potential precursors to anal, vulvar, vaginal, and penile cancers.

Gardasil

Gardasil also known as Gardisil or Silgard, is a vaccine proven to prevent certain types of human papillomavirus (HPV), specifically HPV types 16, 18, 6, and 11. HPV types 16 and 18 are currently associated with about 70 per cent of cervical, 26 per cent of head and neck and many vulvar, vaginal, penile, and anal cancer cases. HPV types 6 and 11 are associated with about 90 per cent of genital warts cases.

Gardasil prevents HPV infections, but does not treat existing infection. Therefore, to be effective it must be given before HPV infection occurs. Some HPV strains are sexually transmitted, and HPV-16 has a 60 per cent per-couple transmission rate.

Influenza vaccine

The influenza vaccine, also known as a Flu Shot, is an annual vaccine to protect against the highly variable influenza virus. Each injected seasonal influenza vaccine contains three influenza viruses: one A (H3N2) virus, one regular seasonal A (H1N1) virus (in 2010 this was replaced by the 2009 pandemic H1N1 virus), and one B virus.

FluMist

FluMist is a nasal spray influenza vaccine manufactured by MedImmune, Inc. that was first introduced in 2003. It was the first and (as of 2007) the only live attenuated vaccine for influenza available outside of Europe. It is also called live attenuated influenza vaccine (LAIV). In September 2009 a LAIV intranasal vaccine for the novel H1N1 influenza virus was approved. Influenza vaccine is a cost-effective counter-measure to the threat of seasonal or pandemic outbreaks of influenza.

Anti-idiotypic vaccine

Anti-idiotypic vaccines comprise antibodies that have three-dimensional immunogenic regions, designated idiotopes, that consist of protein sequences that bind to cell receptors. Idiotopes are aggregated into idiotypes specific of their target antigen.

Cancer Vaccines

Cancer vaccines have been studied for several decades, but advances in this field have been slower than for other forms of immunotherapy. They are still mostly experimental treatments at this time.

Most of us know about vaccines given to healthy people for infectious diseases, such as measles and mumps. These vaccines use weakened or killed viruses, bacteria, or other germs to start an immune response in the body. Getting the immune system ready to defend against these germs helps it keep the germs from making people sick.

Some so-called 'cancer vaccines' are designed to work the same way. For example, new vaccines against the human papilloma virus (HPV) help prevent women from getting cervical, vaginal, and vulvar cancer. Vaccines against hepatitis B virus (HBV) may lower some people's risk of getting liver cancer. But these vaccines don't target cancer cells; they target the viruses that can cause these cancers.

True cancer vaccines are different from the vaccines that work against viruses. Instead of preventing disease, they are meant to get the immune system to attack a disease that already exists.

A true cancer vaccine contains cancer cells, parts of cells, or pure antigens. The vaccine increases the immune response against cancer cells that are already present in the body. It may be combined with other substances or cells called adjuvants that help boost the immune response even further.

Cancer vaccines are thought of as active immunotherapies because they are meant to trigger your own immune system to respond. They are specific because they should only affect the cancer cells. These vaccines do not just boost the immune system in general; they cause the immune system to attack cells with one or more specific antigens. And because the immune system has special cells for memory, it's hoped that the drugs will help keep cancer from coming back.

Although cancer vaccines have shown some promise in clinical trials, none have yet been approved in the United States to treat cancer. Several types of cancer vaccines are now being studied. A few have reached late stage clinical trials.

Tumour cell vaccines

Tumour cell vaccines are made up of actual cancer cells that have been removed during surgery. The cells are treated in the lab, usually with radiation, so they cannot form more tumours. In most cases, doctors also change the cells in certain ways, often by adding chemicals or new genes, to make them more likely to be seen as foreign by the immune system. The cells are then injected into the patient. The immune system recognises antigens on these cells, then seeks out and attacks any other cells with these antigens that are still in the body.

In some cases, doctors give the vaccine along with substances called adjuvants that increase the immune response. The general boost that adjuvants give to the immune system is meant to make the vaccine work better. Some promising newer versions of these vaccines use tumour cells that are fused to dendritic cells, in the hope of further stimulating the immune system.

A possible advantage of tumour cell vaccines over antigen-based vaccines is that not all cancer antigens have been found yet. Using the whole tumour cell may expose the immune system to a large number of important cancer antigens, including some that researchers have not yet recognised. This may make them more effective. Also, dendritic cell-based vaccines may be better than antigen vaccines at recruiting other parts of the immune system to fight the cancer. They seem to be more likely to cause T cells to react against the cancer.

The two basic kinds of tumour cell vaccines are autologous and allogeneic.

Autologous vaccines

Autologous (pronounced aw-TAH-luh-gus) means 'coming from the self'. An autologous tumour cell vaccine is made from killed tumour cells taken from the same person in whom they will later be used. In other words, cells are taken from you (during surgery), the vaccine is made from them in a lab, and the cells are injected back into you. Autologous cancer cells may be reinjected shortly after surgery, or they may be grown in the lab or frozen and given later.

Although autologous tumour cell vaccines are promising, there are some potential drawbacks:

1. It can be expensive to create a new, unique vaccine for each patient.
2. Cancer cells tend to mutate (change) over time, so an autologous tumour vaccine might become less effective later if the cancer cells in your body change.
3. Depending on the surgery and the size of your tumour(s), you may not have enough usable cells in the removed tumour to make a vaccine, or there may not be enough to retreat if the cancer starts growing again.

Because of these problems, researchers are also looking at ways to create tumour cell vaccines that could work in any patient with that particular kind of cancer.

Allogeneic vaccines

Allogeneic means 'coming from another'. These vaccines use cells of a particular cancer type that originally came from someone other than the patient being treated. Allogeneic vaccines are easier to make than autologous vaccines. They are more like off-the-shelf drugs than a vaccine made for just one person. The cells for the vaccine are grown in the lab from a stock of cancer cells kept for that purpose. Some allogeneic tumour vaccines use a mixture of cells which were removed from several patients. The cells are treated and are usually injected along with one or more adjuvant substances to stimulate the immune system.

Types of cancers for which tumour cell vaccines are being studied

Although the FDA has not yet approved any tumour cell vaccines for general use, they are being studied in clinical trials against many types of cancer, including: (i) melanoma, (ii) kidney cancer, (iii) ovarian cancer, (iv) breast cancer, (v) colorectal cancer, (vi) lung cancer, (vii) prostate cancer, (viii) non-Hodgkin lymphoma, and (ix) leukemia.

Antigen vaccines

Antigen vaccines boost the immune system by using only one antigen (or a few), rather than whole tumour cells that contain many thousands of antigens. The antigens are usually proteins or pieces of proteins called peptides. Antigen vaccines may be specific for a certain type of cancer, but they are not made for a unique patient like autologous cell vaccines are.

Scientists have learned how to mass-produce many antigens in the lab. They can also change these antigens to make them more easily recognised by the immune system. This new technology means that large amounts of these very specific antigens can now be given to many patients.

Some antigens cause an immune response only in patients with a certain kind of cancer, while others produce immune reactions to more than one kind of cancer. Scientists often combine several antigens in a vaccine to try to get a stronger immune response. Antigen vaccines are being studied to be used against these cancers, among others: (i) breast cancer, (ii) prostate cancer, (iii) colorectal cancer, (iv) ovarian cancer, (v) melanoma, (vi) kidney cancer, (vii) pancreatic cancer, and (viii) multiple myeloma.

Dendritic cell vaccines

Dendritic cells are special antigen-presenting cells that help the immune system recognise cancer cells. They break down cancer cells into smaller pieces (including antigens), then hold out, or 'present', these antigens to T cells. This makes it easier for the immune system cells to recognise and attack them. Dendritic cells are the most effective antigen-presenting cells known.

Dendritic cell vaccines are autologous vaccines, and must be made individually for each patient. The process used to create them is complex and expensive:

1. Doctors remove some of the cells that grow into dendritic cells (from the blood) and treat them in the lab to make them multiply and turn into dendritic cells. This creates many more dendritic cells than if they just used cells taken from the patient. These dendritic cells are then exposed to cancer cells or cancer antigens.
2. Other methods are to change their genes so that they make their own antigens or to fuse the dendritic cells with tumour cells. These procedures lead to dendritic cells with cancer antigens on their surface.
3. The dendritic cells are then injected back into the body.

The dendritic cells that have cancer antigens on their surface are better able to help the immune system recognise and destroy cancer cells that have those antigens on them.

The dendritic cell vaccine approach has shown promise in tests in lab animals and in some human studies. They are only available through clinical trials at this time. They are being studied for use in people with these and other cancers: (i) prostate cancer, (ii) melanoma, (iii) kidney cancer, (iv) colorectal cancer, (v) lung cancer, (vi) breast cancer, (vii) leukemia, (viii) non-Hodgkin lymphoma.

Anti-idiotype vaccines

Every B cell or plasma cell makes only one kind of antibody. The unique part of each type of antibody is called an idiotype. Antibodies are made when the immune system responds to antigens. But the immune system also makes some antibodies that treat other antibodies like antigens. In other words, sometimes the body makes antibodies against other antibodies. Scientists believe these antibodies against antibodies are important in helping to keep the immune system in check.

Antibodies and antigens fit together like a lock and key. So an antibody to a particular idiotype of another antibody (an anti-idiotype) will usually look like the antigen that triggered cells to make the antibody in the first place (like using the lock itself to make an extra key). Because the anti-idiotype antibodies look like the antigen and appear foreign, injecting them into the body causes the immune system to attack the anti-idiotypes, along with the antigens themselves.

Scientists have learned how to make these anti-idiotype antibodies in the lab. They can be used as part of a cancer vaccine because they look like the antigens on the cancer cells in the patient's body. Therefore, they can trigger an immune response against that specific cancer.

Researchers consider lymphomas to be the most promising targets for anti-idiotype vaccines. This is because all lymphoma cells have unique antigen receptors not present on normal lymphocytes or other normal cells of the body. These unique antigens can be used to make lymphoma vaccines. Early studies of B-cell lymphoma vaccines have been promising.

DNA vaccines

When tumour cells or antigens are injected into the body as a vaccine, they may cause the desired immune response at first, but they may become less effective over time. This is because the immune system recognises them as foreign and quickly destroys them. Without any further stimulation, the immune system often returns to its normal (pre-vaccine) state of activity. To get around this, scientists have looked for a way to provide a steady supply of antigens to keep the immune response going.

DNA is the substance in cells that contains the genetic code for the proteins that cells make. Cells can be injected with bits of DNA that code for protein antigens. This DNA might be taken up by cells and instruct them to keep making more antigens. These types of therapies are called DNA vaccines.

Scientists may be able to do this by removing some of your cells, treating them with DNA that codes for a certain antigen, and then returning them to you. The altered cells would then make the antigen on an ongoing basis to keep the immune response strong.

DNA vaccines are now being studied in clinical trials for use against the following cancers, among others: (i) melanoma, (ii) leukemia, (iii) prostate cancer, and (iv) head and neck cancer.

Not all cancer treatments using DNA focus on the immune system. There are other types of experimental therapy that use DNA to treat cancer cells directly by replacing the damaged genes responsible for the cells' abnormal growth. Some add new genes that make the cancer cells more sensitive to anticancer drugs.

Vector-based vaccines

These vaccines use special delivery systems (called vectors) to make them more effective. They aren't really a separate category of vaccine; for example, there are vector-based antigen vaccines and vector-based DNA vaccines. Vectors are special viruses, bacteria, yeast cells, or other structures that can be used to get antigens or DNA into the body. The vectors are often germs that have been altered to make sure they can no longer cause disease.

Vectors may be helpful in making vaccines for a number of reasons. First, they may be used to deliver more than one cancer antigen at a time, which may make the body's immune system more likely to mount a response. Second, vectors such as viruses and bacteria may trigger their own immune responses from the body, which may help make the overall immune response even stronger. Finally, these vaccines may be easier and less expensive to make than some other vaccines. Many clinical trials of vector-based vaccines are now under way.

NEW GENERATION VACCINES

The advances in the last few years in the knowledge about the immune response and about molecular biology have allowed the identification of a large number of infectious agents and proteins of immunological interest and their expression in different vectors of amplification. The elimination of those proteins that are not of immunological interest or are not related to the virulence of the agent is now possible. Thus, new vaccines have been created which do not contain the whole infectious agent and that, among other advantages, allows the serological discrimination between sick and vaccinated animals.

The basis of these new vaccines is, in the first place, the identification of the protein/s of the infectious agent that are able to induce an immune response in a similar way to that produced by the whole agent. Secondly, the identification of those proteins that are not immunogenic, do not have a role in replication, or that are related to virulence; thus, these proteins are not necessary. Using genetic engineering, the genes coded for these proteins can be selected, cloned and expressed using different vectors; they can also be eliminated by selective deletion. A variation of this system is the chemical production of the selected proteins once they have been identified (Fig. 9.1).

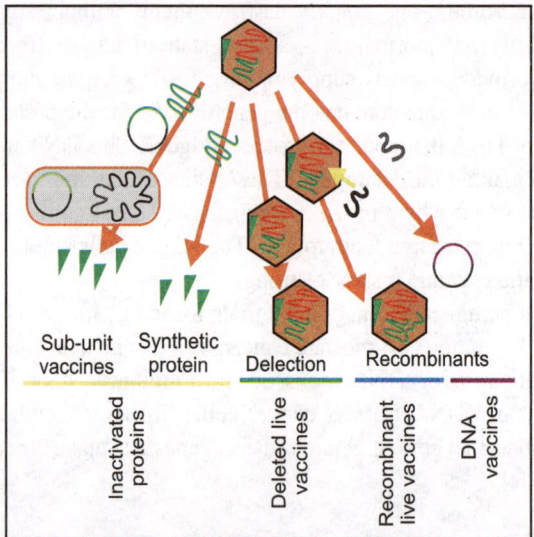

Fig. 9.1. New generation vaccines.

Another interesting aspect, when obtaining these new vaccines, is the possibility of incorporating the immunologically interesting proteins. These would be sequences of other antigens capable of increasing the stimulation of B and T lymphocytes, and even the release of cytokines.

Types of New Generation Vaccines

New generation vaccines can be classified in the following groups based on the different technologies used (inactivated proteins, deleted-attenuated vaccines, recombinant vaccines).

Classification of new generation porcine vaccines:

1. Inactivated proteins:
   (a) Sub-unit vaccines: (i) foot-and-mouth disease, (ii) classical swine fever, and (iii) porcine parvovirus (experimental).
   (b) Synthetic proteins vaccines: (i) foot-and-mouth disease.
2. Deleted live vaccines:
   (a) Aujeszky's disease.
3. Live recombinant:
   (a) Only experimental
4. DNA vaccines:
   (a) Only experimental.

Inactivated proteins

The most commonly used molecular techniques to obtain large quantities of antigenic proteins are:

1. Recombinant DNA technique: Subunit vaccine.
2. Production of synthetic proteins: Synthetic vaccines.

Recombinant DNA technique

This technique is based on the production of proteins from an infectious agent without using the microorganism. Using genetic engineering techniques, DNA is fragmented expressed *in vitro* in different vectors . Thus, large quantities of a protein (subunit) are produced (sometimes more than one protein is produced). This can be used as a subunit vaccine. The different steps of this method are:

Once the relevant protein/s from an etiologic agent has been identified and sequenced, the DNA fragment codifying these proteins is isolated and then inserted into a plasmid that acts as the vector for the transference. Later, this is inserted in the expression vector (the type of plasmid will depend on the vector for expression) (Fig. 9.2).

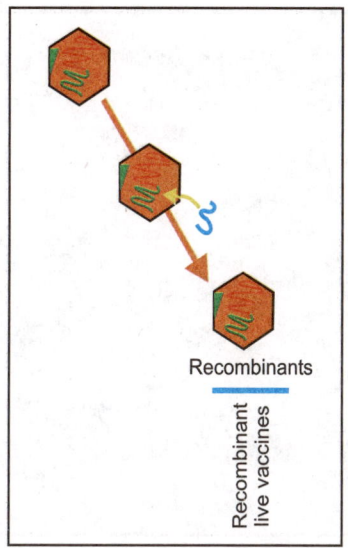

Recombinants

Recombinant live vaccines

Fig. 9.2. Once the fragment of DNA and its sequence are known, (1) this fragment is isolated and (2) inserted into a plasmid. (3) This plasmid is then introduced into an expression vector (*E. coli*, Baculovirus). (4) Some will accept the gene and thus produce the recombinant protein. (5) most of them will not.

Some of these expression vectors will accept the new gene and then produce the protein. Using different labelling techniques the identification of those vectors expressing the new gene will be possible.

The most frequently used vectors for expression are bacteria, especially *E. coli*, yeasts and baculovirus. Bacteria present some problems for adequately glycosilating the produced polypeptides, that's why usually, the obtained proteins have lower immunogenic properties.

Baculovirus are being increasingly used for the production of subunit vaccines due to their great capability of expression. Baculovirus is an insect virus able to replicate in established insect cell lines and whose expression promoter is the gene of polyhydrine. This gene produces up to 60 per cent of the total protein of the virus and can be replaced by foreign genes. Using this system, different proteins against several animal viruses have been produced in insect cells: blue tongue disease, porcine parvovirus, and African equine fever. In some cases, the production of several proteins at the same time simulating the virion particle ('virus like particles' of VLP) (Fig. 9.3), has been possible. This is the case with blue-tongue disease; the obtained product has a high immunogenic capability.

The first sub-unity vaccine against foot-and-mouth disease virus (FMDV) was obtained in the mid-eighties using recombinant DNA techniques. The gene for VP-1 protein was cloned and expressed in *E. coli*, and large quantities of VP were produced.

However, the immune response induced with this vaccine turned out to be much smaller than that produced by the conventional inactivated vaccine. In order to obtain a response similar to that of the conventional vaccine, 1000 times more of VP-1 was necessary. A new sub-unity vaccine against Classical Swine Fever Virus (CSFV) has recently been developed. This vaccine consists of just glycoprotein gp 55, which has been shown to induce immunity and protection against virulent CSFV. The gene of gp 55 has been cloned and expressed using baculovirus. The protein obtained is then inoculated into the pigs which then produce neutralising antibodies that are able to protect against the infection by the virulent virus.

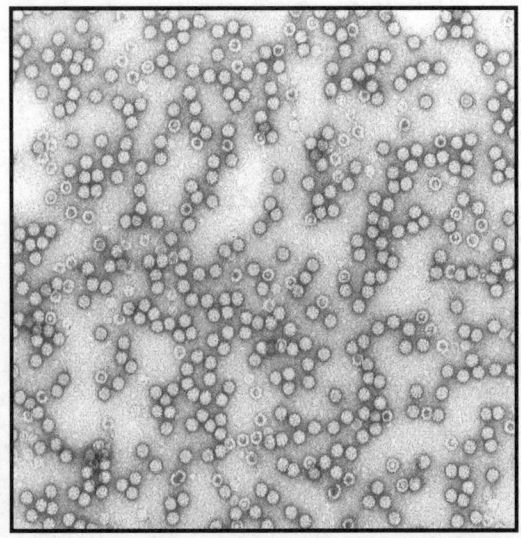

Fig. 9.3. Virus like particles (VLP). Microscropic structure of blue-tongue disease.

Production of synthetic proteins

Synthetic vaccines: When epitopes or antigenic determinants are identified in the complex structure of a protein, as happens with VP-1 of FMD, which is known to be located between aminoacids 140 and 160, it is then possible to chemically synthesise them and then produce a synthetic peptide identical to that of the virus; this is known as a synthetic vaccine. However, the number of protected animals (in the case of foot-and-mouth disease) is less than 50 per cent of the total.

The cause of this lack of protective immunity seems to be due to the fact that the epitope located between aminoacids 140 and 160 is effectively recognised by B lymphocytes, but not by T lymphocytes. The identification of epitopes able to stimulate T lymphocytes is nowadays underway in order to include them in a future vaccine.

SALMONELLA

Salmonella is a genus of rod-shaped, Gram-negative, non-spore forming, predominantly motile enterobacteria with diameters around 0.7 to 1.5 μm, lengths from 2 to 5 μm, and flagella which project in all directions (i.e. peritrichous). They are chemoorganotrophs, obtaining their energy from oxidation and reduction reactions using organic sources, and are facultative anaerobes. Most species produce hydrogen sulphide, which can readily be detected by growing them on media containing ferrous sulphate, such as TSI. Most isolates exist in two phases: a motile phase I and a nonmotile phase II. Cultures that are nonmotile upon primary culture may be switched to the motile phase using a Cragie tube.

Salmonella is closely related to the *Escherichia* genus and are found worldwide in cold- and warm-blooded animals (including humans), and in the environment. They cause illnesses such as typhoid fever, paratyphoid fever, and the foodborne illness salmonellosis.

Salmonella as Disease-causing Agents

Salmonella infections are zoonotic and can be transferred between humans and nonhuman animals. Many infections are due to ingestion of contaminated food. A distinction is made between enteritis *Salmonella* and typhoid/paratyphoid *Salmonella*, where the latter, because of a special virulence factor and a capsule protein (virulence antigen)—can cause serious illness, such as *Salmonella enterica* subsp. *enterica* serovar Typhi, or *Salmonella* typhi). *Salmonella* typhi is adapted to humans and does not occur in animals.

Sources of infection

1. Unclean food, particularly in institutional kitchens and restaurants.
2. Excretions from either sick or infected but apparently clinically healthy people and animals (especially endangered are caregivers and animals).
3. Polluted surface water and standing water (such as in shower hoses or unused water dispensers).
4. Unhygienically thawed fowl (the meltwater contains many bacteria).
5. An association with reptiles (pet tortoises and snakes) (primarily aquatic turtles) is well described.

Salmonella bacteria can survive several weeks in a dry environment and several months in water; thus, they are frequently found in polluted water, contamination from the excrement of carrier animals being particularly important. Aquatic vertebrates, notably birds and reptiles, are important vectors of salmonella. Poultry, cattle, and sheep frequently being agents of contamination, salmonella can be found in food, particularly meats and raw eggs.

MONOCLONAL ANTIBODIES

Antibodies, present in the circulation of all vertebrates, are a body's natural defense against foreign substances. When any substance, such as a disease-causing bacteria or virus, is recognised by the body's immune system as an invader, i.e. an antigen—the body produces proteins that bind to that antigen and help destroy it. These proteins, known as antibodies, are very specific and thus bind only to one particular antigen. Once created in response to an antigen, an antibody continues to resist that foreign molecule. This allows our bodies to fight off diseases that previously afflicted us, without getting sick again. For example, most people will only contract chickenpox once in their lifetime, no matter how often they are exposed to the disease. This phenomenon is also what makes vaccinations possible. A vaccine is an injection of killed or weakened virus that stimulates the production of antibodies when introduced into the body.

Antibodies have many useful purposes, in addition to protection against disease. They can be used to diagnose a wide variety of illnesses, as well as to detect the presence of abnormal substances in the blood, such as drugs, viruses, and bacterial products. In order to be used for diagnostic and detection purposes, antibodies that bind specifically to the virus, bacteria or drug of interest are necessary.

When an antigen is introduced into the body, however, a variety of different antibodies are synthesised. The antigen binds to receptors on the surface of B cells, stimulating those cells to produce antibodies specific to the antigen. When seeking out its target, the antibody binds to a site on the antigen known as the epitope. Although each antibody can only bind to one specific epitope, a single antigen may have several effective epitopes, thereby initiating responses from several different B cells. The antibodies produced are referred to as polyclonal antibodies.

Until the late 1970s, these polyclonal antibodies, obtained from the blood serum of immunised animals, provided the only source of antibodies for research or treatment of disease. Isolation of specific antibodies was essentially impossible, until 1975, when Georges Kohler and Cesar Milstein discovered how to make monoclonal antibodies from hybridomas.

Hybridomas are hybrid cells that have inherited some characteristics of both parent cells. Kohler and Milstein created hybridomas by fusing malignant myeloma cells with antibody-producing B cells (Fig. 9.4). The myeloma cells have the ability to replicate indefinitely and are clonogenic—they will form clones when grown *in vitro*. They selected B cells which produced a specific antibody. By fusing these two cell types, they could obtain cells selected for both immortality and production of the specific antibody of interest.

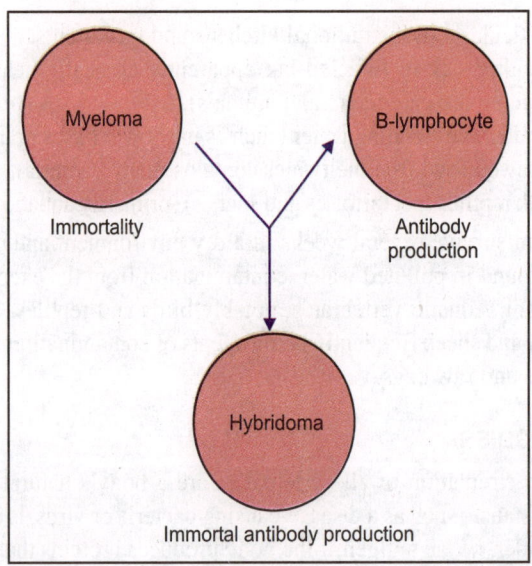

Fig. 9.4. Illustrates the fusion of a myeloma and an antibody-producing cell, resulting in an immortal, antibody-producing hybridoma.

The first step in Kohler and Milstein's technique for production of monoclonal antibodies involves immunising an experimental animal with the antigen of interest. In most of their experiments, Kohler and Milstein injected a mouse with sheep red blood cells. The mouse's body initiates an immune response and begins producing antibodies specific to the antigen. The mouse's spleen is then removed and B cells producing the antibody of interest are isolated. Tumour-producing cells which have been grown in culture are then fused with the B lymphocytes using polyethylene glycol. Only hybridomas resulting from the fusion will survive. The spleen lymphocyte has a limited life span, so any B cells that did not fuse with a myeloma will die in the culture. As well, those cells that lack the antibody-producing aspect of the B cell will not secrete the enzyme HGPRT, which is required for growth in the HAT medium. The hypoxathine-aminopterinthymidine (HAT) medium, on which the cells are grown, inhibits the pathway for nucleotide synthesis. Cells which produce HGPRT can bypass this pathway and continue to grow. By placing the fused cells in a HAT medium, the true hybridomas can be isolated .

The isolated hybridoma cells are then screened for specificity to the desired antigen. Because each hybridoma descends from one B cell, it makes copies of only one antibody. The hybridoma that produces the antibody of interest is grown in culture to produce large amounts of monoclonal antibodies, which are then isolated for further use.

Because of their specificity, monoclonal antibodies are more pure than the polyclonal antibodies of conventional techniques and potentially more effective than contemporary drugs in fighting disease. Drugs often attack the body's own cells in addition to the foreign molecule, producing negative side effects such as nausea. Monoclonal antibodies will bind to only the specific target molecule, without any unwanted side effects (Fig. 9.5).

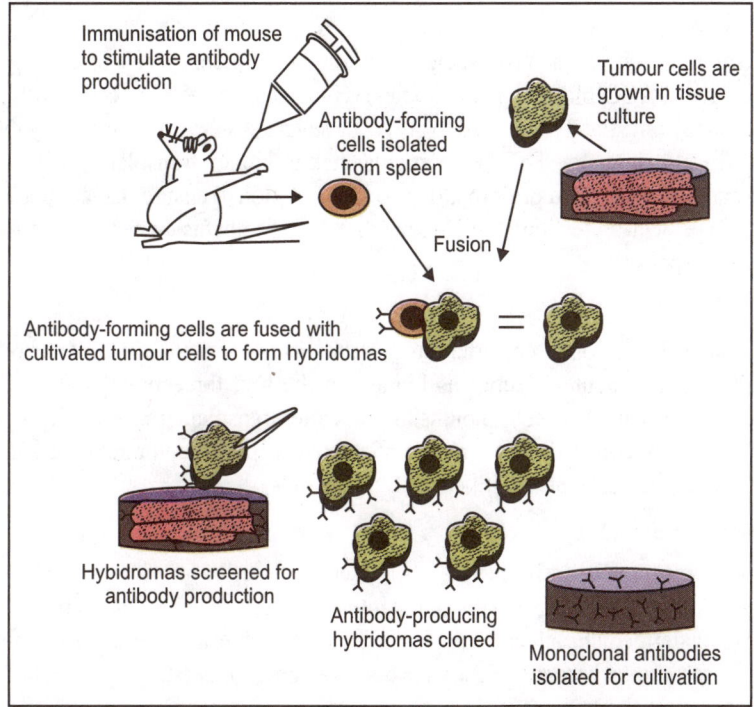

Fig. 9.5. Summarises the production of monoclonal antibodies from a mouse spleen cell.

Monoclonal Antibody Therapy

Monoclonal antibody therapy is the use of monoclonal antibodies (or mAb) to specifically bind to target cells. This may then stimulate the patient's immune system to attack those cells. It is possible to create a mAb specific to almost any extracellular/cell surface target, and thus there is a large amount of research and development currently being undergone to create monoclonals for numerous serious diseases (such as rheumatoid arthritis, multiple sclerosis and different types of cancers). There are a number of ways that mAbs can be used for therapy. For example: mAb therapy can be used to destroy malignant tumour cells and prevent tumour growth by blocking specific cell receptors. Variations also exist within this treatment, e.g. radioimmunotherapy, where a radioactive dose localises on target cell line, delivering lethal chemical doses to the target.

Transplant Rejection

Transplant rejection occurs when a transplanted organ or tissue is not accepted by the body of the transplant recipient. This is explained by the concept that the immune system of the recipient attacks the transplanted organ or tissue. This is expected to happen, because the immune system's purpose is to distinguish foreign material within the body and attempt to destroy it, just as it attempts to destroy infecting organisms such as bacteria and viruses. When possible, transplant rejection can be reduced through serotyping to determine the most appropriate donor-recipient match and through the use of immunosuppressant drugs.

Types of rejection

Hyperacute rejection

Hyperacute rejection is a complement-mediated response in recipients with pre-existing antibodies to the donor (for example, ABO blood type antibodies). Hyperacute rejection occurs within minutes and the transplant must be immediately removed to prevent a severe systemic inflammatory response. Rapid agglutination of the blood occurs. This is a particular risk in kidney transplants, and so a prospective cytotoxic cross-match is performed prior to kidney transplantation to ensure that antibodies to the donor are not present. Hyperacute rejection is analogous to a blood transfusion reaction as it is a humoral-mediated immune response.

Acute rejection

Acute rejection usually begins one week after transplantation (as opposed to hyperacute rejection, which is immediate). The risk of acute rejection is highest in the first three months after transplantation. However, acute rejection can also occur months to years after transplantation. A single episode of acute rejection is not a cause for concern if recognised and treated promptly, and rarely leads to organ failure. But recurrent episodes are associated with chronic rejection.

Chronic rejection

The term 'chronic rejection' was initially a term used to describe a long-term loss of function in transplanted organs, associated with fibrosis of the internal blood vessels of the transplanted tissue. But this pathology is now termed chronic allograft vasculopathy. The term chronic rejection is reserved for cases of transplant rejection where the rejection is due to a poorly understood chronic inflammatory and immune response against the transplanted tissue.

Chronic rejection of the lungs

Chronic rejection after lung transplantation is the leading cause of long-term morbidity and mortality in lung transplant patients. The median survival of lung-transplant patients is approximately 4.7 years— about half that of other major transplanted organ recipients. Histopathologically, the condition is known as *bronchiolitis obliterans*. Clinically, patients present with progressive airflow obstruction often associated with dyspnea and coughing.

Rejection mechanisms

Rejection is an adaptive immune response and is mediated through both T cell mediated and humoral immune (antibodies) mechanisms. The number of mismatched alleles determines the speed and magnitude of the rejection response. Different mechanisms tend to act against different grafts.

Treatment of rejection

Chronic transplant rejection is irreversible and cannot be treated effectively. Treatments with inhaled cyclosporin are being investigated as a means to delay or prevent chronic rejection of the lungs. At present the only definitive treatment is re-transplantation, if patients can be reallocated and if donors are available. Acute transplant rejection can be treated using chemotherapeutic drugs designed to suppress the immune system. Acute rejection is normally treated initially with a short course of high-dose corticosteroids, which is usually sufficient to treat successfully. If this is not enough, the course can be repeated or a triple therapy regimen can be used, consisting of a corticosteroid plus a calcineurin inhibitor and an anti-proliferative agent. Antibodies against specific components of the immune system can be added to this regimen, especially for high-risk patients. mTOR inhibitors can be used in selected patients, where calcineurin inhibitors or steroids are contraindicated. Acute rejection refractory to these treatments may require blood transfusions to remove antibodies against the transplant.

If a bone marrow transplant can be performed, the transplant recipient's immune system can be replaced with the donor's immune system, thus enabling the recipient's body to accept the new organ without risk of rejection. This requires that the bone marrow, which produces the immune cells, be from the same person as the organ donation (or an identical twin or a clone). There is a risk of graft versus host disease (GVHD) in which the lymphoid cells co-injected with the bone marrow transplant recognise the host tissues as foreign and attack and destroy them accordingly.

Sepsis (Blood Infection)

Sepsis is a condition in which the body is fighting a severe infection that has spread via the bloodstream. If a patient becomes 'septic', they will likely be in a state of low blood pressure termed 'shock'. This condition can develop either as a result of the body's own defense system or from toxic substances made by the infecting agent (such as a bacteria, virus, or fungus).

People at risk for sepsis

1. People whose immune systems (the body's defense against microbes) are not functioning well because of an illness (such as cancer or AIDS) or because of medical treatments (such as chemotherapy for cancer or steroids for a number of medical conditions) that weaken the immune system are more prone to develop sepsis. It is important to remember that even healthy people can become septic.
2. Because their immune systems are not completely developed, very young babies may get sepsis if they become infected and are not treated in a timely manner. Often, if they develop signs of an infection such as fever, infants have to receive antibiotics and be admitted to the hospital. Sepsis in the very young is often more difficult to diagnose because the typical signs of sepsis (fever, change in behaviour) may not be present or may be more difficult to ascertain.
3. The elderly population, especially those with other medical illnesses such as diabetes, may be at increased risk as well.

The number of people dying from sepsis has almost doubled in the past 20 years. This is most likely due to the increased number of patients who suffer from sepsis. The number of patients who develop sepsis has increased for many reasons:

1. There has been a large increase in sepsis because doctors have started treating cancer patients and organ-transplant patients, among others, with strong medications that weaken the immune

system. In the past, these patients would have died due to complications of their disease. As we get better at treating the underlying illness, patients survive longer but then sometimes die due to the complications of the therapy.

2. Also, because of our ageing population, the number of elderly people with weak immune systems has grown.

3. Finally, because antibiotic use has increased, many strains of bacteria have become resistant to antibiotics, making the treatment of sepsis more difficult in some cases.

Sepsis causes

Many different microbes can cause sepsis. Although bacteria are most commonly the cause, viruses and fungi can also cause sepsis. Infections in the lungs (pneumonia), bladder and kidneys (urinary tract infections), skin (cellulitis), abdomen (such as appendicitis), and other areas (such as meningitis) can spread and lead to sepsis. Infections that develop after surgery can also lead to sepsis.

Sepsis symptoms and signs

1. If a person has sepsis, they often will have fever. Sometimes, though, the body temperature may be normal or even low.

2. The individual may also have chills and severe shaking.

3. The heart may be beating very fast, and breathing may be rapid. Low blood pressure is often observed in septic patients.

4. Confusion, disorientation, and agitation may be seen as well as dizziness and decreased urination.

5. Some patients who have sepsis develop a rash on their skin. The rash may be a reddish discoloration or small dark red dots throughout the body.

6. You may also develop pain in the joints at your wrists, elbows, back, hips, knees, and ankles.

A person should call the doctor if they or a loved one has signs and symptoms of sepsis. If any of the following are true about the patient's medical history, they need to be especially vigilant regarding possible sepsis symptoms if the person:

1. Is being treated with chemotherapy or radiation.

2. Has had an organ transplant.

3. Has diabetes.

4. Has AIDS.

IMMUNOTHERAPY

Immunotherapy is a medical term defined as 'treatment of disease by inducing, enhancing, or suppressing an immune response'. Immunotherapies designed to elicit or amplify an immune response are classified as activation immunotherapies.

Immunotherapies designed to reduce, suppress or more appropriately direct an existing immune response, as in cases of autoimmunity or allergy, are classified as suppression immunotherapies. The active agents of immunotherapy are collectively called immunomodulators. They are a diverse array of recombinant, synthetic and natural preparations, often cytokines. Some of these substances, such as granulocyte colony-stimulating factor (G-CSF), interferons, imiquimod and cellular membrane fractions from bacterial micro-organisms are already licensed for use in patients. Others including IL-12, various chemokines, synthetic cytosine phosphate-guanosine (CpG), oligodeoxynucleotides and glucans are being currently investigated extensively in clinical and preclinical studies. Immunomodulatory regimens offer an attractive approach as they often have fewer side effects than existing drugs, including less potential for creating resistance in microbial diseases.

Cell based immunotherapies are proven to be effective for cancers, where the immune cells such as lymphocytes, macrophages, dendritic cells, natural killer cells (NK Cell), cytotoxic T lymphocytes (CTL), etc. work together to defend the body against cancers and attacks by 'foreign' or 'non-self' invaders such as bacteria and viruses.

Examples of Activation Immunotherapies

Cancer

Cancer immunotherapy attempts to stimulate the immune system to reject and destroy tumours. In the beginning Immunotherapy treatments involved administration of cytokines such as Interleukin with an aim of inducing the lymphocytes to carry on their activity of destroying the tumour cells. Thereafter the adverse effects of such intravenously administered cytokines lead to the extraction of the lymphocytes from the blood and culture-expanding them in the lab and then injecting the cells alone to enable them to destroy the cancer cells.

Autologous immune enhancement therapy (AIET)

In the multipronged approach to treat cancer, one very useful latest weapon would be AIET. AIET is a treatment method in which some immune cells are taken out of a patient's body which are cultured and processed to be activated or to acquire additional functions until their resistance to cancer is strengthened, then the cells are put back in the body. Researchers have found that the thus activated immune system might also be able to determine the difference between healthy cells and cancer cells to eliminate the cancer cells from the body.

Dendritic cell based immunotherapy

This utilises dendritic cells to activate a cytotoxic response towards an antigen. Dendritic cells, a type of antigen presenting cell, are harvested from a patient. These cells are then either pulsed with an antigen or transfected with a viral vector. The activated dendritic cells are then placed back into the patient; these cells then present the antigens to effector lymphocytes (CD4+ T cells, CD8+ T cells, and in specialised dendritic cells, B cells also).

T cell based adoptive immunotherapy

Adoptive cell therapy (ACT) using autologous tumour-infiltrating lymphocytes is an effective treatment for patients with metastatic melanoma; this is based on adoptive immunity.

Vaccination

Antimicrobial immunotherapy, which includes vaccination, involves activating the immune system to respond to an infectious agent.

Examples of Suppression Immunotherapies

Immune suppression dampens an abnormal immune response in autoimmune diseases or reduces a normal immune response to prevent rejection of transplanted organs or cells.

Immune tolerance

Immune tolerance is the process by which the body naturally does not launch an immune system attack on its own tissues. Immune tolerance therapies seeks to reset the immune system so that the body stops mistakenly attacking its own organs or cells in autoimmune disease or accepts foreign tissue in organ transplantation.

Allergies

Immunotherapy is also used to treat allergies. While other allergy treatments (such as antihistamines or corticosteroids) treat only the symptoms of allergic disease, immunotherapy is the only available treatment that can modify the natural course of the allergic disease, by reducing sensitivity to allergens.

The therapy is particularly likely to be successful if it begins early in life or soon after the allergy develops for the first time. Immunotherapy involves a series of injections (shots) given regularly for several years by a specialist in a hospital clinic. In the past, this was called a serum, but this is an incorrect name. Most allergists now call this mixture an allergy extract. The first shots contain very tiny amounts of the allergen or antigen to which you are allergic. With progressively increasing dosages over time, your body will adjust to the allergen and become less sensitive to it. This process is called desensitisation.

MONOCLONAL ANTIBODY CONJUGATION VIA CHEMICAL MODIFICATION

The most commonly employed method for covalently cross-linking monoclonal antibodies to other molecules is the use of cross-linking reagents. Traditional pharmaceuticals can be linked to monoclonal antibodies to deliver targeted doses, prevent breakdown, and increase bioavailablity in circulation.

Carboxylic Acids (Aspartic Acid, Glutamic Acid)

Proteins contain carboxylic acid groups at the *C*-terminal position and within the side chains of aspartic acid and glutamic acid. The relatively low reactivity of carboxylic acids in water usually makes it difficult to use these groups to selectively modify proteins and other biomolecules. When this is done, the carboxylic acid group is usually converted to a reactive ester by the use of a water-soluble carbodiimide and reacted with a nucleophilic reagent such as an amine, hydrazide, or hydrazine. The amine-containing reagent should be weakly basic in order to react selectively with the activated carboxylic acid in the presence of other amines on the protein. Protein cross-linking can occur when the pH is raised above 8.0.

Sugar Alcohols

Sodium periodate can be used to oxidise the alcohol part of the sugar within the carbohydrate moiety to an aldehyde. Each group can be reacted with an amine, hydrazide, or hydrazine as described for carboxylic acids. Since the carbohydrate moiety is predominantly found on the crystallisable fragment (Fc) region of the antibody, conjugation can be achieved through site-directed modification of the carbohydrate away from the antigen-binding site.

Reagents

This section will briefly describe many of the reagents used in protein modification. In order to understand how to use these reagents, it is necessary to know what reactive group(s) on the protein can be modified; which type of chemical reactions these reactive groups will participate in; and the nature of the chemical bonds that will result (Fig. 9.6).

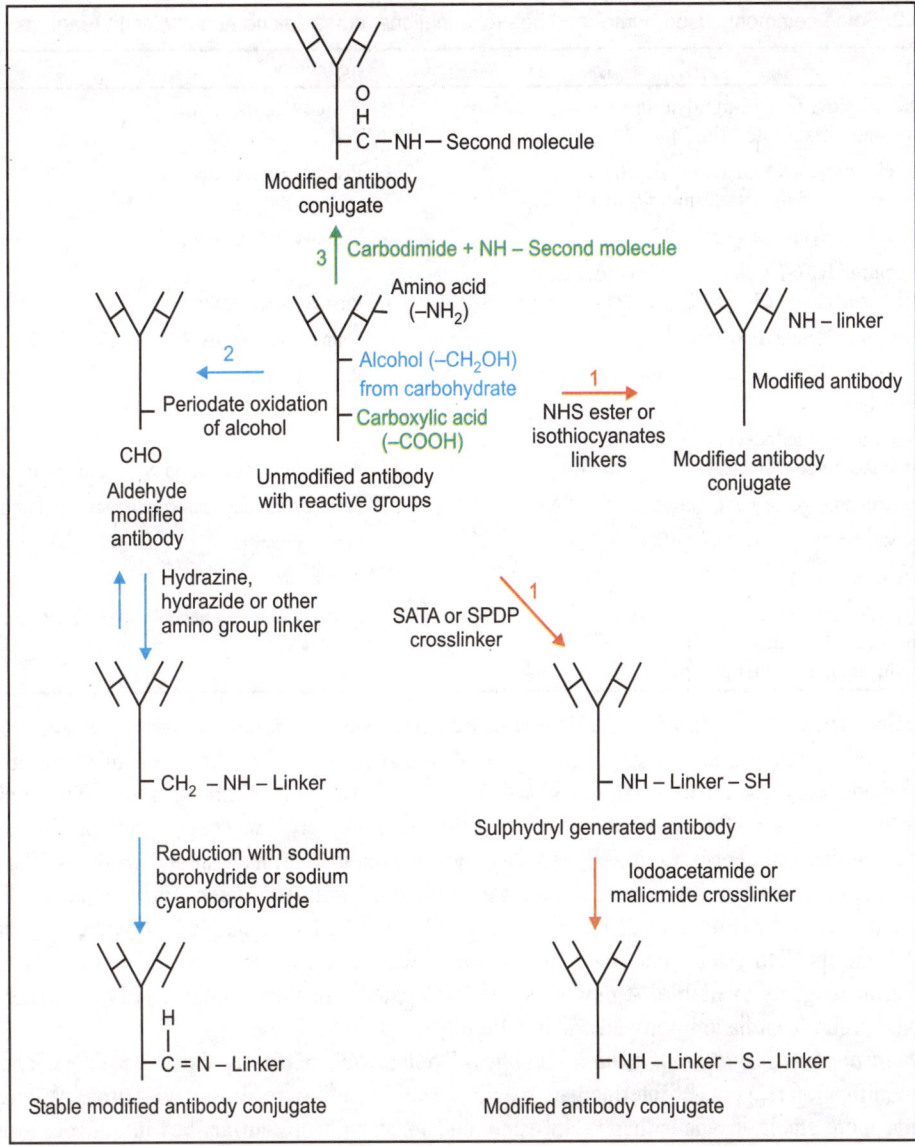

Fig. 9.6. Three side groups provide the major antibody modification pathways. Starting from the unmodified antibody in the center, reactions with the amino group follow the red path (arrows), the alcohol group follows the blue path (arrows), and the carboxylic acid group follows the green path (arrows).

Amine-reactive reagents

These reagents react primarily with lysines and the α-amino groups of proteins. Some amine-reactive reagents are more reactive, and therefore less sensitive, than others. It is necessary to consider reactivity when choosing the best reagent for modification of a specific protein. Table 9.2 lists commercially available amine-reactive reagents.

Table 9.2. Some commonly used homo- and heterobifunctional cross-linking and chelating reagents.

Reagents	Reactivity
Sulphosuccinimidyl 6-[3-(2-pyridyldithio) propionamido]hexanoate (SPDP)	Primary amine, thiol
Sulphosuccinimidyl-4-(N-maleimidylmethyl) cylcohexane-1-carboxylate (Sulpho-SMCC)	Primary amine, thiol
Succinimidyl (acetylthio)acetate (SATA)	Primary amine, thiol
Sulphosuccinimidyl 6-(α-methyl-α-[2-pyridylditio]- toluamido)hexanoate (Sulpho-LC-SMPT)	Primary amine, thiol
2-Iminothiolane (Traut's reagent)	Primary amine, thiol
Sulphosuccinimidyl(4-iodo-acetyl)aminobenzoate (Sulpho-SIAB)	Primary amine, thiol
1,4,7,10-Tetraazacyclododecane-N,N1,N11, N111-tetraacetic acid (DOTA)	Primary amines, carboxylic acid, radionuclides
Diethylenetriamine-pentaacetic anhydride (DTPA)	Primary amines, carboxylic acid, radionuclides
Bis(sulphosuccinimidyl-suberate (BS₃)	Primary amine
6-Hydrazinonicotinamide (SHNH)	Aldehyde
Various polyethylene glycol crosslinkers with maleimide, NHS ester, thioesters, carboxylic acid, and other groups	Primary amine, thiol, aldehyde, other groups

Reactive esters (formation of an amide bond): Reactive esters, particularly N-hydroxy-succinimide (NHS) esters, are among the most commonly employed reagents for modification of amine groups. They are moderately reactive toward amines, with high selectivity toward aliphatic amines. Their reaction rate with aromatic amines, alcohols, phenols, and histidine is relatively low. The optimum pH for reaction in an aqueous environment is 8.0 to 9.0, and they form very stable aliphatic amine products. The NHS esters are slowly hydrolysed by water, but are stable if stored well desiccated. Virtually any molecule that contains a carboxylic acid, or that can be chemically modified to contain a carboxylic acid, can be converted into its NHS ester. That explains why these reagents are among the most powerful protein-modification reagents available. A new class of NHS esters are now commercially available with sulphonate groups that have improved water solubility.

Isothiocyanates (formation of a thiourea bond): Isothiocyanates behave like NHS esters. They are amine-modification reagents of intermediate reactivity and form thiourea bonds with proteins. They are somewhat more stable in water than NHS esters and react with protein amines in aqueous solution (optimally at pH 9.0 to 9.5). Since this is a higher pH than optimal for NHS esters (which undergo competing hydrolysis at pH 9.0 to 9.5), isothiocyanates may not be as suitable as NHS esters when modifying proteins that are sensitive to alkaline conditions.

Aldehydes (formation of imine, Schiff's base, reduction to secondary amine bond): Aldehyde groups react under mild aqueous conditions with aliphatic and aromatic amines, hydrazines, and hydrazides to form an imine intermediate (Schiff's base). A Schiff's base can be selectively reduced with mild or strong reducing agents (such as sodium borohydride or sodium cyanoborohydride) to derive a stable alkyl amine bond. This method of amine modification can successfully be employed in situations in which the antibody is modified away from the antigen-binding site via the oxidation (typically with sodium periodate) of the alcohols on the carbohydrate moiety of the Fc region.

Miscellaneous amine-reactive reagents (anhydrides). Other reagents that have been used to modify amines are acid anhydrides. For example, diethylenetriaminepentaacetic anhydride (DTPA) is a bifunctional chelating agent that contains two amine-reactive anhydride groups. It can react with N-terminal and ε-amine groups of the proteins to form amide linkages. The anhydride rings open to create multivalent, metal-chelating arms able to bind tightly to metals in a coordination complex. This type of reaction is particularly useful in the preparation of radiolabelled immunoconjugates.

Thiol-reactive reagents

Thiol-reactive reagents are those that will couple to thiol groups on proteins, forming thioether-coupled products. These reagents react rapidly at slight acidic to neutral pH and therefore can be reacted selectively in the presence of amine groups.

Haloacetyl derivatives (formation of a thioether bond): These reagents (usually iodoacetamides) are common reagents for thiol modification. In antibodies, the reaction takes place at cysteine groups that are either intrinsically present or that result from the reduction of cystine's disulphides at various positions of the antibody. The thioether linkages formed from any reaction of haloacetamides are very stable. However, iodoacetamide modification reagents are unstable in light, especially in solution. They must be protected from light during reaction and in storage. The level of control to achieve reproducibility required for large scale manufacturing conditions may be difficult to achieve.

Maleimides (formation of a thioether bond): The reaction of maleimides with thiol-reactive reagents is essentially the same as with iodoacetamides. Maleimides react rapidly at slight acidic to neutral pH. Above pH 8.0, maleimides can undergo hydrolysis to form nonreactive maleamic acids.

Aldehyde and carboxylic acid-reactive reagents

Amines, hydrazides, and hydrazines (formation of amide, hydrazone, or alkyl amine bonds). Amines, hydrazides, and hydrazines can be coupled to carboxylic acids of proteins after the activation of the carboxyl group by a water-soluble carbodiimide. As mentioned previously, the amine-containing reagent must be weakly basic so that it reacts selectively with the carbodiimide-activated protein in the presence of the more highly basic e-amines of lysine to form a stable amide bond.

Amines, hydrazides, and hydrazines also can react with aldehyde groups, which can be generated on antibodies by periodate oxidation of the carbohydrate residues on the antibody. In this scenario, a Schiff's base intermediate is formed, which can be reduced to an alkyl amine through the reduction of the intermediate with sodium cyanoborohydride (mild and selective) or sodium borohydride (strong) water-soluble reducing agents.

Bifunctional reagents

Bifunctional cross-linking reagents are specialised reagents that will form a bond between different groups, either on the same molecule or two different molecules. These reagents can be divided into two kinds, homobifunctional reagents (those with the same reactive group at each end of the molecule) and heterobifunctional reagents (those with different reactive groups at each end of the molecule). Recent trends appear to strongly favour the use of heterobifunctional cross-linkers where the bifunctional reagent has two reactive sites, each with selectivity toward different functional groups (for example, an amine reactive and a thiol reactive). Many bifunctional reagents are commercially available with variable chain lengths and water solubility.

Miscellaneous reagents

Photoactive reagents capable of being activated by light can produce a reactive intermediate for coupling to various functional groups on biomolecules. Generation of highly reactive intermediates such as nitrene, carbene, and diradical species employed in photoaffinity labelling is of little value since such species are highly nonspecific and often capable of reaction even with alkyl side-chains. These reagents have not been widely utilised in the modification and coupling of monoclonal antibodies.

Reaction Environment

It is imperative that the scientist understands the practical aspects of reacting with large, complex, conformationally sensitive, water-soluble antibodies and other biomolecules or small organic molecules. The buffers, the cosolvents, and the reaction conditions all must be considered in order to obtain a scalable process that can be validated and used under aseptic, GMP manufacturing conditions.

Buffers

In general, conjugation should be carried out in a well-buffered system at an optimal pH for the reaction. The ionic strength of the buffer in most cases should be around 10 to 100 mM. Phosphate buffers should be well suited for the modification of thiol groups and α-amino groups, because this occurs selectively at physiological pH (7.0 to 7.5). For lysine amines, which require a more alkaline pH (8.0 to 9.2), carbonate-bicarbonate or borate buffers work well. In some cases, the choice of buffer will be dictated by the compatibility of the protein. For example, since many of the conjugations of antibodies involve the utilisation of amine groups, it is necessary to avoid amine-containing buffers like *tris*(hydroxy-methyl)aminomethane (TRIS).

Cosolvents

Many of the available cross-linking reagents are sulphonated and water-soluble at millimolar to micromolar concentrations. These reagents need no cosolvent for solubilisation. If the reagents are not soluble in aqueous medium, water-miscible cosolvent—such as dimethylformamide (DMF), dimethyl-sulphoxide (DMSO), and some alcohols—must be used to dissolve the reagent without causing decomposition. Furthermore, the cosolvent must not cause irreversible denaturation or precipitation of the antibody. DMSO and DMF are the most commonly used cosolvents, usually up to 10 per cent (w/v) concentrations.

Temperature

In general, conjugation reactions involving antibodies (and most other proteins) should be done between room temperature and near-freezing temperature ($\sim$25° to 2°C). Lower temperature tends to slow down the reaction rate and increase the selectivity and control of the reaction. This could result in fewer side reactions and more consistent and reproducible results.

Protein concentration

Typically, a 1 to 10 mg/ml protein concentration is recommended for protein conjugation with an optimum range of 5 to 10 mg/ml.

Concentrations of less than 1 mg/ml have been successfully reported, but these require a longer incubation time to achieve adequate conjugation.

pH

During the modification of primary amines, only the unprotonated form is reactive and, therefore, it is necessary to maintain a pH at which a significant proportion of amines are unprotonated. When working with lysine, it was found that at an average pK_a above 9, the reaction runs at a faster rate. However, some cross-linking reagents may undergo hydrolysis and some antibodies (and other proteins) tend to be unstable at higher pHs. The α-amino groups of the N-terminal amino acids are less basic than lysines and are reactive at pH ~7.0. These amino groups are sometimes preferentially modified when the reaction is run at neutral pH. Thus if the protein and cross-linking reagents are stable, the reaction should be performed close to pH 9.0. For less stable reagents, the reaction should be performed near pH 7.0.

Reaction time

In general, one to two hours should suffice for conjugation reactions to go to completion. Longer reaction times are acceptable, since the degree of labelling is generally limited by the molar ratio of the reagent to antibody, not the reaction time. Many published procedures indicate overnight reaction times and incubations performed at 2° to 8°C. The more reactive the reagent is, the shorter the reaction time.

Molar ratio of the reactants

Antibodies are relatively sensitive to substitution, since there are usually reactive amino acid side chains (amines, thiols) in or near the antigen binding sites. For this reason, a low to moderate degree of labelling is preferable in order to preserve binding specificity. Over-labelling can result in decreased solubility which may reduce the overall activity of the conjugates. In some cases it causes precipitation of the antibody conjugate.

Laboratory Methods

The methods below are widely employed for conjugating amine-reactive and thiol-reactive and other reagents to antibodies. The wide variety of experimental conditions required for activating and coupling antibodies with bifunctional and other reagents make it difficult to generate a simple general procedure. Although the procedures described below are for preparing antibody conjugates, they can also be utilised to prepare many other proteins and biological molecules.

Amine-reactive reagents

Use the following general procedure for the first trial. It is adaptable to amine-reactive molecules such as tags and probes, biotin, homobifunctional and heterobifunctional cross-linkers, haptens, carbodiimides, bifunctional chelating agents (for radioimmunoconjugates), and toxins. The procedure may be modified after the degree of substitution has been determined in analysis of the final product.

For the basic lysine amines, prepare the antibody at 1 to 10 mg/ml in 50 to 100 mM sodium carbonate-bicarbonate (or borate) buffer pH 8.2 to 9.2 at room temperature. For less-basic α-amino groups, which react selectively at physiological pH, prepare the antibody in 10 to 50 mM sodium phosphate buffer, with 150 mM sodium chloride, pH 7.2 to 7.5. Note that amine-containing buffers such as TRIS are not recommended, since these buffers will compete with the antibody in reacting with the modifying reagent.

Add sufficient antibody-modifying reagent from a freshly prepared stock solution, which contains about 5 to 10 mol of isothiocyanate or succinimide ester for each mole of protein. Note that for carboxylic acid-containing reagents such as bifunctional chelating agents DTPA and DOTA, 5 to 10 mols of the chelating agent per mol of antibody should be used in the initial conjugation. These reactions only work through the initial activation of the carboxylic acid–reactive groups of the chelator with a water-soluble carbodiimide reagent such as EDC. Follow up by stabilising the active acylisourea intermediate with NHS ester or immidazole. React the resulting product (activated and stable chelating reagent) with the amino group of the antibody to generate the modified antibody-chelator conjugate. Such conjugates are useful as cancer therapeutic agents through the preparation of radiolabelled antibodies. In general, the preparation of antibody-chelating agent via the reaction of the amino group and carboxylic group is not very efficient. Gosh reported that no more than 0.7 mols of the carboxylic acid containing modification reagent per mol of the proteins were used up.

Most commercially available protein modification reagents have some solubility in water. For insoluble reagents, a stock solution should be prepared immediately before use in a water-miscible solvent such as DMF, DMSO, or dioxane (prepared dry). Prepare a stock solution of the antibody-modifying reagent at about 5 to 10 per cent (w/v) of the volume of conjugation buffer in order to minimise denaturation or precipitation of the antibody. Add the solution of modifying reagent in small amounts to the antibody solution. Gently mix each time to ensure homogeneous reaction mixture over a period of a few minutes at room temperature. Following complete addition of the modifying reagent, ensure that the mixture is homogeneous and incubate at room temperature for one to two hours without further mixing. As a matter of convenience, the reaction mixture can be incubated overnight at 2° to 8°C. Following incubation, quench the reaction mixture using an amine-containing reagent such as excess TRIS buffer. Experience shows that quenching the reaction mixture allows for consistency and reproducibility when preparing the conjugates.

Purify the antibody conjugate from unreacted modifying reagent using the purification device most appropriate to the development and manufacturing scale as described later in this chapter.

Thiol-reactive reagents

Antibody conjugates can be prepared from thiol-reactive reagents such as maleimides, iodoacetates, and homo-bifunctional and heterobifunctional cross-linkers. In general, antibodies exist in their stable oxidised (disulphide) form. As described earlier, the disulphide form is usually converted into the more reactive and relatively unstable free thiol. This is achieved via the reduction of the disulphide bonds with reagents such as DTT, 2-MEA, BME, and TCEP.

If a full-length and intact antibody is needed, several sulphur containing reagents can be attached onto the reactive amino group. Usually a reduction of SATA and SPDP via hydroxyl amine, a reduction of Sulpho-LC-SPDP via DTT, or the hydrolysis of Traut's reagent generates modified antibodies containing multiple, reactive sulphydryl groups. Be aware of the highly reactive nature of some sulphydryl groups that can be oxidised to disulphides. It is best to do all reactions in an oxygen-free environment (for example under an argon or nitrogen blanket) and in the presence of ethylenediamine tetraacetic acid (EDTA) to minimise metal-catalysed oxidation of sulphydryl groups into the more stable and less-reactive disulphide groups.

As with the reactive esters and isothiocyanates, use only freshly prepared reagents. Protection from light (particularly for iodoactamide) is important. Due to the reactive nature of thiol groups, use only filtration to purify the thiolated antibody. Avoid using dialysis since it is time consuming and may result in the conversion of sulphydryl to disulphide.

Step 1: Prepare the antibody at 1 to 10 mg/mL in a suitable conjugation buffer (10 to 100 mM phosphate or TRIS, 150 mM sodium chloride, 1 to 5 mM EDTA at pH 6.5 to 7.5) at room temperature. At this pH range, the thiol groups on the antibody are sufficiently nucleophilic so that they react almost exclusively with the reagent in the presence of the more abundant protein amines, which are protonated and relatively unreactive. At pH 6.5 to 7.0, the reaction of the maleimide group with sulphydryls proceeds at a rate 1000 times greater than its reaction with amines. It is advisable to deoxygenate all buffers to prevent reformation of disulphide.

Step 2: Add sufficient protein modification reagent to the antibody prep from a stock solution to contain 5 to 15 mol of the reagent for each mole of protein. Upon completion of the reaction, quench the reaction mixture with a thiol-containing reagent such as DTT, BME, or glutathione to consume excess modification reagent.

Iodoacetamides

Reactions with iodo-acetamides should be carried out in the dark, since light can cause reagent decomposition. Slowly add the stock reagent solution in small amounts over a period of about one to three minutes with gentle mixing. Once the reaction mixture is homogeneous, let it incubate without further mixing for one to two hours at room temperature.

Maleimides

Reaction conditions for maleimides are essentially the same as with iodoacetamides. The selectivity of maleimides toward thiol groups is greater than iodo-acetamides, thereby allowing somewhat more latitude in the buffer pH. Also, at pH above 8.0, the maleimide group can undergo a competing hydrolysis reaction to form maleamic acid, which is unreactive to thiol groups. As with iodoacetamide, slowly add the stock reagent solution in small amounts with gentle mixing to the antibody solution over approximately one to three minutes and let it incubate without further mixing for one to two hours at room temperature.

Conjugate Purification and Storage

Usually, molar excess of the antibody modifying reagents is used during the preparation of antibody conjugates. It is necessary to remove excess non-covalently bound modifying reagents from the antibody conjugates. There are several techniques and commercially available devices one can utilise in the purification of antibody conjugates.

Dialysis

Dialysis is simple and inexpensive. However, it is the most inefficient and time-consuming method of purifying antibody conjugates. Dialysis may be more appropriate during early conjugation research and small-scale development, but it may not be amenable to large-scale manufacturing. In general, not all molecules dialyse efficiently. The rate of dialysis depends on the relative affinity of the modifying reagent for the protein versus the dialysis solution. Molecules that are sparingly soluble in water or strongly adsorbed to the protein surface will take a long time to dialyse. Dialysis works best when the labelling reagent and its unreacted by-product are hydrophilic. When purifying conjugates by dialysis, a dialysis buffer volume of at least 100 times the volume of conjugate solution should be used, and the dialysis buffer should be changed at least three to five times, allowing at least 4 hours for dialysis between buffer exchanges.

Stirred cell filtration

Stirred cell filtration is a widely used procedure for purification of antibody conjugates. This specialised filtration system (also known as microfiltration, ultrafiltration, and diafiltration) consists of a flat membrane held in place over the outlet of a pressurised reservoir. The device is pressurised to force fluid through the membrane while retaining the macromolecules. A second reservoir contains the final storage buffer for the conjugate product. The membrane material is available in varying pore sizes.

Stirred cell devices have been developed to purify products with volumes from a few millilitres to approximately 2000 ml and are commonly used in research and development laboratories and early manufacturing for clinical study of drug products. This device enables both purification and concentration of the conjugate product.

Tangential flow filtration (TFF)

Tangential flow filtration (TFF) is also a pressure-driven filtration process for purification of antibody conjugates. TFF uses a large membrane surface (commercially available in varying pore sizes). Unlike stirred cell filtration, TFF systems are designed to handle from a few millilitres to hundreds of litres of sample without the concerns associated with pressurised systems. In TFF, the fluid is pumped tangentially along the surface of the membrane. Pressure is applied through the membrane to the filtrate side, allowing macromolecules that are too large to pass through the membrane to be retained on the upstream side. Once it is optimised for flow, flux and transmembrane pressures, a TFF system can be predictably scaled from bench to industrial manufacturing (phase 1 and 2 clinical studies and beyond). Furthermore, the TFF system can use a large surface area while maintaining a minimum hold-up volume. This allows for a shorter processing time than can be achieved with stirred cells. TFF can concentrate the desired product usually with over 90 per cent recovery. Filtration and concentration can be performed in a completely closed system.

Gel filtration chromatography

Gel filtration chromatography is a simple and reliable chromatographic technique for separating molecules by size. The labelled conjugate is separated from the excess noncovalently-bound labelling reagent and other small molecules while allowing the larger antibody conjugate to pass through the void space in the porous gel matrix.

A gel filtration technique is generally faster and more effective in removing most hydrophilic and hydrophobic labelling reagents than other filtration systems.

In order to achieve high-resolution separation, ~5 to 10 per cent of the column's volume should be loaded with the sample. Sometimes up to 30 per cent sample volume can be loaded. There are many sizes of prepacked gel filtration columns available. For development and small-scale purification (<1 ml to ~15 ml), prepacked columns such as PD-10 and HiPrep desalting columns are available. For larger-scale purification (>15 ml), columns such as the XK series or equivalent can be utilised. Generally, you will both pack and qualify such columns with the appropriate gel prior to use. For even higher volume (>100 ml), the sample volume should be reduced (for example, via TFF) to ~10 per cent column volume. We may have to run multiple columns or connect two or more columns in series. It should be noted that the utilisation of gel filtration chromatography produces a relatively low concentration of protein and the product may need more steps to achieve a higher concentration.

Miscellaneous

With the exception of dialysis, all of the separation techniques described above work well if the antibody is significantly larger (>3-fold) than the modifying or coupling reagent. For reagents (mostly protein and other biological molecules) that are similar in size or larger than the antibody, one must resort to other purification techniques such as affinity chromatography, ion-exchange chromatography, and hydrophobic interaction chromatography.

Storage

The researcher must determine the most appropriate buffers to be utilised for both short- and long-term storage of their therapeutic antibody conjugate. From published procedures, buffers close to physiological pH, such as phosphate buffered saline (PBS), are generally recommended.

Immunoconjugate Drugs Today

While only a few immunoconjugate drug products are currently available commercially, many monoclonal antibodies that are conjugated to other biomolecules and pharmaceutical drugs are currently undergoing clinical trials. Table 9.3 listed the latest progress.

Table 9.3. Status of immunoconjugate drug products.

Drug substance	Indicator	Organisation	Clinical trial status	Conjugation chemistry
SGN-15	Lung and ovarian cancer	Seattle genetics	Phase 2	MAb conjugation to doxorubicin
Bexxar	Non-Hodgkin's lymphoma	Corixa Corp.; GlaxoSmithKline	FDA approved	I131 covalently linked to MAb
ETI-104	Systemic lupus erythemalosus	EluSys therapeutics	Phase 2	Thioether (S-C) conjugate product of MAb and double-stranded DNA
Immunotoxin	Acute myelongenous leukemia	MD Anderson cancer center	NA	Disulphide (S-S) conjugate product of MAb and rGelonin conjugate
Zevalin	Non-Hodgkin's lymphoma	IDEC pharmaceuticals	FDA approved	Thiourea conjugate product of MAb and chelator (tuixetan); conjugate labelled with Yttfium-90(therapeutic purposes) or Indium-111

FDA has approved Bexxar and Zevalin for patients with CD20-positive follicular, non-Hodgkin's lymphoma (NHL). The monoclonal antibodies in these drugs recognise and attach to a particular part of a B-cell, the CD20 antigen. This allows Bexxar and Zevalin to specifically target B-cells, destroying the malignant NHL B-cells and also some normal B-cells. Therefore, Zevalin and Bexxar are considered dual-action therapies because they pair the tumour-targeting ability of the monoclonal antibodies with the cancer-killing radioisotope.

It should be noted that tethering a drug molecule to an antibody could dramatically change the biological properties of the drug. Also, because they are large proteins, antibodies do not penetrate cells except under special circumstances (such as with antibody fragments). This can greatly reduce the toxic side effects of a drug—an important goal in many cases. Radiation safety is an important factor when handling and administering Bexxar and Zevalin. The volatile nature of many radiohalogen species (for example, I131) makes handling of these materials somewhat different than other radioactive materials. This is particularly true for handling radioiodine, as it is sequestered by the thyroid gland. Therefore, use a fume hood or vented box or (if large amounts of activity are used) a 'hot cell' when handling these radiolabelled materials. Not enough information is available to adequately assess other immuno-drug conjugates currently undergoing phase 1 and 2 clinical trials.

Through conjugation chemistries, traditional pharmaceutical drugs can be linked to monoclonal antibodies in order to deliver targeted doses, prevent breakdown, and increase bioavailability in circulation. The techniques for coupling drugs to monoclonal antibodies have become more sophisticated with the design of novel linkers and protecting groups that afford unique properties such as stability in the serum. Prior to starting conjugation of biomolecules, it is important to consider the methods used in maintaining the functionality of the antibody, biological properties of the drugs and other biological molecules, and the scalability of the manufacturing process. To date, the majority of drugs used in immunoconjugates has been limited to clinical treatment of cancer and various blood-borne diseases.

Chapter 10

Bioremediation and Biomass Utilisation

INTRODUCTION

Bioremediation can be defined as any process that uses micro-organisms, fungi, green plants or their enzymes to return the natural environment altered by contaminants to its original condition. Bioremediation may be employed to attack specific soil contaminants, such as degradation of chlorinated hydrocarbons by bacteria. An example of a more general approach is the cleanup of oil spills by the addition of nitrate and/or sulphate fertilisers to facilitate the decomposition of crude oil by indigenous or exogenous bacteria. Naturally occurring bioremediation and phytoremediation have been used for centuries. For example, desalination of agricultural land by phytoextraction has a long tradition.

Bioremediation technologies can be generally classified as *in situ* or *ex situ*. *In situ* bioremediation involves treating the contaminated material at the site while *ex situ* involves the removal of the contaminated material to be treated elsewhere. Some examples of bioremediation technologies are bioventing, landfarming, bioreactor, composting, bioaugmentation, rhizofiltration, and biostimulation.

Bioremediation can occur on its own (natural attenuation or intrinsic bioremediation) or can be spurred on via the addition of fertilisers to increase the bioavailability within the medium (biostimulation). Recent advancements have also proven successful via the addition of matched microbe strains to the medium to enhance the resident microbe population's ability to break down contaminants. Micro-organism who perform the function of bioremediation is known as bioremediators (bioaugmentation).

Not all contaminants, however, are easily treated by bioremediation using micro-organisms. For example, heavy metals such as cadmium and lead are not readily absorbed or captured by organisms. The assimilation of metals such as mercury into the food chain may worsen matters. Phytoremediation is useful in these circumstances, because natural plants or transgenic plants are able to bioaccumulate these toxins in their above-ground parts, which are then harvested for removal. The heavy metals in the harvested biomass may be further concentrated by incineration or even recycled for industrial use.

The elimination of a wide range of pollutants and wastes from the environment requires increasing our understanding of the relative importance of different pathways and regulatory networks to carbon flux in particular environments and for particular compounds and they will certainly accelerate the development of bioremediation technologies and biotransformation processes.

GENETIC ENGINEERING APPROACHES

The use of genetic engineering to create organisms specifically designed for bioremediation has great potential. The bacterium *Deinococcus radiodurans* (the most radioresistant organism known) has been modified to consume and digest toluene and ionic mercury from highly radioactive nuclear waste. Most commonly, the process is misunderstood. The microbes are ever-present in any given context—generally referred to as 'normal microbial flora'. During bioremediation (biodegradation) processes, fertilisers/nutrient supplementation is introduced to the environments, in efforts to maximise growth and production potential. Common misbelief is that microbes are transported and dispersed into an unadulterated environment.

MYCOREMEDIATION

Mycoremediation is a form of bioremediation in which fungi are used to decontaminate the area. The term mycoremediation was coined by Paul Stamets and refers specifically to the use of fungal mycelia in bioremediation. One of the primary roles of fungi in the ecosystem is decomposition, which is performed by the mycelium. The mycelium secretes extracellular enzymes and acids that break down lignin and cellulose, the two main building blocks of plant fibre. These are organic compounds composed of long chains of carbon and hydrogen, structurally similar to many organic pollutants. The key to mycoremediation is determining the right fungal species to target a specific pollutant. Certain strains have been reported to successfully degrade the nerve gases VX and sarin. There are a number of cost/efficiency advantages to bioremediation, which can be employed in areas that are inaccessible without excavation. For example, hydrocarbon spills (specifically, petrol spills) or certain chlorinated solvents may contaminate groundwater, and introducing the appropriate electron acceptor or electron donor amendment, as appropriate, may significantly reduce contaminant concentrations after a long time allowing for acclimation.

This is typically much less expensive than excavation followed by disposal elsewhere, incineration or other *ex situ* treatment strategies, and reduces or eliminates the need for 'pump and treat', a common practice at sites where hydrocarbons have contaminated clean groundwater. The process of bioremediation can be monitored indirectly by measuring the oxidation reduction potential or redox in soil and groundwater, together with pH, temperature, oxygen content, electron acceptor/donor concentrations, and concentration of breakdown products (e.g. carbon dioxide). Table 10.1 shows the (decreasing) biological breakdown rate as function of the redox potential.

Table 10.1. Biological breakdown rate as function of the redox potential.

Process	Reaction	Redox potential (E_h in mV)
Aerobic	$O_2 + 4e^- + 4H^+ \rightarrow 2H_2O$	600~400
Anaerobic		
Denitrification	$2NO_3^- + 10e^- + 12H^+ \rightarrow N_2 + 6H_2O$	500~200
Manganese IV reduction	$MnO_2 + 2e^- + 4H^+ \rightarrow Mn^{2+} + 2H_2O$	400~200
Iron III reduction	$Fe(OH)_3 + e^- + 3H^+ \rightarrow Fe^{2+} + 3H_2O$	300~100
Sulphate reduction	$SO_4^{2-} + 8e^- + 10H^+ \rightarrow H_2S + 4H_2O$	0~−150
Fermentation	$2CH_2O \rightarrow CO_2 + CH_4$	−150~−220

This, by itself and at a single site, gives little information about the process of remediation.

1. It is necessary to sample enough points on and around the contaminated site to be able to determine contours of equal redox potential. Contouring is usually done using specialised software, e.g. using Kriging interpolation.

2. If all the measurements of redox potential show that electron acceptors have been used up, it's in effect an indicator for total microbial activity. Chemical analysis is also required to determine when the levels of contaminants and their breakdown products have been reduced to below regulatory limits.

BIOMASS

Biomass, a renewable energy source, is biological material from living, or recently living organisms, such as wood, waste, (hydrogen) gas, and alcohol fuels. Biomass is commonly plant matter grown to generate electricity or produce heat. In this sense, living biomass can also be included, as plants can also generate electricity while still alive. The most conventional way on how biomass is used however, still relies on direct incineration.

Forest residues for example (such as dead trees, branches and tree stumps), yard clippings, wood chips and garbage are often used for this. However, biomass also includes plant or animal matter used for production of fibres or chemicals. Biomass may also include biodegradable wastes that can be burnt as fuel. It excludes organic materials such as fossil fuels which have been transformed by geological processes into substances such as coal or petroleum.

Industrial biomass can be grown from numerous types of plants, including miscanthus, switchgrass, hemp, corn, poplar, willow, sorghum, sugarcane, and a variety of tree species, ranging from eucalyptus to oil palm (palm oil). The particular plant used is usually not important to the end products, but it does affect the processing of the raw material.

Although fossil fuels have their origin in ancient biomass, they are not considered biomass by the generally accepted definition because they contain carbon that has been 'out' of the carbon cycle for a very long time. Their combustion therefore disturbs the carbon dioxide content in the atmosphere.

Plastics from biomass, like some recently developed to dissolve in seawater, are made the same way as petroleum-based plastics. These plastics are actually cheaper to manufacture and meet or exceed most performance standards, but they lack the same water resistance or longevity as conventional plastics.

Chemical Composition

Biomass is carbon based and is composed of a mixture of organic molecules containing hydrogen, usually including atoms of oxygen, often nitrogen and also small quantities of other atoms, including alkali, alkaline earth and heavy metals. These metals are often found in functional molecules such as the porphyrins which include chlorophyll which contains magnesium.

Biomass Sources

Biomass energy is derived from five distinct energy sources: garbage, wood, waste, landfill gases, and alcohol fuels. Wood energy is derived both from direct use of harvested wood as a fuel and from wood waste streams. The largest source of energy from wood is pulping liquor or 'black liquor', a waste product from processes of the pulp, paper and paperboard industry. Waste energy is the second-largest source of biomass energy. The main contributors of waste energy are municipal solid waste (MSW), manufacturing waste, and landfill gas. Biomass alcohol fuel, or ethanol, is derived almost exclusively from corn. Its principal use is as an oxygenate in gasoline.

Biomass can be converted to other usable forms of energy like methane gas or transportation fuels like ethanol and biodiesel. Methane gas is the main ingredient of natural gas. Smelly stuff, like rotting garbage, and agricultural and human waste, release methane gas—also called 'landfill gas' or 'biogas'. Crops like corn and sugar cane can be fermented to produce the transportation fuel, ethanol. Biodiesel, another transportation fuel, can be produced from leftover food products like vegetable oils and animal fats. Also, biomass to liquids (BTLs) and cellulosic ethanol are still under research.

Biomass Conversion Process to Useful Energy

There are a number of technological options available to make use of a wide variety of biomass types as a renewable energy source. Conversion technologies may release the energy directly, in the form of heat or electricity, or may convert it to another form, such as liquid biofuel or combustible biogas. While for some classes of biomass resource there may be a number of usage options, for others there may be only one appropriate technology.

Thermal conversion

These are processes in which heat is the dominant mechanism to convert the biomass into another chemical form. The basic alternatives are separated principally by the extent to which the chemical reactions involved are allowed to proceed (mainly controlled by the availability of oxygen and conversion temperature): combustion, torrefaction, pyrolysis, gasification. There are a number of other less common, more experimental or proprietary thermal processes that may offer benefits such as hydrothermal upgrading (HTU) and hydroprocessing. Some have been developed for use on high moisture content biomass, including aqueous slurries, and allow them to be converted into more convenient forms. Some of the applications of thermal conversion are combined heat and power (CHP) and co-firing. In a typical biomass power plant, efficiencies range from 20–27 per cent.

Chemical conversion

A range of chemical processes may be used to convert biomass into other forms, such as to produce a fuel that is more conveniently used, transported or stored, or to exploit some property of the process itself.

Biochemical conversion

As biomass is a natural material, many highly efficient biochemical processes have developed in nature to break down the molecules of which biomass is composed, and many of these biochemical conversion processes can be harnessed.

Biochemical conversion makes use of the enzymes of bacteria and other micro-organisms to break down biomass. In most cases micro-organisms are used to perform the conversion process: anaerobic digestion, fermentation and composting. Other chemical processes such as converting straight and waste vegetable oils into biodiesel is transesterification. Another way of breaking down biomass is by breaking down the carbohydrates and simple sugars to make alcohol.

MICROBIAL BIODEGRADATION

Interest in the microbial biodegradation of pollutants has intensified in recent years as humanity strives to find sustainable ways to cleanup contaminated environments. These bioremediation and biotransformation methods endeavour to harness the astonishing, naturally occurring, ability of microbial xenobiotic metabolism to degrade, transform or accumulate a huge range of compounds including hydrocarbons (e.g. oil), polychlorinated biphenyls (PCBs), polyaromatic hydrocarbons (PAHs), heterocyclic compounds (such as pyridine or quinoline), pharmaceutical substances, radionuclides and metals. Major methodological breakthroughs in recent years have enabled detailed genomic, metagenomic, proteomic, bioinformatic and other high-throughput analyses of environmentally relevant micro-organisms providing unprecedented insights into key biodegradative pathways and the ability of organisms to adapt to changing environmental conditions.

The elimination of a wide range of pollutants and wastes from the environment is an absolute requirement to promote a sustainable development of our society with low environmental impact. Biological processes play a major role in the removal of contaminants and they take advantage of the astonishing catabolic versatility of micro-organisms to degrade/convert such compounds. New methodological breakthroughs in sequencing, genomics, proteomics, bioinformatics and imaging are producing vast amounts of information. In the field of Environmental Microbiology, genome-based global studies open a new era providing unprecedented *in silico* views of metabolic and regulatory networks, as well as clues to the evolution of degradation pathways and to the molecular adaptation strategies to changing environmental conditions. Functional genomic and metagenomic approaches are increasing our understanding of the relative importance of different pathways and regulatory networks to carbon flux in particular environments and for particular compounds and they will certainly accelerate the development of bioremediation technologies and biotransformation processes.

Aerobic Biodegradation of Pollutants

The burgeoning amount of bacterial genomic data provides unparalleled opportunities for understanding the genetic and molecular bases of the degradation of organic pollutants. Aromatic compounds are among the most recalcitrant of these pollutants and lessons can be learned from the recent genomic studies of *Burkholderia xenovorans* LB400 and *Rhodococcus* sp. strain RHA1, two of the largest bacterial genomes completely sequenced to date. These studies have helped expand our understanding of bacterial catabolism, non-catabolic physiological adaptation to organic compounds, and the evolution of large bacterial genomes. First, the metabolic pathways from phylogenetically diverse isolates are very similar with respect to overall organisation. Thus, as originally noted in pseudomonads, a large number of 'peripheral aromatic' pathways funnel a range of natural and xenobiotic compounds into a restricted number of 'central aromatic' pathways. Nevertheless, these pathways are genetically organised in genus-specific fashions, as exemplified by the β-ketoadipate and Paa pathways. Comparative genomic studies further reveal that some pathways are more widespread than initially thought. Thus, the Box and Paa pathways illustrate the prevalence of non-oxygenolytic ring-cleavage strategies in aerobic aromatic degradation processes. Functional genomic studies have been useful in establishing that even organisms harbouring high numbers of homologous enzymes seem to contain few examples of true redundancy. For example, the multiplicity of ring-cleaving dioxygenases in certain rhodococcal isolates may be attributed to the cryptic aromatic catabolism of different terpenoids and steroids. Finally, analyses have indicated that recent genetic flux appears to have played a more significant role in the evolution of some large genomes, such as LB400's, than others. However, the emerging trend is that the large gene repertoires of potent pollutant degraders such as LB400 and RHA1 have evolved principally through more ancient processes. That this is true in such phylogenetically diverse species is remarkable and further suggests the ancient origin of this catabolic capacity.

Anaerobic Biodegradation of Pollutants

Anaerobic microbial mineralisation of recalcitrant organic pollutants is of great environmental significance and involves intriguing novel biochemical reactions. In particular, hydrocarbons and halogenated compounds have long been doubted to be degradable in the absence of oxygen, but the isolation of hitherto unknown anaerobic hydrocarbon-degrading and reductively dehalogenating bacteria during the last decades provided ultimate proof for these processes in nature. Many novel biochemical reactions were discovered enabling the respective metabolic pathways, but progress in the molecular understanding of these bacteria was rather slow, since genetic systems are not readily applicable for most of them. However, with the increasing application of genomics in the field of environmental microbiology, a new and promising perspective is now at hand to obtain molecular insights into these new metabolic properties.

Several complete genome sequences were determined during the last few years from bacteria capable of anaerobic organic pollutant degradation. The ~4.7 Mb genome of the facultative denitrifying *Aromatoleum aromaticum* strain EbN1 was the first to be determined for an anaerobic hydrocarbon degrader (using toluene or ethylbenzene as substrates). The genome sequence revealed about two dozen gene clusters (including several paralogs) coding for a complex catabolic network for anaerobic and aerobic degradation of aromatic compounds. The genome sequence forms the basis for current detailed studies on regulation of pathways and enzyme structures.

Further genomes of anaerobic hydrocarbon degrading bacteria were recently completed for the iron-reducing species *Geobacter metallireducens* (accession nr. NC_007517) and the perchlorate-reducing *Dechloromonas aromatica* (accession nr. NC_007298), but these are not yet evaluated in formal publications. Complete genomes were also determined for bacteria capable of anaerobic degradation of halogenated hydrocarbons by halorespiration: the ~1.4 Mb genomes of *Dehalococcoides ethenogenes* strain 195 and *Dehalococcoides* sp. strain CBDB1 and the ~5.7 Mb genome of *Desulfitobacterium hafniense* strain Y51.

Characteristic for all these bacteria is the presence of multiple paralogous genes for reductive dehalogenases, implicating a wider dehalogenating spectrum of the organisms than previously known. Moreover, genome sequences provided unprecedented insights into the evolution of reductive dehalogenation and differing strategies for niche adaptation. Recently, it has become apparent that some organisms, including *Desulfitobacterium chlororespirans*, originally evaluated for halorespiration on chlorophenols, can also use certain brominated compounds, such as the herbicide bromoxynil and its major metabolite as electron acceptors for growth. Iodinated compounds may be dehalogenated as well, though the process may not satisfy the need for an electron acceptor.

Bioavailability, Chemotaxis, and Transport of Pollutants

Bioavailability, or the amount of a substance that is physio-chemically accessible to micro-organisms is a key factor in the efficient biodegradation of pollutants. O'Loughlin showed that, with the exception of kaolinite clay, most soil clays and cation exchange resins attenuated biodegradation of 2-picoline by *Arthrobacter* sp. strain R1, as a result of adsorption of the substrate to the clays. Chemotaxis, or the directed movement of motile organisms towards or away from chemicals in the environment is an important physiological response that may contribute to effective catabolism of molecules in the environment. In addition, mechanisms for the intracellular accumulation of aromatic molecules via various transport mechanisms are also important.

Oil Biodegradation

Petroleum oil contains aromatic compounds that are toxic for most life forms. Episodic and chronic pollution of the environment by oil causes major ecological perturbations. Marine environments are especially vulnerable since oil spills of coastal regions and the open sea are poorly containable and mitigation is difficult. In addition to pollution through human activities, about 250 million litres of petroleum enter the marine environment every year from natural seepages. Despite its toxicity, a considerable fraction of petroleum oil entering marine systems is eliminated by the hydrocarbon-degrading activities of microbial communities, in particular by a remarkable recently discovered group of specialists, the so-called hydrocarbonoclastic bacteria (HCB). *Alcanivorax borkumensis* was the first HCB to have its genome sequenced. In addition to hydrocarbons, crude oil often contains various heterocyclic compounds, such as pyridine, which appear to be degraded by similar, though separate mechanisms than hydrocarbons.

Analysis of Waste Biotreatment

Sustainable development requires the promotion of environmental management and a constant search for new technologies to treat vast quantities of wastes generated by increasing anthropogenic activities. Biotreatment, the processing of wastes using living organisms, is an environmentally friendly, relatively simple and cost-effective alternative to physico-chemical clean-up options. Confined environments, such as bioreactors, have been engineered to overcome the physical, chemical and biological limiting factors of biotreatment processes in highly controlled systems. The great versatility in the design of confined environments allows the treatment of a wide range of wastes under optimised conditions. To perform a correct assessment, it is necessary to consider various micro-organisms having a variety of genomes and expressed transcripts and proteins. A great number of analyses are often required. Using traditional genomic techniques, such assessments are limited and time-consuming. However, several high-throughput techniques originally developed for medical studies can be applied to assess biotreatment in confined environments.

Metabolic Engineering and Biocatalytic Applications

The study of the fate of persistent organic chemicals in the environment has revealed a large reservoir of enzymatic reactions with a large potential in preparative organic synthesis, which has already been exploited for a number of oxygenases on pilot and even on industrial scale. Novel catalysts can be obtained from metagenomic libraries and DNA sequence based approaches. Our increasing capabilities in adapting the catalysts to specific reactions and process requirements by rational and random mutagenesis broadens the scope for application in the fine chemical industry, but also in the field of biodegradation. In many cases, these catalysts need to be exploited in whole cell bioconversions or in fermentations, calling for system-wide approaches to understanding strain physiology and metabolism and rational approaches to the engineering of whole cells as they are increasingly put forward in the area of systems biotechnology and synthetic biology.

Fungal Biodegradation

In the ecosystem, different substrates are attacked at different rates by consortia of organisms from different kingdoms. *Aspergillus* and other moulds play an important role in these consortia because they are adept at recycling starches, hemicelluloses, celluloses, pectins and other sugar polymers. Some aspergilli are capable of degrading more refractory compounds such as fats, oils, chitin, and keratin. Maximum decomposition occurs when there is sufficient nitrogen, phosphorus and other essential inorganic nutrients. Fungi also provide food for many soil organisms. For *Aspergillus* the process of degradation is the means of obtaining nutrients. When these moulds degrade human-made substrates, the process usually is called biodeterioration. Both paper and textiles (cotton, jute, and linen) are particularly vulnerable to *Aspergillus* degradation. Our artistic heritage is also subject to *Aspergillus* assault.

BIODEGRADATION OF XENOBIOTIC COMPOUNDS

Xenobiotic compounds are human made chemicals that are present in the environment at unnaturally high concentrations. The xenobiotic compounds are either not produced naturally, or are produced at much lower concentrations.

Micro-organism has the capability of degrading all naturally occurring compounds; this is known as the principle of microbial infallibility proposed by Alexander in 1965. Micro-organisms are also able to degrade many of the xenobiotic compounds, but they are unable to degrade many others. The compounds that resist biodegradation and thereby persist in the environment are called recalcitrant.

The xenobiotic compounds may be recalcitrant due to one or more of the following reasons:

1. They are not recognised as substrate by the existing degradative enzymes.
2. They are highly stable, i.e. chemically and biologically inert due to the presence of substitution groups like halogens, nitro-, sulphonate, amino-, methoxy- and carbamyl groups.
3. They are insoluble in water, or are adsorbed to external matrices like soil.
4. They are highly toxic or give rise to toxic products due to microbial activity.
5. Their large molecular size prevents entry into microbial cells.
6. Inability of the compounds to induce the synthesis of degrading enzymes.
7. Lack of the permease needed for their transport into the microbial cells.

Xenobiotic Metabolism

Xenobiotic metabolism is the set of metabolic pathways that modify the chemical structure of xenobiotics, which are compounds foreign to an organism's normal biochemistry, such as drugs and poisons. These pathways are a form of biotransformation present in all major groups of organisms, and are considered to be of ancient origin. These reactions often act to detoxify poisonous compounds; however, in some cases, the intermediates in xenobiotic metabolism can themselves be the cause of toxic effects.

Xenobiotic metabolism is divided into three phases. In phase I, enzymes such as cytochrome P450 oxidases introduce reactive or polar groups into xenobiotics. These modified compounds are then conjugated to polar compounds in phase II reactions. These reactions are catalysed by transferase enzymes such as glutathione S-transferases. Finally, in phase III, the conjugated xenobiotics may be further processed, before being recognised by efflux transporters and pumped out of cells.

The reactions in these pathways are of particular interest in medicine as part of drug metabolism and as a factor contributing to multidrug resistance in infectious diseases and cancer chemotherapy. The actions of some drugs as substrates or inhibitors of enzymes involved in xenobiotic metabolism are a common reason for hazardous drug interactions. These pathways are also important in environmental science, with the xenobiotic metabolism of micro-organisms determining whether a pollutant will be broken down during bioremediation, or persist in the environment. The enzymes of xenobiotic metabolism, particularly the glutathione S-transferases are also important in agriculture, since they may produce resistance to pesticides and herbicides.

Permeability barriers and detoxification

That the exact compounds an organism is exposed to will be largely unpredictable, and may differ widely over time, is a major characteristic of xenobiotic toxic stress. The major challenge faced by xenobiotic detoxification systems is that they must be able to remove the almost-limitless number of xenobiotic compounds from the complex mixture of chemicals involved in normal metabolism. The solution that has evolved to address this problem is an elegant combination of physical barriers and low-specificity enzymatic systems.

All organisms use cell membranes as hydrophobic permeability barriers to control access to their internal environment. Polar compounds cannot diffuse across these cell membranes, and the uptake of useful molecules is mediated through transport proteins that specifically select substrates from the extracellular mixture. This selective uptake means that most hydrophilic molecules cannot enter cells, since they are not recognised by any specific transporters. In contrast, the diffusion of hydrophobic compounds across these barriers cannot be controlled, and organisms, therefore, cannot exclude lipid-soluble xenobiotics using membrane barriers. However, the existence of a permeability barrier means that organisms were able to evolve detoxification systems that exploit the hydrophobicity common to membrane-permeable xenobiotics. These systems therefore solve the specificity problem by possessing such broad substrate specificities that they metabolise almost any non-polar compound. Useful metabolites are excluded since they are polar, and in general contain one or more charged groups.

The detoxification of the reactive by-products of normal metabolism cannot be achieved by the systems outlined above, because these species are derived from normal cellular constituents and usually share their polar characteristics. However, since these compounds are few in number, specific enzymes can recognise and remove them. Examples of these specific detoxification systems are the glyoxalase system, which removes the reactive aldehyde methylglyoxal, and the various antioxidant systems that eliminate reactive oxygen species.

Phases of detoxification

The metabolism of xenobiotics is often divided into three phases: modification, conjugation, and excretion. These reactions act in concert to detoxify xenobiotics and remove them from cells (Fig. 10.1).

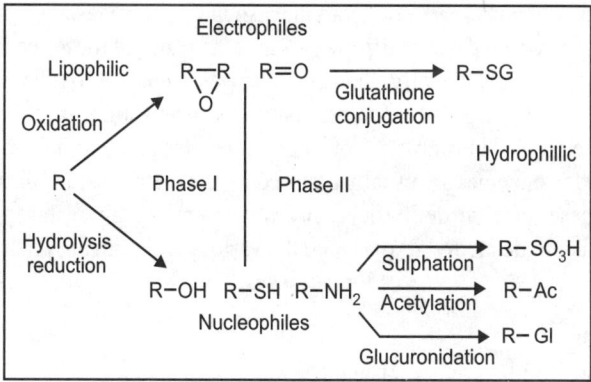

Fig. 10.1. Phases I and II of the metabolism of a lipophilic xenobiotic.

Phase I – modification

In phase I, a variety of enzymes acts to introduce reactive and polar groups into their substrates. One of the most common modifications is hydroxylation catalysed by the cytochrome P-450-dependent mixed-function oxidase system. These enzyme complexes act to incorporate an atom of oxygen into nonactivated hydrocarbons, which can result in either the introduction of hydroxyl groups or N-, O- and S-dealkylation of substrates. The reaction mechanism of the P-450 oxidases proceeds through the reduction of cytochrome-bound oxygen and the generation of a highly-reactive oxyferryl species, according to the following scheme:

$$NADPH + H^+ + RH \rightarrow NADP^+ + H_2O + ROH$$

Phase II – conjugation

In subsequent phase II reactions, these activated xenobiotic metabolites are conjugated with charged species such as glutathione (GSH), sulphate, glycine, or glucuronic acid. These reactions are catalysed by a large group of broad-specificity transferases, which in combination can metabolise almost any hydrophobic compound that contains nucleophilic or electrophilic groups. One of the most important of these groups are the glutathione S-transferases (GSTs). The addition of large anionic groups (such as GSH) detoxifies reactive electrophiles and produces more polar metabolites that cannot diffuse across membranes, and may, therefore, be actively transported.

Phase III - further modification and excretion

After phase II reactions, the xenobiotic conjugates may be further metabolised. A common example is the processing of glutathione conjugates to acetylcysteine (mercapturic acid) conjugates. Here, the γ-glutamate and glycine residues in the glutathione molecule are removed by Gamma-glutamyl transpeptidase and dipeptidases. In the final step, the cystine residue in the conjugate is acetylated.

Conjugates and their metabolites can be excreted from cells in phase III of their metabolism, with the anionic groups acting as affinity tags for a variety of membrane transporters of the multidrug resistance protein (MRP) family. These proteins are members of the family of ATP-binding cassette transporters and can catalyse the ATP-dependent transport of a huge variety of hydrophobic anions, and thus act to remove phase II products to the extracellular medium, where they may be further metabolised or excreted.

Endogenous toxins

The detoxification of endogenous reactive metabolites such as peroxides and reactive aldehydes often cannot be achieved by the system described above. This is the result of these species being derived from normal cellular constituents and usually sharing their polar characteristics. However, since these compounds are few in number, it is possible for enzymatic systems to utilise specific molecular recognition to recognise and remove them. The similarity of these molecules to useful metabolites therefore means that different detoxification enzymes are usually required for the metabolism of each group of endogenous toxins. Examples of these specific detoxification systems are the glyoxalase system, which acts to dispose of the reactive aldehyde methylglyoxal, and the various antioxidant systems that remove reactive oxygen species.

Degradative Plasmids

Some microbes have the ability to degrade 'dead' organic matter resulting from death or excretion. They utilise the organic matter for biosynthesis and energy, and recycle it. Strains of pseudomonads have been isolated which can degrade about a hundred different organic compounds for energy and carbon sources. The degradative enzymes may be coded by the chromosomes or the plasmids. The versatility of pseudomonads is due to the presence of plasmids which code enzymes of catabolic pathways of a number of complex organic substrates.

Some fermentation reactions are specified by plasmids, e.g. the ability to ferment lactose (lac plasmid) and other carbohydrates in strains of the enteric bacteria *Salmonella*, *Proteus* and *Yersinia*. The presence of the lac plasmid can cause confusion in diagnosing medically important bacteria, since the ability or inability to ferment lactose is often used in classifying clinical isolates.

PSEUDOMONAS PUTIDA

Pseudomonas putida is a gram-negative rod-shaped saprotrophic soil bacterium. Based on 16S rRNA analysis, *P. putida* has been placed in the *P. putida* group, to which it lends its name. It is the first patented organism in the world. Because it is a living organism the patent was disputed and brought before the United States Supreme Court in the historic court case Diamond v. Chakrabarty which the inventor, Ananda M. Chakrabarty, won. It demonstrates a very diverse metabolism, including the ability to degrade organic solvents such as toluene. This ability has been put to use in bioremediation, or the use of micro-organisms to biodegrade oil. Use of *P. putida* is preferable to some other *Pseudomonas* species capable of such degradation as it is a safe strain of bacteria, unlike *P. aeruginosa* for example, which is an opportunistic human pathogen.

Uses

Bioremediation

The diverse metabolism of *P. putida* may be exploited for bioremediation; for example, it is used as a soil inoculant to remedy naphthalene contaminated soils. *P. putida* is capable of converting styrene oil into the biodegradable plastic PHA. This may be of use in the effective recycling of Polystyrene foam, otherwise thought to be non-biodegradable.

Biocontrol

P. putida has demonstrated potential biocontrol properties, as an effective antagonist of damping off diseases such as *Pythium* and *Fusarium*.

Method of Production of Ethyl Alcohol from Starch Raw Material

Ethyl alcohol can be produced from a starch raw material consisting in hydrolysation of the starch raw material, for example wheat, barley or rye grain, in the presence of ferments of amylolytic or cellulolytic action. As ferments of cellulolytic action is used a culture preparation of fungus Trichoderma koningiu containing a complex of ferments: C1-ferment, endoglucanase, exoglucanase, cellobioase, xylanase, beta-glucosidase, protease and amylolytic ferments.

Types of modified starch

Modified starch can be divided into three main groups according to the modification process utilised. These three groups are further subdivided according to process and products as shown in Fig. 10.2 and Table 10.2.

Table 10.2. Principal modified starch products and their production process and application.

Product	Production process	Application
Yellow dexterin	Heat for roasting	Casting, construction materials
White dextrin	Heat for roasting	Binding agent in medicines
Pregelatinised starch	Dried and milled by drum	Feed, casting, construction materials

(Contd ...)

Product	Production process	Application
Oxidised starch	Oxidised by oxidising agent	Binding agent for cardboard, textile, food
Acid-hydrolysed starch	Hydrolysed by acid	Food, sizing for textile, paper making
Starch acetate	Esterification by acetic acid	Paper making, textile, casting, food, snack food
Cationic starch	Etherification by trimethyl amine	Paper pulp additive coating
Complex modified starch	–	Paper pulp additive coating
Carboxymethyl starch	Etherification by chloroacetic acid	Lubricant for oil drilling medicine, construction materials
Hydroxy-propyl starch	–	Food, candy
Cross-linked starch	–	Food, medicine, textile, chemical industry
Graft co-polymerised starch	Graft co-polymerised by acrylonitrile	High water-absorbent materials, such as disposable diapers, female napkins, textile sizing material

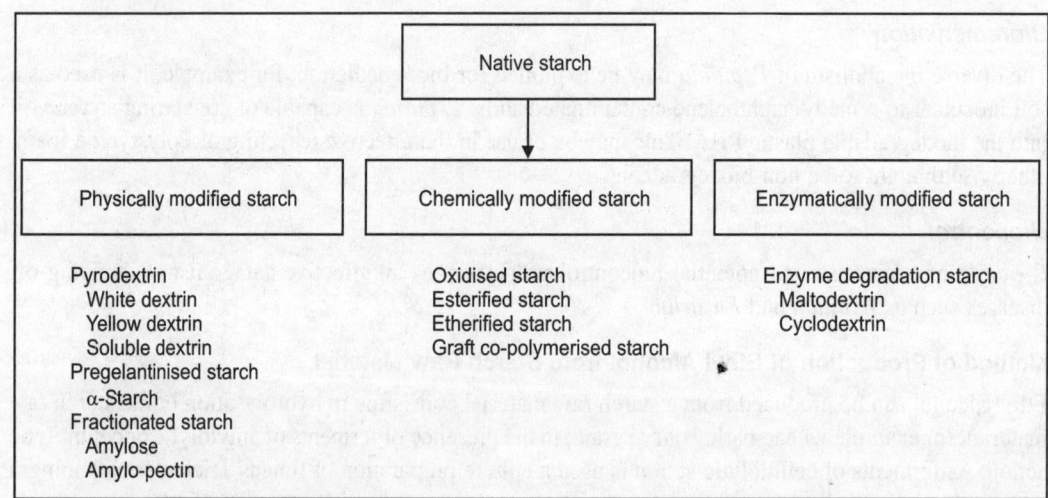

Fig. 10.2. Modified starch processing technologies and products.

Manufacture of Ethanol by Fermentation

Ethanol can be manufactured by the fermentation of: (i) molasses, and (ii) starch.

Slow decomposition of organic compounds is called fermentation. This is the principle behind souring of milk, batter, putrefaction of meat, and preparation of wine and vinegar. Fermentation was the earliest method used for preparing alcohol in industries. This is still used for the manufacture of alcohol and alcoholic drinks like beer, wine, brandy, etc.

Raw materials: Cheap starchy materials like potatoes, maize, barley, rice, etc. or molasses, a by-product of sugar industry.

From molasses: The syrup left after the separation of cane sugar or beet sugar crystals from the concentrated sugar cane juice is called molasses. It is a dark coloured syrupy mass and contains about 30 per cent of uncrystallisable sucrose and about 32 per cent of invert sugar (a mixture of glucose and fructose).

The different steps in the manufacture of ethanol by fermentation of molasses are:

1. Dilution: The molasses is diluted with water until a concentration of 8–10 per cent sugar is obtained in solution. To discourage bacterial growth, this is acidified with a little sulphuric acid. If sufficient yeast (food for the ferment) is not present, a nutritive solution of ammonium salts is added.

2. Alcoholic fermentation: The dilute solution obtained as above is taken in big fermentation tanks and some yeast is added (5 per cent by volume). The temperature is maintained at 330K and the mixture is allowed to stand for a few days. Fermentation sets in and the enzyme (organic catalyst) invertase present in yeast, converts sucrose into glucose and fructose. Zymase, another enzyme present in yeast converts glucose and fructose into ethanol and carbon dioxide.

   The carbon dioxide formed is allowed to escape but air is not allowed to enter. In presence of air ethanol formed would be oxidised to acetic acid.

$$C_{12}H_{22}O_{11} + H_2O \xrightarrow[\text{in yeast}]{\text{Invertase}} \underset{\text{Glucose}}{C_6H_{12}O_6} + \underset{\text{Fructose}}{C_6H_{12}O_6}$$

$$\underset{\substack{\text{Glucose}\\\text{or fructose}}}{C_6H_{12}O_6} \xrightarrow[\text{in yeast}]{\text{Zymase}} \underset{\text{Ethanol}}{2C_2H_5OH} + \underset{\text{Carbon dioxide}}{2CO_2}$$

The fermentation is complete in 3 days. The carbon dioxide obtained as by-product is recovered and can be sold.

3. Distillation: The fermented liquor contains 9–10 per cent of ethanol and is called wash or wort. It is distilled in a Coffey still (distillation of wash in a Coffey still) to remove water and other impurities present in wash. The Coffey still consists of two tall fractionating columns with perforated plates. These columns are called the analyser and the rectifier. This works on the counter-current principle as the steam and alcohol travel in opposite directions through the still. Steam passes up the analyser and takes away the alcohol vapours from the dilute alcohol that is coming down. The mixture leaves the analyser at the top. It then enters the rectifier at the base. The mixture heats the wort flowing through the pipes on its way to the analyser. The steam condenses and the alcohol vapours escaping near the top are condensed in the condenser. The distillate contains about 90 per cent alcohol and the residue left in the still is used as cattle feed.

4. Rectification: The alcohol obtained contains other impurities besides water. These impurities are further removed by fractional distillation. Low boiling impurities like acetaldehyde distil over as first fraction. The middle fraction contains about 93–95 per cent alcohol and is called rectified spirit. Often, distillation and rectification is carried out in the same operation.

From starch: Wheat, barley, rice, maize and potatoes.

Conversion of starch into maltose: Conversion of starch into maltose or saccharification is carried out as follows:

1. Malting: Moist barley is allowed to germinate in dark at 290K. Germinated barley is called Malt and this is heated to 330K (to stop further germination). It is then crushed and extracted with water. This Malt extract contains the enzyme diastase.

2. Mashing: To break the cell walls, starch is reacted with superheated steam. This exposes the starch inside that forms a paste like mass called mash.

3. Hydrolysis: Mash and malt extract are treated together at 320–330K. In about half an hour, hydrolysis is complete and maltose is formed.

$$2(C_6H_{10}O_5)_n + nH_2O \xrightarrow[\text{malt extract}]{\text{Diastase in}} nC_{12}H_{22}O_{11}$$

$$\underset{\text{Starch}}{} \qquad\qquad\qquad\qquad \underset{\text{Maltose}}{}$$

Alcoholic fermentation: Maltose obtained from starch is fermented in the presence of yeast. Maltase present in yeast converts maltose into glucose.

Another enzyme zymase present in yeast, then converts glucose into ethanol and carbon dioxide.

$$\underset{\text{Maltose}}{C_{12}H_{22}O_{11}} + H_2O \xrightarrow{\text{Maltase in yeast}} \underset{\text{Glucose}}{2C_6H_{12}O_6}$$

$$\underset{\text{Glucose}}{C_6H_{12}O_6} \xrightarrow{\text{Zymase in yeast}} \underset{\text{Ethanol}}{2C_2H_5OH} + \underset{\text{Carbon dioxide}}{2CO_2}$$

Subsequent distillation and rectification yields rectified spirit.

LIGNOCELLULOSE BIOTECHNOLOGY: ISSUES OF BIOCONVERSION AND ENZYME PRODUCTION

Lignocellulose is the major structural component of woody plants and non-woody plants such as grass and represents a major source of renewable organic matter. Lignocellulose consists of lignin, hemicellulose and cellulose. The chemical properties of the components of lignocellulosics make them a substrate of enormous biotechnological value. Large amounts of lignocellulosic 'waste' (Table 10.3) are generated through forestry and agricultural practices, paper-pulp industries, timber industries and many agroindustries and they pose an environmental pollution problem. Sadly, much of the lignocellulose waste is often disposed of by biomass burning, which is not restricted to developing countries alone, but is considered a global phenomenon. However, the huge amounts of residual plant biomass considered as 'waste' can potentially be converted into various different value-added products including biofuels, chemicals, cheap energy sources for fermentation, improved animal feeds and human nutrients. Lignocellulytic enzymes also have significant potential applications in various industries including chemicals, fuel, food, brewery and wine, animal feed, textile and laundry, pulp and paper, and agriculture. This review's main focus is to highlight significant aspects of lignocellulose biotechnology with emphasis on demonstrating the potential value from an application rather than basic research perspective. Aspects which will be reviewed in this section include: an overview of some of the major potential lignocellulose derived high-value bioproducts; solid state fermentation processing as a relevant, initial approach to lignocellulose bioconversion relevant for developing countries; some background on lignocellulolytic organisms and their enzymes, and finally looking at cost of enzymes and potential of modern approaches which could be employed to reduce cost.

Table 10.3. Types of lignocellulosic materials and their current uses.

Lignocellulosic material	Residues	Competing use
Grain harvesting		
Wheat, rice, oats barley and corn	Straw, cobs, stalks, husks,	Animal feed, burnt as fuel, compost, soil conditioner
Processed grains		
Corn, wheat, rice, soyabean	Waste water, bran	Animal feed
Fruit and vegetable harvesting	Seeds, peels, husks, stones, rejected whole fruit and juice	Animal and fish feed, some seeds for oil extraction

(Contd ...)

Lignocellulosic material	Residues	Competing use
Fruit and vegetable processing	Seeds, peels, waste water, husks, shells, stones, rejected whole fruit and juice	Animal and fish feed, some seeds for oil extraction
Sugar cane other sugar products	Bagasse	Burnt as fuel
Oils and oilseed plants Nuts, cotton seeds, olives, soyabean, etc.	Shells, husks, lint, fibre, sludge, presscake, waste-water	Animal feed, fertiliser, burnt fuel
Animal waste	Manure, other waste	Soil conditioners
Forestry-paper and pulp		
Harvesting of logs	Wood residuals, barks, leaves, etc.	Soil conditioners, burnt
Saw-and-plywood waste	Woodchips, wood shavings, saw dust	Pulp and paper industries, chip and fibre board
Pulp and paper mills	Fibre waste, sulphite liquor	Reused in pulp and board industry as fuel
Lignocellulose waste from communities	Old newspapers, paper, cardboard, old boards, disused furniture	Small percentage recycled, others burnt
Grass	Unutilised grass	Burnt

Potential Bioproducts and Their Applications

Biomass can be considered as the mass of organic material from any biological material, and by extension, any large mass of biological matter. A wide variety of biomass resources are available (Table 10.3) on our planet for conversion into bioproducts. These may include whole plants, plant parts (e.g. seeds, stalks), plant constituents (e.g. starch, lipids, protein and fibre), processing by-products (distiller's grains, corn solubles), materials of marine origin and animal by-products, municipal and industrial wastes. These resources can be used to create new biomaterials and this will require an intimate understanding of the composition of the raw material whether it is whole plant or constituents, so that the desired functional elements can be obtained for bioproduct production.

There are some excellent and comprehensive literature available on the different potential bioproducts and their many applications but only a few of the high-value products will be reviewed.

Chemicals

Bioconversion of lignocellulosic wastes could make a significant contribution to the production of organic chemicals. Over 75 per cent of organic chemicals are produced from five primary base-chemicals: ethylene, propylene, benzene, toluene and xylene which are used to synthesis other organic compounds, which in turn are used to produce various chemical products including polymers and resins. The aromatic compounds might be produced from lignin whereas the low molecular mass aliphatic compounds can be derived from ethanol produced by fermentation of sugar generated from the cellulose and hemicellulose.

Biofuel

The demand for ethanol has the most significant market where ethanol is either used as a chemical feedstock or as an octane enhancer or petrol additive. Global crude oil production is predicted to decline from 25 billion barrels to approximately 5 billion barrels in 2050. Brazil produces ethanol from the fermentation of cane juice whereas in the US corn is used. In the US, fuel ethanol has been used in gasohol or oxygenated fuels since the 1980s. These gasoline fuels contain up to 10 per cent ethanol by volume. It is estimated that 4540 million litres of ethanol is used by the US transportation sector and that this number will rise phenomenally since the US automobile manufacturers plan to manufacture a significant number of flexi-fuelled engines which can use an ethanol blend of 85 per cent ethanol and 15 per cent gasoline by volume. The production of ethanol from sugars or starch impacts negatively on the economics of the process, thus making ethanol more expensive compared with fossil fuels. Hence the technology development focus for the production of ethanol has shifted towards the utilisation of residual lignocellulosic materials to lower production costs.

Other high-value bioproducts

Currently a number of products such as organic acids, amino acids, vitamins and a number of bacterial and fungal polysaccharides such as xanthan are produced by fermentation using glucose as the base substrate but theoretically these same products could be manufactured from 'lignocellulose waste'. Based upon the predicted catabolic pathway and the known metabolism of *Phanerochaete chrysosporium* of lignin, Ribbons presented a detailed discussion of the potential value-added products which could be derived from lignin. Vanillin and gallic acid are the two most frequently discussed monomeric potential products which have attracted interest. Vanillin is used for various purposes including being an intermediate in the chemical and pharmaceutical industries for the production of herbicides, anti-foaming agents or drugs such as papaverine, L-dopa and the anti microbial agent, trimethoprim. It is also used in household products such as air-fresheners and floor polishes. The high price and limited supply of natural vanillin have necessitated a shift towards its production from other sources. Hemicelluloses are of particular industrial interest since these are a readily available bulk source of xylose from which xylitol and furfural can be derived. Xylitol used instead of sucrose in food as a sweetner, has odontological applications such as teeth hardening, remineralisation, and as an antimicrobial agent, it is used in chewing gum and toothpaste formulations. The yield of xylans as xylitol by chemical means is only about 50–60 per cent making xylitol production expensive. Various bioconversion methods, therefore, have been explored for the production of xylitol from hemicellulose using micro-organisms or their enzymes. Furfural is used in the manufacture of furfuralphenol plastics, varnishes and pesticides.

Enzymes

Cellulases and hemicellulases have numerous applications and biotechnological potential for various industries including chemicals, fuel, food, brewery and wine, animal feed, textile and laundry, pulp and paper and agriculture. It is estimated that approximately 20 per cent of the >1 billion US dollars of the world's sale of industrial enzymes consists of cellulases, hemicellulases and pectinases and that the world market for industrial enzymes will increase in the range of 9–12 billion US dollars by the year 2016. In the baking industry xylanases are used for improving desirable texture, loaf volume and shelf-life of bread. A xylanase, Novozyme 867, has shown excellent performance in the wheat separation process. Hemicellulases are used for pulping and bleaching in the pulp and paper industry where they are used to modify the structure of xylan and glucomannan in pulp fibres to enhance chemical delignification. A patented Lignozyme® process is effective in delignifying wood in a pilot pulp- and paper process. In bio-pulping where lignocellulytic enzymes were used the following was achieved: tensile, tear and burst indexes of the resultant paper improved, brightness of the pulp was increased and an improved energy saving of 30–38 per cent was realised. Laccases can degrade a wide variety of synthetic dyes making them suitable for the treatment of waste-water from the textile industry. Organisms such as the white rot fungi producing lignases could be used for the degradation of persistent aromatic pollutants such as dichlorophenol, dinitrotoluene and anthracene.

There is a huge potential market for fibre-degrading enzymes for the animal feed industry and over the years a number of commercial preparations have been produced. The use of fibre-degrading enzymes for ruminants such as cattle and sheep for improving feed utilisation, milk yield and body weight gain have attracted considerable interest. Steers fed with an enzyme mixture containing xylanase and cellulase showed an increased live-weight gain of approximately 30–36 per cent. In dairy cows the milk yield increased in the range of 4 to 16 per cent on various commercial fibrolytic enzyme treated forages.

Degradation of Lignocellulose

Lignocellulose consists of lignin, hemicellulose and cellulose and Table 10.4 shows the typical compositions of the three components in various lignocellulosic materials. Because of the difficulty in dissolving lignin without destroying it and some of its subunits, its exact chemical structure is difficult to ascertain. In general lignin contains three aromatic alcohols (coniferyl alcohol, sinapyl and pcoumaryl). In addition, grass and dicot lignin also contain large amounts of phenolic acids such as *p*-coumaric and ferulic acid, which are esterified to alcohol groups of each other and to other alcohols such as sinapyl and *p*-coumaryl alcohols.

Table 10.4. Lignocellulose contents of common agricultural residues and wastes.

Lignocellulosic materials	Cellulose (%)	Hemicellulose (%)	Lignin (%)
Hardwood stems	40–55	24–40	18–25
Softwood stems	45–50	25–35	25–35
Nut shells	25–30	25–30	30–40
Corn cobs	45	35	15
Paper	85–99	0	0–15
Wheat straw	30	50	15
Rice straw	32.1	24	18
Sorted refuse	60	20	20
Leaves	15–20	80–85	0
Cotton seeds hairs	80–95	5–20	0
Newspaper	40–55	25–40	18–30
Waste paper from chemical pulps	60–70	10–20	5–10
Primary waste-water solids	8–15	NA	24–29
Fresh bagasse	33.4	30	18.9
Swine waste	6	28	NA
Solid cattle manure	1.6–4.7	1.4–3.3	2.7–5.7
Coastal Bermuda grass	25	35.7	6.4
Switch grass	45	31.4	12.0
S32 rye grass (early leaf)	21.3	15.8	2.7
S32 rye grass (seed setting)	26.7	25.7	7.3
Orchard grass (medium maturity)	32	40	4.7
Grasses (average values for grasses)	25–40	25–50	10–30

Note: NA = data not available.

Lignin is further linked to both hemicelluloses and cellulose forming a physical seal around the latter two components that is an impenetrable barrier preventing penetration of solutions and enzymes. Hemicellulose macromolecules are often polymers of pentoses (xylose and arabinose), hexoses (mostly mannose) and a number of sugar acids while cellulose is a homogenous polymer of glucose.

Of the three components, lignin is the most recalcitrant to degradation whereas cellulose, because of its highly ordered crystalline structure, is more resistant to hydrolysis than hemicellulose. Alkaline and acid hydrolysis methods have been used to degrade lignocellulose. Weak acids tend to remove lignin but result in poor hydrolysis of cellulose whereas strong acid treatment occurs under relatively extreme corrosive conditions of high temperature and pH which necessitate the use of expensive equipment. Also, unspecific side reactions occur which yield nonspecific by-products other than glucose, promote glucose degradation and therefore reduce its yield. Some of the unspecific products can be deleterious to subsequent fermentation unless removed. There are also environmental concerns associated with the disposal of spent acid and alkaline. For many processes enzymes are preferred to acid or alkaline processes since they are specific biocatalysts, can operate under much milder reaction conditions, do not produce undesirable products and are environmentally friendly.

Bioprocessing of lignocellulosic materials

Technologies are currently available for all steps in the bioconversion of lignocelluloses to ethanol and other chemical products. However, these technologies must be improved and new technologies developed to produce renewable biofuel and other bioproducts at prices which can compete with current production costs. The feedstock costs can be minimised by initially focusing on agricultural residues and waste materials. Other process steps, which are particularly expensive, include pretreatments to improve the bioconversion, the production of enzymes for depolymerisation of the complex raw materials and capital costs associated with bioconversions. In general the technology of bioprocessing of raw materials or their constituents into bioproducts entails three steps: process design, system optimisation and model development. Processing involves the use of biocatalysts, whole micro-organisms or their enzymes or enzymes from other organisms to synthesise or bioconvert raw materials into new products; recover/ purify such bioproducts and subsequently any needed downstream modifications.

Bioconversions of lignocellulosic materials to useful, higher value products normally require multi-step processes (Fig. 10.3) which include: (i) pretreatment (mechanical, chemical or biological), (ii) hydrolysis of the polymers to produce readily metabolisable molecules (e.g. hexose or pentose sugars), (iii) bio-utilisation of these molecules to support microbial growth or to produce chemical products, and (iv) the separation and purification. A stirred-tank reactor, widely used for the production of cellulose and other lignocellulosic enzymes, is known to have shear problems which rupture mycelial cells and may deactivate the enzymes. Alternative bioreactors such as the air-lift or bubble-column, which have a lower shear stress, seem to produce better results. For example, studies on cellulase and xylanase production by *A. niger* in various bioreactors showed that in general, better yield and productivity were shown in a bubble-column and an airloop air-lift than in the stirred-tank reactor. However, the relatively high cost of enzyme production has hindered the industrial application of the enzymatic process.

It has been reported that the solid state fermentation (SSF) is an attractive alternative process to produce fungal microbial enzymes using lignocellulosic materials from agricultural wastes due to its lower capital investment and lower operating cost. SSF process, for the reasons stated, will be ideal for developing countries. Solid-state fermentations are characterised by the complete or almost complete absence of free liquid.

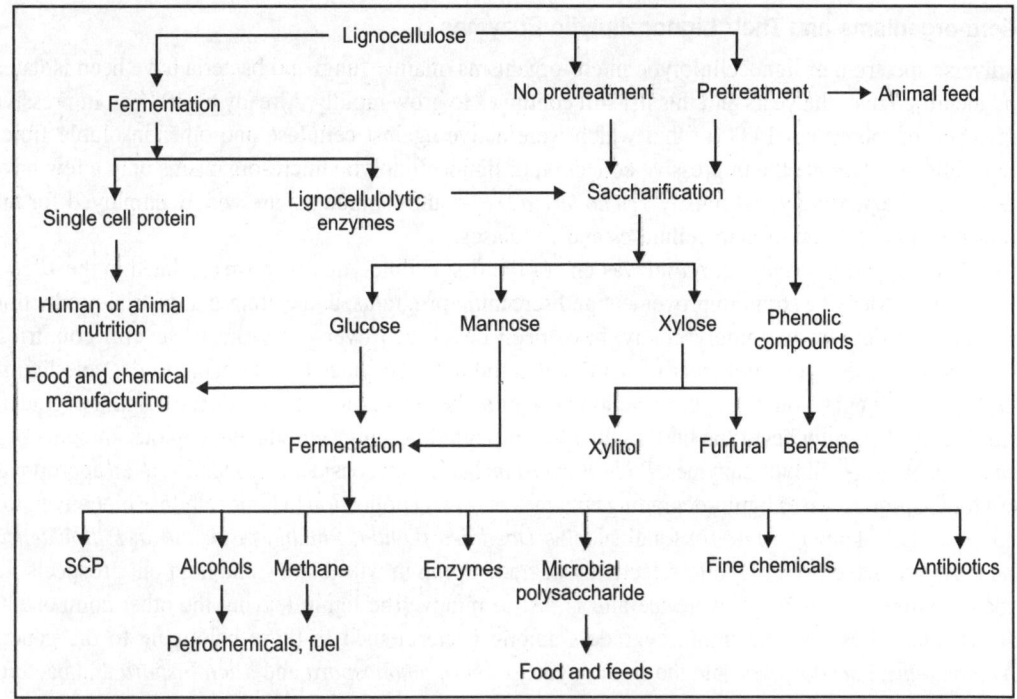

Fig. 10.3. Generalised process stages in lignocellulose bioconversion into value-added bioproducts.

Water, which is essential for microbial activities, is present in an absorbed or in complexed form with the solid matrix and the substrate. These cultivation conditions are especially suitable for the growth of fungi, known to grow at relatively low water activities. As the micro-organisms in SSF grow under conditions closer to their natural habitats they are more capable of producing enzymes and metabolites which will not be produced or will be produced only in low yield in submerge conditions. SSFs are practical for complex substrates including agricultural, forestry and food-processing residues and wastes which are used as carbon sources for the production of lignocellulolytic enzymes. Compared with the two-stage hydrolysis fermentation process during ethanol production from lignocellulosics, Sun and Cheng, reported that SSF has the following advantages: (i) increase in hydrolysis rate by conversion of sugars that inhibit the enzyme (cellulase) activity; (ii) lower enzyme requirement; (iii) higher product yield; (iv) lower requirement for sterile conditions since glucose is removed immediately and ethanol is produced; (v) shorter process time; and (vi) less reactor volume. In a recent review reiterated that the primary objective of lignocellulose treatment by the various industries is to access the potential of the cellulose encrusted by lignin within the lignocellulose matrix. Smith expressed the opinion that a combination of SSF technology with the ability of an appropriate fungus to selectively degrade lignin will make possible industrial scale implementation of lignocellulose-based biotechnologies.

Like all technologies, SSF has its disadvantages and these have received the attention by Mudgett. Problems commonly associated with SSF are heat buildup, bacterial contamination, scale-up, biomass growth estimation and control of substrate content. However, the process has been used for the production of many microbial products and the engineering aspects and the scale-up will depend on bioreactor design and operation. Other lignocellulose bioprocessing strategies include anaerobic treatment, composing, production of single cell protein for ruminant animal feeding and mushroom cultivation.

Micro-organisms and Their Lignocellulytic Enzymes

A diverse spectrum of lignocellulolytic micro-organisms, mainly fungi and bacteria have been isolated and identified over the years and this list still continues to grow rapidly. Already by 1976 an impressive collection of more than 14,000 fungi which were active against cellulose and other insoluble fibres were collected. Despite the impressive collection of lignocellulolytic micro-organisms only a few have been studied extensively and mostly *Trichoderma reesei* and its mutants are widely employed for the commercial production of hemicellulases and cellulases.

This is so, partly because *T. reesei* was one of the first cellulolytic organisms isolated in the 1950's and because extensive strain improvement and screening programs, and cellulase industrial production processes, which are extremely costly, have been developed over the years in several countries. *T. reesei* might be a good producer of hemi-and cellulolytic enzymes but is unable to degrade lignin. The white-rot fungi belonging to the basidiomycetes are the most efficient and extensive lignin degraders with *P. chrysosporium* being the best-studied lignin-degrading fungus producing copious amounts of a unique set of lignocellulytic enzymes. *P. chrysosporium* has drawn considerable attention as an appropriate host for the production of lignin-degrading enzymes or direct application in lignocellulose bioconversion processes. Less known, white-rot fungi such as *Daedalea flavida*, *Phlebia fascicularia*, *P. floridensis* and *P. radiate* have been found to selectively degrade lignin in wheat straw and hold out prospects for bioconversion biotechnology were the aim is just to remove the lignin leaving the other components almost intact. Less prolific lignin degraders among bacteria such as those belonging to the genera *Cellulomonas*, *Pseudomonas* and the actinomycetes *Thermomonospora* and *Microbispora* and bacteria with surface-bound cellulase-complexes such as *Clostridium thermocellum* and *Ruminococcus* are beginning to receive attention as representing a gene pool with possible unique lignocellulolytic genes that could be used in lignocellulase engineering. It is conventional to consider lignocellulose-degrading enzymes according to the three components of lignocellulose (lignin, cellulose and hemicellulose) which they attack but bearing in mind such divisions are convenient classifications since some cross activity for these enzymes have been reported. The exact mechanism by which lignocellulose is degraded enzymatically is still not fully understood but significant advances have been made to gain insight into the micro-organisms, their lignocellulolytic genes and various enzymes involved in the process.

Lignases

Identifying lignin degrading micro-organisms has been hampered because of the lack of reliable assays, but significant progress has been made through the use of a ^{14}C-labelled lignin assay. Fungi breakdown lignin aerobically through the use of a family of extracellular enzymes collectively termed 'lignases'. Two families of lignolytic enzymes are widely considered to play a key role in the enzymatic degradation: phenol oxidase (laccase) and peroxidases (lignin peroxidase (LiP) and manganese peroxidase (MnP). Other enzymes whose roles have not been fully elucidated include H_2O_2-producing enzymes: glyoxal oxidase, glucose oxidase, veratryl alcohol oxidases, methanol oxidase and oxido-reductase.

Enzymes involved in lignin breakdown are too large to penetrate the unaltered cell wall of plants so the question arises, how do lignases affect lignin biodegradation. Suggestions are that lignases employ low-molecular, diffusible reactive compounds to affect initial changes to the lignin substrate.

Hemicellulases

Hemicellulose is a collective term referring to those polysaccharides soluble in alkali, associated with cellulose of the plant cell wall, and these would include non-cellulose β-D-glucans, pectic substances (polygalacturonans), and several heteropolysaccharides such as those mainly consisting of galactose (arabinogalactans), mannose (galactogluco-and glucomannans) and xylose (arabinoglucurono-and glucuronoxylans). However, only the heteropolysaccharides, those with a much lower degree of polymerisation (100–200 units) as compared to that of cellulose (10,000–14,000 units), are referred to as hemicelluloses. The principal sugar components of these hemicellulose heteropolysaccharides are: D-xylose, D-mannose, D-glucose, D-galactose, L-arabinose, D-glucuronic acid, 4-O-methyl-D-glucuronic acid, D-galacturonic acid, and to a lesser extent, L-rhamnose, L-fucose, and various O-methylated sugars.

Rabinovich and Shallom and Shoham, present recent reviews covering the types, structure, function, classification of microbial hemicellulases.

Hemicellulases like most other·enzymes which hydrolyse plant cell polysaccharides are multidomain proteins. These proteins generally contain structurally discrete catalytic and non-catalytic modules. The most important non-catalytic modules consist of carbohydrate binding domains (CBD) which facilitate the targeting of the enzyme to the polysaccharide, interdomain linkers, and dockerin modules that mediate the binding of the catalytic domain via cohesion-dockerin interactions, either to the microbial cell surface or to enzymatic complexes such as the cellulosome. Based on the amino acid or nucleic acid sequence of their catalytic modules hemicellulases are either glycoside hydrolases (GHs) which hydrolyse glycosidic bonds, or carbohydrate esterases (CEs), which hydrolyse ester linkages of acetate or ferulic acid side groups and according to their primary sequence homology they have been grouped into various families.

Xylan is the most abundant hemicellulose and xylanases are one of the major hemicellulases which hydrolyse the β-1,4 bond in the xylan backbone yielding short xylooligomers which are further hydrolysed into single xylose units by β-xylosidase. Most known xylanases belong to the GH 10 and 11 families and β-xylosidases are diustributed in families 3, 39, 43, 52 and 54. Bifunctional xylosidase-arabinosidase enzymes are found mainly in families 3, 43 and 54. β-Mannanases hydrolyse mannan-based hemicellulose and liberate short β-1,4-manno-oligomers which can further be hydrolysed to mannose by β-manno-sidases. About 50 mannases are found in GH families 5 and 26, and about 15 β-mannosidase in families 1, 2 and 5. α-L-Arabinofuranosidases and α-L-arabinanases hydrolyse arabinofuranosyl-containing hemicellulose, and are distributed in GH families 3, 43, 51, 54 and 62. Some of these enzymes exhibit broad substrate specificity, acting on arabinofuranoside moieties at O-5, O-2 and/or O-3 bonds as a single substituent, as well as from O-2 and O-3 doubly substituted xylans, xylooligomers and arabinans. Other xylanases are α-D-glucuronidases which hydrolyse the α-1,2-glycosidic bond of the 4-O-methyl-D-glucuronic acid sidechain of xylans and are found in family 67. Hemicellulolytic esterases include acetyl esterases which hydrolyse the acetyl substitutions on xylose moieties, and feruloyl esterase which hydrolyse the ester bond between the arabinose substitutions and ferulic acid. Feruloyl esterases aid the release of hemicellulose from lignin and renders the free polysaccharide product more amenable to degradation by the other hemicellulases.

Cellulases

In most lignocellulosic materials cellulose forms the major part of the three components (Table 10.4). Cellulose is composed of insoluble, linear chains of β-(1→4)-linked glucose units with an average degree of polymeraisation of about 10000 units but could be as low as 15 units. It is composed of highly crystalline regions and amorphous (non-crystalline) regions forming a structure with high tensile strength that is generally resistant to enzymatic hydrolysis, especially the crystalline regions.

Cellulases, responsible for the hydrolysis of cellulose, are composed of a complex mixture of enzyme proteins with different specificities to hydrolyse glycosidic bonds. Cellulases can be divided into three major enzyme activity classes. These are endoglucanses or endo-1,4-β-glucanase (EC 3.2.1.4), cellobiohydrolase (EC 3.2.1.91) and β-glucosidase (EC 3.2.1.21). Endoglucanases, often called carboxymethylcellulose (CM)-cellulases, are proposed to initiate attack randomly at multiple internal sites in the amorphous regions of the cellulose fibre opening-up sites for subsequent attack by the cellobiohydrolases. Cellobiohydrolase, often called an exoglucanase, is the major component of the fungal cellulase system accounting for 40–70 per cent of the total cellulase proteins and can hydrolyse highly crystalline cellulose. Cellobiohydrolases remove mono- and dimers from the end of the glucose chain. β-Glucosidase hydrolyse glucose dimers and in some cases cello-oligosaccharides to glucose. Generally, the endoglucanases and cellobiohydrolases work synergistically in the hydrolysis of cellulose but the details of the mechanism involved are still unclear. Micro-organisms generally appear to have multiple distinct variants of endo- and exo-glucanases. Similar to hemicellulases most cellulases are multidomain proteins.

Multifunctionality of glucanases

Smith and Collen provide a comprehensive discussion on multifunctional glucanases including some cellulases and hemicellulases, demonstrating that the concept of 'one enzyme one activity' might not hold in all cases, especially with glucanases. A multifunctional protein is a protein consisting of a single type of polypeptide chain, but has multiple catalytic or binding activities. For example, XylA from *Neocallimastrix patriciarum* has two identical catalytic domains. A cellulase with exo-and endo-activities from *Caldocellum saccharolyticum* was identified.

Enzyme cost

Enzyme cost is considered to be a major impediment in extensive commercialisation of enzymatic cellulose hydrolysis. Enzyme cost is estimated to represent approximately 50 per cent of the total hydrolysis process cost.

Screening for organisms with novel enzymes

For more than fifty years one of the main areas of biotechnology research into lignocellulose has been driven by the need to isolate and identify organisms which are either hyper-producers and/or sufficiently robust to withstand conditions of the intended application and/or are producers of novel lignocellulolytic enzymes. In terms of enzyme novelty from an applications perspective, interest is focused on not only finding enzymes which could break down lignocellulose much more rapidly but also enzymes which could withstand pH, temperature and inhibitory agents more resiliently depending on the intended application. Mutant strains of *T. reesei* have been selected that produce extracellular cellulases up to 35 g/l. It has been suggested that cellulase production is probably as high as it would get and it is highly unlikely that it would increase much further and that increasing the specific enzyme activity is the most likely approach to improving the commercial prospects of lignocellulose hydrolysis. Questions have been raised concerning the continued screening of the environment for lignocellulolytic micro-organisms given that on average less than 1 per cent of the potential microbes in the biosphere have been identified using traditional methods of culturing and that genomics and metagenomics might be more productive approaches in biomining for unique lignocellulolytic genes which could then be cloned and expressed in industrial strains. Genomics offer the potential to obtain the complete blueprint of an organism and to assess its genetic potential in a comparative and functional manner. Metagenomics describes genomics associated with the functional analysis of organisms at community level. Although this technology holds out the best opportunity for discovering unique genes, the technology is still in its infancy and issues such as representative cloning, quantitative analysis, and expression still require refining.

Strain improvement of existing industrial organisms and enzyme engineering

Table 10.5 shows the specific activities of commercial cellulase preparations from major USA cellulase manufacturers/suppliers. There is a wider and bigger range of specific activity found in different hemicellulases and cellulases from different organisms thus presenting opportunities for developing industrial commercial enzymes with greater specific activities than commercial enzymes from *T. reesei* which dominate the lignocellulolytic enzyme market. There are a number of possible approaches to creating enzymes with greater activities. This review will only highlight some aspects of these approaches which will dominate the lignocellulolytic research for sometime into the future resulting in a diminishing research focus on screening and isolation of lignocellulytic organisms, which still dominate research in developing countries. These approaches have the potential to create organisms or designer enzymes more rapidly and cost effectively than the continued screening for organisms which are likely to be novel.

Table 10.5. Specific activity of commercial cellulase preparations.

Preparation	Microbial source	FPU*/mg	β-GlucosidaseU/mg	CMCU/mg	Cellobiase U/mg
Biocellulase TRI	T. reesei	0.24	0.72	5.5	0.059
Biocellulase A	A. niger	0.01	1.4	3.6	–
Cellulase 1.5L	T. reesei	0.37	0.16	5.1	0.018
Cellulase TAP10	T. viride	0.13	5.2	14	–
Cellulase AP30K	A. niger	0.03	10	21	–
Cellulase TRL	T. reesei	0.57	1.0	13	0.016
Econase CE	T. reesei	0.42	0.48	8.5	0.038
Multifect CL	T. reesei	0.42	0.20	7.1	0.015
Multifect GC	T. reesei	0.43	0.39	13	0.025
Spezyme #1	T. reesei	0.54	0.35	15	0.026
Spezyme #2	T. reesei	0.57	0.42	15	0.029
Spezyme #3	T. reesei	0.57	0.46	25	0.031
Ultra-low microbial	T. reesei	0.48	0.96	–	–

*FPU (filter paper units), 1 FPU = 1 μmole min^{-1} glucose released.

Enormous amount of data and information have been gathered over the years on the different organism's lignocellulolytic genes and controlling elements, their sequences and organisation, protein sequence data, identification of catalytic amino acids and protein structural data including an increase in three-dimensional modular protein structures obtained from crystallographic studies. Recently, the entire genome of *P. chrysosporium* has been sequenced opening-up new possibilities for a variety of molecular studies. This is the first basidiomycete genome that has been sequenced and is now available for genomic and proteomic studies. All of this information is useful from a biotechnology applications approach for engineering lignocellulolytic enzymes with different properties for various industrial commercial applications.

Optimising cellulase mixtures

Enzyme mixtures with interesting properties including a possible increase in enzyme specific activity could be created by combining purified individual proteins or individual domains either from the producing organisms or from recombinant organisms expressing a single cloned lignase, hemicellulase or cellulase encoding gene. These combinations could either consist of pure enzymes from different organisms or the supplementation of crude enzymes with a pure enzyme or supplementing the pure enzyme with a purified cellulose-binding domain from another organism or with specific co-factors. Addition of pure *T. reesei* cellobiohydrolase I to a *Thermonospora fusca* crude cellulase preparation increased the rate of filter paper hydrolysis approximately two-fold greater than when each component was used separately. A laccase-mediator system (lignozyme®-process) consisting of a combination of laccase and mediators with either NO, NOH or HRNOH groups effectively delignify wood in a pilot pulp and paper process. CBDs have been found in a wide range of hydrolase proteins as part of the mutidomian complex. The CBD exerts nonhydrolytic disruption of cellulose. More than 200 putative sequences in over 40 different organisms have been identified. CBDs from the same organism or different organism can differ in their binding specificity and even two CBDs located on the same enzyme may differ. A pure CBD derived from CBHII of *T. reesei* added to the *T. harzianum* chitinase increased the hydrolytic activity of the insoluble substrate. Replacing the CBD of endo-1,4-β-glucanase from *B. subtilis* with the CBD of the *T. viride* exoglucanase resulted in higher binding and enhanced hydrolytic activity on microcrystalline cellulose.

Genetics and recombinant DNA technology

The initial work on the genetics of lignocellulolytic organisms was dominated by random mutagenesis, and selection of hyper-cellulase producing mutants and mutants insensitive to catabolite repression. Most of the *T. reesei* mutants such as RUT C 30, CL-847, VTT-D which are used for commercial production of cellulases were derived from the wild strain *T. reesei* QM 6a that was originally isolated by the US Army Laboratories. The first catabolite repressed *Bacillus pumilus* with cellulase yield four times higher than the wild type strain was created through mutagenesis.

Attempts have also been made to identify genomic heterogeneticity within individual strains of *P. chrysosporium* and between different strains classified as belonging to this species with the expectations that their genetic differences may also translate into variations in their lignocellulolytic genes and efficiency in lignocellulose degradation. These different strains could then be used for breeding purposes to generate novel hybrids strains.

While significant progress has been made using physical and chemical mutagens to increase production of lignocellulolytic enzymes, recombinant DNA technology and protein engineering used apart or in combination are powerful modern approaches holdingout the greatest potential for making significant improvements in several aspects of lignocellulolytic enzymes such as increased production, increased specific activity, pH and temperature stability and also creating 'synthetic' designer enzymes for specific applications.

Computer programs permit the researcher to identify catalytic-sites, residues which are essential for protein stability under various pH and temperature conditions and protein folding patterns. This accumulated knowledge is then used to simulate enzymatic behaviour upon any changes in any one or a combination of sites. Then a specific gene is cloned, subjected to site-directed mutagenesis to give rise to a protein with properties similar to the simulated model. The gene-product's enzymatic behaviour is then experimentally verified.

Equally so DNA technology offers the possibility of fusing different lignocellulolytic genes or sections of genes from different organisms to give rise to novel chimeric gene-products with altered properties. A few examples will briefly be discussed to demonstrate the value and potential of these approaches in lignocellulolytic enzyme improvement. Unique lignocellulolytic enzymes with multiple activities can be created by artificial gene-fusion. A bifunctional exoglucanase-endoglucanase and a chimeric xylanases-endoglucanase were successfully constructed. A novel thermostable hybrid (1,3-1,4)-β-glucanases expressed from a gene fusion consisting of the beta-glucanase encoding genes from *Bacillus amyloliquefaciens* and *Bacillus macerans* was created. A heterologously expressed *Neocallimastrix patriciarum* CelD encoding a multi-domain, multi-functional enzyme possessing endoglucanase, cellobiohydrolase and xylanase activity exhibited higher specific activities on Avicel than two *T. reesei* cellobiohydrolase and a *T. reesei* endoglucanase.

A number of designer enzymes, also called glycosynthases, including cellulases and hemicellulases have been engineered by replacing the nucleophilic residue thus resulting in higher yields of different oligosaccharides. Substituting two tryptophan residues in the heme cavity by two phenylalanines in a cytochrome-c peroxidase resulted in improved activity. Increasing the thermostability of recombinant manganese peroxidase has been attempted by engineering a disulphide bridge contiguous to the distal Ca^{+2} binding site. Attempts have also been made to create a bifunctional hybrid of manganese-lignin peroxidase.

Using a combination of genetic and DNA technology approaches, a few strains with increased specific activities have been reported. A *T. reesei* strain KY 746 showed a 50 per cent increase in filter paper activity with only a 25 per cent increase in endoglucanase activity over the wild type QM 9414, while *T. reesei* RUT-P 37 showed a doubling of specific activity in both filter paper and endoglucanse units compared with the wild type QM 6a. A genetically improved *T. reesei* mutant strain CL 847, resistant to catabolite repression, was generated that exhibited a four-fold increase in cellulose productivity compared with QM 9414 and increased β-D-glucosidase specific activity. A heterologous expressed *Cellulomonas fimi* exoglucanase with increased specific activity from *E. coli* was overproduced. Although some strides have been made in increasing lignocellulolytic activity, there is an enzyme activity ceiling beyond which it would not be possible to move since the rate and extent of breakdown of lignocellulose is influenced by the complex structural nature of the substrate, as previously discussed, including structural features which prevent enzyme access and binding.

SINGLE CELL PROTEIN

The term single cell protein (SCP) was coined at Massachusetts Institute of Technology (MIT) by a group of scientists in 1966. The term, as used today, is rather misleading, since it refers to not only the isolated cell protein but to 'any microbial biomass from either uni- and multicellular bacteria, yeasts, filamentous fungi or algae which can be used as food or feed additives'. On an average, the microbial biomass contains about 45 to 55 per cent protein, although in some bacteria the protein content is as high as 80 per cent. The biomass also contains other essential nutrients as well, and as such it is an ideal supplement to conventional food supply.

However, in many countries, use of microbial biomass as a supplement to diet has met with scepticism because of certain psychological barriers. But even in these countries, it will play a major role via SCP feeding to animals which will be then consumed by the humans. As compared with traditional methods of producing proteins for food or feed, large scale production of microbial biomass has the following advantages: (i) micro-organisms in general have a high rate of multiplication, (ii) microbes have high protein content, (iii) they can utilise a large number of different carbon sources, some of which are waste products, (iv) strains with high yield and good composition can be selected or produced relatively easily, and (v) microbial biomass production is independent of seasonal and climatic variation.

Hydrolysis involves the use of waste materials as feedstock to produce single-cell protein and ethanol. Strictly speaking, two concepts are involved, the first of which is the production of a nutritious food for consumption by livestock or by humans. The second concept is the production of ethanol that can serve as a fuel in the production of energy. However, both concepts have a distinguishing characteristic — namely, the use of a carbonaceous waste as the major source of carbon for the micro-organisms that are involved. The implementation of the first concept is a one-step process that consists of the use of waste as substrate in the culture of the single-cell micro-organisms that collectively constitute an edible feedstuff that is highly nutritious for humans and livestock. Micro-organisms that constitute the feedstuff are varieties or strains of the yeast, *Saccharomyces cerevisae*, or of some other comparable species. The implementation of the second concept is an integrated two-part process that consists first in the culture of micro-organisms capable of fermenting sugars to ethanol, followed by harvesting the micro-organisms and mixing them with sugar to produce ethanol. The micro-organisms may be a particular yeast or bacterial species noted for its ethanol fermentation capability.

Although in the preceding sections, reference is made to the concepts as one- or two-part processes, both must begin with a pretreatment process in which the carbon in the waste is made available to the micro-organisms. Pretreatment is essential because, with rare exception, most of the carbon in waste is bound in highly complex molecules and, thus, is unavailable to all but a few highly specialised micro-organisms. Fortunately, the bound carbon can be made accessible to the desired micro-organisms through a process that disrupts the complex molecules — namely, hydrolysis. Thus, hydrolysis is an essential step. Because of its importance, the greater part of this section is concentrated on hydrolysis and its various aspects. The principal source of cellulose and related complex carbohydrates in developing nations is agricultural residue; another source would be paper in municipal solid waste, although availability could be limited. This alternative to the management of some of the organic residues generated in economically developing countries may be too costly and sophisticated to be applicable to only but a few specific situations.

Hydrolysis

Principles of hydrolysis

Role of hydrolysis

As stated earlier, hydrolysis is an essential element in the waste to food and energy concepts, because it is through hydrolysis that the cellulose and carbohydrates in wastes are split into their constituent sugars. For example, the cellulose molecule may consist of more than 5000 glucose units. The carbon in the glucose and other simple sugars is readily available to most micro-organisms. Without the intervention of hydrolysis, the carbon in the cellulose and the complex carbohydrates are not available to micro-organisms, particularly to those associated with single-cell protein or with ethanol fermentation. (The term 'complex carbohydrates' will be referred to as 'carbohydrates'.) It is through hydrolysis that the carbon in the glucose units that make up cellulose, and in the simple sugars that make up other carbohydrate molecules, are rendered available to yeasts and any other micro-organisms that may be responsible for fermentation. ('Hydrolysis' often is termed 'saccharification' when used in reference to the concept.)

Factors

An especially influential factor in the hydrolysis of cellulosic waste is the ratio of crystalline to paracrystalline (amorphous) cellulose. The ratio has a major bearing on the practicality of using a particular waste as a feedstock to the process. The crystalline region of cellulose molecules is marked by a very closely packed structure and, hence, strong internal forces of attraction. On the other hand, the paracrystalline region is more randomly oriented. The high degree of order in the crystalline region renders the region more resistant than the amorphous (paracrystalline) region to hydrolysis. Therefore, the higher the ratio of crystalline to paracrystalline cellulose in a waste, the more difficult it is to hydrolyse the waste. The surface-to-mass ratio of the waste particles exerts an important impact on hydrolysis, in that the smaller the particle, the more rapid is the physical or biological hydrolytic reaction. Another rate-related factor is the partial or complete masking of the cellulose molecules by lignin or some other resistant substance. The masking inhibits access of the hydrolytic mechanisms to the cellulose.

Classification of methods of hydrolysis

The various methods of hydrolysis can be classified into three classes on the basis of the mechanism or process of splitting, i.e. disrupting cellulose and carbohydrate molecules. The classes are: chemical, physical-chemical, and enzymatic. In the literature, the terms 'chemical hydrolysis' and 'acid hydrolysis' are often used synonymously. Even though physical disruption does not fully fit the classic definition of 'hydrolysis', in this section 'acid hydrolysis' includes physical and physical-chemical disruption. Enzymatic hydrolysis is mostly biological in nature. Yet another class could be formed by integrating enzymatic hydrolysis with chemical hydrolysis.

Acid hydrolysis

Basically, acid hydrolysis is a process in which the cellulosic fraction of a waste is suspended in an acidified aqueous medium that is maintained under pressure at an elevated temperature. It shares with other hydrolysis systems the general substrate and operational factors described in the preceding section. Other factors of particular significance to acid hydrolysis are liquids-to-solids ratio, acid concentration, and temperature. The rate of acid hydrolysis increases with increase in liquids-to-solids ratio.

Minimum particle size is determined by economic practicality, because energy and monetary costs of size reduction increase almost exponentially when the intended particle size is less than 5 cm. The permissible upper limit of the liquids-to-solids ratio also is determined by economic practicality. The consensus apparently places the upper ratio at 10 parts liquid to 1 part solids. Cost of acid, percentage of acid recovery, and rate of acceleration of corrosion establish the maximum permissible acid concentration. For sulphuric acid, the concentration would be about 0.5 per cent in most situations. Yield of sugar is highest at the higher temperature levels and acid concentrations.

System design

Acid hydrolysis can be carried out on either a batch basis or a continuous basis. Not unexpectedly, the batch approach is more appropriate for smaller operations, i.e. processing on the order of 120 mg or less per day. In a batch operation, the entire hydrolysis process takes place in a single reactor. It proceeds in a sequence of steps: hydrolysis, flash vapourisation, neutralisation, and centrifugation. A 110 mg/day operation would be based on two 70 mg/day reactors operating in parallel, and involve the use of the same storage tanks and same centrifuge.

As in a batch system, the process steps in a continuous system are hydrolysis, flash vapourisation, neutralisation, and centrifugation. In a continuous system, however, a series of reactors is involved, the design of which differs from that of the single reactor in a batch operation. Each reactor in the series is followed by a screw press. The first reactor is designed to hydrolyse only the hemicellulose fraction of the waste. Sugars released by the hydrolysis are harvested by passing the reactor discharge through the screw press. Liquid discharge from the press contains the sugars. Sugars in the alphacellulosic fraction are in the solids (pulp) residue from the press. These sugars are obtained by re-acidifying the pulp and then passing it successively through a second and a third reactor. These two reactors are designed to hydrolyse the alphacellulose fraction of the waste. The yield of sugars produced in acid hydrolysis is equal to about 35 to 45 per cent of the incoming cellulose.

Recent developments in technology

Most of the recent developments in hydrolysis seem to centre on the improvement and broadening of conventional chemical hydrolysis. This is accomplished by way of conditioning cellulosic and carbonaceous waste components, particularly fibres, such that sugar recovery efficiency is substantially improved. Thus, one approach involves exploding cellulosic fibres through the application of liquid anhydrous ammonia to biomass under pressure at 30° to 80°C for a few minutes, and then rapidly releasing the pressure. This blows individual fibres apart, thereby greatly increasing the surface area and accessibility of the cellulosic component. The ammonia is removed and the resulting material can be hydrolysed by weak acid or enzymes. Another innovation involves the use of a coaxial feeder and extruder to process biomass at 250°C and 3.2 MPa pressure.

The exploded product is a moist fibre that is partially hydrolysed to permit easy fermentation. In a third innovation, concentrated acid (sulphuric, hydrochloric, or hydrofluoric acid) at 140° to 160°C results in approximately a 90 per cent conversion of cellulose to sugar. (Compensating for the use of weaker acid by elevating the temperature to 180° to 200°C results in the production of undesirable by-products, and sugar conversion drops to 50 to 60 per cent.)

Enzymatic hydrolysis

Principles

In keeping with the descriptive term, 'enzymatic', hydrolysis of cellulosic and carbonaceous wastes is accomplished through the agency of the enzyme, cellulase. The process is essentially biological in that the hydrolytic enzyme is produced by micro-organisms genetically capable of synthesising it. Cellulase is an enzyme that specifically splits cellulose molecules into their constitutive sugars (hexoses and pentoses).

Types of cellulases and their relative effectiveness

Constitutive vs. induced

The presence of cellulase is continuous in some microbes and is continuously synthesised. It is not continuously present in certain other microbes, and its synthesis must be triggered, i.e. induced by an external stimulus, usually the presence of cellubiose or other reducing agent. Enzymes in the first class are termed 'constitutive', and those in the second class are termed 'induced'.

Extracellular vs. intracellular cellulase

The microbial origin of cellulase necessitates a two-stage process in enzymatic hydrolysis. In stage-1, cellulases are produced and harvested. In stage-2, the harvested enzymes are introduced into a waste. In the waste, the enzymes split, i.e. hydrolyse, cellulose and carbohydrate molecules into fermentable sugars, which are then harvested. Generally, the harvested sugars are used as the carbon source in ethanol fermentation. Harvesting is facilitated by the fact that the cellulases involved in enzymatic hydrolysis are synthesised extracellularly by the cellulolytic micro-organisms that produce them. Because they are extracellular, the cellulases are in the culture medium. If necessary, they can be extracted from the medium. Some cellulolytic bacteria synthesise their enzymes intracellularly. For example, the cytophage have their enzymes system bound in the cell wall or membrane. With such an arrangement, hydrolysis depends upon the existence of a close contact between the cellulose and the cell wall or membrane. Access to the bound enzyme would necessarily be by way of disrupting the individual microbes. Obtaining a cell-free enzyme extract would be an expensive operation.

Enzymatic systems

The various cellulolytic enzyme (cellulase) systems can be divided into two groups—namely, C_1 and C_X. The C_1 groups are effective on highly crystalline forms of cellulose (e.g. cotton fibre). They split crystalline cellulose into linear anhydroglucose. The anhydrous glucose chains are then split into soluble carbohydrates by C_X enzymes. This sequence has an important bearing on rate of hydrolysis of cellulosic waste because the first step in the hydrolysis must be the splitting of crystalline, i.e. resistant forms into simpler forms that are accessible by a wider array of enzymes. Thus, the higher the concentration of C_1 enzymes and hence the greater the concentration of microbes that synthesise them, the faster is the rate of hydrolysis. The fungus, *Trichoderma reesei*, has long been recognised as being an especially active synthesiser.

Factors

The factors discussed in this section are specific to enzymatic hydrolysis. Chief among them are: (i) concentration of inducing agent (i.e. reducing sugar), (ii) concentration of hydrolysis product (glucose), and (iii) pretreatment of waste.

Concentration of inducing agent

The required concentration of cellubiose is minute, i.e. about 0.5 per cent. Activity usually is assured because cellubiose generally is found in minute amounts with cellulose. However, it should be noted that cellulase production is repressed and activity is curtailed at cellubiose concentrations greater than about 1.9 per cent.

Concentration of hydrolysis product

Cellulase formation also is inhibited and repressed in the presence of high concentrations of glucose. Inhibition resulting from a concentration of cellubiose above the critical level can be counteracted by simultaneously imposing an inhibitory situation. It has been reported that the concentration of enzymatic hydrolysis reducing sugars increases with the increase in concentration of solids in the substrate. The report states that using a 25 per cent solids charge of compression-milled paper and a 10 IU/g enzyme-to-substrate ratio, it is possible to produce a reducing sugar syrup that has a concentration of 11 per cent. Practical ethanol production is possible with such a syrup.

Pretreatment

Ideally, pretreatment at a reasonable cost decreases cellulose crystallinity, disrupts the physical structure of lignin, and curtails cellulose polymerisation. The various proposed forms of pretreatment may involve one or all of following three major steps: particle size reduction, heating, and perhaps, chemical treatment.

Most pretreatment methods are based on the assumption that the cellulosic waste has been separated from the municipal solid waste stream and that all contaminants have been removed to the maximum extent permitted by economic feasibility. Maintaining the temperature of the cellulose at 218°C during milling renders the inner surface of the cellulose more accessible and modifies the structure of the cellulose. Structure is modified through the oxidation that takes place during heating. Cellulose can be heated either in a rotary kiln or preferably in an indirect-heat calciner dryer.

One of the several proposed forms of pretreatment involves the induction of mild swelling and the partial solubilisation of lignin through exposure to an alkali (e.g. NaOH). Succeeding the exposure to alkali is a period of air oxidation, which depolymerises the cellulose to a lower degree of crystallinity.

Another proposed form of pretreatment calls for exposure to steam and compression milling (two-roll). Steaming is done by exposing moist solids to temperatures of 195° to 200°C for 15 to 30 min. in a pressure vessel. The problem is that, although steaming increases the reactivity of agricultural residues and hardwoods, urban wastes lose 40 per cent of their reactivity.

Another of the several proposed methods calls for compression or two-roll milling of newspaper for 6 to 10 min. Apparently, this innovation results in substantial increases in rates of enzymatic hydrolysis and yields of sugar. Another benefit attributed to compression milling is an increase in bulk density of the paper great enough to permit slurries of 20 to 30 per cent to be used in hydrolysis. The treatment is equally effective with all types of cellulosic materials. The additional expenditure of energy involved in compression milling reportedly is less than 0.60 kWh/kg newspaper.

Technology

Advances in the technology of enzymatic hydrolysis of urban solid wastes took place in the 1970s. Since then, advance has been very slow and largely confined to refinements in equipment. Thus, the basic technology current in the 1970s is, with minor modifications, pertinent to present conditions. One of the more active centres of research into practical application of hydrolysis to municipal solid waste, i.e. the paper fraction, was at the Berkeley campus of the University of California (UC), and is fairly typical. Hence, the process developed there is used to exemplify hydrolysis technology and the complexities associated with it. The UC process incorporates the following five major steps: (1) feedstock preparation, (2) enzyme production, (3) the actual hydrolysis, (4) collection of the sugar (glucose) product, and (5) drying the residue. The entire flow pattern is diagrammed in Fig. 10.4.

The detailed description begins with step-2, because step-1 (feedstock) was essentially covered in the preceding section, pretreatment. The first of the two stages that constitute step-2, enzyme production, involves fungal growth followed by enzyme synthesis. Separation of the enzyme solution is the second stage. Fungal growth is accomplished by using standard industrial fermenters and a medium, and applying cultural conditions that favour the growth of the desired fungus (e.g. *Trichoderma*). Among these conditions are: (i) a medium that includes 0.3 per cent superphosphate, 0.5 per cent glucose, and the essential trace elements; and (ii) a dilution rate of 0.2 per day. The medium should be sterilised. Sterilisation can be done by way of steam injection or heat exchange. Within the first stage, pure cellulose is introduced into the rapidly growing culture to induce enzyme synthesis. The introduction of pure cellulose initiates enzyme synthesis. Separation of the enzyme is the second of the two main stages of step-2 of the UC process. The three methods available for separation are ultracentrifugation, precipitation by adding ammonium sulphate, and precipitation by adding acetone. Ultracentrifugation is very costly. Of the two precipitation methods, only the acetone method is practical because it is not always possible to separate the ammonium sulphate from the precipitate. A disadvantage of the acetone method is a

14 per cent loss of enzymatic activity with each reuse of the enzyme solution. The precipitate (cellular material and unhydrolysed cellulose) is removed from the enzyme solution by pressure filtration. The precipitate may then be dried and used as a cattle feedstuff.

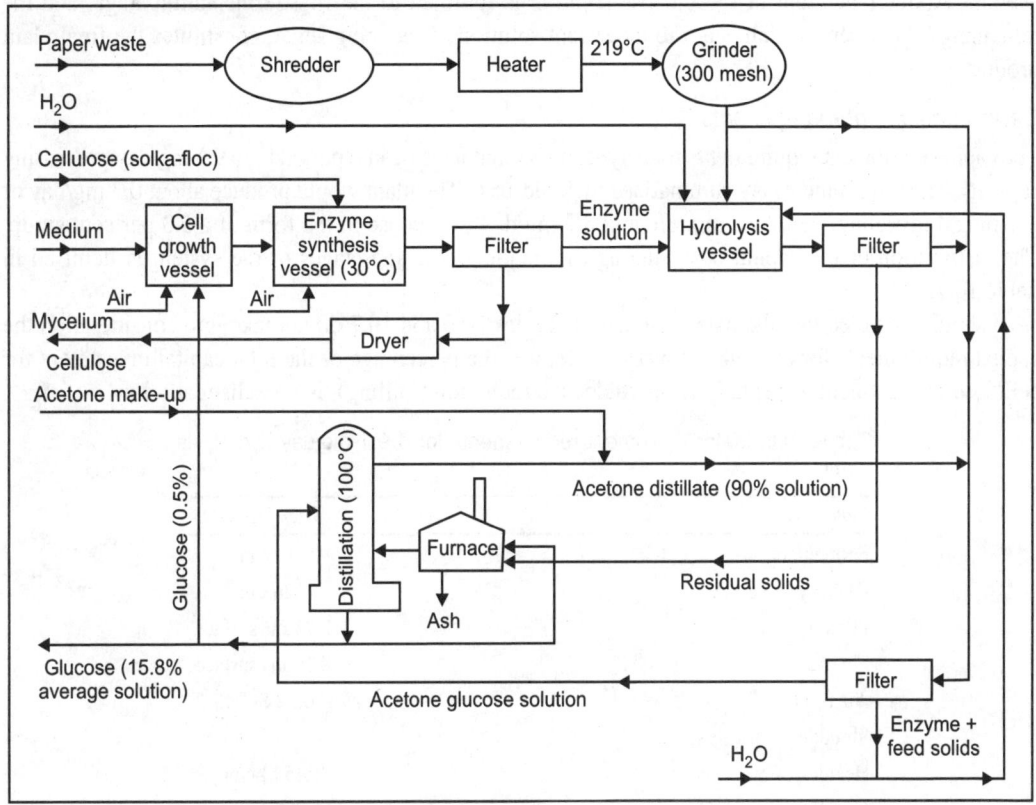

Fig. 10.4. Diagram of the UC hydrolysis process.

Production system

Hydrolysis is the step in which the cellulose waste to be hydrolysed is introduced. Introduction is by way of suspending the waste in the enzyme solution produced in step-1. The enzymes in the solution catalyse the conversion of the cellulose into sugars.

Specifications

The specifications and conditions are: (i) solids concentration of suspension, 11.5 per cent, (ii) retention time, 40 hr, and (iii) suspension temperature, 50°C (this renders conditions relatively aseptic). Solids remaining in the suspension after hydrolysis is completely removed by passing hydrolysed effluent through a pre-coated vacuum filter. The solids residue can be burned and the resulting heat energy used to generate steam and distil acetone from the effluent. Acetone from the distillation system (combined with a small make-up stream) is added to the aqueous enzyme-glucose solution in a volumetric ratio of 2:1. An almost complete precipitation of protein results. The precipitate may contain as much as 85 per cent of the original enzyme activity. The enzyme solution is recovered by means of a pressure filter and returned to the hydrolysis units. Acetone is recovered by passing the filtrate through acetone distillation columns. Heat for the distillation columns comes from the combustion of the residual solids. The distillate is 90 per cent acetone. The glucose solution remaining after the distillation contains only a trace of acetone. About 1 per cent of the glucose solution is returned to the first fermentation stage, and the remaining 99 per cent, which is a 5 to 6 per cent solution of reducing sugar, constitutes the final plant product.

Capital equipment requirements

The capital equipment requirements for a hydrolysis plant have been reported for a 9.1 mg/day processing capacity. The requirements are summarised in Table 10.6. The plant would produce about 0.3 mg/day of dry fungal mycelium-cellulose mixture and 8.3 mg/day of glucose in the form of a 5.3 per cent syrup. The distribution of the capital costs among the major processing stages of the system is itemised in Table 10.7.

It should be noted that the lists presented in Tables 10.6 and 10.7 do not take into consideration the capital requirements for acetone recovery. Moreover, the percentage of the total capital investment for cellulose pretreatment, especially for particle size reduction (milling), is unrealistically low.

Table 10.6. Major equipment requirements for a 9.1 mg/day hydrolysis plant.

Item	Size/Capacity
Fermenters	197 m^3
Hydrolysis vessel	263 m^3
Filter 1	2.23 m^2 surface
Filter 2	8.36 m^2 surface
Air filter	0.22 SCMS
Shredder	454 kg/hr
Heater	454 kg/hr
Grinder	817 kg/hr
Dryer 1	13.9 m^2 surface
Dryer 2	118 m^2 surface
Heat exchanger 1	7.9 m^2
Heat exchanger 2	4.7 m^2
Heat exchanger 3	18.6 m^2
Heat exchanger 4	2.8 m^2
Air compressor	0.234 SCMS
Medium supply tanks	37.9 m^3
Fermenter motors	10 hp
Hydrolysis unit motor	20 hp
Medium supply motors	5 hp
Solids feeder	817 kg/hr
Screw conveyors	454 kg/hr
Centrifugal pumps	189 l/min

Table 10.7. Distribution of fixed capital costs for a 9.1 Mg/day hydrolysis plant.

Item	(%)
Cellulose pretreatment	11.1
Shredding	
Heating	
Grinding	
Enzyme production	52.6
Fermentation	
Air and medium sterilisation	
Medium supply system	
Cellulose hydrolysis	12.4
Cellulose recycle and product recovery	23.9
Filtration	
Drying	
Total	100

Selection of an Appropriate Micro-organism in Single-cell Protein

Selection of an appropriate micro-organism is essential to the success of any single-cell protein production undertaking. The micro-organism must be one that is edible and can serve as a feedstock for humans and/or livestock. Of course, its culture must be technologically and economically feasible. To satisfy the second condition: (i) the organisms must grow rapidly and vigorously, (ii) culture of the organism should involve the use of relatively simple growth units and inexpensive nutrient sources (e.g. commercial crop fertilisers), (iii) ideally, the organism could be grown in open culture, or at least as an enrichment culture, and (iv) because single-cell protein production is only marginally economically feasible, the least 'permissible' condition is the need to culture the organism under sterile conditions, i.e. as a completely pure culture. However, competition with other organisms is eliminated in sterile culture and rapidity of growth is thereby increased. Moreover, contamination with possibly toxic organisms is avoided. Most of the work on single-cell protein production has been focused on the yeast, *Candida utilis* (*Torula utilis*). The yeast meets most of the requirements named in the preceding paragraph. Not only is the yeast easily grown, it also is a good food and fodder yeast. Although sterility is necessary, purity of culture is not essential.

The high nucleic acid content of bacterial proteins renders them less desirable as feedstuff for man and animal. Additionally, some groups of bacteria are characterised by the possession of endotoxins. The endotoxins could be incorporated in the feedstuff product. There is also a possibility that certain bacterial feedstuffs can promote allergenic reactions in humans who handle or ingest them. Finally, the much smaller size of bacteria makes them more difficult to harvest than yeasts.

Indirect vs. direct production

The relation of single-cell protein production to the reclamation of useful nutrient elements in waste is by way of the utilisation of sugars formed through hydrolisation of cellulosic substances in municipal waste. However, a separate hydrolysis step may be bypassed by culturing the yeast directly on the cellulosic waste. For convenience, in this presentation, the two approaches are respectively designated by the terms 'indirect' and 'direct'.

Indirect production

The production of *C. utilis* is an example of the indirect approach. The sequence of events in the production is diagrammed in Fig. 10.5. With respect to nutritional requirements, the sugars (glucose) satisfy the carbon needs. The other required essential nutritional elements are nitrogen, phosphorus, and potassium, which must come from an external source. Usually, nitrogen is added as an ammonium compound (e.g. ammonium sulphate); a phosphate is used for phosphorus; and a potassium sulphate or hydroxide compound for potassium. Generally, it is not necessary to add the essential trace elements.

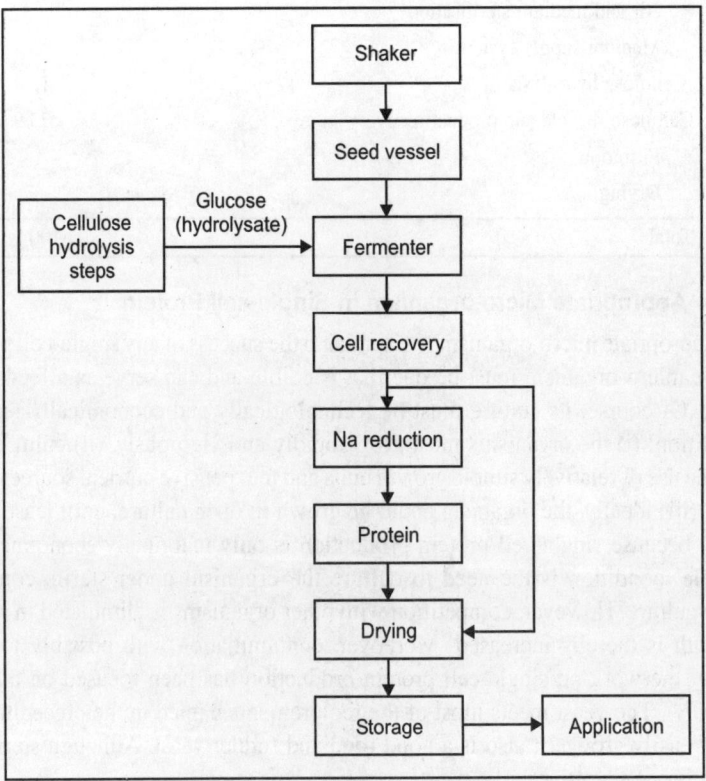

Fig. 10.5. Indirect production of single-cell protein.

Principal cultural conditions are a temperature at 20° to 35°C; and O_2, about 1.02 kg/kg cell mass-produced. The necessarily aerobic conditions are attained by continuously agitating the culture. The volume of air applied to meet the oxygen demand would be a rate of about 120 millimoles O_2 absorbed per L-hr (3.84 g/L-hr). The yield to be expected at such a rate is 3.66 g yeast per L-hr.

Under proper cultural conditions, the yield of the cell mass should be from 45 to 55 per cent of the sugar consumed. The production rate under continuous conditions depends upon a combination of cell mass and hydraulic detention time (culture volume/volume feed medium/day). Maximum cell concentration is a function of the hydrolysate sugar concentration multiplied by the sugar conversion efficiency of the yeast.

Direct production

Direct production differs from indirect production in that organisms are cultured upon unhydrolysed wastes. Indirect production involves two discrete steps (hydrolysis and cell production); whereas in direct production, the two steps are neither spatially nor always temporally discrete. Although of necessity, the steps are sequential (hydrolysis must precede utilisation for cellular growth; both may involve the same micro-organism). In other words, an organism can degrade a cellulosic molecule and utilise the constituent sugars to synthesise cellular mass. All sequences are not occurring simultaneously and, collectively, they constitute a single unit process. Therefore, at least some of the micro-organisms must be cellulolytic, i.e. capable of breaking down cellulose molecules. Preferably, most should be cellulolytic. A disadvantage is the inability to use submerged culture in the absence of special adaptations.

Most of the experience with single-cell production from waste has been at the laboratory- and pilot-scale levels and has been with paper and bagasse. Paper is from 40 to 80 per cent cellulose, 20 to 30 per cent lignin, and 10 to 30 per cent hemicellulose and xylosans. Bagasse is the residue remaining after the juice has been extracted from sugar cane by milling. Inasmuch as the studies were limited to laboratory- and pilot-scale levels, projections and estimates based on the studies must be considered in that light. Among the cellulolytic micro-organisms that have been studied are the yeasts, *C. utilis* and *Myrothecium verrucaria*, and the bacteria, *Cellulomonas flarigena*. In a study that involved the culture of *M. verrucaria* on a substrate composed of ball-milled newspaper, a yield of crude protein amounting to 1.42 g/l was obtained. A pilot-scale study involved the application of a system such as is diagrammed in Fig. 10.6. The organism used in the investigation was *C. utilis*.

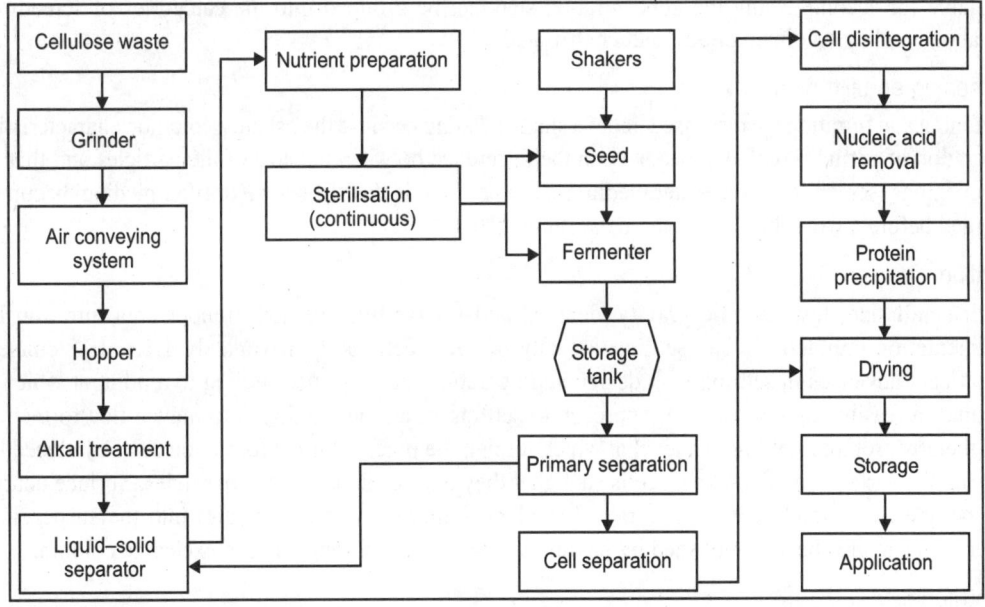

Fig. 10.6. Direct production of single-cell protein.

The bagasse was pre-treated because experience had shown that without pretreatment, the soluble carbohydrate content of untreated bagasse is only about 2 per cent; whereas after treatment, it is almost 18 per cent. Pretreatment reduces the cellulose crystallinity of the bagasse from almost 50 per cent to only 10 per cent. As stated earlier, pretreatment generally takes one or a combination of the following forms: fine milling and exposure to moderately elevated temperature under either acid or alkaline conditions. The bacteria *C. flavigena* and *C. uda* constituted the product in a pilot study in which the feedstock was bagasse. The study confirmed the need to pre-treat bagasse—specifically, alkaline pretreatment. Moreover, in the study, extent of conversion of feedstock to cell mass was very modest despite a continuous fermenter efficiency of 75 per cent and an approximate 90 per cent solubilisation of bagasse. Supplementary nutritional needs could be supplied by fertiliser and industrial chemicals. From 50 to 55 per cent of the product is crude protein that has a good amino acid balance. Another pilot-scale study involved a mixed culture of *Cellulomonas* and *Alcaligenes faecalis*. The cell density was 6.24 g/l. The crude protein composition was as follows (in g/100 g protein): arginine, 9.21; histidine, 2.30; isoleucine, 4.74; leucine, 11.20; lysine, 6.84; methionine, 1.86; phenylalanine, 4.36; tyrosine, 2.67; threomine, 5.37; and valine, 10.71.

Harvesting

Harvesting usually is done in two main stages: a concentration stage and a concentrate processing stage.

First-stage concentration

This stage results in the formation of a concentrate that has a sludge-like consistency and is in need of further processing. The need for the concentration step arises from the relatively low concentration of cells and large volumes of material that must be processed. The sludge (concentrate) is dewatered and dried. The concentration step is beset with many and grave difficulties due to the microscopic size and the physical characteristics of the cells, as well as their modest monetary value. The several technologies available for accomplishing the concentration step can be grouped into the categories of screening, filtration, settling (sedimentation), and centrifugation.

Screening and filtration

Screening and filtration are discussed under a single heading because they share a common characteristic: separation of particles (cells) depends upon the difference between the size of the particles and that of the openings (screen) or pores (filter medium). The problem is that the screen or filter medium becomes clogged before a workable 'cake' can be accumulated.

Settling

Their small size, low specific gravity, density, and low settling velocity render concentration by sedimentation impractical. The settling velocity of yeast cells is approximately 1.1×10^{-5} cm/sec. Significant advances in settling tank design and operation may enhance settling to a point at which it becomes a feasible option. Another approach to settling or a modification is to induce floc formation and thereby promote settling to a level at which it might be practical. Floc formation can be induced by altering the surface charge of yeast cells such that they agglomerate into floc particles. Surface charge can be altered by introducing a polymer flocculant (either anionic or cationic) into the suspension. Alteration can also be accomplished by passing the suspension through an ion exchange column.

Centrifugation

Centrifugation is an effective concentration method. Unfortunately, it is expensive in terms of equipment and power, and requires skilled personnel. A high-velocity rotor is necessary because of the microscopic size and low specific gravity and density of the cells and viscosity of the medium. A putative advantage is that the two separation stages can be accomplished in a single operation.

Second stage—concentrate (sludge) processing

Treatment consists of dewatering and drying. Flash drying is a good approach. It is rapid and is amenable to mass production and is successfully used in food and feedstuff preparation. Moreover, it removes threats to human and animal health posed by chance pathogens. Other options include pressure filtration and vacuum drying, such as is used in sewage sludge conditioning. The data listed in Table 10.8 provide an indication of the equipment that might be required in commercial production of single-cell protein.

Table 10.8. Equipment requirements and relative costs for the production of single-cell protein.

Cost element	Direct production		Indirect production	
	Equipment (500-L base)	% of total cost	Equipment (1200-L base)	% of Total cost
Pretreatment line	6 units	18	5 units	15
Sterilisation system	2 units	3	2 units	3
Enzyme production line	–	–	5 units[a]	11
Syrup manufacturing line	–	–	4 units	3
Cell (metabolite) line	2 units[b]	22	2 units[c]	11
Cell recovery line	2 units	5	2 units	5
Protein recovery	3 units	7	3 units	6
Drying distillation	1 unit	10	1 unit	10
Instrumentation – interface	–	15	–	18
Computer hardware – program (software)	–	20	–	18
Total		100		100

[a] 350-L seed vessel; 1200-L fermenter; two storage tanks; one ultrafiltration system.
[b] 100-L seed vessel; 500-L fermenter.
[c] 550-L seed vessel, 1200-L fermenter.

The Table 10.8 includes data that indicate the relation of the cost of individual types of equipment to the total cost. The basic flows for minimum size versions of direct and indirect production of single-cell protein are presented in Table 10.9.

Table 10.9. Basic annual flows of a minimum-size commercial single-cell protein plant.

Parameter	Direct production (mg)	Indirect production (mg)
Raw material input	8100	17000
Intermediate output	–	6000
SC output	1200	1200
Liquid flow rate for cell separation	20,000	20,000
Average cell mass (g/l)[a]	25	25

[a] Assuming 20 per cent loss during recovery.

Chapter 11

Plant Growth Promoting Bacteria and Nitrogen Fixation

INTRODUCTION

Bacteria that 'invade' trees are there to cause certain destruction. But like the helpful bacteria that live within our guts, some microbes help plants thrive. To find out what makes these microbe-plant interactions 'tick', scientists at the U.S. Department of Energy's (DOE) Brookhaven National Laboratory decoded the genome of a plant-dwelling microbe they'd previously shown could increase plant growth by 40 per cent.

To fuel and feed the planet for the future, we need new approaches, 'Biofuels derived from plants are an attractive alternative energy source, but many biofuel feedstock crops are in direct competition with food crops for agricultural resources such as land, water, and fertilisers'. Among the bacterial genes identified are ones that code for proteins that help the microbe survive and compete with other species for resources in the soil; take up nutrients released by plant roots; and move toward, adhere to, and colonise poplar root tissues. The microbes also have genes that provide benefits for the plant, including: genes that may help confer drought resistance and the ability to coexist with toxic metals; genes that produce antimicrobial agents that protect plants from fungal and bacterial infections; and genes that produce plant-growth enhancing 'phytohormones' and precursors that poplar cannot produce on its own.

PLANT GROWTH PROMOTING BACTERIA: PROSPECTS FOR NEW INOCULANTS

Root colonising bacteria (rhizobacteria) that exert beneficial effects on plant development via direct or indirect mechanisms have been defined as plant growth promoting rhizobacteria (PGPR). Although significant control of plant pathogens or direct enhancement of plant development has been demonstrated by PGPR in the laboratory and in the greenhouse, results in the field have been less consistent. Because of these and other challenges in screening, formulation, and application, PGPR have yet to fulfill their promise and potential as commercial inoculants. Recent progress in our understanding of their diversity, colonisation ability, mechanisms of action, formulation, and application should facilitate their development as reliable components in the management of sustainable agricultural systems.

Plant growth in agricultural soils is influenced by a myriad of abiotic and biotic factors. While growers routinely use physical and chemical approaches to manage the soil environment to improve crop yields, the application of microbial products for this purpose is less common. An exception to this is the use of rhizobial inoculants for legumes to ensure efficient nitrogen fixation; a practice that has been occurring in North America for over 100 years. The region around the root, the rhizosphere, is relatively rich in nutrients, due to the loss of as much as 40 per cent of plant photosynthates from the roots. Consequently, the rhizosphere supports large and active microbial populations capable of exerting beneficial, neutral, or detrimental effects on plant growth. The importance of rhizosphere microbial populations for maintenance of root health, nutrient uptake, and tolerance of environmental stress is now recognised. These beneficial micro-organisms can be a significant component of management practices to achieve the attainable yield, which has been defined as crop yield limited only by the natural physical environment of the crop and its innate genetic potential.

The prospect of manipulating crop rhizosphere microbial populations by inoculation of beneficial bacteria to increase plant growth has shown considerable promise in laboratory and greenhouse studies, but responses have been variable in the field. The potential environmental benefits of this approach, leading to a reduction in the use of agricultural chemicals and the fit with sustainable management practices, are driving this technology. Recent progress in our understanding of the biological interactions that occur in the rhizosphere and of the practical requirements for inoculant formulation and delivery should increase the technology's reliability in the field and facilitate its commercial development.

Plant growth-promoting rhizobacteria (PGPR) were first defined by Kloepper and Schroth to describe soil bacteria that colonise the roots of plants following inoculation onto seed and that enhance plant growth. The following are implicit in the colonisation process: ability to survive inoculation onto seed, to multiply in the spermosphere (region surrounding the seed) in response to seed exudates, to attach to the root surface, and to colonise the developing root system. The ineffectiveness of PGPR in the field has often been attributed to their inability to colonise plant roots. A variety of bacterial traits and specific genes contribute to this process, but only a few have been identified. These include motility, chemotaxis to seed and root exudates, production of pili or fimbriae, production of specific cell surface components, ability to use specific components of root exudates, protein secretion, and quorum sensing. The generation of mutants altered in expression of these traits is aiding our understanding of the precise role each one plays in the colonisation process. Progress in the identification of new, previously uncharacterised genes is being made using nonbiased screening strategies that rely on gene fusion technologies. These strategies employ reporter transposons and *in vitro* expression technology (IVET) to detect genes expressed during colonisation. Using molecular markers such as green fluorescent protein or fluorescent antibodies it is possible to monitor the location of individual rhizobacteria on the root using confocal laser scanning microscopy (Fig. 11.1). This approach has also been combined with an rRNA-targeting probe to monitor the metabolic activity of a rhizobacterial strain in the rhizosphere and showed that bacteria located at the root tip were most active.

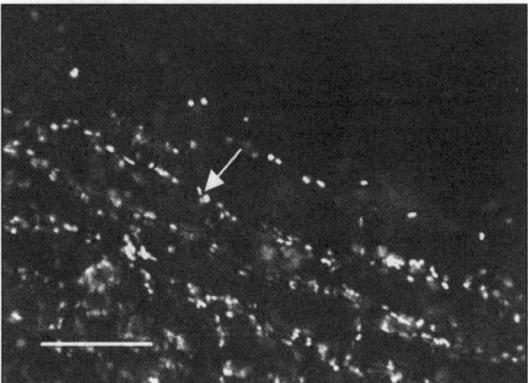

Fig. 11.1. Confocal laser scanning micrograph of a 5-day old canola root colonised by *Pseudomonas putida* strain 6–8 labelled with white fluorescent protein (as indicated by the arrow). The bar is equal to 60 µm.

An important aspect of colonisation is the ability to compete with indigenous micro-organisms already present in the soil and rhizosphere of the developing plant. Our understanding of the factors involved in these interactions has been hindered by our inability to culture and characterise diverse members of the rhizosphere community and to determine how that community varies with plant species, plant age, location on the root, and soil properties. Phenotypic and genotypic approaches are now available to characterise rhizobacterial community structure. Phenotypic methods that rely on the ability to culture micro-organisms include standard plating methods on selective media, community level physiological profiles (CLPP) using the BIOLOG system, phospholipid fatty acid (PLFA), and fatty acid methyl ester (FAME) profiling. Culture-independent molecular techniques are based on direct extraction of DNA from soil and 16S-rRNA gene sequence analysis, bacterial artificial chromosome or expression cloning systems. These are providing new insight into the diversity of rhizosphere microbial communities, the heterogeneity of the root environment, and the importance of environmental and biological factors in determining community structure. These approaches can also be used to determine the impact of inoculation of plant growth-promoting rhizobacteria on the rhizosphere community.

Mechanisms of Action

PGPR enhance plant growth by direct and indirect means, but the specific mechanisms involved have not all been well-characterised. Direct mechanisms of plant growth promotion by PGPR can be demonstrated in the absence of plant pathogens (Fig. 11.2) or other rhizosphere micro-organisms, while indirect mechanisms involve the ability of PGPR to reduce the deleterious effects of plant pathogens on crop yield. PGPR have been reported to directly enhance plant growth by a variety of mechanisms: fixation of atmospheric nitrogen that is transferred to the plant, production of siderophores that chelate iron and make it available to the plant root, solubilisation of minerals such as phosphorus, and synthesis of phytohormones.

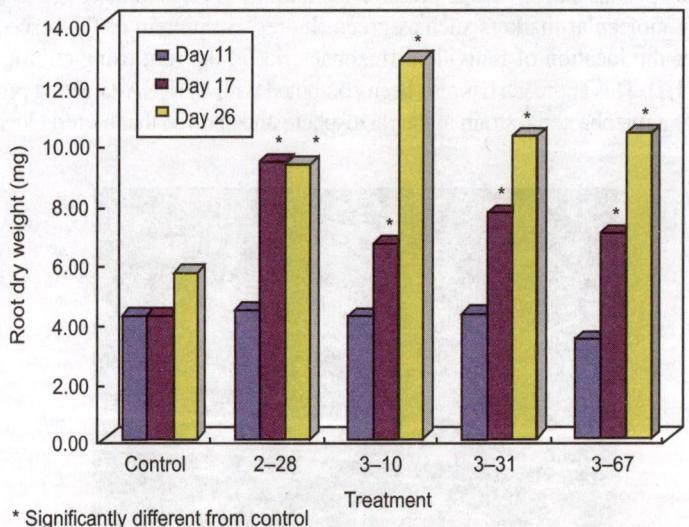

Fig. 11.2. Example of growth promotion of lentil following inoculation with PGPR isolates, 2–28, 3–10, 3–31, and 3–67. Plants were grown in cone-tainers at 80°C in a growth chamber and sampled 11, 17, and 26 days following inoculation.

Direct enhancement of mineral uptake due to increases in specific ion fluxes at the root surface in the presence of PGPR has also been reported. PGPR strains may use one or more of these mechanisms in the rhizosphere. Molecular approaches using microbial and plant mutants altered in their ability to synthesise or respond to specific phytohormones have increased our understanding of the role of phytohormone synthesis as a direct mechanism of plant growth enhancement by PGPR. PGPR that synthesise auxins and cytokinins or that interfere with plant ethylene synthesis have been identified.

PGPR that indirectly enhance plant growth via suppression of phytopathogens do so by a variety of mechanisms. These include the ability to produce siderophores that chelate iron, making it unavailable to pathogens; the ability to synthesise anti-fungal metabolites such as antibiotics (Fig. 11.3), fungal cell wall-lysing enzymes, or hydrogen cyanide, which suppress the growth of fungal pathogens; the ability to successfully compete with pathogens for nutrients or specific niches on the root; and the ability to induce systemic resistance. Biochemical and molecular approaches are providing new insight into the genetic basis of these traits, the biosynthetic pathways involved, their regulation, and importance for biological control in laboratory and field studies.

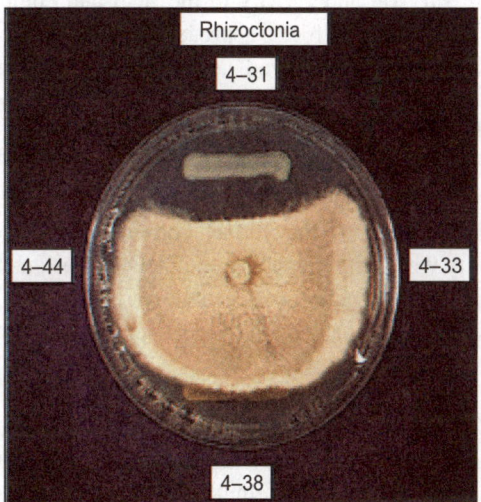

Fig. 11.3. Example of *in vitro* assay for inhibition of fungal growth. Different bacterial isolates were tested for their ability to inhibit the growth of *Rhizoctonia* spp., a soil-borne plant pathogen of legumes. A zone of inhibition can be observed around isolate 4-31 in the upper quadrant of the plate.

Challenges in Selection and Characterisation of PGPR

One of the challenges in developing PGPR for commercial application is ensuring that an effective selection and screening procedure is in place, so that the most promising organisms are identified and brought forward. In the agricultural chemical industry, thousands of prospective compounds are screened annually in efficient high-throughput assays to select the best one or two compounds for further development. Similar approaches are not yet in place for PGPR. Effective strategies for initial selection and screening of rhizobacterial isolates are required. It may be important to consider host plant specificity or adaptation to a particular soil, climatic conditions or pathogen in selecting the isolation conditions, and screening assays. The spermosphere model, an enrichment technique that relies on seed exudates as the nutrient source, has been used for selection and isolation of promising N_2-fixing rhizosphere bacteria from rice. One approach for selection of organisms with the potential to control soil-borne phytopathogens is to isolate from soils that are suppressive to that pathogen. Other approaches involve selection based on traits known to be associated with PGPR such as root colonisation, 1-aminocyclopropane-1-carboxylate

(ACC) deaminase activity, and antibiotic and siderophore production. The development of high throughput assay systems and effective bioassays will facilitate selection of superior strains.

Challenges in Field Application of PGPR

The application of PGPR for control of fungal pathogens in greenhouse systems shows considerable promise, due in part to the consistent environmental conditions and high incidence of fungal disease in greenhouses. Achieving consistent performance in the field where there is heterogeneity of abiotic and biotic factors and competition with indigenous organisms is more difficult. Knowledge of these factors can aid in determination of optimal concentration, timing and placement of inoculant, and of soil and crop management strategies to enhance survival and proliferation of the inoculant. The concept of engineering or managing the rhizosphere to enhance PGPR function by manipulation of the host plant, substrates for PGPR, or through agronomic practices, is gaining increasing attention. Development of better formulations to ensure survival and activity in the field and compatibility with chemical and biological seed treatments is another area of focus; approaches include optimisation of growth conditions prior to formulation and development of improved carriers and application technology.

Challenges in Commercialisation of PGPR

Prior to registration and commercialisation of PGPR products, a number of hurdles must be overcome. These include scale up and production of the organism under commercial fermentation conditions while maintaining quality, stability, and efficacy of the product. Formulation development must consider factors such as shelf life, compatibility with current application practices, cost, and ease of application. Health and safety testing may be required to address such issues as non-target effects on other organisms including toxigenicity, allergenicity and pathogenicity, persistence in the environment, and potential for horizontal gene transfer.

Future Prospects

As our understanding of the complex environment of the rhizosphere, of the mechanisms of action of PGPR, and of the practical aspects of inoculant formulation and delivery increases, we can expect to see new PGPR products becoming available. The success of these products will depend on our ability to manage the rhizosphere to enhance survival and competitiveness of these beneficial micro-organisms. Rhizosphere management will require consideration of soil and crop cultural practices as well as inoculant formulation and delivery. Genetic enhancement of PGPR strains to enhance colonisation and effectiveness may involve addition of one or more traits associated with plant growth promotion. Genetic manipulation of host crops for root-associated traits to enhance establishment and proliferation of beneficial micro-organisms is being pursued. However, regulatory issues and public acceptance of genetically engineered organisms may delay their commercialisation. The use of multi-strain inocula of PGPR with known functions is of interest as these formulations may increase consistency in the field. They offer the potential to address multiple modes of action, multiple pathogens, and temporal or spatial variability.

PGPR offer an environmentally sustainable approach to increase crop production and health. The application of molecular tools is enhancing our ability to understand and manage the rhizosphere and will lead to new products with improved effectiveness.

NITROGEN FIXATION

Nitrogen fixation generally refers to the natural process, either biological or abiotic, by which nitrogen (N_2) in the atmosphere is converted into ammonia. This process is essential for life because fixed nitrogen is required to biosynthesise the basic building blocks of life, e.g. nucleotides for DNA and amino acids for proteins. Formally, nitrogen fixation also refers to other abiological conversions of nitrogen, such as its conversion to nitrogen dioxide.

Nitrogen fixation is utilised by numerous prokaryotes, including bacteria, actinobacteria, and certain types of anaerobic bacteria. Micro-organisms that fix nitrogen are called diazotrophs. Some higher plants, and some animals (termites), have formed associations (symbioses) with diazotrophs. Nitrogen fixation also occurs as a result of non-biological processes. These include lightning, industrially through the Haber-Bosch Process, and combustion.

Biological Nitrogen Fixation

Biological nitrogen fixation (BNF) occurs when atmospheric nitrogen is converted to ammonia by an enzyme called nitrogenase. The formula for BNF is:

$$N_2 + 6H^+ + 6e^- \rightarrow 2NH_3$$

The process is coupled to the hydrolysis of 16 equivalents of ATP and is accompanied by the co-formation of one molecule of H_2. In free-living diazotrophs, the nitrogenase-generated ammonium is assimilated into glutamate through the glutamine synthetase/glutamate synthase pathway.

Enzymes responsible for nitrogenase action are very susceptible to destruction by oxygen. (In fact, many bacteria cease production of the enzyme in the presence of oxygen). Many nitrogen-fixing organisms exist only in anaerobic conditions, respiring to draw down oxygen levels, or binding the oxygen with a protein such as Leghemoglobin.

Plants that contribute to nitrogen fixation include the legume family — Fabaceae — with taxa such as clover, soyabeans, alfalfa, lupines, peanuts, and rooibos. They contain symbiotic bacteria called *Rhizobia* within nodules in their root systems, producing nitrogen compounds that help the plant to grow and compete with other plants. When the plant dies, the fixed nitrogen is released, making it available to other plants and this helps to fertilise the soil. The great majority of legumes have this association, but a few genera (e.g. *Styphnolobium*) do not. In many traditional and organic farming practices, fields are rotated through various types of crops, which usually includes one consisting mainly or entirely of clover or buckwheat (family *Polygonaceae*), which were often referred to as 'green manure'.

Symbiotic Nitrogen Fixing Bacteria

Symbiotic bacteria are protected from oxygen by inhabiting a plant host. Bacteria of the genus *Rhizobium* and *Bradyrhizobium* inhabit the root nodules of leguminous plants (e.g. peas, beans, clover, alfalfa, soyabeans). Other symbiotic associations occur but are less important. *Anabaena azollae*, a nitrogen fixing cyanobacterium, lives in pores on the fronds of a water fern called *Azolla*. This symbiotic partnership is used to enrich rice paddies with organic nitrogen (Fig. 11.4).

Rhizobium is also found free in the soil but only fixes N_2 when inside the root nodules of its host plant, in a strictly controlled microaerophilic environment. Oxygen is required to generate sufficient respiratory energy to drive N_2 fixation. But too much oxygen inactivates nitrogenase.

In root nodules the O_2 level is regulated by a special haemoglobin-leghemoglobin. The globin protein is encoded by plant genes but the heme cofactor is made by the symbiotic bacteria. This is produced only when the plant is infected with *Rhizobium*. The plant root cells convert sugar to organic acids which they supply to the bacteroids. In exchange, the plant receives amino-acids (rather than free ammonia).

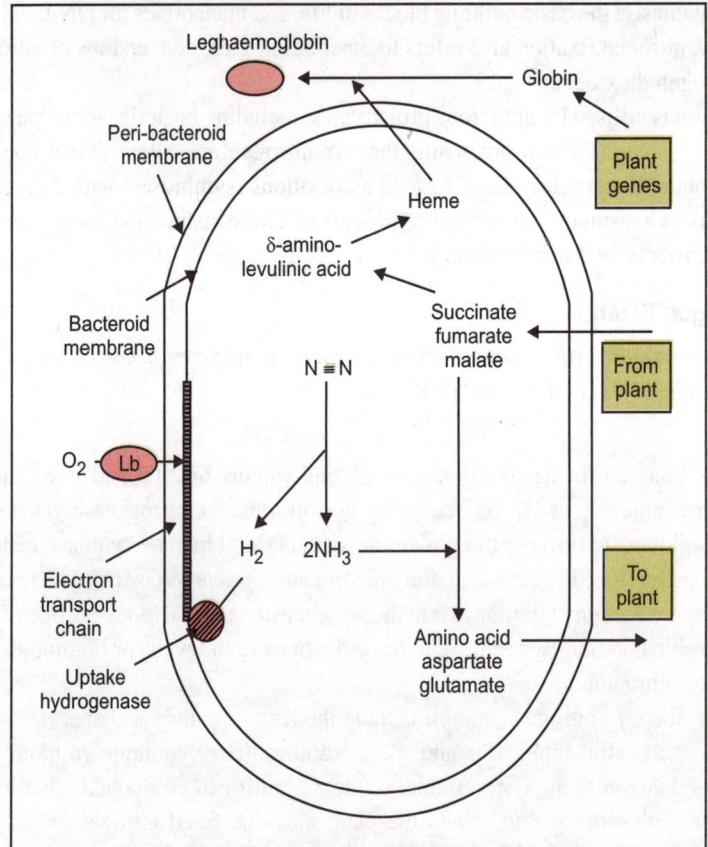

Fig. 11.4. Rhizobium bacteriod performing symbiotic nitrogen fixation.

Specific strains of bacteria are found inhabiting specific plant species. For example, a carbohydrate binding protein (lectin) on the surface of root cells of clover (*Trifolium*) specifically binds to lipopolysaccharide of *Rhizobium trifolii* which contains 2-deoxyglucose. The bacteria then enter and produce cytokinins (a type of plant hormone) which promote the division of plant cells to form nodules. The bacteria lose their outer membranes and become irregular in shape-'bacteroids'.

Structure and Operation of Nitrogenase

Nitrogenase contains the two proteins molybdoferredoxin and azoferredoxin. These must be supplied with reducing equivalents by other proteins that vary. Here we consider nitrogenase from *Klebsiella*, a close relative of *E. coli* where the accessory proteins are flavodoxin and pyruvate flavodoxin reductase. In most bacteria electrons are passed from NAD(P)H or pyruvate to ferredoxin, an FeS protein. If iron is in short supply ferredoxin is replaced by flavodoxin, a flavoprotein. In *Klebsiella* there is no ferredoxin and flavodoxin (NifF protein) is used all the time. Azoferredoxin transfers electrons from reduced flavodoxin (or ferredoxin) to molybdoferredoxin (Fig. 11.5).

Molybdoferredoxin is an alpha2/beta2 tetramer. The alpha and beta subunits are similar but distinct and are encoded by genes *nifK* and *nifD*. Each tetramer contains 2 Mo and several FeS groups. The molybdenum is part of a low molecular weight cofactor containing Mo bound to an Fe7S8 cluster and to homocitrate. This MoFe cofactor is unique to nitrogen fixation and distinct from the Mo-pterin cofactor of other Mo proteins (e.g. nitrate reductase, xanthine oxidase). Azoferredoxin is a dimer of identical subunits encoded by *nifH* and contains a single Fe4S4 group per dimer. Azoferredoxin is modified by the NifM protein. Molybdoferredoxin from one genus can often interact with azoferredoxin from another genus to give active enzyme.

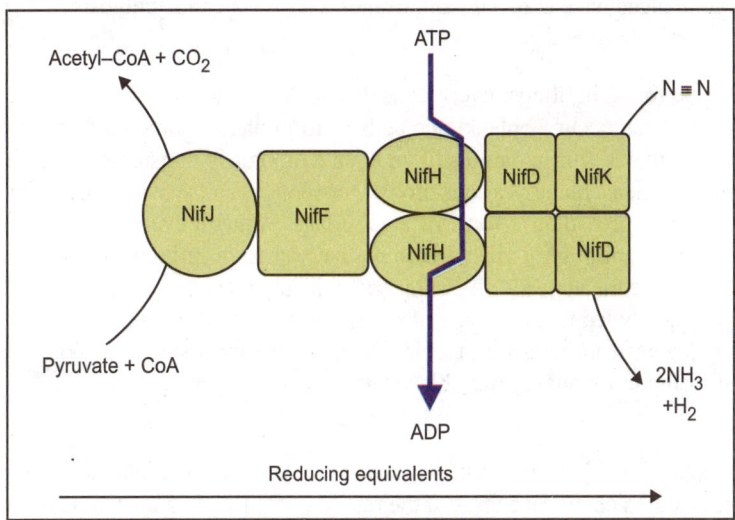

Fig. 11.5. Nitrogenase.

Micro-organisms that Fix Nitrogen

Diazotroph

Diazotrophs are bacteria that fix atmospheric nitrogen gas into a more usable form such as ammonia. A diazotroph is an organism that is able to grow without external sources of fixed nitrogen. Examples of organisms that do this are rhizobia and *Frankia* (in symbiosis) and *Azospirillum*. All diazotrophs contain iron-molybdenum nitrogenase systems. Two of the most studied systems are those of *Klebsiella pneumoniae* and *Azotobacter vinlandii*. These systems are used because of their genetic tractability and their fast growth.

Diazotrophs are scattered across bacterial taxonomic groups (mostly in the Bacteria but also a couple of Archaea). Even within a species that can fix nitrogen there may be strains that do not fix nitrogen. Fixation is shut off when other sources of nitrogen are available, and, for many species, when oxygen is at high partial pressure.

Cyanobacteria

Cyanobacteria is a phylum of bacteria that obtain their energy through photosynthesis. The name 'cyanobacteria' comes from the colour of the bacteria. They are a significant component of the marine nitrogen cycle and an important primary producer in many areas of the ocean, but are also found in habitats other than the marine environment; in particular cyanobacteria are known to occur in both freshwater, hypersaline inland lakes and in arid areas where they are a major component of biological soil crusts.

Stromatolites of fossilised oxygen-producing cyanobacteria have been found from 2.8 billion years ago, possibly as old as 3.5 billion years ago. The ability of cyanobacteria to perform oxygenic photosynthesis is thought to have converted the early reducing atmosphere into an oxidising one, which dramatically changed the composition of life form on earth by stimulating biodiversity and leading to the near-extinction of oxygen-intolerant organisms. According to endosymbiotic theory, chloroplasts in plants and eukaryotic algae have evolved from cyanobacteria via endosymbiosis.

Ecology

Cyanobacteria can be found in almost every conceivable environment, from oceans to fresh water to bare rock to soil. They can occur as planktonic cells or form phototrophic biofilms in fresh water and marine environments, they occur in damp soil, or even temporarily moistened rocks in deserts. A few are endosymbionts in lichens, plants, various protists, or sponges and provide energy for the host. Some live in the fur of sloths, providing a form of camouflage. Aquatic cyanobacteria are probably best known for the extensive and highly visible blooms that can form in both freshwater and the marine environment and can have the appearance of blue-green paint or scum. The association of toxicity with such blooms has frequently led to the closure of recreational waters when blooms are observed. Marine bacteriophage are a significant parasite of unicellular, marine cyanobacteria. When they infect cells they lyse them releasing more phages into the water.

Photosynthesis

Cyanobacteria account for 20–30 per cent of Earth's photosynthetic productivity and convert solar energy into biomass-stored chemical energy at the rate of ~450 TW. Cyanobacteria utilise the energy of sunlight to drive photosynthesis, a process where the energy of light is used to split water molecules into oxygen, protons, and electrons. While most of the high-energy electrons derived from water are utilised by the cyanobacterial cells for their own needs, a fraction of these electrons are donated to the external environment via electrogenic activity. Cyanobacterial electrogenic activity is an important microbiological conduit of solar energy into the biosphere.

Cyanobacteria have an elaborate and highly organised system of internal membranes which function in photosynthesis. Cyanobacteria get their name from the bluish pigment phycocyanin, which they use to capture light for photosynthesis. Photosynthesis in cyanobacteria generally uses water as an electron donor and produces oxygen as a by-product, though some may also use hydrogen sulphide as occurs among other photosynthetic bacteria. Carbon dioxide is reduced to form carbohydrates via the Calvin cycle. In most forms the photosynthetic machinery is embedded into folds of the cell membrane, called thylakoids. The large amounts of oxygen in the atmosphere are considered to have been first created by the activities of ancient cyanobacteria. Due to their ability to fix nitrogen in aerobic conditions they are often found as symbionts with a number of other groups of organisms such as fungi (lichens), corals, pteridophytes (Azolla), angiosperms (*Gunnera*), etc.

Cyanobacteria are the only group of organisms that are able to reduce nitrogen and carbon in aerobic conditions, a fact that may be responsible for their evolutionary and ecological success. The water-oxidising photosynthesis is accomplished by coupling the activity of photosystem (PS) II and I (Z-scheme). In anaerobic conditions, they are also able to use only PS I—cyclic photophosphorylation—with electron donors other than water (hydrogen sulphide, thiosulphate, or even molecular hydrogen) just like purple photosynthetic bacteria. Furthermore, they share an archaeal property, the ability to reduce elemental sulphur by anaerobic respiration in the dark. Their photosynthetic electron transport shares the same compartment as the components of respiratory electron transport. Actually, their plasma membrane contains only components of the respiratory chain, while the thylakoid membrane hosts both respiratory and photosynthetic electron transport. Attached to thylakoid membrane, phycobilisomes act as light harvesting antennae for the photosystems. The phycobilisome components (phycobiliproteins) are responsible for the blue-green pigmentation of most cyanobacteria. The variations to this theme is mainly due to carotenoids and phycoerythrins which give the cells the red-brownish colouration. In some cyanobacteria, the colour of light influences the composition of phycobilisomes. In green light, the cells accumulate more phycoerythrin, whereas in red light they produce more phycocyanin. Thus the bacteria appear green in red light and red in green light. This process is known as complementary chromatic adaptation and is a way for the cells to maximise the use of available light for photosynthesis.

A few genera, however, lack phycobilisomes and have chlorophyll *b* instead (*Prochloron*, *Prochlorococcus*, *Prochlorothrix*). These were originally grouped together as the prochlorophytes or chloroxybacteria, but appear to have developed in several different lines of cyanobacteria. For this reason they are now considered as part of the cyanobacterial group.

Azotobacteraceae

The family Azotobacteraceae contains aerobic diazotrophs with two Genera, Azomonas and Azotobacter, distinguished by the ability to form cysts. The family is also characterised by variable cell shape, the classic shape being ovoid while many are pleomorphic. With an adequate supply of Mo the Azotobacteraceae are able to fix at least 10 mg of molecular nitrogen per gram of carbohydrate consumed under aerobic conditions. Like most Pseudomonadacea, the Azotobacteraceae are able to utilise a wide variety of carbon sources, including sucrose. Recent analysis of the unannotated genome of Azotobacter vinelandii has shown that this bacterium is most appropriately grouped in the family Pseudomonadaceae. The original familial distinction was based on the ability to fix nitrogen, but a few Pseudomonadaceae have been found to fix nitrogen as well. The relation is not surprising given the ability of many Azotobacteraceae to fluoresce due to the production of Pyoverdine, a nonribosomal peptide siderophore typical of many Pseudomonadaceae.

Rhizobia

Rhizobia are soil bacteria that fix nitrogen (diazotrophy) after becoming established inside root nodules of legumes (Fabaceae). Rhizobia require a plant host; they cannot independently fix nitrogen. Morphologically, they are generally gram negative, motile, non-sporulating rods (Fig. 11.6).

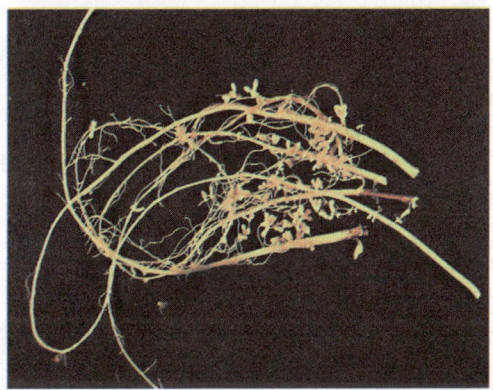

Fig. 11.6. Soyabean root nodules, each containing billions of *Bradyrhizobium* bacteria.

The first species of rhizobia, *R. leguminosarum*, was identified in 1889, and all further species were initially placed in the *Rhizobium* genus. However, more advanced methods of analysis have revised this classification, and now there are many other genera. Most research has been done on crop and forage legumes such as clover, alfalfa, beans, and soy; recently, more work is occurring on North American legumes.

These groups include a variety of non-symbiotic bacteria. For instance, the plant pathogen *Agrobacterium* is a closer relative of *Rhizobium* than the *Bradyrhizobium* that nodulate soyabean (and may not really be a separate genus). The genes responsible for the symbiosis with plants, however, may be more closely related than the organisms themselves, acquired by horizontal transfer (via bacterial conjugation) rather than vertical gene transfer.

Although much of the nitrogen is removed when protein-rich grain or hay is harvested, significant amounts can remain in the soil for future crops. This is especially important when nitrogen fertiliser is not used, as in organic rotation schemes or some less-industrialised countries. Nitrogen is the most commonly deficient nutrient in many soils around the world and it is the most commonly supplied plant nutrient. Supply of nitrogen through fertilisers has severe environmental concerns.

Rhizobia are unique because they live in a symbiotic relationship with legumes. Common crop and forage legumes are peas, beans, clover, and soy.

Infection and signal exchange

The symbiotic relationship implies a signal exchange between both partners that leads to mutual recognition and development of symbiotic structures. Rhizobia live in the soil where they are able to sense flavonoids secreted by the root of their host legume plant. Flavonoids trigger the secretion of Nod factors, which in turn are recognised by the host plant and can lead to root hair deformation and several cellular responses such as ion fluxes. The best known infection mechanism is called intracellular infection, in this case the rhizobia enter through a deformed root hair in a similar way to endocytosis, forming an intracellular tube called the infection thread. A second mechanism is called 'crack entry', in this case no root hair deformation is observed and the bacteria penetrate between cells, through cracks produced by lateral root emergence. Later on bacteria become intracellular and an infection thread is formed like in intracellular infections.

The infection triggers cell division in the cortex of the root where a new organ, the nodule appears as a result of successive processes.

Nodule formation and functioning

Infection threads grow to the nodule, infect its central tissue and release the rhizobia in these cells where they differentiate morphologically into bacteroids and fix nitrogen from the atmosphere into a plant usable form, ammonium (NH_4^+), utilising the enzyme nitrogenase. In return the plant supplies the bacteria with carbohydrates, proteins, and sufficient oxygen so as not to interfere with the fixation process. Leghaemoglobins, plant proteins similar to human haemoglobins help to provide oxygen for respiration while keeping the free oxygen concentration low enough not to inhibit nitrogenase activity. Recently, it was discovered that a *Bradyrhizobium* strain forms nodules in *Aeschynomene* without producing Nod factors, suggesting the existence of alternative communication signals other than Nod factors.

The legume—rhizobium symbiosis is a classic example of mutualism—rhizobia supply ammonia or amino acids to the plant and in return receive organic acids (principally as the dicarboxylic acids malate and succinate) as a carbon and energy source—but its evolutionary persistence is actually somewhat surprising. Because several unrelated strains infect each individual plant, any one strain could redirect resources from nitrogen fixation to its own reproduction without killing the host plant upon which they all depend. But this form of cheating should be equally tempting for all strains, a classic tragedy of the commons. There are two competing hypotheses for the mechanism that maintains legume-rhizobium symbiosis (though both may occur in nature). The sanctions hypothesis suggests that plants police cheating rhizobia. Sanctions could take the form of reduced nodule growth, early nodule death, decreased carbon supply to nodules, or reduced oxygen supply to nodules that fix less nitrogen. The partner choice hypothesis proposes that the plant uses pre-nodulation signals from the rhizobia to decide whether to allow nodulation and chooses only non-cheating rhizobia. There is evidence for sanctions in soyabean plants, which reduce rhizobium reproduction (perhaps by limiting oxygen supply) in nodules that fix less nitrogen. Similarly, wild lupine plants allocate less resources to nodules containing less-beneficial rhizobia, limiting rhizobial reproduction inside.

Other diazotrophs

Many other species of bacteria are able to fix nitrogen (diazotrophs), but few are able to associate intimately with plants and colonise specific structures like Legume nodules. Bacteria that do associate with plants include the actinobacteria *Frankia*, which form symbiotic root nodules in actinorhizal plants, and several cyanobacteria (*Nostoc*) associated with aquatic ferns, *Cycas* and *Gunneras*. Free-living diazotrophs are often found in the rhizosphere and in the intercellular spaces of several plants including rice and sugarcane, but in this case the lack of a specialised structure results in poor nutrient transfer efficiency compared to legume or actinorhizal nodules.

Frankia

Frankia is a genus of nitrogen fixing filamentous bacteria that live in symbiosis with actinorhizal plants, similar to *Rhizobia*. Bacteria of this genus form root nodules (Fig. 11.7).

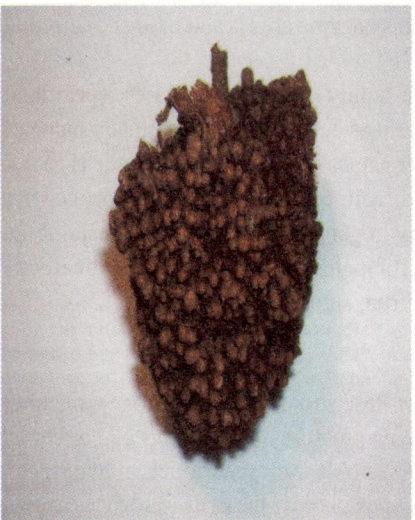

Fig. 11.7. *Frankia.*

Frankia sp. strains are filamentous bacteria that convert atmospheric N_2 gas into ammonia. This process is known as nitrogen fixation. *Frankia* fix nitrogen while living in root nodules on 'actinorhizal plants' *frankia* thus can supply most or all or the host plants nitrogen needs. Consequently, actinorhizal plants colonise and often thrive in soils that are low in combined nitrogen. The recent availability of three *frankia* genomes may help clarify the volution of prokaryote/plant symbioses. Environmental and geographical adaptation, metabolic diversity and horizontal gene flow among symbiotic prokaryotes.

HYDROGENASE

A hydrogenase is an enzyme that catalyses the reversible oxidation of molecular hydrogen (H_2). Hydrogenases play a vital role in anaerobic metabolism.

Hydrogen uptake (H_2 oxidation) (Eq. 11.1) is coupled to the reduction of electron acceptors such as oxygen, nitrate, sulphate, carbon dioxide, and fumarate, whereas proton reduction (H_2 evolution) (Eq. 11.2) is essential in pyruvate fermentation and in the disposal of excess electrons. Both low-molecular weight compounds and proteins such as ferredoxins, cytochrome c_3, and cytochrome c_6 can act as physiological electron donors (D) or acceptors (A) for hydrogenases:

$$H_2 + A_{ox} \rightarrow 2H^+ + A_{red} \qquad \text{... (11.1)}$$

$$2H^+ + D_{red} \rightarrow H_2 + D_{ox} \qquad \text{... (11.2)}$$

Hydrogenases were first discovered in the 1930s, and they have since attracted interest from many researchers including inorganic chemists who have synthesised a variety of hydrogenase mimics. Understanding the catalytic mechanism of hydrogenase might help scientists design clean biological energy sources, such as algae, that produce hydrogen.

Ferredoxin Hydrogenase

In enzymology, a ferredoxin hydrogenase (EC 1.12.7.2) is an enzyme that catalyses the chemical reaction

$$H_2 + 2 \text{ oxidised ferredoxin} \rightleftharpoons 2 \text{ reduced ferredoxin} + 2 \text{ H}^+$$

Thus, the two substrates of this enzyme are H_2 and oxidised ferredoxin, whereas its two products are reduced ferredoxin and H^+.

This enzyme belongs to the family of oxidoreductases, specifically those acting on hydrogen as donor with an iron-sulphur protein as acceptor. The systematic name of this enzyme class is hydrogen: ferredoxin oxidoreductase. Other names in common use include H_2 oxidising hydrogenase, H_2 producing hydrogenase [ambiguous], bidirectional hydrogenase, hydrogen-lyase [ambiguous], hydrogenase (ferredoxin), hydrogenase I, hydrogenase II, hydrogenlyase [ambiguous], and uptake hydrogenase [ambiguous]. This enzyme participates in glyoxylate and dicarboxylate metabolism and methane metabolism. It has 3 cofactors: iron, sulphur, and nickel.

Hydrogen Metabolism

Here we will only give a short description of the hydrogen metabolism of *Scenedesmus obliquus*. Depending on the partial hydrogen pressure *Scenedesmus* can either take up or produce hydrogen gas. Hydrogen uptake occurs in an anaerobic atmosphere rich in hydrogen and carbon dioxide, and is light dependent. The hydrogen taken up is used by the cells to reduce carbon dioxide to carbohydrates. Since hydrogen-rich atmospheres are very uncommon and unlikely habitats for green algae one can assume that the hydrogen uptake reactions are only laboratory artifacts but do not resemble nature. Hydrogen production occurs under anaerobic conditions both in the dark and in the light. Dark hydrogen production is believed to be connected to fermentation. The following graphic shows the anaerobic hydrogen and oxygen production as measured by gas chromatography. In the dark hydrogen is produced by fermentation. In the light hydrogen production ceases directly and oxygen is produced by photosynthesis (Fig. 11.8).

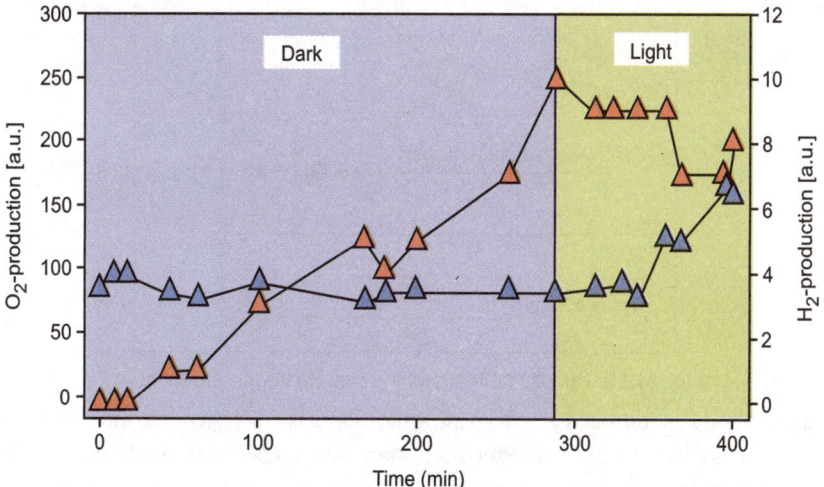

Fig. 11.8. Anaerobic hydrogen and oxygen production as measured by gas chromatography.

If only dim light is used to illuminate anaerobically adapted Scenedesmus cells, both hydrogen and oxygen are produced simultaneously (Fig. 11.9).

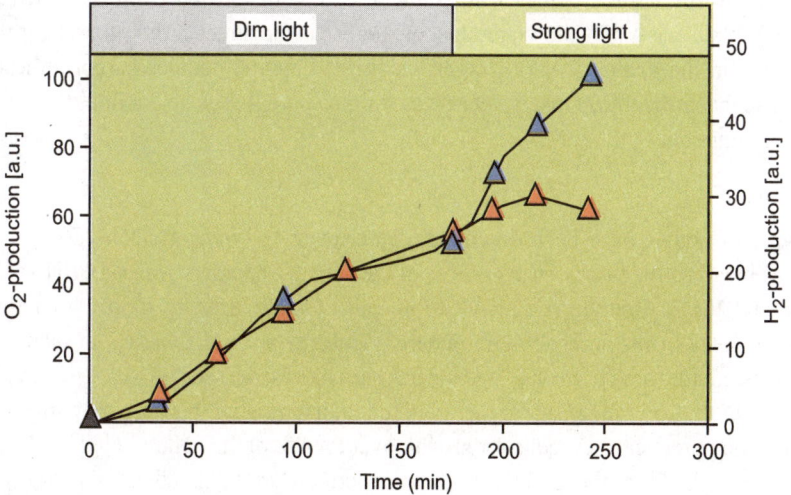

Fig. 11.9. Anaerobically adopted *scenedesmus* cells, both hydrogen and oxygen.

In the strong light normal photosynthesis takes over again and only oxygen is produced. The reactions involved in photohydrogen production are summarised as in Fig. 11.10.

Root Nodule

Root nodules occur on the roots of plants that associate with symbiotic nitrogen-fixing bacteria. Under nitrogen-limiting conditions, capable plants form a symbiotic relationship with a host-specific strain of bacteria known as rhizobia. This process has evolved multiple times within the Fabaceae, as well as in other species found within the Rosid clade.

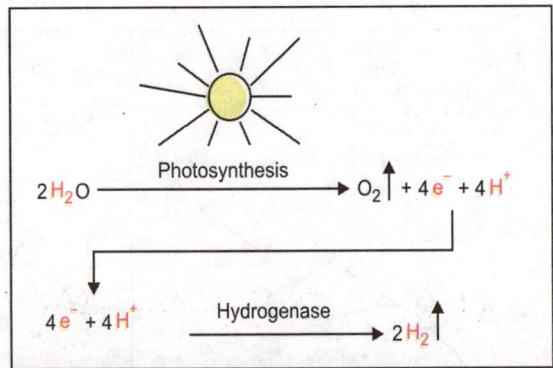

Fig. 11.10. Reactions involved in photohydrogen production.

Within legume nodules, nitrogen gas from the atmosphere is converted into ammonia, which is then assimilated into amino acids (the building blocks of proteins), nucleotides (the building blocks of DNA and RNA as well as the important energy molecule ATP), and other cellular constituents such as vitamins, flavones, and hormones. Their ability to fix gaseous nitrogen makes legumes an ideal agricultural organism as their requirement for nitrogen fertiliser is reduced. Indeed high nitrogen content blocks nodule development as there is no benefit for the plant of forming the symbiosis. The energy for splitting the nitrogen gas in the nodule comes from sugar that is translocated from the leaf (a product of photosynthesis). Malate as a breakdown product of sucrose is the direct carbon source for the bacteroid. Nitrogen fixation in the nodule is very oxygen sensitive. Legume nodules harbor an iron containing protein called leghaemoglobin, closely related to animal myoglobin, to facilitate the conversion of nitrogen gas to ammonia.

Classification

Two main types of nodule have been described: determinate and indeterminate. Determinate nodules are found on tropical (sub)legumes, such as those of the genera *Glycine* (soyabean), *Phaseolus* (common bean), *Lotus*, and *Vigna*. Determinate nodules lose meristematic activity shortly after initiation, thus growth is due to cell expansion resulting in mature nodules which are spherical in shape.

Indeterminate nodules are found on temperate legumes like *Pisum* (pea), *Medicago* (alfalfa), *Trifolium* (clover), and *Vicia* (vetch). They earned the moniker 'indeterminate' because they maintain an active apical meristem that produces new cells for growth over the life of the nodule. This results in the nodule having a generally cylindrical shape. Because they are actively growing, indeterminate nodules manifest zones which demarcate different stages of development/sybmiosis (Fig. 11.11):

1. Zone I: The active meristem. This is where new nodule tissue is formed which will later differentiate into the other zones of the nodule.
2. Zone II: The infection zone. This zone is permeated with infection threads full of bacteria. The plant cells are larger than in the previous zone and cell division is halted.
   (a) Interzone II–III: Here the bacteria have entered the plant cells, which contain amyloplasts. They elongate and begin terminally differentiating into symbiotic, nitrogen-fixing bacteroids.

3. Zone III: The nitrogen fixation zone. Each cell in this zone contains a large, central vacuole and the cytoplasm is filled with fully differentiated bacteroids which are actively fixing nitrogen. The plant provides these cells with leghemoglobin, resulting in a distinct pink colour.

4. Zone IV: The senescent zone. Here plant cells and their bacteroid contents are being degraded. The breakdown of the heme component of leghemoglobin results in a visible greening at the base of the nodule.

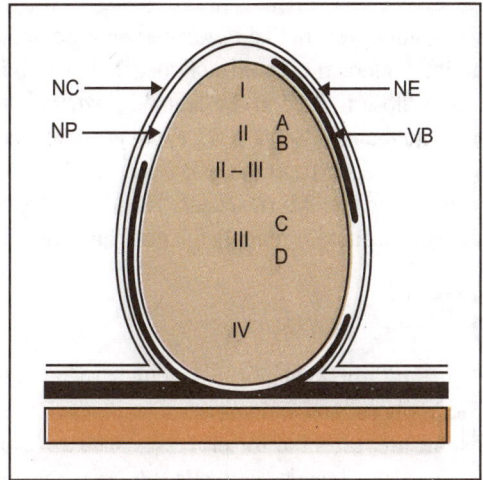

Fig. 11.11. Illustrating the different zones of an indeterminate root nodule.

Nodulation

Legumes release compounds called flavonoids from their roots, which trigger the production of nod factors by the bacteria. When the nod factor is sensed by the root, a number of biochemical and morphological changes happen: cell division is triggered in the root to create the nodule, and the root hair growth is redirected to wind around the bacteria multiple times until it fully encapsulates 1 or more bacteria. The bacteria encapsulated divide multiple times, forming a microcolony. From this microcolony, the bacteria enter the developing nodule through a structure called an infection thread, which grows through the root hair into the basal part of the epidermis cell, and onwards into the root cortex; they are then surrounded by a plant-derived membrane and differentiate into bacteroids that fix nitrogen.

Nodulation is controlled by a variety of processes, both external (heat, acidic soils, drought, nitrate) and internal (autoregulation of nodulation, ethylene). Autoregulation of nodulation controls nodule numbers per plant through a systemic process involving the leaf. Leaf tissue senses the early nodulation events in the root through an unknown chemical signal, then restricts further nodule development in newly developing root tissue. The Leucine rich repeat (LRR) receptor kinases (NARK in soyabean (*Glycine max*); HAR1 in *Lotus japonicus*, SUNN in *Medicago truncatula*) are essential for autoregulation of nodulation (AON). Mutation leading to loss of function in these AON receptor kinases leads to supernodulation or hypernodulation. Often root growth abnormalities accompany the loss of AON receptor kinase activity, suggesting that nodule growth and root development are functionally linked. Investigations into the mechanisms of nodule formation showed that the ENOD40 gene, coding for a 12–13 amino acid protein, is up-regulated during nodule formation.

Connection to root structure

Root nodules apparently have evolved three times within the Fabaceae but are rare outside that family. The propensity of these plants to develop root nodules seems to relate to their root structure. In particular, a tendency to develop lateral roots in response to abscisic acid may enable the later evolution of root nodules.

In other species

Root nodules that occur on non-legume genera like *Parasponia* in association with Rhizobium bacteria, and those that arise from symbiotic interactions with Actinobacteria *Frankia* in some plant genera such as *Alnus*, vary significantly from those formed in the legume-rhizobia symbiosis. In these symbioses the bacteria are never released from the infection thread. *Frankia* nodulates approximately two hundred species in the following orders (families in parentheses): Cucurbitales (Coriariaceae and Datiscaceae), Fagales (Betulaceae, Casuarinaceae, and Myricaceae), Rosales (Rhamnaceae, Elaeagnaceae and Rosaceae). Actinorhizal symbioses account for roughly the same amount of nitrogen fixation as rhizobial symbioses.

SIDEROPHORE

Siderophores are small, high-affinity iron chelating compounds secreted by micro-organisms such as bacteria, fungi and grasses. Siderophores are amongst the strongest soluble Fe^{3+} binding agents known.

Iron is essential for almost all life, essential for processes such as respiration and DNA synthesis. Despite being one of the most abundant elements in the Earth's crust, the bioavailability of iron in many environments such as the soil or sea is limited by the very low solubility of the Fe^{3+} ion. This is the predominant state of iron in aqueous, non-acidic, oxygenated environments. It accumulates in common mineral phases such as iron oxides and hydroxides (the minerals that are responsible for red and yellow soil colours) hence cannot be readily utilised by organisms. Microbes release siderophores to scavenge iron from these mineral phases by formation of soluble Fe^{3+} complexes that can be taken up by active transport mechanisms. Many siderophores are nonribosomal peptides, although several are biosynthesised independently.

Siderophores are also important for some pathogenic bacteria for their acquisition of iron. In mammalian hosts, iron is tightly bound to proteins such as haemoglobin, transferrin, lactoferrin and ferritin. The strict homeostasis of iron leads to a free concentration of about 10^{-24} mol L^{-1}, hence there are great evolutionary pressures put on pathogenic bacteria to obtain this metal. For example, the anthrax pathogen *Bacillus anthracis* releases two siderophores, bacillibactin and petrobactin, to scavenge ferric iron from iron proteins. While bacillibactin has been shown to bind to the immune system protein siderocalin, petrobactin is assumed to evade the immune system and has been shown to be important for virulence in mice.

Siderophores are amongst the strongest binders to Fe^{3+} known, with enterobactin being one of the strongest of these. Because of this property, they have attracted interest from medical science in metal chelation therapy, with the siderophore desferrioxamine B gaining widespread use in treatments for iron poisoning and thalassemia. Besides siderophores, some pathogenic bacteria produce *hemophores* (heme binding scavenging proteins) or have receptors that bind directly to iron/heme proteins. In eukaryotes, other strategies to enhance iron solubility and uptake are the acidification of the surrounding (e.g. used by plant roots) or the extracellular reduction of Fe^{3+} into the more soluble Fe^{2+} ions.

Structure and Identification

Siderophores usually form a stable, hexadentate, octahedral complex with Fe^{3+} preferentially compared to other naturally occurring abundant metal ions, although if there are less than six donor atoms water can also coordinate. The most effective siderophores are those that have three bidentate ligands per molecule, forming a hexadentate complex and causing a smaller entropic change than that caused by chelating a single ferric ion with separate ligands.

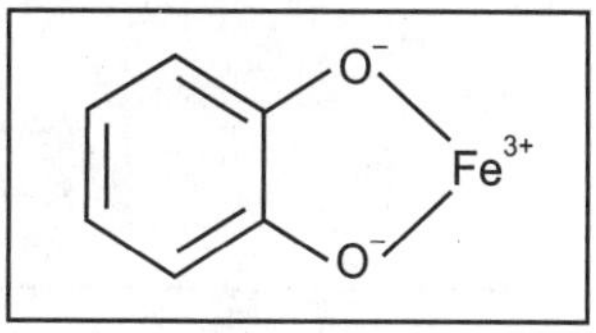

Catecholate-iron complex

Fe^{3+} is a hard Lewis acid, preferring hard Lewis bases such as anionic or neutral oxygen to coordinate with. Microbes usually release the iron from the siderophore by reduction to Fe^{2+} which has little affinity to these ligands.

Siderophores are usually classified by the ligands used to chelate the ferric iron. The major groups of siderophores include the catecholates (phenolates), hydroxamates and carboxylates (e.g. derivatives of citric acid). Citric acid can also act as a siderophore. The wide variety of siderophores may be due to evolutionary pressures placed on microbes to produce structurally different siderophores which cannot be transported by other microbes' specific active transport systems, or in the case of pathogens deactivated by the host organism.

Diversity

Examples of siderophores produced by various bacteria and fungi (Fig. 11.12 and Table 11.1)

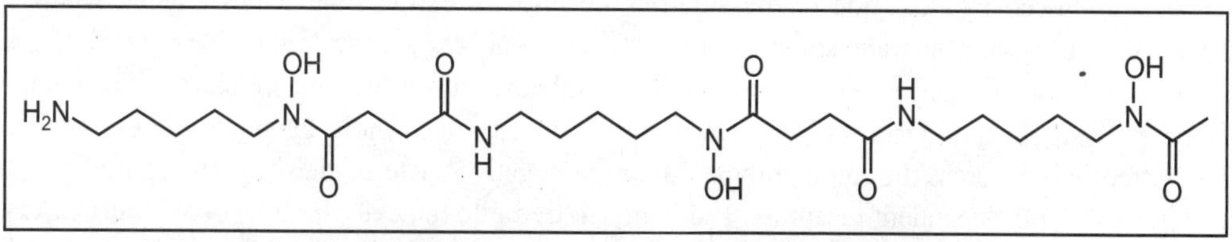

Fig. 11.12. Desferrioxamine B, a hydroxamate siderophore.

Table 11.1. Hydroxamate siderophores.

Siderophore	Organism
Hydroxamate siderophores	
Ferrichrome	*Ustilago sphaerogena*
Desferrioxamine B	*Streptomyces pilosus*
(Deferoxamine)	*Streptomyces coelicolor*
Desferrioxamine E	*Streptomyces coelicolor*
Fusarinine C	*Fusarium roseum*
Ornibactin	*Burkholderia cepacia*

(Contd...)

Siderophore	Organism
Catecholate siderophores	
Enterobactin	*Escherichia coli*
	enteric bacteria
Bacillibactin	*Bacillus subtilis*
	Bacillus anthracis
Vibriobactin	*Vibrio cholerae*
Mixed ligands	
Azotobactin	*Azotobacter vinelandii*
Pyoverdine	*Pseudomonas aeruginosa*
Yersiniabactin	*Yersinia pestis*

Some poaceae (grasses) including wheat and barley produce a class of siderophores called phytosiderophores or mugineic acids.

Biological Function

In response to iron limitation in their environment, genes involved in microbe siderophore production and uptake are derepressed, leading to manufacture of siderophores and the appropriate uptake proteins. In bacteria, Fe^{2+}-dependent repressors bind to DNA upstream to genes involved in siderophore in high intracellular iron concentrations. At low concentrations, Fe^{2+} dissociates from the repressor, which in turn dissociates from the DNA, leading to transcription of the genes. In gram-negative and AT-rich gram-positive bacteria, this is usually regulated by the *Fur* (ferric uptake regulator) repressor, whilst in GC-rich gram-positive bacteria (e.g. Actinobacteria) it is *DtxR* (diphtheria toxin repressor), so-called as the production of the dangerous diphtheria toxin by *Corynebacterium diphtheriae* is also regulated by this system.

This is followed by excretion of the siderophore into the extracellular environment, where the siderophore acts to sequester and solubilise the iron. Siderophores are then recognised by cell specific receptors on the outer membrane of the cell. In fungi and other eukaryotes, the Fe-siderophore complex may be extracellularly reduced to Fe^{2+}, whilst in many cases the whole Fe-siderophore complex is actively transported across the cell membrane. In gram-negative bacteria, these are transported into the periplasm via TonB-dependent receptors, and is transferred into the cytoplasm by ABC transporters.

Once in the cytoplasm of the cell, the Fe^{3+}-siderophore complex is usually reduced to Fe^{2+} to release the iron, especially in the case of 'weaker' siderophore ligands such as hydroxamates and carboxylates. Siderophore decomposition or other biological mechanisms can also release iron, especially in the case of catecholates such as ferric-enterobactin, whose reduction potential is too low for reducing agents such as flavin adenine dinucleotide, hence enzymatic degradation is needed to release the iron.

Iron in Yeasts

Yeasts take up iron by three main mechanisms. In the reductive uptake mechanism, specialised flavo-hemoproteins (Fre) dissociate extracellular ferric complexes by reduction involving trans-plasma membrane electron transfer. The resulting free iron is then imported by a high-affinity permease system (Ftr), coupled to a copper-dependent oxidase (Fet), which channels iron through the plasma membrane. As a consequence, iron uptake by this mechanism is dependent on the availability of copper. In the siderophore-mediated mechanism, siderophores excreted by the cells or produced by other bacterial or fungal species are taken up without prior dissociation, via specific, copper-independent high-affinity receptors. The iron is then dissociated from the siderophores intracellularly, probably by reduction. In the heme uptake mechanism, free heme or heme bound to haemoglobin is taken up as such, probably by endocytosis. Iron is released intracellularly after hydrolysis of the porphyrin ring catalysed by heme oxygenase. Within the cell, iron is stored in vacuoles or in siderophores.

Iron can be mobilised from vacuoles by a reductive mechanism homologous to that found at the plasma membrane. Regulation of iron uptake and iron use are mediated by transcriptional regulators acting either as activators in iron-deficient conditions or as repressors in iron-rich conditions, according to the yeast species; these regulators thus adjust the iron uptake flux to the cell's requirements. In the baker's yeast, *Saccharomyces cerevisiae*, a post-transcriptional mechanism is active under low iron conditions, involving the degradation of RNAs encoding in essential iron-utilising proteins. Other fungi have mechanisms serving a similar purpose at the transcriptional level. Studies in *S. cerevisiae* show that mitochondria are central to regulating cellular iron homeostasis, through the synthesis of iron-sulphur clusters.

Iron in *Staphylococci*

Staphylococcus aureus causes a significant amount of human morbidity and mortality. The ability of *S. aureus* to cause disease is dependent upon its acquisition of iron from the host. *S. aureus* can obtain iron from various sources during infection, including heme and transferrin. The most abundant iron source in humans is heme-iron bound by haemoglobin contained within erythrocytes. *S. aureus* is known to lyse erythrocytes through secretion of pore-forming toxins, providing access to host haemoglobin.

Proteins of the iron-regulated surface determinant (Isd) system bind host haemoproteins, remove the heme cofactor, and shuttle heme into the cytoplasm for use as a nutrient iron source. Deletion of Isd system components decreases staphylococcal virulence, underscoring the importance of heme-iron acquisition during infection. In addition to heme, *S. aureus* can utilise transferrin-iron through the secretion of siderophores. Several staphylococcal siderophores have been described, some of which have defined roles during the pathogenesis of staphylococcal infections. A greater understanding of staphylococcal iron acquisition may lead to the development of novel therapeutic strategies that target nutrient uptake and decrease the threat of this increasingly drug-resistant bacterial pathogen.

Iron in *Bacillus*

Bacillus subtilis is a metabolically versatile soil microbe and Gram-positive model organism that displays a sophisticated adaptive response to conditions of iron limitation. The endogenous siderophore of *B. subtilis* is bacillibactin, a trimeric catecholate siderophore similar in structure to enterobactin. In addition to bacillibactin, *B. subtilis* can obtain iron from several xenosiderophores, ferric citrate, heme, and through a newly discovered elemental iron permease.

The regulation of iron homeostasis in *B. subtilis* is complex and involves a ferric uptake regulator (Fur) protein as master regulator and at least two subsidiary regulatory systems. The most significant of these is an iron-sparing/prioritisation response controlled by the small RNA FsrA and three auxiliary proteins (FbpABC). In addition, the bacillibactin uptake system is transcriptionally activated by an AraC family activator, Btr that directly senses bacillibactin. Iron uptake and homeostasis systems in *B. anthracis* and related organisms are largely similar to those in *B. subtilis* with some additional components. These include a second siderophore synthesis operon for petrobactin, which is important for virulence, and a more elaborate (or at least better understood) heme uptake system.

Iron in *Cyanobacteria*

Cyanobacteria are dependent on but can also be compromised by metals such as iron. On the one hand the demand for iron for photosystem functionality represents a challenge for the iron uptake machinery in iron limiting environments. On the other hand intoxication by iron causes a severe problem for growth and reproduction. To overcome this dilemma cyanobacteria have developed a regulatory network controlling iron uptake. They produce siderophores, which are distinct from that of other bacteria. Furthermore, the iron metabolism is linked to the nitrogen metabolism as documented for example in *Anabaena* sp. PCC 7120.

Iron in *Bordetella*

Upon colonisation of the mammalian respiratory epithelium by mucosal pathogens of the genus *Bordetella*, the host-pathogen interaction causes inflammatory changes, immune activation, and host cell injury. In this dynamic environment, *Bordetella* cells scavenge the nutritional iron necessary for growth. The three classical *Bordetella* species produce the siderophore alcaligin. In addition, they can utilise xenosiderophores that could be produced by commensals or other microbes that transiently inhabit the nasopharynx.

As infection progresses, extravasation of immune cells, erythrocytes and serum to the mucosal surface can occur, exacerbated by the damaging action of *Bordetella* toxins, thus providing iron sources such as transferrin and heme compounds to the microbe. The three characterised *Bordetella* iron systems for utilisation of alcaligin, enterobactin and heme are each inducible by the cognate iron source. The ability to sense and respond to the presence of available iron sources allows these pathogens to adapt to temporal changes in iron source availability, and this ability is important for successful *in vivo* growth.

PLANT HORMONE

Plant hormones (also known as phytohormones) are chemicals that regulate plant growth, which, in the UK, are termed 'plant growth substances'. Plant hormones are signal molecules produced within the plant, and occur in extremely low concentrations. Hormones regulate cellular processes in targeted cells locally and when moved to other locations, in other locations of the plant. Hormones also determine the formation of flowers, stems, leaves, the shedding of leaves, and the development and ripening of fruit. Plants, unlike animals, lack glands that produce and secrete hormones, instead each cell is capable of producing hormones. Plant hormones shape the plant, affecting seed growth, time of flowering, the sex of flowers, senescence of leaves and fruits. They affect which tissues grow upward and which grow downward, leaf formation and stem growth, fruit development and ripening, plant longevity, and even plant death. Hormones are vital to plant growth and lacking them, plants would be mostly a mass of undifferentiated cells.

Plant hormones affect gene expression and transcription levels, cellular division, and growth. They are naturally produced within plants, though very similar chemicals are produced by fungi and bacteria that can also effect plant growth. A large number of related chemical compounds are synthesised by humans, they are used to regulate the growth of cultivated plants, weeds, and *in vitro*-grown plants and plant cells; these manmade compounds are called Plant growth regulators or PGRs for short. Early in the study of plant hormones, 'phytohormone' was the commonly used term, but its use is less widely applied now.

Plant hormones are not nutrients, but chemicals that in small amounts promote and influence the growth, development, and differentiation of cells and tissues. The biosynthesis of plant hormones within plant tissues is often diffuse and not always localised. Plants lack glands to produce and store hormones, because, unlike animals, which have two circulatory systems (lymphatic and cardiovascular) powered by a heart that moves fluids around the body, plants use more passive means to move chemicals around the plant. Plants utilise simple chemicals as hormones, which move more easily through the plant's tissues. They are often produced and used on a local basis within the plant body, plant cells even produce hormones that affect different regions of the cell producing the hormone.

Hormones are transported within the plant by utilising four types of movements. For localised movement, cytoplasmic streaming within cells and slow diffusion of ions and molecules between cells are utilised. Vascular tissues are used to move hormones from one part of the plant to another; these include sieve tubes that move sugars from the leaves to the roots and flowers, and xylem that moves water and mineral solutes from the roots to the foliage.

Not all plant cells respond to hormones, but those cells that do are programmed to respond at specific points in their growth cycle. The greatest effects occur at specific stages during the cell's life, with diminished effects occurring before or after this period. Plants need hormones at very specific times during plant growth and at specific locations. They also need to disengage the effects that hormones have when they are no longer needed. The production of hormones occurs very often at sites of active growth within the meristems, before cells have fully differentiated. After production they are sometimes moved to other parts of the plant where they cause an immediate effect or they can be stored in cells to be released later. Plants use different pathways to regulate internal hormone quantities and moderate their effects; they can regulate the amount of chemicals used to biosynthesise hormones. They can store them in cells, inactivate them, or cannibalise already-formed hormones by conjugating them with carbohydrates, amino acids or peptides. Plants can also break down hormones chemically, effectively destroying them. Plant hormones frequently regulate the concentrations of other plant hormones. Plants also move hormones around the plant diluting their concentrations. The concentration of hormones required for plant responses are very low (10^{-6} to 10^{-5} mol/l). Because of these low concentrations, it has been very difficult to study plant hormones, and only since the late 1970s have scientists been able to start piecing together their effects and relationships to plant physiology. Much of the early work on plant hormones involved studying plants that were genetically deficient in one or involved the use of tissue-cultured plants grown *in vitro* that were subjected to differing ratios of hormones, and the resultant growth compared. The earliest scientific observation and study dates to the 1880s; the determination and observation of plant hormones and their identification was spread-out over the next 70 years.

Classes of Plant Hormones

In general, it is accepted that there are five major classes of plant hormones, some of which are made up of many different chemicals that can vary in structure from one plant to the next. The chemicals are each grouped together into one of these classes based on their structural similarities and on their effects on plant physiology. Other plant hormones and growth regulators are not easily grouped into these classes; they exist naturally or are synthesised by humans or other organisms, including chemicals that inhibit plant growth or interrupt the physiological processes within plants. Each class has positive as well as inhibitory functions, and most often work in tandem with each other, with varying ratios of one or more interplaying to affect growth regulation.

Abscisic acid

Abscisic acid also called ABA, was discovered and researched under two different names before its chemical properties were fully known, it was called *dormin* and *abscicin II*. Once it was determined that the two latter compounds were the same; it was named abscisic acid. The name 'abscisic acid' was given because it was found in high concentrations in newly abscissed or freshly fallen leaves.

Auxins

Auxins are compounds that positively influence cell enlargement, bud formation and root initiation. They also promote the production of other hormones and in conjunction with cytokinins, they control the growth of stems, roots, and fruits, and convert stems into flowers. Auxins were the first class of growth regulators discovered. They affect cell elongation by altering cell wall plasticity. Auxins decrease in light and increase where it is dark. They stimulate cambium cells to divide and in stems cause secondary xylem to differentiate. Auxins act to inhibit the growth of buds lower down the stems (apical dominance), and also to promote lateral and adventitious root development and growth.

The auxin indoleacetic

Cytokinins

Cytokinins or CKs are a group of chemicals that influence cell division and shoot formation. They were called kinins in the past when the first cytokinins were isolated from yeast cells. They also help delay senescence or the ageing of tissues, are responsible for mediating auxin transport throughout the plant, and affect internodal length and leaf growth. They have a highly synergistic effect in concert with auxins and the ratios of these two groups of plant hormones affect most major growth periods during a plant's lifetime. Cytokinins counter the apical dominance induced by auxins; they in conjunction with ethylene promote abscission of leaves, flower parts and fruits.

The cytokinin zeatin , *Zea*, in which it was first discovered in immature kernels.

Gibberellins

Gibberellins, or GAs, include a large range of chemicals that are produced naturally within plants and by fungi. They were first discovered when Japanese researchers, including Eiichi Kurosawa, noticed a chemical produced by a fungus called *Gibberella fujikuroi* that produced abnormal growth in rice plants. Gibberellins are important in seed germination, affecting enzyme production that mobilises food production used for growth of new cells. This is done by modulating chromosomal transcription. In grain (rice, wheat, corn, etc.) seeds, a layer of cells called the aleurone layer wraps around the endosperm tissue. Absoption of water by the seed causes production of GA. The GA is transported to the aleurone layer, which responds by producing enzymes that break down stored food reserves within the endosperm, which are utilised by the growing seedling. GAs produce bolting of rosette-forming plants, increasing internodal length. They promote flowering, cellular division, and in seeds growth after germination. Gibberellins also reverse the inhibition of shoot growth and dormancy induced by ABA.

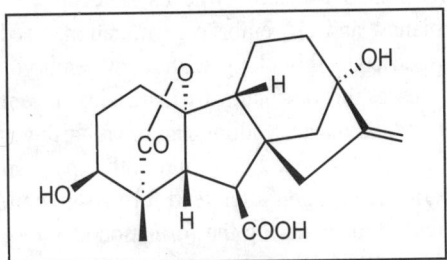

Gibberellin A1

Other known hormones

Other identified plant growth regulators include:
1. Salicylic acid: Activates genes in some plants that produce chemicals that aid in the defense against pathogenic invaders.
2. Jasmonates: Jasmonates are produced from fatty acids and seem to promote the production of defense proteins that are used to fend off invading organisms. They are believed to also have a role in seed germination, and affect the storage of protein in seeds, and seem to affect root growth.
3. Plant peptide hormones: Encompasses all small secreted peptides that are involved in cell-to-cell signaling. These small peptide hormones play crucial roles in plant growth and development, including defense mechanisms, the control of cell division and expansion, and pollen self-incompatibility.
4. Polyamines: Polyamines are strongly basic molecules with low molecular weight that have been found in all organisms studied thus far. They are essential for plant growth and development and affect the process of mitosis and meiosis.
5. Nitric oxide (NO): Serves as signal in hormonal and defense responses.
6. Strigolactones, implicated in the inhibition of shoot branching.
7. Karrikins, a group of plant growth regulators found in the smoke of burning plant material that have the ability to stimulate the germination of seeds.

Hormones and Plant Propagation

Synthetic plant hormones or PGRs are commonly used in a number of different techniques involving plant propagation from cuttings, grafting, micropropagation, and tissue culture.

The propagation of plants by cuttings of fully developed leaves, stems, or roots is performed by gardeners utilising auxin as a rooting compound applied to the cut surface; the auxins are taken into the plant and promote root initiation. In grafting, auxin promotes callus tissue formation, which joins the surfaces of the graft together. In micropropagation, different PGRs are used to promote multiplication and then rooting of new plantlets. In the tissue-culturing of plant cells, PGRs are used to produce callus growth, multiplication, and rooting.

Seed dormancy

Plant hormones affect seed germinations and dormancy by affecting different parts of the seed. Embryo dormancy is characterised by a high ABA/GA ratio, whereas the seed has a high ABA sensitivity and low GA sensitivity. To release the seed from this type of dormancy and initiate seed germination, an alteration in hormone biosynthesis and degradation towards a low ABA/GA ratio, along with a decrease in ABA sensitivity and an increase in GA sensitivity needs to occur.

ABA controls embryo dormancy, and GA embryo germination. Seed coat dormancy involves the mechanical restriction of the seed coat, this along with a low embryo growth potential, effectively produces seed dormancy. GA releases this dormancy by increasing the embryo growth potential, and/or weakening the seed coat so the radical of the seedling can break through the seed coat. Different types of seed coats can be made up of living or dead cells and both types can be influenced by hormones; those composed of living cells are acted upon after seed formation while the seed coats composed of dead cells can be influenced by hormones during the formation of the seed coat. ABA affects testa or seed coat growth characteristics, including thickness, and effects the GA-mediated embryo growth potential. These conditions and effects occur during the formation of the seed, often in response to environmental conditions. Hormones also mediate endosperm dormancy. Endosperm in most seeds is composed of living tissue that can actively respond to hormones generated by the embryo. The endosperm often acts as a barrier to seed germination, playing a part in seed coat dormancy or in the germination process. Living cells respond to and also affect the ABA/GA ratio, and mediate cellular sensitivity; GA thus increases the embryo growth potential and can promote endosperm weakening. GA also affects both ABA-independent and ABA-inhibiting processes within the endosperm.

Chapter 12

Microbial Insecticides and Pesticides

INTRODUCTION

Microbial insecticides are a new form of pesticide that work by infecting selected insect populations with bacteria, viruses, amoebas or fungi. Though this sounds potentially dangerous, many argue that it is actually quite safe, since the application of microbial insecticides is specific to the species one is trying to kill. Microbial insecticides usually have no effect on animal populations, unless diminishing a certain bug in the area interrupts the food chain. Each type usually works against only one type of insect.

Bacterial microbial insecticides may be used to control certain types of caterpillars that eat crops. They will kill caterpillars of both moths and butterflies, though, and should only be used where one will not diminish a butterfly population. Normally, this preparation is sprayed directly on crops.

One bacterial microbial insecticide works specifically on mosquito populations. It is considered extremely beneficial in eliminating populations that might spread the potentially deadly West Nile virus.

Several viral microbial insecticides work to first sicken and kill some insect species. They may affect moths, and sawflies, depending upon the virus used. Fungal microbial insecticides may be used on cockroaches, and create disease among a whole population. Amoebic insecticides may not kill an insect but may shorten the lifespan of an insect or cause it not to reach sexual maturity.

While microbial insecticides may be fantastic at killing a single type of insect, those with infestations of several different types of insects may require the use of several different sprays. Since microbial insecticides are so species specific, they are unlikely to harm any other bugs eating up or infesting crops, so they may not reduce all bug infestations at the same time. Microbial insecticides also tend to be more vulnerable to outdoor elements. For example, long exposure to the sun, or heavy rains can kill certain bacteria. Therefore those attempting to control insect populations must be careful as to when it is appropriate to spray crops to achieve the maximum effect desired.

The revival of interest in microbial insecticides over the last 20 years, has led to large-scale production of *Bacillus thuringiensis* [Berliner], a promising fungi candidate, and to the marketing of the first bacterio-insecticides 'dipel, thuricide, bactospeine, vectobac, tecnar, bactimos, baturin 82' and myco-insecticides 'mycotal, vertalex' based on the formulation of *Verticillium lecani* and metaquino which is based on the formulation of *Metarhizium anisopliae*. While, the production of bacterio-insecticides is common worldwide, there is little information available on the biotechnology of entomopathogenic fungi, and their industrial production is still relatively unsophisticated.

A microbial toxin can be defined as a biological poison derived from a micro-organism, such as a bacterium or fungus. Pathogenesis by microbial entomopathogens occurs by invasion through the integument or gut of the insect, followed by multiplication of the pathogen resulting in the death of the host, e.g. insects. Studies have demonstrated that the pathogens produce insecticidal toxin important in pathogenesis. Most of the toxins produced by microbial pathogens which have been identified are peptides, but they vary greatly in terms of structure, toxicity and specificity. Toxins of *Bacillus thuringiensis* are the most widely investigated example. Many compounds, such as *Beauvericin*, and the destruxin of *Metarhizium anisopliae, aphidicolin* of *Verticillium lecanii* are highly toxic to insects.

PROCESS DEVELOPMENT AND PRODUCTION

Before one can sell a live micro-organism as a pest control agent, a reliable method of production must be developed which yields large quantities for which a product specification can be drawn up.

Organism Storage

The first problem in producing a micro-organism is storing it in a way that ensures the retention of desirable features. The most obvious feature to be retained is pathogenicity; the second is productivity in terms of yield in the commercial production process. This is typically measured either by total biomass, or by number of infective propagules, i.e. spores or fragments of mycelium, produced per litre-hour of fermentation time. Many micro-organisms are known to lose desirable features either on storage or after repeated sub-culturing. Among insect pathogens, *Beauveria bassiana* has been reported to have reduced virulence after subculturing whereas both *Verticillium lecanii* and *Metarhizium anisopliae* are reported as being undiminished in virulence after many passages. Organisms which lose virulence may sometimes be restored to their former potency by passing them through their normal host, i.e. the target insect; however, such a technique would be cumbersome as a routine part of a production process and always presents the risk of contamination. Therefore the problem is often avoided by storing a large number of elements of a single spore isolate in a deep frozen or freeze-dried condition. Samples are checked periodically to make certain that virulence and productivity have not diminished with time.

Fermentation Method

The standard method of production of micro-organisms is the process of fermentation. There are many types of fermentation; the two most common are 'submerged' and 'semisolid'.

Submerged or deep-tank fermentation is, as the name implies, a growth of micro-organisms in a fully liquid system. There are a number of advantages to fully liquid systems which include the ability to hold temperature and pH constant, the ability to pump large quantities of air into the system and disperse it by means of stirring impellers, and the ability to generate reasonably homogeneous conditions to maximise the growth of micro-organism.

Despite the many advantages of submerged fermentation some fungi will not yield a satisfactory product by this technique. Semisolid fermentation offers an alternative in which the fungi grow primarily on the wet surface of a solid material, often some form of processed cereal grain to which nutritional adjuvants have been added, though attempts are made frequently to use "waste" materials or media of low value, such as straw. This allows fungi to grow in conditions more similar to those found in nature; spores, the infective propagules by which the fungus survives and infects insects, are produced in the air and are consequently more durable. Semi solid fermentations are relatively easy to develop on a small scale. Scaling them up to the sizes necessary for commercial product presents numerous problems; aeration becomes a major difficulty as the volume of a semisolid mass increases more rapidly than the available surface area. This requires either a very large area of relatively shallow media, e.g. on trays, or in a vessel which can agitate or tumble the media. On any scale, trays are very difficult to sterilise and keep sterile. The development of large vessels for semisolid media fermentation requires the invention of a number of techniques or pieces of equipment for:

1. Keeping the media friable after sterilisation. Its tendency is to set solid when it cools, rather like oatmeal.
2. Inoculation with the desired fungus without contamination.
3. Aeration and agitation during fermentation.
4. Drying the material prior to opening the fermenter in order to avoid contamination.

Medium development: Which ever type of fermentation is chosen, nutrients must be provided so that the micro-organism can grow. Which nutrients are chosen will markedly affect how fast the organism grows, how much is produced and often, how infective the final product is. Nutrients to be provided include a carbon source, e.g. glucose or molasses, nitrogen source, e.g. soyabean meal or yeast extract, and a 'defined', in which case the precise nature and quantity of every nutrient is known, or, alternatively, they can contain ingredients of an indeterminate and occasionally variable nature e.g. molasses; most commercial media are latter type.

Theoretical Background of Industrial Processing in Biotechnology

The two main disciplines which determine the trends of small and large-scale industrial microbiology are theoretical microbiology (including microbial genetics, physiology and biochemistry) which forms the theoretical ground, and microbial engineering which creates the basis for the application of engineering aspects in microbial processes. A successful microbial process on a small or large scale requires the research and development [R&D] of methods satisfying providing for the following demands:

Maintenance of stability of the production culture, both in its initial form (preservation) and as subcultures infrequently propagated via sporulation or vegetative generations.

Maintenance of suitable conditions ensuring reproducible yields. This entails the use of raw materials of appropriate quality, especially complex organic compounds, and the development of analytical methods for controlling both culture processes and the quality of the raw materials used.

Application of the technology for maintaining strictly aseptic conditions; this factor is important in the biotechnology of most products, in the isolation steps, and in the conversion of the product to the final form. Increase in production yields of a particular product by modifying the medium composition and the genetic properties of the production strain.

Small scale production

The first task in small scale production is the development of a basic culture procedure affording reproducible results. Absolute production yields are of secondary importance, the main emphasis being put on the expected standard course of the microbial process with the attendant changes in growth, pH, consumption of nutrients, production of metabolites, and in the physiological state of the micro-organisms. On attaining reproducible results the search for individual optimum conditions can begin.

The first factors to be explored are usually aeration and stirring. Next to be examined is the effect of changes in the ratio of individual components of the nutrient medium, with special reference to the source of carbon and nitrogen and their mutual proportions. The effect of different types and amounts of antifoam agents is also studied since the physical action of these agents can affect the dispersion of air in the culture and respiration of the micro-organisms; some antifoam agents (vegetable oils, lard oil) can be utilised by the micro-organisms, thus changing the metabolism of the culture. Fluid from laboratory and small scale fermenters can be used for tentative isolation of metabolites and preliminary tests of their quality (Fig. 12.1).

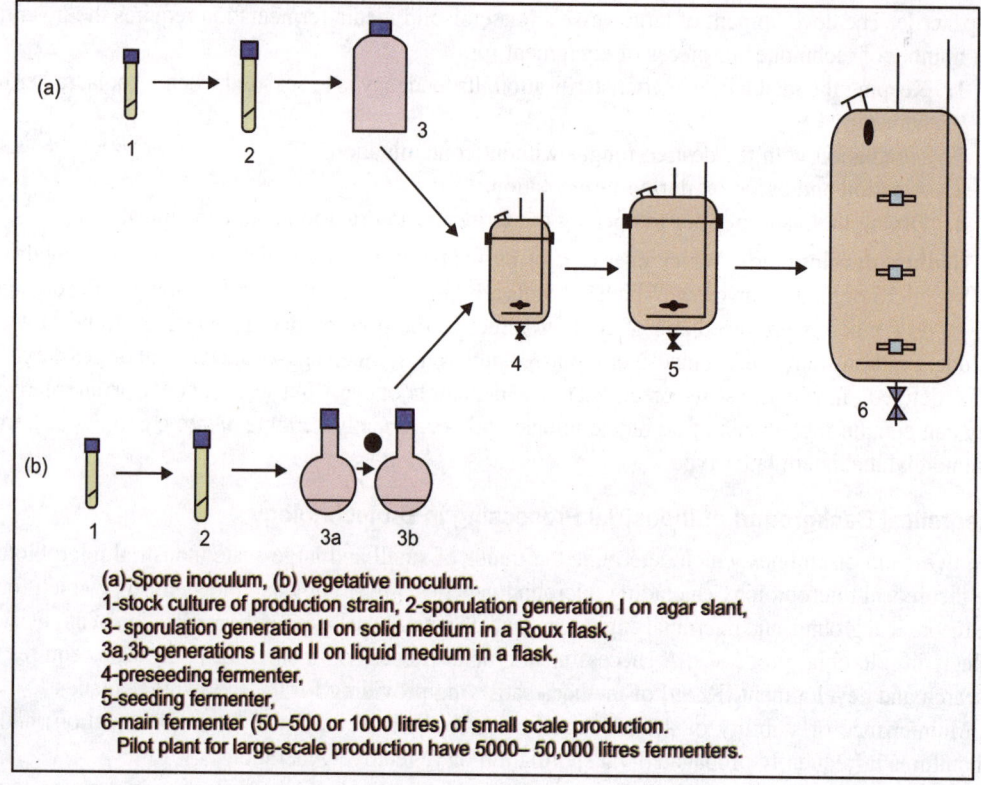

(a)-Spore inoculum, (b) vegetative inoculum.
1-stock culture of production strain, 2-sporulation generation I on agar slant,
3- sporulation generation II on solid medium in a Roux flask,
3a,3b-generations I and II on liquid medium in a flask,
4-preseeding fermenter,
5-seeding fermenter,
6-main fermenter (50–500 or 1000 litres) of small scale production.
Pilot plant for large-scale production have 5000– 50,000 litres fermenters.

Fig. 12.1. Preparation of a microbial product.

Problems of contamination of microbial processes

Microbial contamination of fermentation processes and principles and techniques for its elimination should be appraised from several viewpoints:

1. Type of the metabolite produced.
2. Specific properties of the culture.
3. Machinery and equipment used in the process.
4. Nutrient medium and the raw materials used for its preparation.
5. Technology adopted in the process.

Contaminating micro-organisms affect negative the microbial process by:
1. Destroying the cells of the production strain.
2. Inactivating the synthesised metabolites.
3. Producing substances affecting the producer's metabolism and thus decreasing the production of the required metabolite.
4. Exhausting compounds crucial for growth and product synthesis from the medium.

However, the presence of a contaminating micro-organism need not always results in a drop in metabolite or spores production; in the absence of this drop, it is often difficult to detect contamination. In semisolid fermentation process, contamination need not always lead to failure. The term 'protected fermentation' is used for such processes in which foreign contamination is suppressed by the presence of an antimicrobial agent. This agent is added to the medium in suitable form.

Sterility of microbial process

Checks of the absence of alien micro-organisms are required during all crucial stages of the process, culture, product isolation, and its final formulation. Identification of microbial contamination is done by microscopic and culture methods. Microscopic examination represents a useful tool for immediate detection of massive contamination of cultures with an alien microflora. In most cases viable cells are difficult to distinguish from dead ones. The differentiation is somewhat aided by the so-called vital test which, however, is not always fully reliable. The most reliable method for identification of alien micro-organisms is by culturing. The following procedure is currently used in laboratories: Samples are transferred under aseptic conditions into sterile flasks. A volume of 1 ml serves to inoculate two tubes with 5 ml broth each and, using a loop, blood, blood agar in a Petri dish. Incubation is then carried out for 24–48 hours at 37°C. Both microscopic and macroscopic counts of alien micro-organisms are then taken. If the results are not unequivocal then 1 ml of culture from the test tubes and colonies on the Petri dishes is used to inoculate another four test tubes (2 + 2) and counts are taken again after 24 hours of incubation at 37°C. A macroscopic indication of the presence of contaminating micro-organisms is often a different growth form.

Sensitivity of microbial processes to and protection against contamination

From this viewpoint, microbial processes can be divided into:
1. Processes that do not require stringent control and protection against the proliferation of a foreign microflora in the medium.
2. Processes requiring strictly aseptic conditions—the so-called aseptic processes—microbial insecticides.

STANDARDISATION OF PRODUCTS

Standardisation is the most important process and is based on theoretical background of industrial microbiology. The selection of a fungal strain, or a species in the case of a target pest susceptible to several pathogens, is a critical step since the aggressiveness of a fungus is highly dependent on it. The assessment of pathogenicity is usually based on the results of pest, or progeny (in the case of fast reproducing insects), mortality obtained from laboratory tests. It should be stressed, however, that bioassays conducted under laboratory conditions invariably optimise the potentialities of the fungus and thus the data should be interpreted carefully. For example, bioassays are run in the absence of any microbial competitors, in ambient conditions ideally chosen for the pathogen and with *in vitro* reared insects, the physiology of which may be different from that of the wild types. These bioassays, which are useful to compare strains or species, should represent, therefore, only the preliminary step before field experimentation. The latter is essential in order to determine if the microclimatic requirements of the pathogen and the host coincide and thereby to assess the true potential of an entomopathogenic fungus as a biocontrol agent. The pathogenic stability of a strain during repetitive transfers should also be checked. The media used for these transfers and for subsequent production should be chosen with care since it is known that nutrients can markedly influence conidial viability. Preferably, the strain selected should not have too narrow and specific, it being commercially advantageous if a product has a relatively wide host range within an insect group containing several pest genera. However, the host range within an insect group of several pest genera cannot be too wide and obviously must exclude beneficial insects as well as other invertebrates and vertebrates. Experiments have been carried out with several entomopathogenic fungi to test their effects on vertebrates, specifically to evaluate any allergic, irritation or toxic properties. Only minor allergic responses have been detected amongst a few of the entomopathogenic fungi screened so far.

Strains with the highest sporulation capacities should be selected since variations both in the amount of spores produced and in their mode of production have been reported. Industry will also screen for strains with the simplest nutritional requirements.

Most strain selections have been made from wild isolates of entomopathogenic fungi from naturally infected hosts. However, recent developments in fungal genetics suggest that the natural properties of a strain can be improved through genetic manipulation. In the past, mutagenesis has been used to enhance the virulence or sporulation of *Metarhisium anisopliae*. Conceivably, this process could also be exploited to produce mutants resistant to the pesticides normally encountered in the crop habitat of the target pest. Recombination of selected strains, markers, has been attempted amongst the *Deuteromycetes*. Parasexual recombinants from heterozygous diploids, produced by hyphal anastomosis, have also been identified in *M. anisopliae*. Recombination by protoplast fusion has been investigated in *Beauveria brongniartii*, *M. anisopliae* and *Verticillium lecanii*. One of the problems typically encountered in recombination is the poor stability of the highly sporulating strain and this is why the spectrum of insecticide activity to the target must be continuously monitored. The aggressiveness or the sporulation potential of a fungal strain should be controlled by numerous genes. Thus, genetic improvement, either by classical techniques or the new methods of genetic engineering, is fraught with difficulties. Nevertheless, it is feasible that the genes responsible for toxin excretion could be cloned and that their reinsertion into genome of another strain or species would be a method of increasing the efficiency of a mycoinsecticide.

Propagule

All entomopathogenic fungi are characterised by a biphasic biological cycle: a mycelium vegetative phase and reproductive phase. Two spore types are usually found: asexual spores 'anamorpha', for promoting rapid dissemination of the fungus and resting spores (sexual spores 'telomorpha' or vegetative chlamydospores), responsible for survival of the pathogen during adverse conditions or in absence of suitable hosts. Theoretically, any of these fungal propagules could be considered for the production of mycoinsecticides.

Because of their primary role in the infection process, spores have been considered since the beginning of biological control history as the most adapted fungal propagule to produce. Conidia of the *Deuteromycetes* are readily mass-produced on solid media under aerated conditions. Conidia can also be obtained in liquid media, being produced on typical conidiophores arising from hyphal filaments or directly from the spore through a sporulation microcycle. This microcycle, typically induced by nutrient and/or temperature manipulation, has been developed as a model to study the biochemical events occurring during sporulation of the conidial fungi. This potential for microcyclic sporogenesis has been of particular interest in the case of entomopathogenic fungi since it shortens the culture time and increases spore yields. The other type of mass producible spore is the resting spore of the *Mastigomycotina* and *Zygomycotina* which have a role in disease carryover. These spores offer the advantage of being highly resistant and can survive for several months both *in vitro* and in nature. They can also be produced in liquid culture as well as on solid media. However, these spores, like the mycelium, are not directly infectious; their pathogenicity is dependent upon their potential to produce infective spores by germination.

The production of mycelium has been also contemplated especially in the case of *Oomycetes* and *Zygomycetes* for the reasons explained above. Mycelium propagules of entomopathogenic fungi are noninfective and thus the successful use of a mycelium formulation in biological control is dependent upon the ability of the mycelium to sporulate under natural conditions. On solid media, a continuous segmented mycelium is usually produced, whilst in shake-liquid cultures, as in the insect body, fungal development is most often characterised by the formation of yeast-like cells able to reproduce by fission. The terminology applied to these propagules depends on the fungal group under consideration, being termed: blastospores (*Deuteromycetes*); hyphal bodies (*Entomophthorales, Coleomomyces*); hyphal segments or subthalli (*Lageniales*).

The yeast-like cells are often produced by hyphal constriction and thus their wall structure is mycelial. The fungal dimorphism exhibited by entomopathogenic fungi needs to be investigated more thoroughly *in vitro* since the multiplication of yeast-like forms would facilitate not only mass production but would also be an indication of the virulence of a strain as these cells are responsible for the rapid colonisation of the insect haemolymph.

Microbial Insecticide Based on *Bacillus Thuringiensis*

Cultures of this species now-a-days serve as the basis for large-scale production of microbial insecticides. Worldwide production now constitutes a few thousand tons annually. The cultures of *B. thuringiensis* are closely related to those of *B. cereus*, which are widely distributed in nature. They differ from the former only by the formation of crystalline inclusions.

For the purpose of systematics and identification of *B. thuringiensis* cultures, an efficient method is serotyping by H-antigen along with some biochemical properties of the cultures. Up to now 23 serotypes have also been differentiated within some of the species. From a practical point of view it is essential that there exist certain correlations in the spectrum and activity of entomocide effect between the various subspecies as well as subserotypes.

There are three basic questions that can be asked in any study of production of toxin by *B. thuringiensis*.

What toxins are produced?

In what quality?

How reproducible is the fermentation?

In this discussion of our program which follows we will direct most of our attention to ask what toxins are produced. However, our interpretation must not be confused by the quantities of toxin present in product powders. This is important to remember. We will use several concepts, ratios, distributions of toxicities, crystal-types, H-types, etc. It is impossible to eliminate quantity as a variable. The quantity of toxin produced in a fermentation can be influenced by the isolate of *B. thuringiensis* used and by medium on which it is grown. Thus two powders may differ many-fold in toxicity yet still contain the same toxin. All analyses will be made in the light of this factor and will attempt to pinpoint type as differentiated from quantity of toxin.

The basic active agent, called δ-endotoxin, is produced in the form of crystalline parasporal inclusions during sporulation and liberated in the medium after its completion.

Principally important especially for production purposes is that the level of endotoxin insecticide activity is not correlated with its size and quantity but is defined by subspecies and the strain. For example: the strain HD-1 belonging to the subserotype kurstaki of the subspecies alesti and having the same mass of crystalline inclusions reveals 100 times more insecticide activity than these of other strains. Industrial production of more than 30 preparations has been developed in different countries and the products have been introduced in the market under different trade names since the sixties.

The main sources for the production of *Bt* preparations are strains of the subspecies *kurstaki, galeriae* and *dendrolimus*. The cultures of serotype-I berliner, *thuringiensis* and some other subspecies also produce soluble termostabile α-exotoxin of a nucleotide nature, beside crystalline inclusions. A number of preparations manufactured from exotoxin producing strains are characterised by a broad spectrum of entomopathogenous action. Some producers exclude exotoxin in ready-made preparative forms because of possible side effects.

Morphology of Bacillus thuringiensis

Bacillus thuringiensis (Bt) is a Gram-positive bacterium forming elliptical spores, contained in unswollen sporangia, and a parasporal body (or crystal) which appears mainly as a bipyramidal shape. *B. thuringiensis* is a complex species divisible into subspecies and H-serotypes by serological and biochemical tests. These produce several insecticidal toxins, two of which are used in agriculture.

The relative activity of each isolate against different insect species 'spectrum activity' arrives partly from the combined effects of the potencies of the varying concentrations of the different insecticides that it produces. The δ-endotoxin of different isolates of *Bt* can kill different insect species or differ in the degree of their activity toward them. This variation of activity spectrum according to the *Bt* isolate is very important. Failure to control a pest insect with a particular *Bt* preparation does not mean that all preparations will fail; it mean just that the wrong isolate was selected for use against the target insect. Similarly, even though a pest species may be satisfactorily controlled by the toxins in the present commercial preparations, it is possible that a different isolate may be more effective and thus cheaper to use. The picture is further complicated because different isolates can produce more or less of the same δ-endotoxin than other. Also maximum toxin production can be achieved only by careful attention to the interaction of fermentation conditions, media and the isolates involved—there is, for example, no one medium best suited to all isolates.

Insecticidal toxins produced by Bacillus thuringiensis

The β-exotoxin, 'heat-stable exotoxin', is a water soluble toxin highly toxic to larvae of several species of flies, while alfa-exotoxin 'heat-unstable' is toxic *per os* to mice and to the diamond moth, Plutella xylostella (maculipennis). α-Exotoxin has been defined chemically as an adenine nucleotide and ATP analogue and given the name 'thuringiensin'. Many regulatory authorities opted to prevent its use in agriculture, because it has a terratogenic effect in insects and has mutagenic activity.

The δ-endotoxin in crystals of *Bt* has a limited infectivity spectrum limited, to certain Lepidoptera, mosquitoes, chiromonids and blackflies. The crystalline glycoprotein is formed during sporulation, it is variously called the crystal, parasporal body or δ-endotoxin. There is evidence that plasmids are related to crystal formation. Different numbers of plasmids are found in most serotypes of *Bt*. The plasmids DNA (CCC—covalently closed circular DNA) has different values from 2 to 32 Mda and depend on subspecies and serotype. The strains which loss the large plasmid >32 Mda, loss insecticide activity. There are two categories of plasmids:

Role of bacteriophages

The role of phages in *Bt* genetics is most important. They provide a mechanism for a specialised and generalised transduction which constitute functional genetic transmission systems. The discovery of lysogeny in *Bt* has also opened the possibility that one of the toxins is coded by a prophage.

Three types of phages lyse *Bt*, and these are virulent, pseudolysogenic and temperate. They respectively lyse cells immediately, or form temporary or permanent associations with mitomycin C or UV light, but none have formed a lysogenic relationship with the host.

Mode of action

The crystals from various subspecies are composed of up to four proteins with molecular weights ranging from 26 to 140 kDa. In the case of the lepidopteran-specific subspecies, the major components of this crystal is a 130–140 kDa protein referred to as the protoxin. Upon dissolution at alkaline pH in the mitgut of targeted larvae, the protoxin is further 'activated' by specific proteolysis and the toxic moiety released. Upon its attachment to specific receptors of the columnar cells in the midgut epithelium, the cells swell and are released from the basement membrane and finally burst. The insect (larvae) stops feeding, becomes rapidly dehydrated and generally dies within the next 48 hours.

Taxonomy

Many strains of *Bt* have now been isolated and classified upon biochemical, enzymatic and serological criteria. The generally accepted key for the taxonomic division of the species of *B. thuringiensis* is based on the antigenic properties of the flagella as developed by de Barjac and Bonnefoi. However, *Bt* strains can also be allocated to different subspecies or varieties based on their pathotypes or insecticidal activity for different insects.

For the purpose of the systematics and identification of *Bt* cultures, an efficient method is serotyping by H-antigen along with determining some biochemical properties of the cultures. Up to now 23 serotypes have been described. Subspecies and a number of serotypes have also been differentiated within some of the species. From a practical point of view it is essential that there exist certain correlations in the spectrum and activity of insecticide effect between the various subspecies as well as subserotypes.

The cultures of a majority of serotypes of these species *Bt* var. *kurstaki* are characterised by strong entomocide activity to *Lepidoptera*, products DIPEL (Abbott), *Bactospeine* (Philips Duphar), THURICIDE, JAVELIN (Sandoz). Some differences in the spectrum have also been observed. Thus, the cultures of serotype 5 (*galleriae*) are very active to *Galleria mellonella,* while representatives of serotype 10 (*darmstadiensis-caucasicus*) do not reveal any insecticide activity towards this insect. The cultures of serotype 4 are very active to Siberian silkworm and comparatively less virulent to silkworm Bombyx mori. Of great interest was serotype 14 that was describes in 1978 as *Bt* subsp. *israelensis*. Cultures of this serotype thus produce crystalline parasporal toxin with strong larvicide activity to mosquitoes, black fly and other insect of the *Simallidae*. It is worth mentioning that they are characterised by specific larvicide pathogenicity and are practically harmless to mammals, plants and useful hydrobionts. A number of countries have organised industrial production of larvicide preparations on the basis of *Bt* subsp. *israelensis* cultures.

Of special practical interest was the description of cultures named as *Bt* var. *tenebrionis* with activity to *Coleoptera*. Other pathotype of *Bt* var. *san diego* with insecticide activity to Coleoptera products like TRIDENT (Sandoz) and M-ONE (Mycogen) and pathotype of *Bt* var. *aizawai* with insecticide activity to Lepidoptera and Diptera products like CERTAN (Sandoz).

In the case of *Bt*, the subspecies (varieties) and H-serotypes as well as biotypes with different enzymatic features are defined on a biological and serological basis. This is the case with the serotypes H4a4b and H6, these biotypes have a different spectrum of pathogenic properties, the discovery of antigenic subfactors (fractions) in five of the serotypes of H3, H4, H5, and H11 allows for further differentiation of various subtypes or biotypes. The first three letters of the subspecies name can be used as an abbreviation of the strain name. For instance, KUR H-3a3b (serotype) kurstaki isolated from *Ephestia kuhniella*; KUR H-3a3b HD-1 *kurstaki* isolated from *Pectinophora gossipiella*; ISR H14-*israelensis*.

Lepidoptera Bt var. *aizawai* Certan (Sandoz) *Coleoptera thuringiensis* var. *kurstaki* (mainly HD1 and HD12 isolates) has been used for some years on a limited scale in both agriculture and forestry. It is well known that *Bt* is very selective in its biological action, and kills only a limited range of insects; birds, mammals and fish are not affected. This selectivity is a key to marketable product; very favourable toxicology and environmental profile, zero pre-harvest interval on vegetable crops, 'biorational' registration like in North America. Table 12.1 lists pathotypes of *Bacillus thuringiensis*.

However *B. thuringiensis* var. *kurstaki* has drawbacks including speed and mode of action, and solar radiation sensitivity which have limited its usage. Combining these problems, *Bt* application on foliage remains a challenge in most agricultural situations. Anti-feeding effects observed in various *Bt* formulations combined with non-optimised application rates and spray technology especially in agriculture have decreased significantly its attractiveness to farmers.

Isolation of β-exotoxin

Exotoxin formulations of sufficient purity can be obtained by rechromatography on DEAE-cellulose or silicagel. The purification process which does not use any adsorption on carbon makes use of the supernatant of the *Bt* cultivation medium which is thickened to 1/10 of its original volume by boiling. The inactive material is then precipitated out by stepwise ethanol additions. At 90 vol. per cent of ethanol an active precipitate is obtained which can be further purified on cellulose or ion exchange columns. The β-exotoxin, called thuringiensin, is a nucleotide composed of adenine, ribose, glucose, and phosphorylated allaric acid.

Table 12.1. Pathotypes of *Bacillus thuringiensis*.

Pathotype example commercial products and subspecies
Specific to:
Lepidoptera Bt var. *kurstaki Dipel* (Abbott)
Bactospeine (Philips Duphar)
Thuricide, Javelin (Sandoz)
Bathurin 82 (Slulovice) *Diptera Bt* var. *israelensis*
Vectobac (Abbott)
Bactimos (Philips Duphar)
Teknar (Sandoz)
Moskitur (Slulovice)
Coleoptera Bt var. *san diego Trident* (Sandoz)
M-One (Mycogen)

Mode of action of β-exotoxin

It inhibits the synthesis of ribonucleic acid by stopping off the polymeration catalysed by DNA-dependent RNA-polymerase. The toxicity of β-exotoxin to caterpillars. Galleria mellonella is $LD_{50} = 0.5$ µg/g, that to mice is $LD_{50} = 18$ µg/g. The spectrum of effectiveness of β-exotoxin is much broader than that of delta-endotoxin and it is lethal to insects of *Lepidoptera*, *Coleoptera*, *Isoptera*, and *Orthoptera* groups. Effectiveness varies depending on dose, time, and mode of application.

Application of β-exotoxin in practice

Autoclaved preparation was effective against two-spotted mite (*Tetranychus urticae*), citrus mite (*Panonychus citri*), and Nematode Meloidogyne. Formulations containing β-exotoxin are prohibited in Europe and the USA formulation called Bitoxibacillin containing 0.5–0.8 per cent exotoxin is in use in the USSR. In production where the bacterial mass is separated from the liquid of the cultivation medium by centrifugation, the exotoxin is removed.

Growth cycle

Living cycle of *B. thuringiensis* has two phases: vegetative and sporogenic (Fig. 12.2).

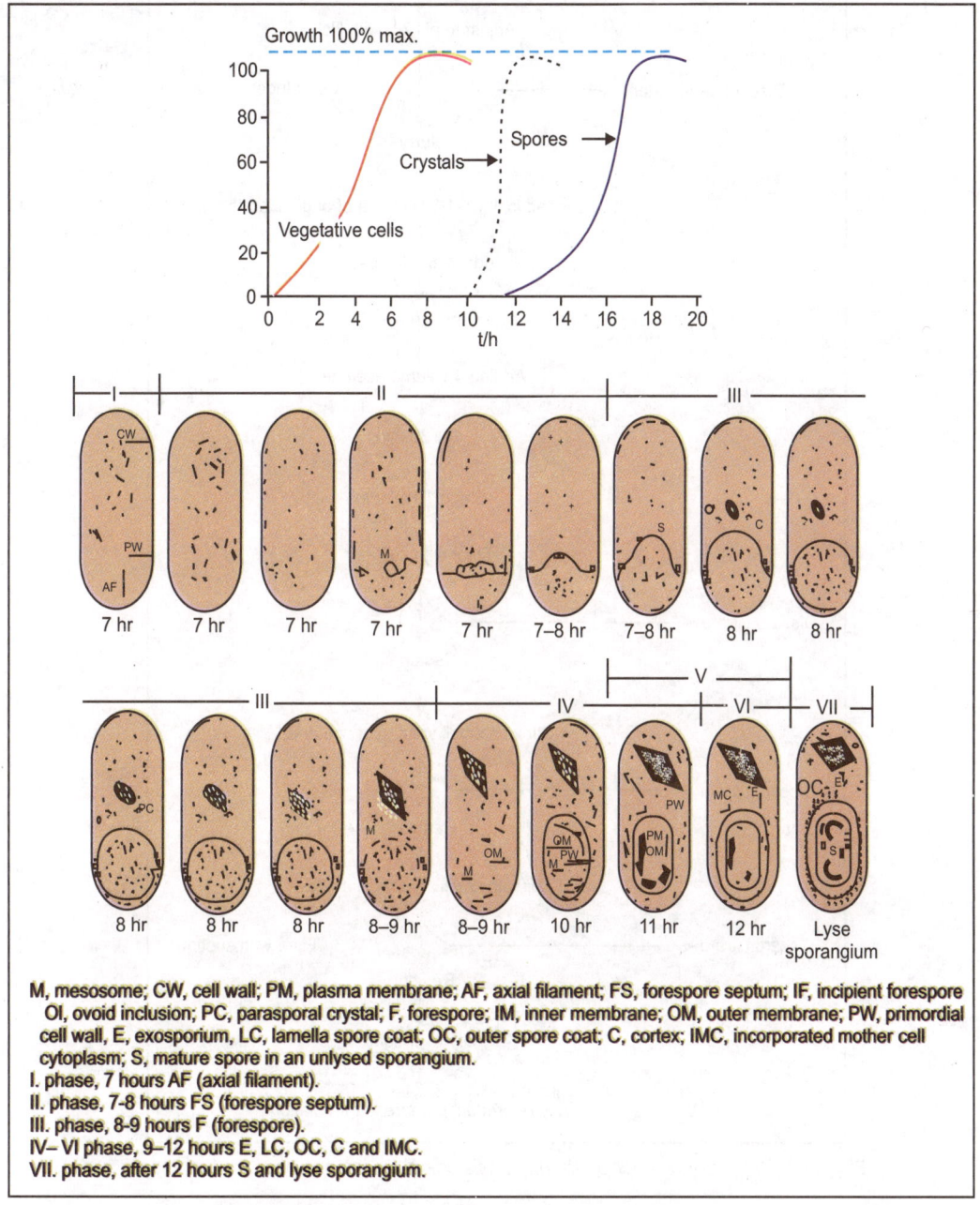

M, mesosome; CW, cell wall; PM, plasma membrane; AF, axial filament; FS, forespore septum; IF, incipient forespore
OI, ovoid inclusion; PC, parasporal crystal; F, forespore; IM, inner membrane; OM, outer membrane; PW, primordial
cell wall, E, exosporium, LC, lamella spore coat; OC, outer spore coat; C, cortex; IMC, incorporated mother cell
cytoplasm; S, mature spore in an unlysed sporangium.

I. phase, 7 hours AF (axial filament).
II. phase, 7-8 hours FS (forespore septum).
III. phase, 8-9 hours F (forespore).
IV– VI phase, 9–12 hours E, LC, OC, C and IMC.
VII. phase, after 12 hours S and lyse sporangium.

Fig. 12.2. Diagram of sporulation in *B.thuringiensis* I.

Recovery of Bacillus thuringiensis

Recovery of *Baccillus thuringiensis* can be made using the lactose-acetone technique as shown in Fig. 12.3.

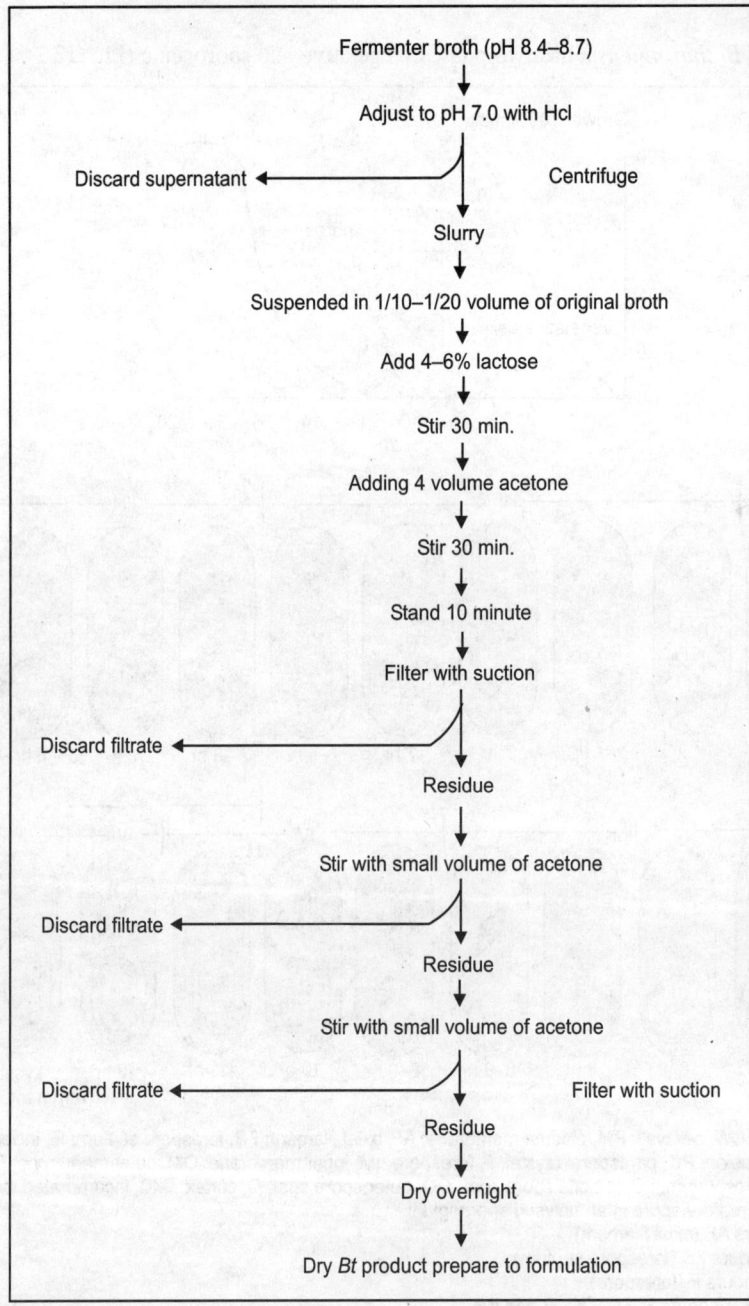

Fig. 12.3. Recovery of *Bacillus thuringiensis* using the lactose-acetone technique.

Bioassay procedures

In all assays, the powder is administrated to the insects by mixing it into their diet, with larvae being allowed to feed adlibitum on the powder-diet mixtures. The effect of this exposure is judged by a single criterion: death. A severely retarded or moribund larva is considered alive if it could move. The assays measured only per cent dead. Preliminary assays determined kill at two levels, usually 500 µg and 50 µg powder/unit of diet. If activity is sufficient, repeat assays with an appropriate series of dilutions to determine the LC_{50}.

Microbial Insecticide Based on *Metarhizium Anisopliae*

The first attempt at using *Metarhizium anisopliae* = *Ma* for biological control was by Krassilstchik. He was successful in destroying 55–80 per cent of clones punctiventris insects in small areas. Varied results have also been obtained when *Ma* was used against other insects. Presently *Ma* were applied successfully against insect pests of several crops, including pests of rice in the tropics. In this region annually treated about several hundred thousand hectares, and using around 2.5×10^{12} viable spores/ha.

Ma 'Metaquino' is produced in Brazil by some five commercial companies as well as grower cooperatives and individual plantation owners. It is used for control of the sugarcane spittle bug, *Mahanarva postica*. *M. anisopliae* var. *majus* is also used for control in parts of the Pacific and SE-Asia to augment *baculovirus* at high larval densities.

According to Zimmermann and Simmons it is possible to recommend *Ma* against *Otiorrhynchus sulcatus* in greenhouse and to lesser degree in the field. Bayer AG produce Bio 1020 granule, Chabchoul and Táborsky have also been used *Ma* against Colorado beetle *Leptinotarsa decemlineata*.

Mode of action

Adhesion of the spore to the cuticle

Adhesion appears to be a prerequisite for successful invasion as noted for hypovirulent strains of *M. anisopliae*. Dillon and Charnley showed that germination of *Ma* is initiated by water but progress to the first overt stage of germination (swelling) is depended on an exogenous nutrient. Prior exposure to water 'soaking' synchronised and accelerated swelling, germ tube and appressorial formation when a nutrient was finally provided. Soak spores were significantly more pathogenic than the controls. Vegetative spores 'conidia' are strong hydrophobic and keep their viability for more than two weeks after spraying on target insects.

For example; larvae of *L. decemlineata* are compleat bay destroyed in the soil by green muscardine. For germination of conidia *Ma* by the test of viability is possible put into drop on microscopy slides special nutrients like orange juice (0.05 per cent). Current evidence for *Ma* suggests that differentiation of appressoria is strictly governed by the concentration of low molecular weight nitrogen compounds on a conductive surface.

Penetration of the host cuticle

Penetration of host exosceleton appears to involve both mechanical and enzymic components (Fig. 12.4).

In soft cuticles, e.g. caterpillars growth across the cuticle is more or less direct, in hard cuticles, e.g. wireworms the fungus proceeds in a stepwise fashion. The production of cuticle-degrading endoproteases with similar modes of action by all Deuteromycetes studied suggests that it is unlikely that they contribute to host specific or virulence, though the common occurrence implies an indispensable fungi differ only in charge. However, this does have practical significance as binding to cuticle with different charge may be favourable or unfavourable to binding by individual enzymes, with consequences for the parts of the body which can be invaded by enzymic action. This can influence the speed of penetration and thus virulence.

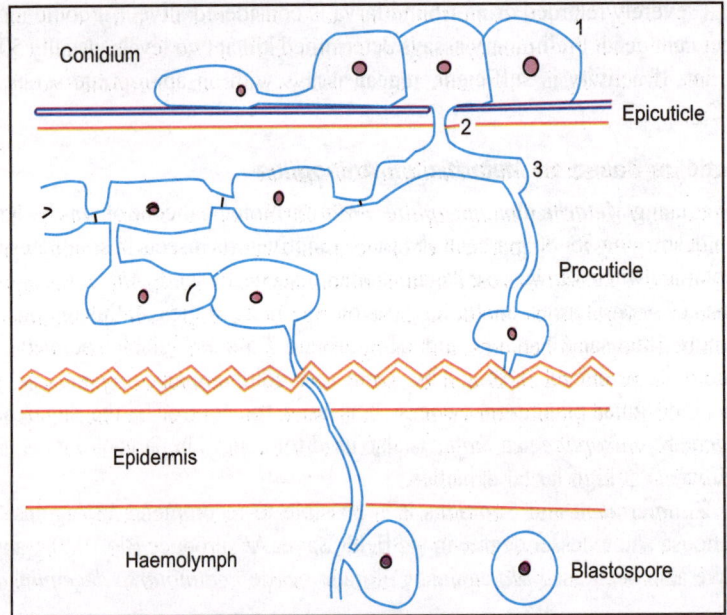

Fig. 12.4. Penetration of host cuticle by a Deuteromycetes entomopathogens 1 = appressorial complex, 2 = penetration peg, 3 = penetration plate.

Host defence

Deposition of oxidised phenols (melanin) in cuticle by host phenoloxidase is the first overt response to infection. Antimicrobial effects of phenols are well established, but in insect cuticles melanisation appears to be primarily an effective defense against more virulent pathogens. Protease inhibitors within the cuticle may serve to restrict pathogen enzyme activity. Within the haemocoel the main cellular response of the insect is a multihaemocytic encapsulation of the fungal element following initial recognition of the fungus by the haemocytes. The yeast like blastospores, produced by Deuteromycetes in the insect haemolymph, reduce the effectiveness of the cellular defences by sheer weigh of numbers and not being as antigenic as the mycelium. Finally the cyclodepsipeptide toxins, destruxin produced by *Ma* appear to interfere with haemocyte function, specially by suppressing prophenoloxidase activation. However, recent evidence is consistent with destruxins being a determinant of virulence for *Ma*. *Destruxins* are active in causing symptoms, principally by paralysing muscles of caterpillars, while in other insect hosts of *Ma* such as *Orthoptera*, whose muscles are not susceptible to destruxins, and in susceptible insects infected with low destruxins producing strains, the toxin may act indirectly to assist the pathogen to overcome host defences perhaps as stated earlier by interfering with haemocyte activity.

Strain improvement

Deuteromycetes do not have a sexual cycle and thus recombination can only be achieved either by use of the parasexual cycle or by direct genetic manipulation. Recombinants from heterozygous diploids produced by hyphal anastomosis or protoplast fusion have been identified from *Ma* and *V. lecanii*. Frequently parasexual recombinants exhibit reduced pathogenicity in comparison with the wild-type parents due to the possibility to disrupt of clusters of pathogenicity genes. The recent demonstrations of transformation in a number of filamentous fungi have indicated that molecular cloning techniques could be used to investigate pathogenicity determinants of entomo-pathogenic fungi, isolate genes coding for specific pathogenicity determinants and produce organisms with enhanced virulence. At the present time *Ma* seems to be the most appropriate fungus for this approach as there are two putative pathogenicity/ virulence determinants like endoprotease, chymoelastase and destruxins. The development of a transformation system and cloning vectors for *Ma* is an essential prerequisite for such approach. For the future once recombinant plasmids containing genes coding for virulence factors have been identified. It may be possible to use them in a programme of strain improvement, particularly as transformation in filamentous fungi is frequently accompanied by gene amplification.

Small-scale production

Ma is possible to produce like local product in plastic fermenters. The isolate *Ma* must be passed through target host and then be cultivated on Sabouraud's liquid medium. As far as the concentration of conidia was very high and reached after 8 days 3.19×10^{10} conidia/1 g. Light and darkness have not any decisive effect on mass production of conidia. The temperature is most important for the yield of conidia. At first 6 days is the best temperature 24°–25°C and then it is possible to decrease temperature to 22°–20°C. Submersed culture produce through 3–4 days blastospores, which are suitable like seed culture with medium for plastic fermenters.

Harvesting and formulation

Process harvesting must be done with Tween 80 or Triton 100, and then is used Siloxyd 125–150 g per 1 litre mud and dry during 24 hours. Formulation WP is suitable for conidia *Ma* and shelf life during storage is good at 4°–10°C.

Standardisation

100 g of conidia powder (2.5×10^{10} conidia/1 g) must be mix with Siloxyd and diluent so, that the total weight will be 500 g. The recommended dose per ha is in this case 500 g of formulated product (e.g. 2.5 $\times 10^{12}$ of conidia).

Microbial Insecticide Based on *Beauveria Bassiana*

Beauveria bassiana = Bb is best known as the causal agent of the disastrous muscardine in silkworms. It is the most widely distributed species of the genus and is generally found forming white dusty raised tufts on Coleoptera, Lepidoptera, Diptera and other insects in both temperate and tropical areas. *Bb* is sensitive to soil-mycostatic factors. Survival in soil is favoured by darkness and reductions in both temperature and soil moisture; at 8°C and under dry conditions, 90 per cent of the conidia survive for over 635 days; on silica gel conidia survived up to 36 months of storage at –20°C. After spraying on the crops conidia survival only 3 days on the same level of germination before application.

Biological control experiments with it are numerous and have been directed particularly to the Colorado beetle and other Coleoptera and Lepidoptera. Various species of mosquito larvae can be killed by dusting conidia on the water surface; conversely, bees larvae were not susceptible while adult bees succumbed. It has also been isolated from the lungs of giant tortoises and box turtles affected with a pulmonary disease; an increase in the air spore has also led to allergic responses in man. *Bb* is employed on a large scale in the People's Republic of China to control pine caterpillars *(Dendrolimus punctatus)*, green leaf hoppers *(Nephotettix* spp.) and corn borer *(Ostrinia nubilalis)*. In the USSR *Bb* like 'Boverin' is produced for the control of the Colorado beetle *(Leptinotarsa decemlineata)* and the codling moth

(*Laspeyresia pomonella*), in CSRF 'Boverol' against Colorado beetles, Whiteflies (*Trialeurodes vaporariorum*) and black vine beetle *Otiorhynchus sulcatus*.

Small-scale production

On agar media conidiogenesis starts after six days, while in liquid culture this takes only 3–4 days. In stirred liquid cultures employed in mass production of this fungus, so-called 'blastospores' developed which are thin-walled, larger (3–5 × 2–3 mm) and less resistant than conidia; blastospores germinated in 6–10 hours at 18°–24°C, while conidia require 15–20 hours. The germination of conidia requires a saturated atmosphere and the optimal temperature for growth is in the range 25°–30°C, minimum 10°C, and maximum 32°C apparently depending on the geographic origin of the isolate; no germination occurs either below 10°C or above 35°C; the thermal death point of conidia has been determined as 50°C for 10 min. in water. The optimal pH for growth is 5.7–5.9, and for conidia formation 7–8.

Culture medium

Good growth occurs on maltose and sucrose and, among others, on the N sources glutamic and aspartic acids, and ammonium oxalate, citrate or tartrate. A medium recommended for optimal growth contains 2 per cent corn steep liquor, 2.5 per cent glucose, 2.5 starch, 0.5 per cent NaCl, and 0.2 per cent $CaCO_3$. The fungus produces lipase, protease, urease, amylase, chitinase, cellulase and 1,2-α-glucanase. Chitinase can be realised into the medium during autolysis, but was also found to act jointly with other enzymes in decomposing insect integuments. The production of a toxic substance is proteins complex consisting of two fractions with different molecular weights. This toxic metabolite is produced most abundantly on complex media (e.g. cornmeal, yeast or beef extract); inorganic N sources are ineffective. A red bibenzoquinone pigment, oosporein, with antifungal properties and the yellow pigments tenellin and bassianin have been found.

Microbial Insecticides Based on *Verticillium Lecanii*

Verticillium lecanii is a well documented entomopathogen of insect order homoptera, most commonly aphids, scale insects and whiteflies in tropical and subtropical regions. Also, *V. lecanii* sometimes hyperparasitises phytopathogenic fungi, mostly rusts and powdery mildews.

Laboratory culture is possible on all conventional mycological media, but the best growth is on Sabouraud's agar. On solid media, conidia are produced and in submerged culture are produced blastospores. Colonial growth rate was optimal at 23°–24°C. Both germination and growth declined steeply above 25°C and ceased above 30°C. Sporulation responded over slightly narrower temperature range than growth or germination, ceasing at 30°C.

Effect of humidity

Virtually all fungi require humidity for spore germination, growth and sporulation. Thus, to ensure maximum germination of spores and hence highest possible levels of infection of insects, spore sprays should be synchronised with optimal humidity, which for most crops should occur in the evening as ambient temperature falls.

Virulence and strain specific

Virulence of *V. lecanii* spores can be measured by bioassay LD_{50} for a 100 per cent viability conidia suspension in which adult, apterous *Macrosiphoniella sanborni* are immersed briefly in to the concentrations ca. 10^5 spores/ml and that blastospores is slightly lower. However, when untreated aphids are placed on still wet spore-treated chrysanthemum leaves, the LD_{50} is increased by a factor of 100. Furthermore, after drying, spores are preasumatly not readily dislodged from the leaves by the aphids. This suggests that a prophylactic spore-spray applied to an aphid-free crop may be wasted and ineffective when aphids invade. Virulence of single and multi-spore isolates of the strain remained remarkably stable on most artificial media. Passaging of *V. lecanii* through an aphid host did not increase virulence, but there are many data, according passaging through an aphid host or white fly increased virulents.

Longevity spores

The half-life of conidia in distilled water varies, both at 2°C (110–160 days) and –17°C (60–120 days), blastospores on the whole are even shorter-lived and more variable (100–150 days at 2°C). When conidia were equilibria at a range of humidities at 20°C, only high humidity permitted good survival. In contrast, dried conidia (whether in slime-heads separated from their parent mycelium or washed) at 58 per cent RH died in less than 24 hours. However, conidia in slime heads still attached to the parent mycelium on aphids or on culture mycelium (without agar) survived for up to 13 days at 58 RH. A favourable microclimate humidity was probably responsible for good survival of spores on aphid bodies killed by *V. lecanii* in glasshouses; 80/90 of conidia survived for at least 30 days after death of aphids despite daytime air temperatures of well over the upper temperature limit for growth.

Spread of infection

Fungal spores in slime/heads adhere firmly to the mycelium when dry *V. lecanii* conidia did not become airborne from dried cultures or from *V. lecanii* killed aphids. Presumably, infection of a new aphid population on a new crop originates from soil.

Control of aphids

Control of aphids and scale insect 0.02 per cent Triton X-100 or Tween 20 in the same concentration are used as wetting agent with concentration (5×10^7 blastospores/ml). Concentrations (10^7–10^8 blastospores/ml) died 2–3 times faster (LD_{50} 1.9-2.3 days) than those treated with a lower concentration, 10^5 spores/ml (LD_{50} 4.8–6.2 days). *Aphis gossypii* is controlled within 14 days.

Mode of action penetration of the host integument

Once the spore has attached to the insect, it must germinated to produce a germ tube which will then penetrated the host cuticle. However, highly pathogenic strains germinate quicker and penetrate the epicuticle directly whilst strains of low pathogenicity took longer to germinate and grew extensively over the cuticle surface with only limited penetration. Virulence of *V. lecanii* has been associated with high *extracelluar chitinase* activity.

Development of the fungus inside the host

Most entomopathogenics are also able to excrete toxins; mycelium of *V. lecanii* can contain a cyclodepsipeptide.

Production and storage of V. lecanii

The choice of infectious material is between conidia and blastospores. Production of conidia on agar is too expensive and it is also difficult to ensure culture purity. Alternatively, conidia can be produced on a cheap granular solid media such as grain, jack seeds (*Arthocarpus*) pearl millet or potato extract for 5–6 days in aerated vessels.

Small-scale production

Kybal and Vlèek used polyethylene cushions made of large thin walled, polyethylene tubing sealed into sections which were partially filled (1 cm high layer absolutely horizontal) with submerged culture of *V. lecanii* after 2 + 1 days cultivation and inflated with sterile air. Product was harvested (ca. after 14–16 days) by discarding the medium and retaining the mad. Yield from a 0.8 per cent peptone, 1 per cent sorbitol medium was 1×10^{12} conidia/1 m^2.

Formulated product

Harvesting of mud is done by mixing it with Siloxyd (ca. 100–125 g/1 litre of mad and wetting agent (Tween 80) and, after predrying at 30°C one day, the wet cake is crushed using a meat-mincer, and the product if dry to perfection at 30°C can be stored or milled (Condux Universal Mühle Typ 150/S-D) and packaged like water-dispersable powders which is prepared for dilution with water into a final spray. The application dose per hectare or meter square is determined depending of the conidia content.

Standardisation

Despite theoretical strain stability, a commercial product must be shown to have constant potency. This should be measured by viable spore count and bioassay. The viability of *V. lecannii* conidia and blastospores can easily be assessed by an agar-slide technique. Pathogenicity of production batches of spores should be measured by bioassay in comparison with a standard since variation between consecutive assays is often significant. *V. lecanii* is a clearly promising biological control agent against aphids, scales, thrips under glass, humid tropic and as mycofungicide against rust diseases.

Small-scale Processing of Submerged Fermentation

Growth kinetics in submerged culture

The use of stirred fermenters with automatic control of the culture environment is the most suitable technique to evaluate bacterial or fungal kinetics. Cultures can be discontinuous (batch cultures).

The batch culture growth curve of a micro-organism can be divided into six phases (Fig. 12.8); log phase; accelerating growth; exponential growth; declearing growth; stationary; lytic decline phase. Growth has been often represented by mathematical models. In the case of media limitation, the equation of Monod is most often used (Fig. 12.5).

$$\mu = \mu_m \frac{S}{Ks + S}$$

$\mu_m = \mu$ maximum specific growth rate.
K = Saturation constant.

If $Ks \ll S, \dfrac{S}{K+S} \sim 1$ and the growth is exponential; if the value of Ks is relatively high in comparison to S, when S decrease, a decelerating growth phase is reached. Values of μ are dependent on the combination media-fungus but are most often between 0.1 and 0.4 h^{-1}.

Values Ksa can be determined by plotting 1/m against 1/S. The equation becoming 1/m = Ks/mm. 1/S + 1/mm. In the case of nonexponential growth the Ks value can be approximated from the curve $m = f(s)$ (Fig. 12.6). Within fungi in batch culture, it is difficult to observe exponential increases in biomass for more than five doubling times. After a certain growth time, the fungus will eventually modify the physicochemical condition of its environment and corresponding growth slow down will occur due to limitation in nutrient concentration or oxygen transfer or accumulation of staling products. Morphologically, linear growth can be correlated with a blockage of the branching whereas branching of the mycelium or the fermentation of blastospores 'yeast-like cells' induce an exponential increase of the biomass.

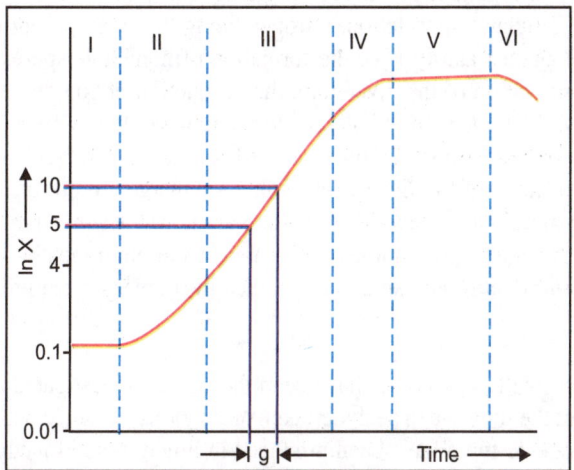

Fig. 12.5. Batch growth curve with six phases; g = generation time.

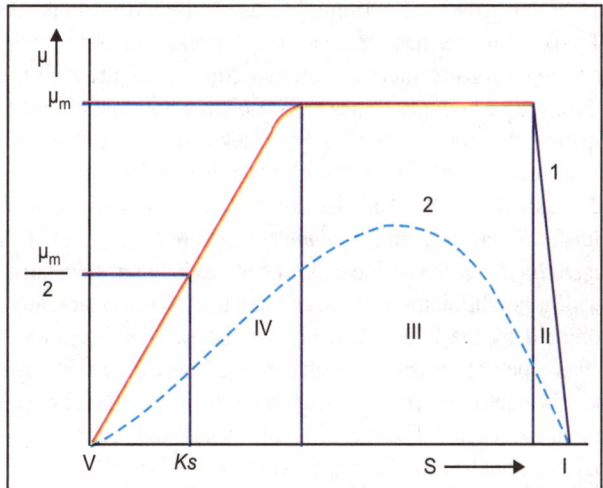

Fig. 12.6. Nonexponential growth, the *Ks* value can be approximated from the curve *m* = *f*(*s*).

Factors Governing Sporulation

It is well documented that conditions favouring spore formation are usually different and more restricted than those controlling mycelial growth. Although spores are the main target propagule in the production of mycoinsecticides, the environmental factors governing the sporulation of entomopathogenic fungi have been poorly studied. In particular, the optimum conditions for sporulation and for enhancing the pathogenicity or viability of the spores produced need to be determined, since it has been established that the environmental factors during fermentation influence both the aggressiveness of the spores and their survival. A period of vegetative growth invariably precedes sporulation and the production of a large number of spores normally requires a well-nourished mycelium. The nutrient concentration and quality that favour sporogenesis are often highly specific. For *Beauveria bassiana*, maximum sporulation is attained with glucose and vegetable oil plus either glutamine, lysine or serine. Starvation or reduction in food supply usually stimulates sporulation, nitrogen being the first nutrient to be exhausted, which appears to be a defence against autolysis or the formation of nonviable spores. However, sporulation can occur without any starvation of the mycelium, the production of conidia of *Hirsutella thompsonii* and blastospores of *Verticillium lecanii* in batch culture being parallel to mycelia growth.

A sexual spores are formed predominantly in aerated conditions and this has led to classic two-step production procedure for most of the *Deuteromycotina*: submerge culture of the mycelium and solid media fermentation for sporulation. Nevertheless, there are no rules concerning the degree of aeration in order to reach a satisfactory sporulation level amongst the entomopathogenic fungi. Conidia of *B. bassiana* and *Hirsutella thompsoni* can all be obtained in submerged culture.

Mass Production

After the growth and sporulation processes have been thoroughly investigated and tested at laboratory level, mass production of the fungus can be undertaken on an industrial scale with various raw materials. Until now, entomopathogenic fungi have been produced in liquid or solid media.

Production in liquid media

Three types of reactors or fermenters are commonly used: the stirred tank; the tower and the loop fermenters. The stirred tank fermenter has the form of a vertical cylinder with the agitator mechanism centrally placed. These reactors produce a violent agitation of the culture medium with good homogenisation of the broth and a high gas transfer coefficient whilst at the same time avoiding mycelial aggregation and subsequent pellet formation. One drawback is damage to the mycelium on contact with the stirring mechanism. Stirred tank fermenters have been employed for the production of the production of both mycelium and yeast-like cells of all the common entomopathogenic fungi. Blastospores of Deuteromycotina, conidia of *B. bassiana* and *H. thompsoni* and resting spores of *Conidiobolus obscurus*, *C. thromboides* and *Lagenidium giganteum* have also been produced in such tanks. The tower fermenter is a vertical cylinder with a height/diameter ratio greater than six and lack any mechanical agitation. Nutrient mixing is promoted by the injection of gas at the base of the reactor. Most fungi produce mycelial aggregates in this type of fermenter, which can also be used for those species producing spores by conjugation. The loop fermenter is a modification of the latter in which the culture medium is forced back down to the bottom of the reactor. The recycling of the medium is achieved by the incorporation of a draught tube (internal recirculating or by a pipe (external recirculating), in the design. The mass transfer at the gas-liquid interface can be as efficient as the stirred tank fermenter but with an important saving of energy. Resting spores of *C. obscurus* can be produced in this type of fermenter. The presence of oxygen could not be detected more than 0.2 mm from the pellet surface.

Production of *Bacillus thuringiensis*

Bt is an ideal micro-organism for large scale cultivation. Present commercial production turns out *Bt* based formulations in submerged cultivation conditions, in fermenter or chemostats.

Storage of production strain

Conserved cultures of *Bt* can be kept in lyofilised condition in sealed ampoules for decades. The culture is suspended into sterile skimmed milk, is filled into ampoules drop by drop (cc 0.2 ml), and is lyofilised. The sealed ampoule is vacuum tested. When revitalising the culture the outside of the ampoule is wiped with disinfectant solution (e.g. 70 per cent ethyl alcohol) to prevent possible contamination on opening the ampoule. Then the ampoule is cut to facilitate rupture, and 1–2 ml of sterile nutrient medium is added into it. The suspension obtained is transfer redonto the surface of slanted agar or of Petri dish agar, and is allowed to cultivate for 24–48 hours at 28°C.

Cultivation media

The selection of nutrients for cultivation depends on availability, price, and suitability for *Bt*. The media used, however, represent only a small share of the costs of equipment, servicing, and utilities required for operation.

Source of carbon

When formulating the nutrient medium, carbon is provided by mono, di, and polysaccharides such as glucose, starch, molasses, etc. If their concentration is too high the pH will drop below 5.6–5.8, and acidity may prevent growth. It depends on balancing the level of saccharides and the sources of nitrogen, in as much as *Bt* is producing alkaline components from the nitrogen-bearing material and these can neutralise the acidic products. As long as the medium is properly chosen the initial pH will drop from neutral to 5.8–6.0 and then will rise slowly toward 8.0–8.3.

Sources of nitrogen

In the fermentation of *Bt* there are variegated sources of nitrogen; these can include albuminous materials containing vitamins and various factors such as yeast autolysate, yeast extract, dried yeasts, peptone, soya meal, maize meal, maize extract, residues from the production of alcoholic beverages, fish meal, etc.

Trace elements

Some ions which supplement nutrition are indispensable for the growth and sporulation of *Bt*.

Cultivation in fermentation tanks

In the beginning of small scale processing the fermenters used are the seed fermenters of 20-40 litres capacity which contain 10–25 litres of nutrient medium. Culture from the shaker or from laboratory fermenter (1–3 litres), to the amount of 1–3 per cent of volume of the medium, serves for inoculation.

The seed tanks can be made of glass or stainless steel; the fermentation tanks are made of stainless. An aeration ring is used to aerate the culture, together with an agitator or an air outlet under a propeller. The air volume used for aeration should correspond to between 1/2 and full volume of the cultivation medium. The changes of pH during fermentation depend on the composition of the medium used. After sterilisation of the fermentation medium the pH should be 6.8–7.2. After inoculation, with acids being formed from the saccharides, pH will drop to 5.8–6.0 (after 10-12 hours) and then will rise again to about 7.5 (25 hours) and further on to 8.0 (ca. 30 hours) and, ultimately, 8.8 (50–60 hours).

Defoaming

Unless foam suppressing agents are used, the fermentation liquid will be subject to intensive foaming at the beginning of fermentation and also at the sporulation time (after about 24 hours). Silicone defoaming agents can be used to mitigate foam formation.

Growth phases

After *Bt* inoculation and the lag phase there follows the exponential phase where an intensive growth and separation of the culture takes place. This phase persists up to the 16–18th hour. At the end of the exponential phase, spores start appearing within the cells, together with inclusions of crystalline toxin. Sporulation is complete after 20–24 hours. Subsequently, the sporangia become subject to lysis, liberating spores and crystalline inclusions of the fermentation liquid. Some 90–98 per cent of all spores and inclusions are liberated after 32–42 hours. Prior to stopping the fermentation, it is recommended to add another 10–12 hours in order to maximise toxin production.

Harvesting of active biomass

Separation and drying

The sporulated culture of *Bt* consisting of spores and crystal inclusions must be separated from the fermentation media with its residues of nutrients, dissolved metabolites, enzymes and possibly exotoxins. From small volumes the *Bt* can easily be separated by precipitation with acetone, using a procedure described by Dulmage. The biomass is centrifuged from the fermentation liquid and is suspended in 1/10–1/20 of volume of 4–6 per cent lactose. Under constant stirring, 4–5 parts of acetone are added and the mix is blended in dish for 30 minutes. The product is kept on hold for 10–30 minutes and is filtered by suction (using a water vacuum pump) in a Buchner filter using filtering paper. The biomass on the paper filter is triply flushed with acetone. The second and third filtrations with acetone serve to remove water from the biomass. Then the biomass is allowed to dry on the filter overnight. On the next day the dry powder is transferred into a dish and aggregates are removed by slight wiping action. The culture grown and sporulated on solid agar medium can be processed in the same way after being transferred into acetone by a wire scraper. From large volumes the *Bt* is separated by spray drying. This drying can be preceded by thickening of the fermentation liquid with the biomass, in order to reduce volume. The solution can be thickened by centrifugation or by evaporation. In either process the temperature must not be allowed to rise above 80°C. In the spray drier the liquid is sprayed in droplets onto heated walls of the drying chamber, and the dry particles are collected at the bottom. The drying time on the walls is no more than several seconds, so that no overheating occurs even with entry temperatures of 150°–200°C. The outlet temperature should be less than 80°C.

Final adjustment

The final product, a microbial insecticide of *Bt*, is of the form of wettable powder, aqueous or oil concentrate (flowable), spraying powder, or granulate. The formulation is so prepared as to afford optimum efficiency toward a specific pest on a specific host (crop).

The formulations contain inert filler for adjustment to the desired activity level. Further, they contain wetting agents and adhesives. The wettable powders contain wetting agents such ascasein, gelatine, lactose, NaCl, Triton-100, soaps, and modern detergents. In as much as these substances also accelerate flushing of the preparations by rainfall or dew, adhesives must also be added such as molasses, syrups, methyl cellulose dried milk, dried blood, latexes, dextrins, etc. The objective is to form a water-resistant film on the plant. In no case must these substances repel the pests as this would impair the pathogenicity of the bioinsecticide. Substances added for taste include glucose, lactose, gustol, molasses, etc.

The emulsified preparations are either water concentrates or oil concentrates. On completion of the fermentation, the spores and crystal are thickened and stabilised by addition of various protective and conserving such as sorbitol, sodium benzoate, xylol, etc. The oil emulsions are suitable for low-volume spray apparatuses. These oil formulations make use of edible oils which are harmless when sprayed onto vegetables and fruits. Granulates represent yet another form of the *Bt* formulations. Granulates are made by impregnation of organic or inorganic granules with a thick suspension of bacteria, with or without emulsifier. In water or dew the bacteria will liberate from the granules and exert a long term effect. The media for organic granules can be grains or coarse particles of maize; as mineral granules are used crushed polystyrene or polypropylene or sifted zeolites (bentonite, diatomaceous earth).

In case of field application, the granules will fall into leaf troughs and there they will serve as a permanent source of infection to caterpillars (e.g. corn borer) which tend to penetrate the stalk near the bottom of a walled-in leaf. When applied against mosquitoes, the preferred granules are those anorganic media which will stay on the surface of water for a period of time and later, at the bottom, is used for nutrition by larvae which will thus become infected. Quality inspection, in the form of an assay of biological effectiveness, e.g. against *Trichoplusia caterpillars*, is done prior to separation by centrifugation, at the time when the semi-product is scaled-down for standard efficiency, i.e. prior to formulating the final product.

PRODUCT HARVESTING AND FORMULATION OF MICROBIAL INSECTICIDES

Product Harvesting

Harvesting micro-organisms from submerged fermentation is often difficult due to the low concentration of the products, their thermolabile nature and in some cases their poor stability. Stabilising adjuvants may have to be incorporated immediately post-harvest to prevent spore death and/or germination. Rapid drying or the addition of specific biocidal chemicals may be required to prevent growth of microbial contamination in the broth or centrifuge slurry.

Spore-forming *Bacillus thuringiensis* are usually concentrated prior to drying by centrifugation or filtration. Centrifugation using a continuous centrifuge concentrates the product from 2–3 per cent suspended solids to 15–20 per cent. Centrifugation may result in some loss of suspended solid as well as loss of dissolved materials. Such losses may not be acceptable and concentration using this technique can often be omitted. Following concentration, one of the technique mixes the crystal/spores slurry with lactose, adjuvants such as wetting agents, spreader-stickers or dispersing agents, and the whole product is spray-dried at 175°C. The dry product is blended and/or mixed with additional formulation adjuvants before packaging and/or use. The lactose added may act as a cryoprotectant or it may help to prevent clumping Dulmage and Rhodes. Dulmage developed an alternative drying technique for laboratory preparations where spray drying facilities are not available; this technique of recovery of *B. thuringiensis* is based on the lactose-acetone processing. Many patents exist such as a foam flotation process for separating *Bt* sporulation products. Fungal blastospores obtained in submerged culture are much less stable than conidia and are consequently difficult to process after harvesting. Laboratory cultures are frequently freeze-dried with or without protectants, but even dried product may have short viability. *Verticillium lecanii* freeze-dried blastospores, for example, have a half-life at 5, 20 and 30°C of 11, 4 and 2 days, respectively. Blachere harvested *Beauveria brongniartii* by centrifugation before mixing with silica powder, osmotically active materials (such as sucrose and sodium glutamate), anti-oxidising agents (sodium ascorbate) and a mixture of liquid paraffin-polyoxyethylene glycerin oleate. The resultant paste was then dried at 4°C in ventilated drying closet. Blastospores dried in this fashion were viable for 8 months at 4°C.

Belova dried *Beauveria bassiana* product in five different ways: vacuum, freeze, spray-drying, drying by mixing with an inert filler, and in a fluidised bed with an inlet temperature of 40°C and an outlet of 30°C. The virulence of the fluidised bed-dried material is enhanced and the process accelerated by precipitation using a calcium carbonate, surfactant, silica gel mixture. In addition, a sulphite liquor is mixed in. Drying in a vacuum desiccator produced samples of high viability and virulence, some remaining active for 1 year at 4°C storage. Spray-dried *B. bassiana* spores together with the culture media led to a complete loss of viability. However, using a 2 per cent molasses mixture as a protective medium permitted retention of viability and efficacy, although to a lesser extent than for the freeze-dried product. Globa recovered *Beauveria bassiana* from fermenter broth by precipitation with calcium carbonate. Fargues spray-dried *B. brongniartii* conidiospores coated with bentonite clay, yielding 50–70 per cent viable spores. However, blastospores were too sensitive for this technique and these were lyophilised with powdered milk and glycerine. The spray-dried conidia showed no loss of viability after 18 months storage at 5°C: lyophilised blastospores were still viable after 8 months.

Formulation

Angus and Luthy, Couch and Ignoffo mentioned that the development of microbial insecticide formulation closely paralleled that of chemical insecticides. Pesticide formulation is the process of transforming a pesticide chemical into a product which can be applied by practical methods to permit its effective, safe and economic use. Important specific differences, of course, do exist because microbial insecticides do not directly depend on the effect of a poisonous chemical but exploit the activity of living (or self-replicating) entities. An exception is the enterotoxinosis caused by *Bacillus thuringiensis* where a preformed toxic glycoprotein is essential for infection to occur. The aim of the formulator then is to avoid practices that might inhibit or harm the pathogen and wherever possible to enhance the possibility of infection. Thus, not only must one avoid agents in any way antimicrobial but also, with *B. thuringiensis*, any compounds capable of denaturing the glycoprotein comprising the toxic crystal. Any attempts to utilise a particular species of micro-organism in an insecticide formulation should be based on an intimate knowledge of the host-parasite relationships. Generally, however it is the multiplication of a micro-organism in the host tissues that leads to disease and death. A microbial pesticide formulation is a physical mixture of living entities with inert ingredients which provides effective and economic control of pests. Formulation of a pathogen product with an extensive shelf-life (>18 month) is critical to industrialisation. In commercial development of a basic formulation of an entomopathogen, technology concerns maintaining pathogen viability and virulence during the production process and developing a product form which preserves or enhances these properties. To do this, knowledge of the biology of pathogen and target insect is essential. Effect of temperature, humidity and media (inert carrier) on the entomopathogen can turn out to be the most important.

Additives

Spreaders or wetting agents are added to the water diluent to ensure 'wetting' of the surface to be sprayed. Many materials have been used including dried milk, powdered casein, gelatine, saponins, soaps etc. In so far as microbial insecticides are concerned, it is essential that the compound used should encourage premature growth or germination and that it should not inhibit successful establishment of the pathogen. Some factors are likely to be rather subtle, e.g. although detergents such as sodium dodecyl sulphate do not inactive the crystal toxin of *Bt*, they open up the structure of the crystal and make it more sensitive to destruction by other means.

Chapter 13

Production of Proteins from Recombinant Micro-organisms

INTRODUCTION

Proteins have many essential roles in living organisms and so the study of proteins is central to molecular biology, while their production is important in many industries. Generally, proteins are best studied in pure form. It is a central concept of much molecular biology that living processes can be broken down into individual steps that are much easier to study than entire processes. This means that studying the properties of individual proteins can help us to understand the processes in which they participate. Examples of the kinds of studies that can be done with purified or partially purified proteins are many and, while some of these studies were possible long before molecular biology came along, cloning techniques have greatly enhanced our ability to study and understand proteins. This is mostly because we can now express and purify them in high quantities in organisms which are easily grown in the laboratory.

Experiments on purified cellular components such as proteins or DNA are referred to as *in vitro* experiments (as opposed to experiments on living cells or organisms, which are called *in vivo* experiments). Our ability to study proteins *in vitro* depends on two things: the availability of a suitable assay, and the availability of the pure protein. The activity may be a relatively straightforward one such as an enzyme activity, or a more complex one such as binding to DNA and regulating gene expression, or membrane transport or signalling. Protein purification can vary from easy to difficult depending on the particular protein, but our ability to express many proteins at high levels by cloning the genes that encode them is very helpful in devising successful ways of purifying them.

Proteins have many practical uses in the laboratory. With molecular biology itself, of course, most of the key reagents are proteins: restriction enzymes, DNA ligase, various DNA polymerases such as the thermostable polymerases used in the polymerase chain reaction (PCR), and so on. These enzymes were originally purified from a diverse range of organisms, but now nearly all of them have been cloned and expressed in *Escherichia coli*, and are purified from there.

Proteins also have numerous applications, many of which produce goods with which we are all familiar. Enzymes, in particular, are widely used: in brewing and wine making, in paper manufacture, in the production of detergents, in making cheese, in making soft-center mints, and in many other examples. Proteins also have very important roles as pharmaceuticals. Insulin for diabetics, factor VIII for hemophiliacs, and the active component of the vaccine against the hepatitis B virus for children, are some of the many examples of proteins which are drugs. Many more drugs are active against particular proteins. The search for compounds which are active against particular proteins is helped enormously by having the pure proteins available for study in the laboratory. (To give an example, the anticancer drug Glivec is a highly specific inhibitor of a protein called bcr-abl tyrosine kinase which itself is implicated in the development of chronic myeloid leukemia. The availability of this protein, expressed from the cloned gene, was essential in the development of the drug.) Again, in the vast majority of cases, the proteins in these examples are produced by cloning the gene for the protein from its original organism and expressing it in a different (heterologous) organism, often *E. coli*. Thus, there are numerous examples stretching from pure research, through the production of mundane and everyday items, to the development of advanced pharmaceuticals, which illustrate the use of different proteins. In this sections we are going to look at how proteins can be produced in both bacterial and eukaryotic cells, focusing on cases where the proteins are needed in reasonably large amounts and in an active form.

Requirements for protein production from cloned genes: The basic concept of protein production in a heterologous organism (one which is not where the gene for the protein first originated) is simple. The aim is usually to get the organism to produce as much of that protein as possible. To do this, the processes which lead to the production of the protein (transcription and translation) must be made to occur at as high a level as possible. The gene for the protein has to be placed downstream from a strong promoter, to maximise the amount of mRNA which is produced for translation into protein. Ideally, there will be many copies of this gene present in each cell, which will increase the amounts of mRNA and hence of protein which are produced. This is done by placing the gene and its promoter into a suitable vector, typically a plasmid. The protein needs to be produced in such a way that it does not harm the host, at least until high levels of the protein have accumulated. Finally, the protein ideally needs to be in a soluble, active form which can be easily purified away from the other components of the organism, such as other proteins, lipids, metabolites and nucleic acids, all of which might interfere with the uses to which the protein is going to be put.

The commonest organism used for the expression of proteins is *E. coli*. Many of the issues that arise with getting high protein expression from *E. coli* can also occur with other expression systems, and one should bear this in mind while reading the description of protein production in *E. coli* that follows. *E. coli* is an easy organism to grow: it grows rapidly and in very large numbers in fairly cheap media. The strains used for protein production are not harmful to humans or to the environment—indeed, most of them have been grown in the laboratory for so long that they would struggle to survive outside the laboratory or production plant. Most importantly, a large number of biological 'tools' have been developed for maximising the efficiency of protein production in *E. coli*.

FERMENTATION

A process, which employs micro-organisms, animal cells and/or plant cells for the production of materials, is a bioprocess. Most biotechnical products are produced by fermentation. In fermentation, the products are formed by catalysts that catalyse their own synthesis. Enzymes are biological catalysts and are produced as secondary metabolites of enzyme fermentation.

There are many aspects that complicate the modelling of the bioprocesses. A fermentation process has both nonlinear and dynamic properties. The metabolic processes of the micro-organisms are very complicated and cannot be modelled precisely. Because of these reasons, traditional modelling methods fail to model bioprocesses accurately. The modelling is further complicated because the fermentation runs are usually quite short and large differences exist between different runs.

Fermentations can be operated in batch, fed-batch or continuous reactors. In batch reactor all components, except gaseous substrates such as oxygen, pH-controlling substances and antifoaming agents, are placed in the reactor in the beginning of the fermentation. During process there is no input nor output flows. In fed-batch process, nothing is removed from the reactor during the process, but one substrate component is added in order to control the reaction rate by its concentration. There are both input and output flows in a continuous process, but the reaction volume is kept constant.

Cells

Every cell in nature has a finite lifetime and in order to maintain the species the continuous growth of the organisms is needed. A bacterial cell is able to duplicate itself. The duplication process is quite complicated and includes as many as 2000 different chemical reactions. The generation time, that is the time needed for the cells to double the mass or the number of the cells, depends on the number of factors, both nutritional and genetic. For *Escherichia coli* in ideal conditions the doubling time can be as short as 20 min. but usually it takes a longer time.

To be able to live, reproduce and make products, a cell must obtain nutrients from its surroundings. Heterotrophic micro-organisms, which include most of the bacteria, require an organic compound as the carbon source. A cell can use either light or chemicals as its energy source. A chemotroph obtains energy by breaking high-energy bonds of chemicals. Most organisms that are used in industrial processes are chemoheterotrophs, i.e. organisms that use an organic carbon source and a chemical source of energy.

A view of a cell as an open system is presented in Fig. 13.1. A cell produces more cells, chemical products and heat from chemical substrates. A cell requires many different kinds of substrates to function. In most cases carbon is supplied as sugar or some other carbohydrate. Glucose is often used. In aerobic processes oxygen is a vital component. Oxygen can be fed into the process by continuous aeration. The most common source of nitrogen is ammonia or an ammonium salt. In some cases the growth rate of the organisms increases if amino acids are supplied. Required amounts of hydrogen can be derived from water and organic substrates. Other compounds that are needed for growth include P, S, K, Mg and trace elements, which are added in the growth media as inorganic salts.

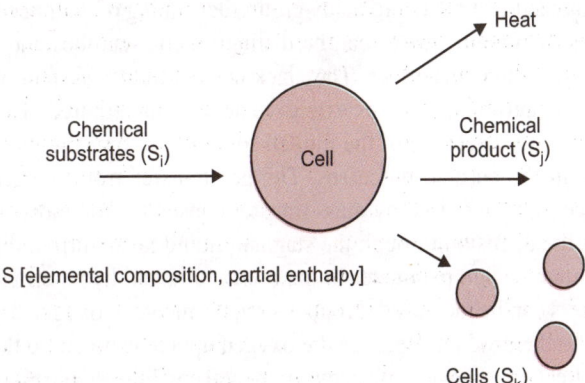

Fig. 13.1. A view of a cell as an open system.

When micro-organisms are grown in a batch reactor certain phases of growth can be detected. A typical growth characteristic is shown in Fig. 13.2. The appearance and the length of each phase depend on the type of organisms and the environmental conditions.

The first phase in the growth, where the growth rate stays almost constant, is the lag phase. The lag phase is caused for many reasons. For example, when the cells are placed in fresh medium, they might have to adapt to it or adjust the medium before they can begin to use it for growth. Another reason for the lag phase might be that the inoculum is composed partly of dead or inactive cells. If a medium consists of several carbon sources, several lag phases might appear. This phenomenon is called diauxic growth. Micro-organisms usually use just one substrate at a time and a new lag phase really results when the cells adapt to use the new substrate.

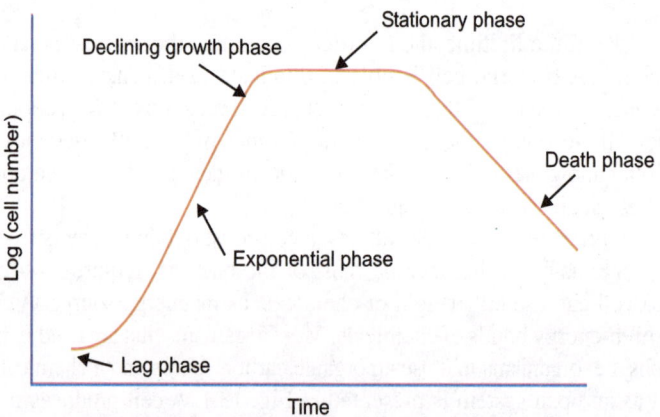

Fig. 13.2. Growth phases in a batch process.

When a substrate begins to limit the growth rate the phase of the declining growth begins. The growth rate slows down until it reaches zero and the stationary phase begins. In the stationary phase the number of the cells remains practically constant, but the phase is important because many products are only produced during it. The last phase is called the death phase. During the death phase the cells begin to lyse and the growth rate decreases.

The micro-organisms can be divided into many groups depending of their need for oxygen. Although there are several groups, two main classes can be distinguished—aerobes and anaerobes. Organisms that cannot use oxygen are called anaerobes. They lack the respiratory system. Aerobes are capable of using oxygen and in many aerobic processes extensive aeration is required. The cells can usually use only waterdissolved substrates. Because of the limited solubility of oxygen into water, oxygen transfer can become a problem in the aerobic processes. The gas transfer from oxygen bubble into the cell includes many resistances, characterised by mass transfer constants. The most significant resistance in a well-stirred reactor is the diffusion through the stagnant liquid layer surrounding the air bubble.

Aeration is an important design parameter in the bioreactors and by its efficient control the overall productivity of the process can be increased. Product's requirements of oxygen depend on the energetics of the pathway leading to the product. Because the oxygen uptake is linked to the cellular metabolism, the oxygen dynamics reflect the changes in the environmental conditions. The rate of change of dissolved oxygen concentration is about 10 times faster than the cell mass or substrate concentrations.

Enzyme Production

Since 1980's a large increase has occurred in the range of commercial fermented products, particularly secondary metabolites and recombinant proteins. In the past, only the fermentation of extracellular enzymes, such as amylases and proteases, was industrially possible. The release of intracellular enzymes has become possible by largescale mechanical techniques. Also chemical or physical methods can be used in the cell disintegration. Recombinant organisms will likely be used for producing a large proportion of enzymes in the future, because this approach enables the production of many different enzymes in substantial quantities and minimises the production costs by using a small number of host/vector systems. In many cases only low levels of protein can be produced by natural hosts. Systems, which have the gene of interest cloned and inserted in the expression vector, have been developed to achieve the abundant expression of the functional protein.

The active form of an enzyme is a folded globular structure. If enzymes are subjected to stress, either *in vitro* or *in vivo*, they might unfold partially or completely. The stress can be provided by denaturants, high (or low) temperature or ionic composition of medium. When protein is overproduced in a recombinant micro-organism, the local concentration of protein is raised and aggregation may occur. Denatured proteins may form bodies that cannot be recovered.

Fed-batch Fermentation

Fed-batch reactors are widely used in industrial applications because they combine the advantages from both batch and continuous processes. Figure 13.3 presents biomass concentration as the function of time in a typical fed-batch process. Process is at first started as a batch process, but it is exhibited from reaching the steady state by starting substrate feed once the initial glucose is consumed. The fermentation is continued at a certain growth rate until some practical limitation inhibits the cell growth.

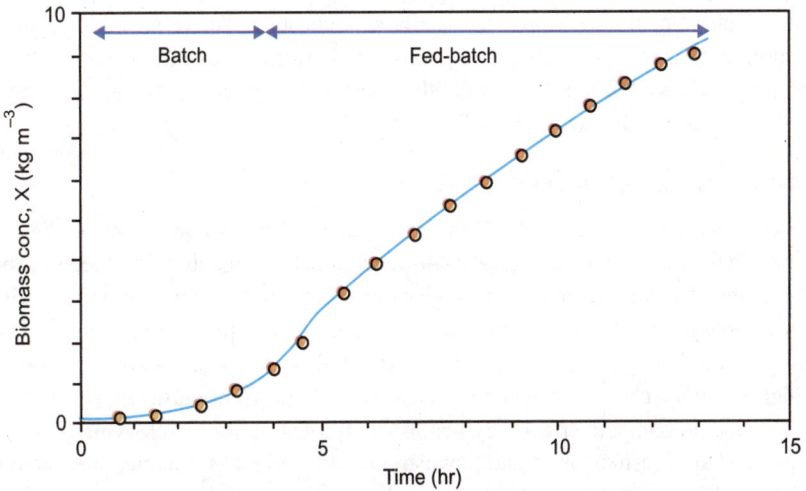

Fig. 13.3. Biomass vs. time in a fed-batch process.

The inlet substrate feed should be as concentrated as possible to minimise dilution and to avoid process limitation caused by the reactor size. In a fed-batch process the dilution rate means the components rate of dilution because of the volume increase caused by the inlet feed. The main advantages of the fed-batch operation are the possibilities to control both reaction rate and metabolic reactions by substrate feeding rate. The limitations caused by oxygen transfer and cooling can be avoided by controlling the reaction rate. In industrial fermentation systems, consistent operation is achieved by manual monitoring and control by process operators. The operators detect potential problems and make necessary modifications to the process based on their experience and knowledge of the process together with the information provided by supervisory control systems. Because the models for model-based control are rare, fermentation processes are usually run with a predetermined feed profile.

A typical operation procedure is presented. The fermentation is started with a small amount of biomass and substrate in the fermenter. The substrate feed is started when most of the initially added substrate has been consumed. This procedure enables the maintaining of a low substrate concentration during fermentation, which is necessary for achieving a high product formation rate. The growth rate can be controlled by the substrate concentration to avoid catabolite repression and sugar-overflow metabolism. The sugar-overflow metabolism, or glucose effect, occurs when glucose concentration exceeds a critical value and leads to excretion of partially oxidised products, such as acetic acid and ethanol. Most micro-organisms exhibit some kind of overflow metabolism and that is often detrimental to the process. Catabolite repression is a repression of the respiration on the enzyme synthesis level. It occurs during the long-term exposure of the cell to the high glucose concentration.

Different types of substrate limitations can be used in the fed-batch processes. The repression of the growth rate can be achieved for example by sugar, nitrogen or phosphate sources. If no reaction rate control is used, and the cells are growing exponentially, the reaction will eventually be limited by oxygen or by heat. The metabolism control with the fed-batch process is useful also for the production of the secondary metabolites such as antibiotics, because the synthesis of them is repressed during the unrestricted growth.

While in continuous fermentation the key variables are held constant, in fed-batch technique almost every key variable is changing as the process progresses. In order to give the best possible growing conditions the pH and temperature levels are usually kept constant. The fermentation systems are very sensitive to abnormal changes in operating conditions. The performance of fermentation depends greatly on the ability to keep the system operating smoothly. A smoothly operated process is likely to be more productive than one that is subjected to significant disturbances.

FERMENTATION ON LARGE SCALE

Trend toward environmental sustainability and development of renewable resources has significantly increased interest in the recovery of fermentation products, such as organic acids, feed or food additives, and industrial chemicals. Consequently, the range of products produced by fermentation is expanding beyond the traditional high-value low-volume compounds, such as pharmaceuticals, and is beginning to compete with traditional synthetic production of commodity chemicals. As fermentation moves into lower-value higher volume chemicals, it becomes necessary to maximise efficiency, and minimise costs and waste byproducts to compete effectively against traditional options. Achieving these goals means approaching the design of fermentation and downstream separations as a single, integrated process. As stated by Williams: 'The bioreactor should be regarded as an integrated unit operation with both upstream and downstream unit operations.'

However, all too often, the design of fermentation and downstream separations are regarded separately in process development. Typically, a separation specialist takes on the challenge of designing steps to separate the various components of a complex fermentation broth that the fermentation-process designers included to maximise fermentation performance. Hence, if the required separation becomes complex and costly, the most efficient fermentation may not necessarily yield the optimum overall process.

Typically, 50–70 per cent of the total production cost in classical processes is due to downstream processing, whereas in fermentation that employs recombinant DNA, the fraction can reach up to 80–90 per cent. This large percentage is often due to separation and purification of the fermentation product.

Fermentation broths are complex aqueous mixtures of cells, soluble extracellular products, intracellular products, and converted substrate or unconvertible components. The particular separation techniques useful for any given bioprocess depend not only on the location of the product (intracellular vs. extracellular) and its size, charge and solubility, but also on the scale of the process itself and the product value. For example, chromatography is generally useful for high-value pharmaceuticals or biologicals, such as hormones, antibodies and enzymes, but is expensive and difficult to scale up.

As with other chemical processes, fermentation for producing commodity chemicals and products is also aimed at minimising production costs. Due to the significant impact of raw substrate materials and downstream processing on the total production cost, process optimisation is primarily focused on finding new, competitive and, above all, sustainable production technologies.

In addition, many fermentation processes are hampered by the accumulation of products in the fermenter. The recovery cost as a percent of the total production cost can vary from as low as 5–10 per cent in, for example, the production of single-cell protein (SCP) and extracellular enzymes such as proteases, amylases, etc. to as much as 90 per cent for the bacterial production of poly(3-hydroxyalkanoates) used to produce biodegradable thermoplastics. The high cost of recovery is due to the generally low product concentrations in aqueous fermentation broths; the complexity of the broth mixture, especially when liberating intracellular products by cell disruption; and the multiple, discrete separation and purification steps in purifying the product. The latter steps lead to high capital and operating costs, as well as multiple operations that each can result in significant product yield losses and generation of waste streams that must be disposed of or recycled.

Therefore, fermentation development is bound by the overall recovery strategy chosen for a certain product. This depends on the required product purity, which can be as high as 99.99 per cent for diagnostic and therapeutic proteins. In addition, economic consideration must be given to the feasibility of minimising unit-operation complexity and waste production, while maximising yield and productivity.

The impact of fermentation on the overall production economics strongly depends on the type of product made, i.e. industrial vs. therapeutic proteins; and specialty vs. bulk chemicals. This depends on the desired vs. achievable product concentration in the final broth. According to the economy of scale, the selling price of a product is inversely correlated with its achievable concentration at the end of fermentation, and can range by 9–10 orders of magnitude.

Regardless of the product, the highest purity in the final broth is the most desirable. Since, for bulk chemical and biomass routes, fermentation already represents a large fraction of the total production costs, it is here that so-called 'clean' fermentation development (i.e. integration of fermentation and separation to reduce the environmental footprint) can have a major impact on the overall economics. There is continual pressure for technical improvement on the upstream bioreactor section to yield a final broth of higher-product concentration to lower the cost of separation and recovery.

The most obvious benefits that can be achieved from integrating fermentation and downstream processing are minimising waste, raw materials, capital and energy. An often-forgotten and more-challenging-to-achieve benefit is environmental sustainability. The same materials have been recycled for billions of years. The new industrial revolution is all about absorbing the lessons we should have learned from nature long ago. Efficient use of energy and materials and a reduction in waste can help the bottom line. In general, large-scale fermentation development comprises of the following steps:

1. Organism selection, with regard to
   (a) Substrate versatility.
   (b) Byproduct formation characteristics.
   (c) Robustness of the organism, e.g. to process upsets.
   (d) Viability with regard to cell recycling.

    (e) Physiological characteristics (maximum growth rate, aeration requirements, etc.).

    (f) Genetic accessibility.

2. Metabolic and cellular engineering

    (a) Improve existing properties of the organism.

    (b) Introduce novel functions, for example, by simplifying product recovery, expanding substrate and product ranges, and enabling fermentation to occur under nonstandard conditions.

3. Fermentation process development

    (a) Culture and media optimisation (from complex to defined minimal media).

    (b) Optimisation of cultivation parameters that take into account product recovery and purification (minimise byproduct formation, minimise chemical inputs, and develop high-cell-density cultivation).

    (c) Incorporation of cell retention/recycling.

4. Introduction of downstream unit operations within a fermentation process

    (a) Examples are extractive fermentation, electrodialysis and in-line membrane separation technologies.

INTEGRATION TIPS

Integration can be approached from different angles. The following examples by no means comprise a comprehensive list, but relate to the steps involved in large-scale fermentation development.

Simplify the fermentation broth: In principle, any ingredient added to the broth that does not end up as product will have to be removed. It therefore behooves the fermentation-process designer to eliminate any unnecessary ingredients from the broth. For example, many fermentation processes employ complex media, such as yeast extract or corn steep liquor (initial waste stream of corn wet milling operation; generally used as a rich source for nitrogen in fermentation media). These media are inexpensive and ample in nutrients. Designing defined fermentation media from salts and vitamins requires a considerable development effort to provide a recipe capable of supporting microbial production at the desired levels. However, it is sometimes worth considering the tradeoff between slightly reduced fermentation performance and a greatly simplified downstream process. In addition, if a complex medium component must be used, the component may contain elements that do not directly benefit the fermentation, yet provide a separation challenge downstream. In some cases, it may be feasible to separate out these non-beneficial nutrients before they reach the broth.

Ease separation by altering the product form: In some cases, different forms of the product are easier to separate downstream than others. A common example of this is organic acids, where the free-acid form of the product may be easily extracted from a fermentation broth, while the salt is not easily removed. If fermentation is designed separately from downstream processes as is usually the case, an acidification step will be required downstream. However, this requires that a neutralising base be added to the broth, which must later be removed by adding an acid, with both base and acid becoming a waste salt that must then be disposed of. This inefficiency can be avoided if the fermentation can be carried out at a low enough pH to provide the product predominantly as the acid. The resulting savings in acid, base and waste disposal costs may offset a considerable amount of decline in fermentation performance resulting from the more unfavorable acidic fermentation conditions.

Reuse the fermentation broth components: Significant improvements in fermentation raw-material yield and production rate can be effected by reusing components of the broth. For example, recycling cells, although a technical challenge, holds promise for improving fermentation efficiency. Separation of the biomass from the broth requires that the cell fraction be treated cleanly to prevent contamination of subsequent fermentations, and that the cells not be subjected to unnecessary stresses to maintain their viability. However, any live biomass that can be reused reduces the amount of new substrate that is required for biomass growth, as well as reducing the challenges of biomass disposal. Also, an increased concentration of cells can increase the production rate in the fermenter, which will reduce fermentation capital costs. Even if the biomass cannot be recycled viably, if it can at least be recycled cleanly, it can become a nutrient source for later biomass production. Another strategy is reusing some or all of the broth after product separation. Often, optimum product synthesis and biomass growth take place when medium nutrients are present in excess. However, this results in nutrients being left over at the end of fermentation. Reuse of the broth allows a reduction of nutrient addition to the next batch, as well as avoiding the cost of treating a high biochemicaloxygen-demand (BOD) waste stream.

Remove the product during fermentation: In many fermentations, the product acts as an inhibitor to the production reactions. This can limit the concentration that can be achieved in the fermenter. However, as said above, the product concentration in the finished fermentation broth is a clear inverse indicator of cost. Removing the product during fermentation increases the yield by allowing more to be produced from a given amount of biomass, plus increases the production rate by reducing the accumulation of an inhibitory product. Using continuous extraction, a side-stream can be pumped out of the unit and the extracted broth returned to it. Further, two-phase fermentations have been developed to extract the product from a biomass-containing aqueous phase into an organic phase, which can then be removed on-line.

Reduce the water content of the broth: Typically, as much as 90 per cent or more of the broth is water, which must be removed. This is not only costly to separate, but also produces a large aqueous stream that must then be disposed of or recycled. Integrative approaches to water reduction include increasing the biomass concentration [i.e. high-cell-density (HCD) fermentation], engineering the organism to tolerate higher product concentrations, and removing inhibitory elements from the fermentation recipe. Several examples will now illustrate how costs can be kept down. The large-scale fermentation for the production of lactic acid, baker's yeast, and recombinant human albumin embody an integrated approach to process design that integrates the steps listed above to reduce waste-management and production costs.

CRITICAL ISSUES IN FERMENTATION DEVELOPMENT

Irrespective of producing proteins or biomass, HCD yeast biomass production requires aerobic conditions. Due to the low oxygen solubility in aqueous solutions and limited oxygen transfer/cooling capacity in large-scale fermenters, it is necessary to control the specific growth rate of biomass by controlling the carbohydrate feedstock addition-rate to maintain fully aerobic conditions in the fermenter. Concomitant with extremely low specific growth rates, a large amount of consumed sugar carbon is simply burned by the yeast biomass to carbon dioxide to provide energy for cell maintenance. This is a general observed phenomenon with many organisms that reduces the overall product yield in biomass and protein-production processes. In baker's yeast production, low, specific growth rates result in low doughleavening capacity of the final product. Therefore, the focus in the baker's yeast production industry is to improve this parameter at low, specific growth rates.

In heterologous protein production, the specific rate of protein production, q_p, is a key parameter that is rarely reported in the scientific literature. Values of pp generally range from 0.5–2.5 mg/g.h at a growth rate of 0.1 lh and represents generally less than 10 per cent of the overall cellular production rate. Efforts are on understanding the relationship between the specific growth rate of the culture and the specific rate of protein production. This relationship is needed to further optimise the protein expression system with respect to factors such as the stability of expression constructs (over a large number of cell generations), selection markers (cost stability), constitutive vs. inducible promoters, and the dependency on expression conditions, among other factors. As with baker's yeast production, work on HCD protein-production systems also focuses on improving expression levels in slowly growing cultures. Over the past few years, research in this field has been directed towards innovative fermentation process design that can reduce downstream processing costs significantly or even eliminate them completely (as in baker's yeast production). Further, designing new-generation bioprocesses increasingly depend on engineering process-compatible micro-organisms. The latter, whether through genetic or physiological manipulations, can be greatly assisted by metabolic engineering. To achieve these goals, more fundamental knowledge is needed about metabolic pathways, control mechanisms and process dynamics to optimally design integrated systems. This knowledge will enable industry to select the right biocatalyst in clean fermentation processes, as well as introduce and express new or improved properties of the biocatalyst via genetic engineering to facilitate and/or improve downstream processing. Chemical engineers, metabolic/genetic engineers and microbial physiologists will have to work together on this journey.

MICROBIAL GROWTH

Micro-organism require desirable physical chemical and nutritional conditions for their growth. They grow in number as well as in their size. The micro-organism take nutrients from the medium and they use it for the energy production. Partly it is used for the biosynthesis and formation of products.

Microbial cells + substrate $\rightarrow$ more of microbial cells + products (extracellular)

$$X + \Sigma S \rightarrow nX + \Sigma P \qquad \qquad ... (13.1)$$

The growth rate is proportional to the concentration of the cell. Specific growth rate depicts, rate of microbial growth and is represented by:

$$\mu_{net} X = \frac{dx}{dt} \qquad \qquad ... (13.2)$$

where,

X = cell mass concentration (g/l).

t = time (hr).

μ_{net} = specific growth rate (hr^{-1}).

During the growth of microbial cells, they consume material from cells environment and convert them to metabolic end products. Unlike the chemical reactions which depends on only reactants, microbial reactions depend on various like type of cell, their growth, etc. The microbial cells or their unicellular organisms or moulds affect the cell growth and physical and chemical characteristics of reacting medium (Fermentation broth). During the process of microbial growth, nutrients and substrate are consumed simultaneously to convert them into metabolic products and on the different ages of the microbial cells.

Microbial Cell Growth Phases

After inoculation, micro-organism grow in the liquid medium, by consuming the nutrients present in the medium. The growth cure consists of following phases: (i) lag phase, (ii) logarithmic, (or) exponential phase, (iii) stationary phase, and (vi) death phase.

Lag phase

The lag phase starts immediately after inoculating the microbial cells to the growth medium, At this time the microbial cells adjusts themselves to the new environment. Their molecular constituents are reorganised during their transfer to the new medium. The microbial cells synthesise new enzymes suiting to the new-medium while the synthesis of some other enzymes is repressed. During this time the cell mass may be increased and there will not be any change in the number of cells.

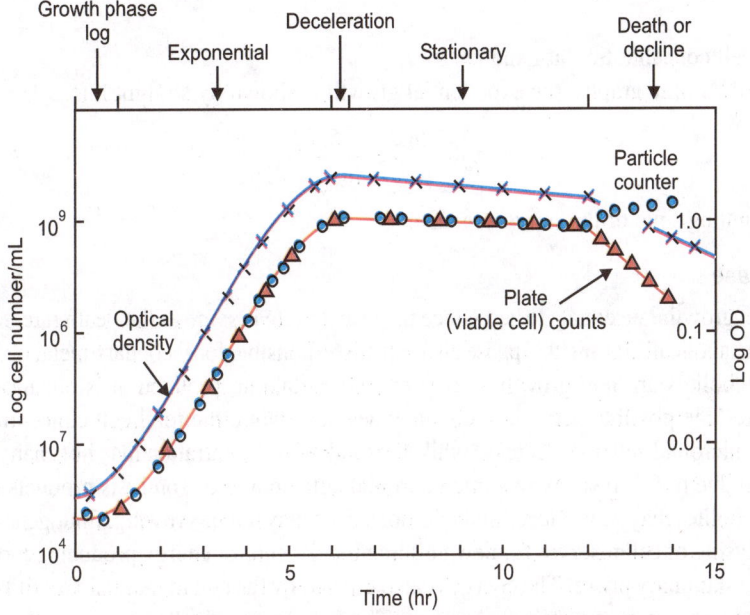

Fig. 13.4. Growth curve for micro-organism (bacteria).

The long lag phase may be caused by the low concentration of nutrients or growth factors. The Inoculum cultures age plays an important role on the lag phase period. Normally the lag phase is proportional to the Inoculum age. The lag phase period may be by adopting the microbial cells to the growth medium prior inoculation. Preferably the microbial cells must by young and active. Also the incoulum size may be sufficient large, i.e. 5–10 per cent by volume. Some growth factors medium be added and optimisation of nutrient medium may be adopted to reduce the lag phase.

Exponential growth phase

During this phase microbial cells which are already adapted to the new environment, start multiplying rapidly. The cells multiply rapidly resulting in increase of cell mass as well as cell number. Interestingly most of the components of the cell grow at the same rate during this phase. Also the net specific growth rate based on cell number or cell mass may be equal. The growth rate is not dependent upon the concentration of nutrients since their concentration is large. The growth rate of organism during this phase follows first order.

$$\frac{dx}{dt} = \mu_{net} X \qquad \qquad ...\,(13.3)$$

$$x = x_0 \text{ at } t = 0$$

upon integration we get,

$$\ln \frac{x}{x_0} = \mu_{net} t \qquad \qquad ... (13.4)$$

or

$$x = x_0 \; e^{\mu_{net}{}^t}$$

where, x, x_0 = cell concentration at t and $t = 0$

In the $\ln x/x_0$ Vs time graphs, the exponential growth is shown by straight line:

$$\tau_d = \frac{\ln 2}{\mu_{net}} = \frac{0.693}{\mu_{net}} \qquad \qquad ... (13.5)$$

where, τ_d = doubling time of the micro-organisms.

Stationary phase

In this phase net growth rate equals to zero since the growth rate is same as the death rate. Microbial cells will be active metabolically during this phase also and are responsible for secondary metabolites production. Secondary metabolites are non-growth associated and metabolic production is enhanced during this stationary phase. The possible activities cells may decrease while the total cell concentration may not change. Viable microbial cell may decrease while the total cell concentration may not change. Viable cells may be reduced due to cell lysis. Also some microbial cells may grow on lysis products of lysed cells. Secondary metabolites may be produced and microbial cells may not be growing. Endogenous metabolism namely catabolysing of cell reserves for new building blocks and for energy producing monomers, takes place during the stationary phase. The energy is also utilised by the cell to maintain motility and repair of damaged structures as a part of metabolic function. The conversion of cell mass into maintenance energy, during stationary phase, can be described by the following equation:

$$\frac{dx}{dt} = -k_d x \qquad \qquad ... (13.6)$$

or

$$X = X_0 \; e^{-kdt}$$

where,

k_d = decay constant or first order rate constant for endogenous metabolism.

X_0 = cell mass concentration at the onset of stationary phase.

The growth of cells may be reduced either due to depletion of essential nutrients or accumulation of toxic compounds or products. The product, which is produced or accumulated in the medium, may inhibit the growth and the inhibitor may stop the growth of cells at an increase to certain level. For example, the ethanol produced during sugar fermentation will inhibit the growth of yeast.

Death phase or decay phase

Even though the decay of cells may be started during stationary phase, the distribution between stationary and decay phase is not always possible. The death or decay phase starts at the end of stationary phase, either due to accumulation of toxic compounds or due to depletion of nutrients which are required for the growth of cells.

The death or decay rate follows first order kinetics and is represented by the following equations:

$$\frac{dN}{dt} = -K_d' N \qquad \qquad \text{... (13.7)}$$

or

$$N = N_s e^{-K' dt}$$

where,

N_s = concentration of cells at the end of stationary phase.

K_d = first order death rate constant.

It is interesting to note that during the onset of death phase, if nutrient rich medium is provided, the same cells may grow again. The cell will die if it is not replenished with nutrient rich medium.

Yield coefficient

Yield coefficient are defined based on consumption of a material:

$$Y_{x/s} = \frac{-\Delta X}{\Delta S} \qquad \qquad \text{... (13.8)}$$

The pattern of-substrate utilisation in a cell can be expressed as given below:

$$\Delta S = \Delta S \quad + \quad \Delta S \quad + \quad \Delta S \quad + \quad \Delta S \qquad \text{... (13.9)}$$

| (Assimilation into biomass) | (assimilated into an extracelluar product) | (growth energy) | (Maintenance energy) |

Yield coefficient based on substrates and products formed.

$$Y_{x/O_2} = -\frac{\Delta X}{\Delta O_2} \qquad \qquad \text{... (13.10)}$$

$$Y_{P/s} = -\frac{\Delta P}{\Delta S} \qquad \qquad \text{... (13.11)}$$

Some typical values of yield coefficient are given in Table 13.1.

Table 13.1. Partial list of yield factors of some microorganism.

Organism	Substrate	Yx/s (g/g)	Y_{x/O_2}(g/g)
Candida	Glucose	0.51	1.32
Penicllium chrysogemum	Glucose	0.43	1.35
Saccharomyces cerviase	Glucose	0.50	0.70
Candida utilis	Acetate	0.36	0.70
Pseudomonoas sp.	Methanol	0.41	0.44
Pseudomonas sp.	Methane	0.80	0.20

Y_{x/O_2} = Yield factor gram of cell formed per gram of O_2 formed.

Specific rate of substrate uptake for cellular maintenance is described by maintenance coefficient:

$$m = -\frac{[ds/dt]_m}{x} \qquad \qquad \text{... (13.12)}$$

Endogenous metabolism of biomass components will be used for maintenance energy during stationary phase since little substrate is available. Microbial products can be basically categorised into three major types (Fig. 13.5).

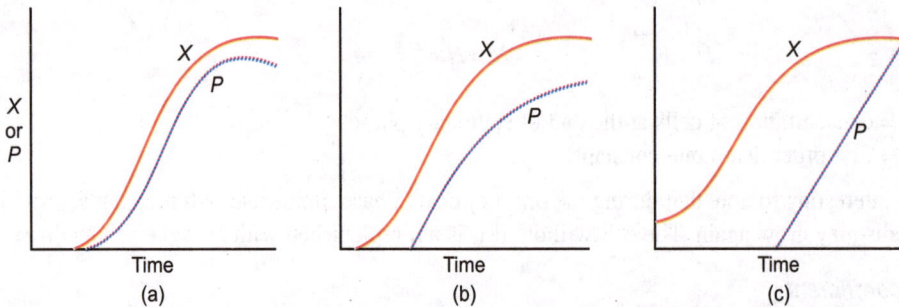

Fig. 13.5. Batch fermentations–Kinetics patterns of growth and product formation: (a) growth associated product formation, (b) mixed growth associated product formation, (c) non-growth associated product formation.

Growth of Filamentous Organism

Growth associated products
The products are formed simultaneously along with microbial growth the specific rate of product formation is directly proportional to specific growth rate μ_g.

μ_g (specific growth rate) differ from μ_{net} (net specific growth rate) when endogenous metabolism is non zero (>0).

$$q_p = \frac{1}{X}\frac{dP}{dt} = Y_{P/X}\mu_g \qquad \qquad \text{... (13.13)}$$

Non-growth associated products
The product formed during stationary phase when there is no growth rate. At time the specific rate of product formation remain constant.

$$q_p = \beta = \text{constant} \qquad \qquad \text{... (13.14)}$$

Mixed growth associated products
These products are formed during slow growth and stationary phase. Here the specific rate of product formation is given by:

$$q_p = \alpha\,\mu g + \beta \qquad \qquad \text{... (13.15)}$$

Examples are lactic acid fermentation and Xanthan gum production. Growth and product formation patterns in fermentations:
1. Growth associated product formation.
2. Mixed growth associated product formation.
3. Non-growth associated product formation.

Luedking–piret equation
If $\alpha = 0$, the product is only non-growth associated and if $\beta = 0$, the product would be only growth associated and consequently a would be equal to $Y_{p/x}$.

Growth Kinetics

The growth of microbial cultures at various stages depends upon the nutrient and also on the inhibition. Various models are used to describe the growth kinetic depending on the available environment to the cells. Models can be: (i) structured and segregated, (ii) structured and non-segregated, and (iii) unstructured and segregated, and (iv) unstructured and non-segregated. Out of all the models, structured and segregated models are realistic but these models are complex in nature. Unstructured and non-segregated models are described here.

Unstructured and non-segregated models:

Substrate limited growth

The specific growth rate and substrate concentration are related to each other as given in the Fig. 13.6

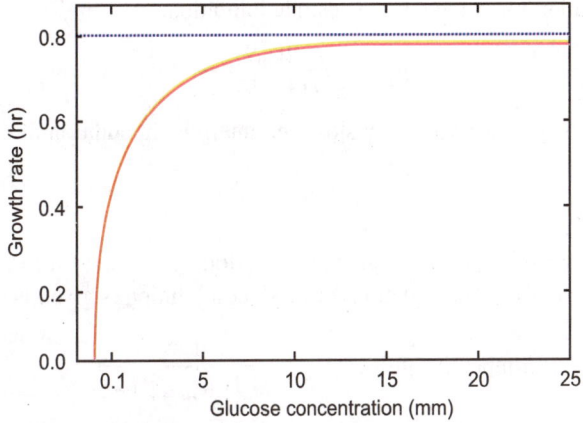

Fig. 13.6. Effect of substrate concentration on specific growth rate.

The growth kinetics can be depicted by Monod equation:

$$\mu_g = \frac{\mu_m S}{K_s + S} \qquad \qquad ... (13.16)$$

where,

$$\mu_m = \text{Maximum specific growth}$$

when $\qquad S >> K_s$

if endogenous metabolism is neglected

then $\qquad \mu_g = \mu_{net}$

K_s is known as saturation constant and it is equal to the concentration of rate limiting substrate when the specific growth rate is equal to the equal one half of the maximum specific growth rate so $K_s = S$

when $-\mu_g > \dfrac{\mu_{max}}{2}$.

Monod equation is often used for many systems satisfactorily and it is the unstructured and non-segregated model. Particularly when the cell growth is slow and population density is low, the Monod equation describes substrate limited growth only. The toxic waste products will be released when the consumption of a carbon-energy substrate is rapid. Also the build up of toxic metabolic by-products becomes very important, at high population levels.

So for rapidly growing dense cultures, the following rate expressions may be used.

$$\mu_g = \frac{\mu_m S}{K_{s0} + S} \qquad \ldots (13.17)$$

$$\mu_g = \frac{\mu_m S}{K_{s1} + K_{s0} s_0 + S} \qquad \ldots (13.18)$$

where,

s_0 = initial concentration of substrate

K_{s0} = dimensional less

Monod equation is often used for many systems satisfactorily and it is the unstructured and non-segregated model. Equation for competitive substrate inhibition.

$$\mu_g = \frac{\mu_m S}{K_s (1 + s/K_1) + S} \qquad \ldots (13.19)$$

Substrate inhibition may be alleviated by slow and intermittent addition of substrate to the growth medium.

Production inhibition

Microbial growth may be inhibited by high concentrations of product. Product inhibition may be competitive or non-competitive. The equation for product inhibition is given here:

$$\text{Competitive product } \mu_g = \frac{\mu_m S}{K_s (1 + p/K_p) + S} \qquad \ldots (13.20)$$

$$\text{Non-competitive inhibition } \mu_g = \frac{\mu_m}{(1 + K_s/S)(1 + P/K_p)} \qquad \ldots (13.21)$$

The example for non-competitive product inhibition is fermentation of glucose by yeast for ethanol production. The product ethanol at more than 5 per cent inhibits the growth yeast.

Toxic compounds inhibition

The equation used for descriptive of toxic compounds inhibition are given here:

$$\text{Competitive inhibition} = \mu_g = \frac{\mu_m S}{K_s (1 + I/K_I) + S} \qquad \ldots (13.22)$$

$$\text{Non-competitive inhibition } \mu_g = \frac{\mu_m}{(1 + K_s/S)(1 + I/K_I)} \qquad \ldots (13.23)$$

The presence of toxic compounds in medium may result in the cell death. The equation for such condition is given here.

$$\mu_g = \frac{\mu_m S}{K_s + S} - k_d \qquad \ldots (13.24)$$

where, k_d = decay rate constant (hr^{-1}).

DISTILLERY YIELDS

Just as in a sugar factory there are a number of measures of operational efficiency in a distillery. In the sugar industry ratios like extraction, boiling house recovery, and overall recovery are well defined and universally understood. Sadly in the alcohol industry things are a little more disorderly. To help bring a little order the following is offered.

Theory

There are four commonly used measures of yield:
1. Fermentation yield.
2. Fermentation efficiency.
3. Alcohol recovery.
4. Overall conversion efficiency.

Fermentation Yield

Fermentation yield is measured in litres of absolute alcohol in beer per ton of sugars in molasses, and is calculated by the formula below:

$$Y_f = V_b \cdot a_b / (M_m \cdot {}_f s_m)$$

where,

Y_f = fermentation yield.
V_b = volume of beer [litre].
a_b = alcohol content of beer (v/v).
M_m = mass of molasses [tonne].
${}_f s_m$ = fermentable sugars content of molasses (m/m).

Fermentation Efficiency

Fermentation efficiency is an expression of how much alcohol was actually produced in beer relative to the amount that could be theoretically produced, and is given by

$$E_f = Y_f \cdot 0.794/0.5111 \times (100/1000)$$

The factor 0.794 corresponds to the specific gravity of absolute alcohol and the factor 0.5111 is best explained as follows:

If one kilogram of sugar was completely fermented (using theoretical 100 per cent efficient yeast); 511.1 grams of alcohol and $1000 - 511.1 = 488.9$ grams of carbon dioxide would result.

Alcohol Recovery

Alcohol recovery is a measure of how much alcohol was finally produced relative to the amount that was in the beer. It shows the amount of losses in the evaporation and distillation sections combined. Alcohol recovery is calculated as follows:

$$E_{de} = ({}_{aa}V_p + {}_{ss}V_f)/{}_{aa}V_b \cdot 100$$

where,

E_{de} = Alcohol recovery (or distillation and evaporation efficiency).
${}_{aa}V_p$ = volume of potable alcohol as litres absolute alcohol.
${}_{ss}V_f$ = volume of feints as litres absolute alcohol.
${}_{aa}V_b$ = volume of beer as litres absolute alcohol.

Overall Conversion Efficiency

Overall conversion efficiency is a measure of how much alcohol is finally produced relative to the amount that could be theoretically produced, and is given by:

$$E_o = E_f \cdot E_{de} \cdot 100$$

Values of Yield

Table 13.2 gives values of yield that one would expect in a well run distillery.

Table 13.2. Values of yield.

Parameter	Value
Alcohol Recovery	98.5%
Fermentation Yield	57.3%
Fermentation Efficiency	89%
Overall Conversion Efficiency	87%

BIOREACTOR

Bioreactor design is essential for developing a product of commercial significance. The laboratory reactors are operated at optimum conditions like mixing and flow characteristics. The reactor size and scale will be considered here and its effect on flow, mixing, mass and heat transfer patterns with the bioreactor.

The bioreactor systems need special attention due to the involvement of micro-organisms as biocatalysts and free enzymes of microbial origin.

The kinetics of the bioreactions depend on the cell growth of micro-organisms and rate of substrate consumption. The morphology of the cells also gives the overall reaction. Bioenergetics, stoichiometry, batch and continuous sterilisation also play an important role during the design of bioreactors.

Types of Bioreactors

The different types of bioreactors are used in biotechnology process include, batch bioreactors, continuous stirred tank reactors, fed batch bioreactor, air lift bioreactor and fluidised bed bioreactor. The general description of each type is given here.

Batch bioreactor

All the reactants are fed to the batch bioreactor initially during startup of the bioreactors. During the reaction there will not be any in-flow or out-flow from the system. These batch bioreactors are frequently used for small scale operations, for producing expensive chemicals and for developing new products. However, most of the pharmaceutical products are made by using batch type bioreactors only.

Continuous reactors

Continuous reactors normally mean continuous flow stirred tank reactors (Fig. 13.7). The mixing will be good due to vigorous stirring and uniform temperature could be maintained. The in-flow and out-flow will be continuous and, product can be withdrawn continuously. Product quality could be controlled by online analysis of the out-flow stream, Mostly for continuous cultivation of organisms, these types of bioreactors are used.

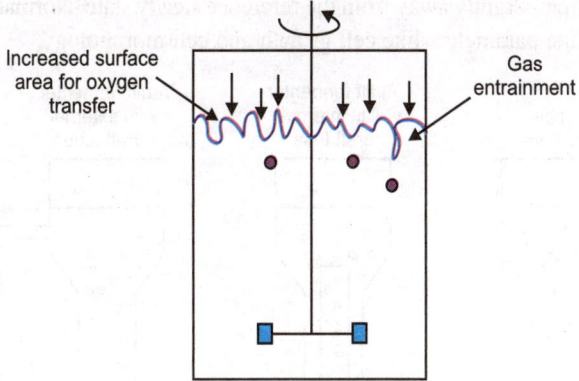

Fig. 13.7. Continuous stirred tank reactor.

Fed batch bioreactors

These types of bioreactors are used frequently for improving yields of various products. The nutrients, substrates are depleted during biochemical reactions. So, if the nutrients and substrate are fed continuously to the bioreactor, probably the product yield may be enhanced. The product will be removed after the batch is over. One of the advantages of these types of reactors is that the concentration of the limiting substrate may be maintained at a very low level, thus avoiding the repressive effects of high substrate concentration. The production of bakers yeast was achieved by using fed batch bioreactors.

Airlift bioreactors

In these reactors (Fig. 13.8), mixing and internal circulation is achieved by passing air through the reactor contents. Air is passed through the spargers at high velocities into the riser. The difference of density between the liquid column in the riser and the liquid column in the down comer, will be the driving force for circulation of the medium in the airlift bioreactor. Circulation times in loops of 45 m height may be 120 seconds. These types of bioreactors may be used for producing SCP (single cell protein).

Bubble column bioreactors

The bioreactors with large aspect ratio that is height to diameter ratio may be known as bubble column bioreactors. Mixing in these types of bioreactors is achieved by forcing compressed gas through the reactor contents. The operating costs of these reactors are low due to low energy requirement. These bioreactors may be operated either in batch mode or in continuous mode.

Fluidised bed bioreactors

Solid fluid contact may be achieved in these types of bioreactors. The fluid is pumped from the bottom from perforations and the solid particles are taken in the reactor. When the fluid velocity is increased the solid particles will get fluidised. The gravitational force, acting down on the particle, is counter acted by the buoyancy forces by the fluid going up. Mostly the fluidised bed bioreactors are used in waste-water treatment systems.

Stability of bioreactors

The designing and control of bioreactor systems involves the stability of the bioreactor. When a steady state is locally stable, the system concentration will return to the steady state even after a small distance moves those concentrations slightly away from the reference steady state. Normally the stable bioreactor system is governed by the parameters like cell growth and cell morphology.

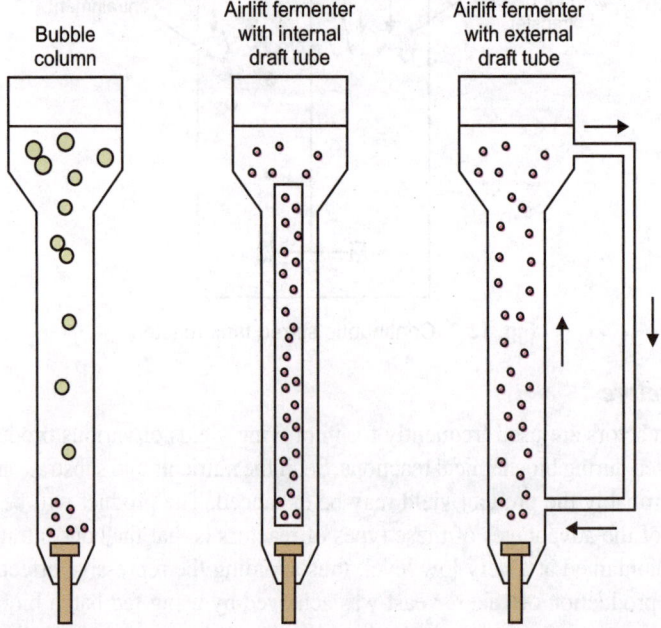

Fig. 13.8. Airlift fermenter.

Bioreactor Dynamics

The dynamic characteristics of the bioreactors are considered here. The dynamics of continuous stirred tank reactor (CSTR) are considered which may be further extrapolated to other type's reactors. Initially, for unsteady state reactor performance the equations are developed. The dynamic model proposed by Bailey and Ollis for unsteady state is d/dt (total amount in the reactor) = rate of addition to reactor- rate of removal from reactor + rate of formation within the reactor.

So in a CSTR,

$$\frac{d(Vc_i)}{dt} = v(c_{io} - c_i) + vr_{fi} \qquad \dots (13.25)$$

where,

V = volume of the reactor.

v = volumetric feed rate.

r_{fi} = rate of formation of component 'i' in the reactor.

c_i = local concentration of component 'i' in the reactor.

c_{io} = concentration of component 'i' in the feed.

(Equation 13.25), dividing by v and where D (dilution rate) = v/V, becomes,

$$\frac{d(c_i)}{dt} = D(c_{io} - c_i) + r_{fi} \qquad \dots (13.26)$$

In the above material balance, it is assumed that the feed stream and reactor contents have equal density and inlet and out-let volumetric flow rates are equal. The unsteady state material balance will be the starting point for reactor dynamics characterisation. The dynamic characteristics of bioreactor are a function of concentration changes fc_i and function of parameter changes.

Now we will consider the situation where single substrate limits the growth cells and the performance of a bioreactor. Upon application of unsteady state mass balance to growth of cells and substrate consumption and by using Monod expression, gives:

$$\frac{dx}{dt} = D(x_o - x) + \frac{\mu_{max} s x}{k_s + s} \qquad \qquad \text{... (13.27)}$$

$$\frac{ds}{dt} = D(s_o - s) - \frac{1}{y_{x/s}} \frac{\mu_{max} s_x x}{x + k_s} \qquad \qquad \text{... (13.28)}$$

In the (Eq. 13.27), for sterile feed $x_o = 0$. There are two possible states.

1. Non-initial steady state solution.

$$X_{ss} = Y_{x/s}(s_R - s_{ss})$$

$$s_{ss} = \frac{k_s(D)}{\mu_{max} - D}$$

2. Washout steady state situation.

$$X = 0, s = s_o$$

The Monod-Chemostate study results for steady state washout condition are given as for:

1. $D \geq \dfrac{\mu_{max} s_o}{K_s + s_o}$ Chemostat performance is stable.

2. $D \leq \dfrac{\mu_{max} s_o}{K_s + s_o}$ Chemostat performance is unstable.

Biomass Production

Considering the cell balance across the reactor.
We have,

$$\frac{dx}{dt} = D(x_o - x) + \frac{\mu_{max} s x}{k_s + s}$$

At steady state condition, $dx/dt = 0$
So,

$$\left[\frac{\mu_{max} s}{K_s + s}\right] x + D x_o = 0 \qquad \qquad \text{... (13.29)}$$

The balance on substrate gives:

$$\frac{dx}{dt} = D(s_o - s) - \frac{1}{y_{x/s}} \frac{\mu_{max} s x}{k_s + s} \qquad \qquad \text{... (13.30)}$$

At steady state $ds/dt = 0$

$$0 = D(s_o - s) - \frac{1}{y_{x/s}} \frac{\mu_{max} s\, x}{k_s + s} \qquad \text{... (13.31)}$$

Equations 13.29 and 13.31 are called as monod chemostat model.

For a sterile feed $x_o = 0$, Eqs 13.29 and 13.31 can be solved to yield equation.

$$X_{ss} = Y_{x/s}(s_R - s_s) \qquad \text{... (13.32)}$$

$$s_{ss} = \frac{K_s D}{\mu_{max} - D}$$

Hence the steady state condition depends on dilution rate 'D'. For very slow flows at a given volume when dilution rate tends to zero S_{ss} tends to zero. The cell mass concentration X_{ss} will be equal to $= Y_{x/s}(S_R)$.

It is seen that with the increase of 'D', s initially increase linearly (Fig 13.9). After a point 'P' in the Figure, since increase rapidly as dilution rate approaches μ_{max} and as s_{ss} become very high, X_{ss} and this condition is known as 'washout'.

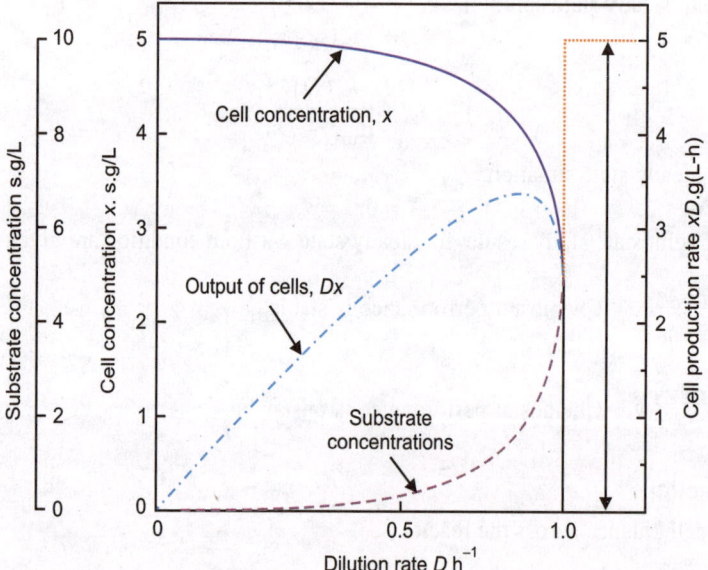

Fig. 13.9. Dependence of effluent substrate concentration s, cell concentration x, and cell production rate xD on continuous culture dilution rate D (Monod Chemostat).

Thus, D_{max} becomes:

$$D_{max} = \frac{\mu_{max}\, s_R}{K_s + s_R} \qquad \text{... (13.33)}$$

Also the cell output, i.e. x. D will be increased rapidly till the point P and decelerating sharply. Bailey and Ollis predict maximum value of cell production to avoid the region of large sensitivity.

Batch Reactors

In biochemical processes, it is always essential to add liquid streams to batch reactor during the process. Mostly, liquid streams such as nutrients, precursors, inducers, etc. are added so as to minimise catabolic repression. The liquid streams may be added in the process to extend stationary phase and to obtain additional products by adding nutrients. The culture volume altered when a liquid feed stream is added to the reactor, and described in equations.

$$\frac{d}{dt}[V_R.C_i] = V_R.r_{fi} + F(t) \qquad \text{... (13.34)}$$

where,

$F(t)$ = volumetric flow rate of entering feed stream.

C_i = stream moles i/unit volume of cells.

$C_{i_f}(t)$ = concentration of components 'i' in the entering stream.

r_{fi} = molar rate of formation of component 'l'.

V_R = culture volume.

It is assumed that the density will be 'ρ' for entering liquid stream and culture liquid.

$$\frac{d}{dt} = [\rho.V_R] = \rho.F(t) \qquad \text{... (13.35)}$$

Now if 'ρ' does not change with time during batch process.

$$\frac{dV_R}{dt} = F(t) \qquad \text{... (13.36)}$$

Carrying out differentiation of equation and upon dividing (Eq. 13.34) by V_R and substituting in (Eq. 13.36) given:

$$\frac{dC_i}{dt} = \frac{F(t)}{V_R}(C_{if} - C_i) + r_{fi} \qquad \text{... (13.37)}$$

Equations 13.36 and 13.37 are mass and component balance equation respectively.

Enzyme catalysed reactions in CSTRS

The enzyme catalysed reaction can be carried out in a variety of CSTRs (Fig 13.10). The various configurations are given below.

In a simple system: (i) enzymes are added to reactor and removed from the reactor through feed at out let streams. This is applied when the enzymes are cheaply available. Different configuration of CSTRs will be used for costly enzymes, (ii) ultra filtration membrane is used in the effluent stream which retains the enzymes in the reactor, (iii) a screen is filled in the effluent line which prevents the escape of enzymes, (iv) enzymes are attached to the agitated shafts in screen baskets, and (v) enzymes are fixed in packed column through which the reactor contents are circulated.

The main objective of the various reactor configuration is to maintain desired enzymes concentration inside the reactor. Applying the basic principles of material balances, substrate and product concentration could be estimated. Considering the basic equation,

$$S \rightarrow P$$

If 1 mol of product P is for each mole of substrate 'S' and the feed (S_0, P_0) and effluent concentration. (S, P) are depicted as,

$$S_0 - S = P - P_0 \qquad \text{... (13.38)}$$

The substrate mass balance considering reaction rate expression $v(s,p)$ can be written as,

$$F(s_0 - s) - V_R v(s, P_0 + s_0 - s) = 0 \qquad \text{... (13.39)}$$

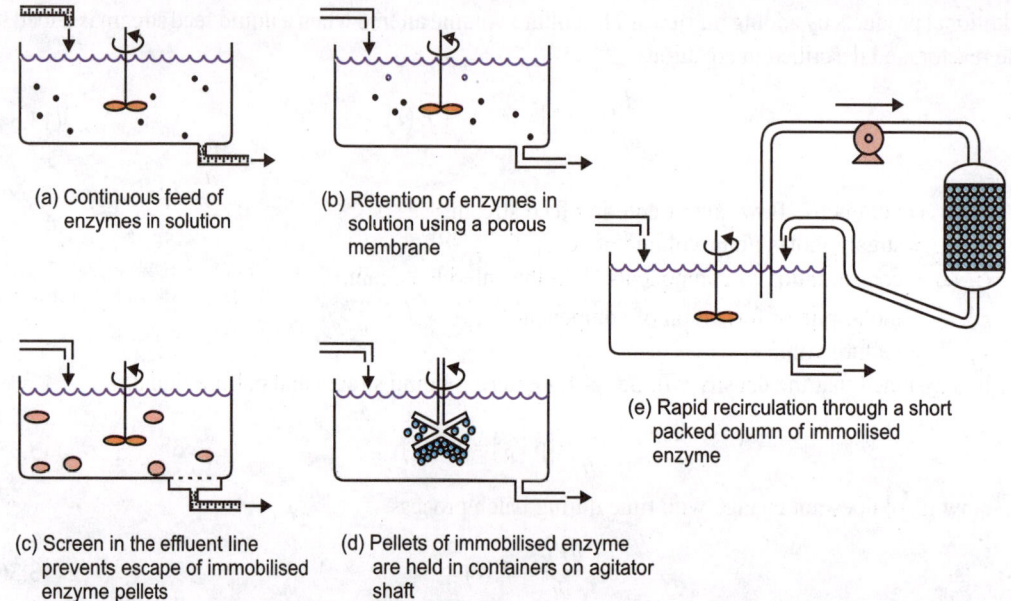

(a) Continuous feed of enzymes in solution

(b) Retention of enzymes in solution using a porous membrane

(c) Screen in the effluent line prevents escape of immobilised enzyme pellets

(d) Pellets of immobilised enzyme are held in containers on agitator shaft

(e) Rapid recirculation through a short packed column of immoilised enzyme

Fig. 13.10. CSTR systems for immobilised reactions.

CSTR with cell cycle and cell growth

The CSTR with a separator at out let stream and recycle from separator to feed will enhance biomass in reactor and results in increase in product yield. This shown in the (Fig. 13.11).

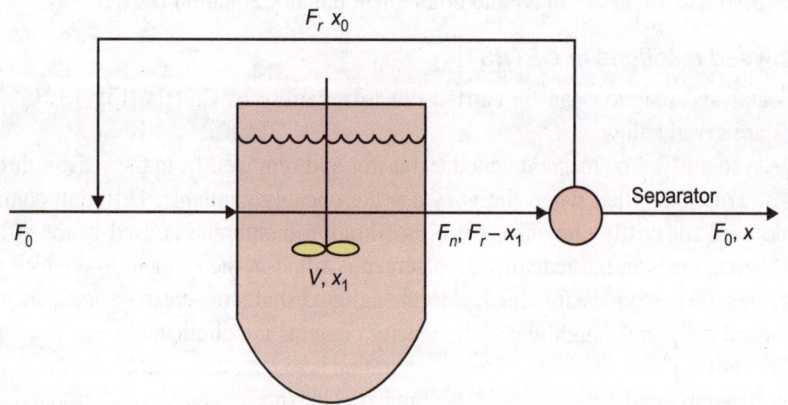

Fig. 13.11. CSTR with recycle.

where,

F_0, F_r = feed and recycle volumetric flow rates.

x_1, x_0, x = reactor, recycle stream and products streams biomass concentrations.

The steady state biomass considerations equation for recycle is given as,

$$F_r x_0 + \mu x_1 V_R - (F_0 + F_r) x_1 = 0 \qquad \dots (13.40)$$

where,

$A = F_r/F_0$

$b = x_0/x_1$

The dilution rate is separated as,

$$D = \frac{\mu}{1 - a(b-1)}$$ ... (13.41)

The micro-organism in recycle liquid is more concentrated than the micro-organisms in the effluent and b>1.

It is known from the Eq. 13.41 that dilution rate D is larger than organism specific growth rate μ.

It can be visualised that reactor with recycle can process more feed material than the reactor without recycle. The substrate balance upon assumption of constant yield factor is:

$$D = (S_0 - S) - \frac{\mu x_1}{Y} = 0$$ ... (13.42)

After combining Eqs 13.41 with 13.42 the biomass production rate per unit reactor volume μ_x, is:

$$\mu x_1 = \frac{\mu Y(S_0 - S)}{1 - a(b-1)}$$ ... (13.43)

Recycle production rate is greater by $[1 - a(b-1)]^{-1}$ than non-recycle production rate.

During cell cultivation, it is observed that the dilution rates are high without washout, than observed ideal CSTR. This is possible because of growth of cells on the wall.

The organism will be seen as solid films on the reactor wall. Now-considering cells on the film at the reactor, may be above reactor liquid level as x_f. The cells reproduced on solid films at the reactor-could fall back into the reactor.

The steady state continuous reactor mass balance will be in the form,

$$D_x = \mu_x + \mu_f x_f$$ ... (13.44)

$$D(s_0 - s) = \frac{1}{\tau}\mu x + \frac{1}{Y_f}\mu_f x_f$$ ... (13.45)

where,

μ_f = specific growth in the film.

Y_f = yield factor in the film.

This may offer from μ and Y for various reasons including diffusion reactions.

Ideal plug flow reactors

The plug flow is expected when fluid moves in large channel or in pipe with high Reynolds number, i.e. more than 2100 in a pipe and there is no variation of axial velocity over the cross-section. In contrast to ideally mixed bioreactor, there is no mixing in, plug flow reactor (Fig 13.12). The length to diameter ratio is high in plug flow reactor. Substrate enters from one side and leaves process other side while the reaction takes place by microbial population within the reactor. The concentration of substrate decreases as it flows along the bioreactor since there is no mixing in the bioreactor. However the substrate concentration will be uniform in the completely mixed bioreactor. The packed bed immobilised bioreactor behave like plug flow bioreactor.

It is assumed that plug flow prevails in the bioreactor; the mass balance can be made by differential section approach in plug flow reactor.

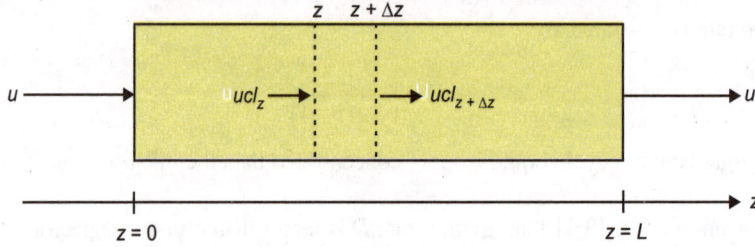

Fig. 13.12. Ideal plug flow reactor.

The mass balance on the section can be taken as,

$$Avc|_z - Avc|_{z+\Delta z} + A\Delta_z r_{fc}|_z = 0 \qquad (13.46)$$

where,

r_{fc} = rate of formation of species.

c = amount/unit volume . time

Rearranging and dividing by $A\Delta_z$ we get,

$$\frac{Vc|_{z+\Delta z} - V|_z}{\Delta z} = r_{fc} \qquad \ldots (13.47)$$

Taking limits

$$\frac{d}{dz}(vc) = r_{fi} \qquad \ldots (13.48)$$

Upon assuming no change in density during reaction, the axial velocity will be constant and Eq. 13.48 changes to,

$$\frac{dc}{dz} = r_{fc} \qquad \ldots (13.49)$$

The time required to move one fluid section from entry point of reactor to position of z is z/v.

Is

$$t = \frac{z}{v} \qquad \ldots (13.50)$$

The mass balance Eq. 13.49 can be written as,

$$\frac{dc}{dt} = r_{fc} \qquad \ldots (13.51)$$

Equation 13.51 is same as the mass balance equation of batch reactor. The plug flow with constant velocity and each segment moves with no interaction, with neighboring segments. The system is totally segregated and each segment behaves as a batch bioreactor. Also if the initial feed to batch reactor and feed at entry point of plug flow reactor are same and L/v the residence time of PFR is same as batch time, then the tube effluent will be same as batch reactor effluent.

So the boundary condition for this will be:

$$C|_{z=0} = C_0 \qquad \ldots (13.52)$$

where,

Z = 0 inlet to reactor.

C_0 = concentration of feed at inlet.

If Monod Chemostat is applicable to PFR,

The mass balance on cells and substrate would be,

$$\frac{dx}{dt} = \frac{\mu_{max} \, x_s}{s + k_s}$$ ... (13.53)

$$\frac{ds}{dt} = \frac{1}{Y} \frac{\mu_{max} \, x_s}{s + k_s}$$ ... (13.54)

Applying initial conditions

$$x(0) = x_0$$
$$s(0) = s_0$$ ... (13.55)

Equation 13.53 and 13.54 upon computations and substrate and cell concentration, can be stoichiometrically written as,

$$X + Y_s = x_s + Y_{so}$$ ... (13.56)

Using Eq. 13.56 and expression x in terms of s, and substituting in Eq. 13.53, we get

$$\frac{ds}{dt} = \frac{\mu_{max \, s}}{Y} \frac{\left[x_0 + Y(s_0 - s) \right] s}{s + k_s}$$ ... (13.57)

Integration of this and applying initial conditions, we get,

$$x_0 + Y(s_o + K_s) \ln \frac{x_0 + Y(s - s_0)s}{x_0} - K_s Y \ln \frac{s}{s_0} = \mu_{max} t (x_0 + Y_{so})$$ ... (13.58)

The outlet substrate concentration will be s value with respect to $t = L/v$ and then x is formed with Eq. 13.56.

Residence Time Distribution Concept

What would be the fate of small segment of fluid which enters the continuous flow bioreactor? This small segment of fluid will be further reduced to smaller particle due to mixing in the reactor and disperse throughout the bioreactor. Of course, some part of these smaller particles will reach effluent stream. Nevertheless the remaining particles would be spending various times before actually reaching the effluent stream. Hence the effluent stream would be the mixtures of various particles that have resided for different length of time inside the bioreactor. Now the determination of residence times of the particles at the effluent stream will give the information about mixing and flow patterns in the bioreactor.

Stimulus—response studies are conducted by introducing tracer as stimulus to know the extent of stay of elements inside the bioreactor. The tracer is selected such that, it has the following characteristics.

1. It will not react with the reactants.
2. It will be easily detected.
3. It will not disturb the flow pattern

Tracers like salts, acids or base or hydrocarbon gas are introduced either as step input or as pulse input. The stimulus and response features are depicted in the Fig. 13.13

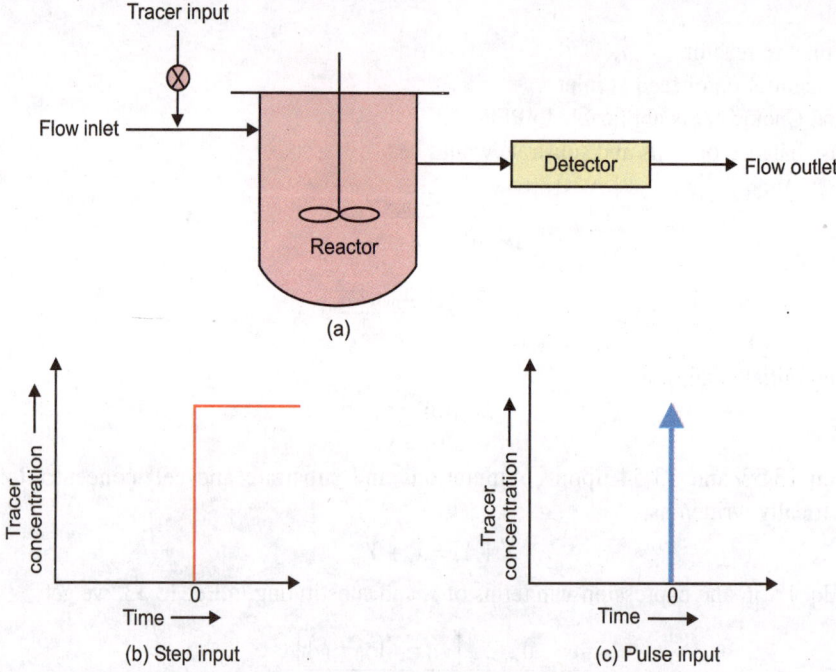

Fig. 13.13. Stimulus response studies on CSTR.

MICROBIAL FUEL CELL

A microbial fuel cell (MFC) or biological fuel cell is a bioelectrochemical system that drives a current by mimicking bacterial interactions found in nature. Mediator-less MFCs are a much more recent development and due to this the factors that affect optimum operation, such as the bacteria used in the system, the type of ion membrane, and the system conditions such as temperature, are not particularly well understood. Bacteria in mediatorless MFCs typically have electrochemically active redox enzymes such as cytochromes on their outer membrane that can transfer electrons to external materials. A typical microbial fuel cell consists of anode and cathode compartments separated by a cation (positively charged ion) specific membrane. In the anode compartment, fuel is oxidised by micro-organisms, generating electrons and protons. Electrons are transferred to the cathode compartment through an external electric circuit, and the protons are transferred to the cathode compartment through the membrane. Electrons and protons are consumed in the cathode compartment, combining with oxygen to form water. In general, there are two types of microbial fuel cells: mediator and mediator-less microbial fuel cells.

Mediator Microbial Fuel Cell

Most of the microbial cells are electrochemically inactive. The electron transfer from microbial cells to the electrode is facilitated by mediators such as thionine, methyl viologen, methyl blue, humic acid, neutral red and so on. Most of the mediators available are expensive and toxic.

Mediator-less Microbial Fuel Cell

Mediator-less microbial fuel cells can, besides running on waste-water, also derive energy directly from certain aquatic plants. These include reed sweetgrass, cordgrass, rice, tomatoes, lupines, and algae.

These microbial fuel cells are called plant microbial fuel cells (Plant-MFC). Given that the power is thus derived from a living plant (*in situ* energy production), this variant can provide extra ecological advantages.

Generating Electricity

When micro-organisms consume a substrate such as sugar in aerobic conditions they produce carbon dioxide and water. However when oxygen is not present they produce carbon dioxide, protons and electrons as described below:

$$C_{12}H_{22}O_{11} + 13H_2O \rightarrow 12CO_2 + 48H^+ + 48e^- \qquad \ldots (13.59)$$

Microbial fuel cells use inorganic mediators to tap into the electron transport chain of cells and steal the electrons that are produced. The mediator crosses the outer cell lipid membranes and plasma wall; it then begins to liberate electrons from the electron transport chain that would normally be taken up by oxygen or other intermediates. The reduced mediator exits the cell laden with electrons that it shuttles to an electrode where it deposits them; this electrode becomes the electro-generic anode (negatively charged electrode). The release of the electrons means that the mediator returns to its original oxidised state ready to repeat the process. It is important to note that this can only happen under anaerobic conditions, if oxygen is present then it will collect all the electrons as it has a greater electronegativity than the mediator.

In a microbial fuel cell operation, the anode is the terminal electron acceptor recognised by bacteria in the anodic chamber. Therefore, the microbial activity is strongly dependent on the redox potential of the anode. In fact, it was recently published that a Michaelis-Menten curve was obtained between the anodic potential and the power output of an acetate driven microbial fuel cell. A critical anodic potential seemed to exists at which a maximum power output of a microbial fuel cell is achieved.

A number of mediators have been suggested for use in microbial fuel cells. These include natural red, methylene blue, thionine or resorfuin.

This is the principle behind generating a flow of electrons from most micro-organisms (the organisms capable of producing an electrical current are termed Exoelectrogens. In order to turn this into a usable supply of electricity this process has to be accommodated in a fuel cell.

In order to generate a useful current it is necessary to create a complete circuit, not just shuttle electrons to a single point.

The mediator and micro-organism, in this case yeast, are mixed together in a solution to which is added a suitable substrate such as glucose. This mixture is placed in a sealed chamber to stop oxygen entering, thus forcing the micro-organism to use anaerobic respiration. An electrode is placed in the solution that will act as the anode as described previously.

In the second chamber of the MFC is another solution and electrode. This electrode, called the cathode is positively charged and is the equivalent of the oxygen sink at the end of the electron transport chain, only now it is external to the biological cell. The solution is an oxidising agent that picks up the electrons at the cathode. As with the electron chain in the yeast cell, this could be a number of molecules such as oxygen. However, this is not particularly practical as it would require large volumes of circulating gas. A more convenient option is to use a solution of a solid oxidising agent.

Connecting the two electrodes is a wire (or other electrically conductive path which may include some electrically powered device such as a light bulb) and completing the circuit and connecting the two chambers is a salt bridge or ion-exchange membrane. This last feature allows the protons produced, as described in Eq. 13.59 to pass from the anode chamber to the cathode chamber.

The reduced mediator carries electrons from the cell to the electrode. Here the mediator is oxidised as it deposits the electrons. These then flow across the wire to the second electrode, which acts as an electron sink. From here they pass to an oxidising material.

Uses

Microbial fuel cells have a number of potential uses. The first and most obvious is harvesting the electricity produced for a power source. Virtually any organic material could be used to 'feed' the fuel cell. MFCs could be installed to waste-water treatment plants. The bacteria would consume waste material from the water and produce supplementary power for the plant. The gains to be made from doing this are that MFCs are a very clean and efficient method of energy production.

DOWNSTREAM PROCESSING

Recombinant proteins synthesised by bacterial, animal, plant or fungal cells are either stored in or secreted from these cells. For easy downstream processing, the secretion of proteins from cells is preferred since the proteins can be harvested fairly easily from the simpler extracellular environment. It is common for animal and fungal cells to secrete recombinant proteins. However, in simple prokeryotic bacterial cells and in plants recombinant proteins are generally stored inside the cell in some sort of storage space, a vesicle, granule or vacuole for example. This results in the relatively more difficult isolation and purification of protein from the more complicated cytoplasm of the cell.

If isolating and purifying recombinant proteins from bacterial cells, the cell must be treated in various ways to release the recombinant proteins from their storage sites in the cytoplasm. Once released the protein can be separated from the rest of the cellular contents by centrifugation or by filtration. Human proteins made in bacterial cells may not be folded or may be improperly folded so a refolding step or steps might be necessary before final isolation and purification. Proteins made in transgenic plants would present similar technical problems.

Proteins made in animal and fungal cells are, by-in-large, secreted so they are easier to separate from the surrounding medium. The first step in downstream processing of such secreted proteins would be to separate the medium containing the proteins from the cells that secreted them. In downstream processing using bioreactors and suspension cells this would usually be effected by centrifugation or filtration. In downstream processing of recombinant proteins secreted by transgenic animals the fluid containing human proteins is often ascites fluid or milk. If the protein is in ascites fluid secreted by a hybridoma in a mouse, a syringe could draw off the 10 ml or so of fluid rich in human protein; if the protein is in the milk of a goat or sheep, a simple mechanical milking could remove the fluid containing the human protein. Liquid chromatography and membrane filtration processes are then used to removed the desired human protein from other proteins and contaminants in the medium and to concentrate the desired human protein.

In liquid chromatography a solid support is used to trap a desired protein. The desired protein in its fluid medium is loaded onto a column, is trapped by the solid support, the column is washed, and the desired protein is bumped off the column using an eluting buffer with a predetermined pH and ionic strength. Today, the types of chromatography most often used to separate a desired human protein from other materials are ion exchange and affinity chromatography. Another type of liquid chromatography that is gaining more interest is gel filtration (also known as molecular sieving or size exclusion) chromatography. Ion exchange chromatography, based on electrostatic interactions between the solid support and the molecular species to be separated, is used extensively because it is fairly inexpensive. Affinity chromatography is very expensive. However, it is the most selective medium because it is based on lock and key interactions between the solid support and the molecular species to be separated.

Preparative chromatography is carried out during research and development. During preparative chromatography, methods are worked out to ensure that the protein of interest will be separated at the lowest cost with the highest yield and purity. Bench scale liquid chromatography systems and fraction collectors, along with protein standards, are employed to isolate the protein of interest from the medium and determine the best separation conditions. Protein electrophoresis is used as a companion to liquid chromatography and the fractions are electrophoresed with standards to confirm the location of a particular protein in a particular fraction, to determine the purity of the protein of interest and to determine the protein's molecular weight. The isoelectric point (pI) of the protein can also be determined using a protein gel box and a technique known as isoelectric focusing (IEF). The isoelectric porint is the point at which the protein carries equal numbers of negative and positive charges. Knowing the pI can be helpful in separating a protein by liquid chromatography. A 'rule of thumb' is that the protein can be most easily separated at a pH a little above or below its isoelectric point.

Preparative chromatography and electrophoresis would be accompanied by bench-scale methods development, followed by large scale column chromatography using the same or a slightly modified process that would be validated. Among other things, the expected yield would be calculated for the protein of interest for each batch of medium of a certain size received from fermentation or upstream processing. A measure of the efficiency of column packing or (HETP) would also be made each time the column is packed to help to ensure reproducibility of the chromatographic process.

There could be many contaminants in the medium which must be removed during the chromatographic process or before or after chromatography used to isolate the protein of interest. Contaminants of animal cells might include: prions, viruses, micro-organisms such as *Mycoplasma* species, and DNA. There do not seem to be many contaminants of yeast cells and other fungi.

Chapter 14

Genetic Engineering of Plants

INTRODUCTION

Genetic engineering can be used to introduce specific traits into plants. It will not replace conventional breeding but can add to the efficiency of crop improvement. It is possible due to the fact that plants are totipotent, enabling regeneration of a new plant from an isolated cell. Transformation of dicots is usually carried out using the bacterium, *Agrobacterium tumefaciens*. Genes are cloned into plant expression vectors that carry the right and left border sequences. They are introduced into plants with the aid of a disarmed Ti plasmid whose virulence gene products allow the genes to be transferred to the plant nucleus where they are integrated into the genome. Monocots are usually transformed by a biolistic process, using a 'gene gun'. In both cases callus tissue is regenerated on media containing an antibiotic or herbicide to select for transformants. The exception is transformation of the common wall cress, *Arabidopsis thaliana*, where tissue culture is not required. Gene silencing, whereby plants shut off the expression of multiple copies of a gene, can be a problem when attempting to introduce a new trait into a plant. Although the process is not fully understood it can, at the level of transcription, be due to methylation or ectopic DNA pairing. At the post-transcriptional level, the transgene RNA could be specifically degraded if tagged by a small complementary RNA molecule. It is often advantageous for plants to express the introduced transgenes in specific tissues or under specific conditions. As a result many genes are cloned downstream of tissue-specific or inducible promoters. High expression of a transgene may be required under certain circumstances. The 35S promoter of the cauliflower mosaic virus is commonly used in dicots while the maize ubiquitin promoter is the monocot promoter of choice. Targetting genes to organelles such as chloroplasts can also enhance expression. Little is understood of the way in which genes are integrated into the plant chromosomes. In many cases multiple inserts occur at one locus. The field of plant genetic engineering is a fascinating one and will continue to grow in efficiency and sophistication in the years to come.

Conventional plant breeding has succeeded in producing a wide variety of commercial plants and crops with a range of important agronomic traits. It has succeeded in converting a Mexican grass into maize and Middle East grass into wheat. However, it is to a large extent a hit-or-miss process, combining large parts of parental genomes in a rather uncontrolled fashion, although this is currently being improved due to the modern technique of marker assisted breeding. Genetic engineering, on the other hand, allows scientists to transfer very specific genes into plants, resulting in the introduction of one or more defined traits into a particular genetic background. This process is called transformation and the genes involved are expressed to form a protein responsible for the particular trait. The traits involved include herbicide and drought tolerance, and resistance to viral, bacterial and fungal pathogens as well as to herbivorous insects. The added advantage is that the transferred gene(s), or transgene(s), can come from any organism as long as its expression is compatible with its new host.

Plant transformation is possible due to the fact that plants are totipotent, enabling regeneration of a new plant from an isolated cell. Thus if a gene is transferred to a plant genome in a cell the regenerated plant will contain that gene in every cell. In practice the gene(s) of interest are introduced together with a selectable marker such as resistance to a herbicide or antibiotic to which the plant is sensitive. Cells and regenerating plants are grown in gel-like media containing that herbicide or antibiotic and only plants expressing the genes for resistance will grow. The hormone auxin is used to initiate and maintain callus. Once cells have been transformed, cytokinin hormones are incorporated into the medium to allow shoot development. Withdrawal of cytokinin promotes root growth. Once plants are fully developed they are taken out of the media and planted in soil for 'hardening off'. The process is shown diagrammatically in Fig. 14.1.

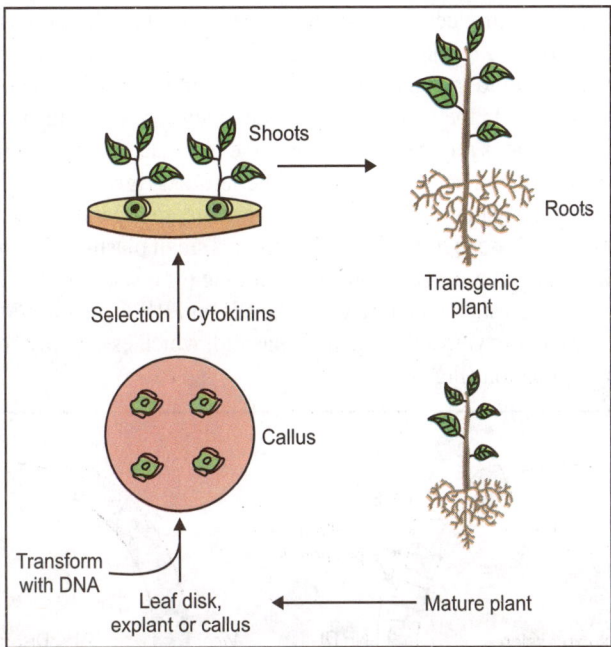

Fig. 14.1. Plant transformation. Plant material is transformed with DNA carrying a selectable marker and the gene of interest. Callus tissue develops on selective media. Shoots develop on the addition of cytokinins. Withdrawal of cytokinins promotes root development.

TRANSFORMATION OF DICOTYLEDONOUS PLANTS

Dicotyledonous plants are those which develop from two cotyledons in the seed. They can be recognised by the branching veins in their leaves. Dicots of commercial value include many horticultural plants such as petunias, and crops such as tobacco, tomatoes, cotton, soyabean and potatoes. Petunias have been engineered to produce a range of attractive flower colours and patterns. Tobacco, due to its ease of transformation, initially became the workhorse of plant genetic engineering, but more recently the common wall or thale cress, *Arabidopsis thaliana*, has become very popular. It has the advantage of not requiring tissue culture during its transformation. Tomatoes have been transformed to delay their ripening, cotton to insect resistance and herbicide tolerance, soyabeans to improved oil quality and herbicide tolerance, and potatoes to resist viruses.

Transformation Using *Agrobacterium Tumefaciens*

Agrobacterium tumefaciens is a plant pathogenic soil bacterium. It makes (tumefacient = swollen: Latin = tumefacere) a tumor on plants it infects and as these are often on the crown region where the stem meets the roots, the disease is called Crown Gall. Scientists were amased to discover that the bacteria transfer part of their DNA to the plant nucleus where it becomes integrated into the plant genetic material. The transferred DNA, or T-DNA, is part of a large tumor-inducing (Ti) plasmid. The T-DNA carries an *onc* (oncogenic) region, which, by coding for the production of plant growth hormones, results in the proliferation of plant cells forming a tumor or gall. It also codes for the production of unusual derivatives of arginine, such as nopaline or octopine, which the bacteria can use as growth substances. This bacterial-plant interaction is known as genetic colonisation. It was not long after this discovery that scientists realised that the introduction of a foreign gene into the T-DNA would enable its transfer to the plant cell nucleus. This led to the development of plant transformation using a disarmed, *onc-*, version of the Ti plasmid that could transfer DNA into plants without causing the production of a tumor.

The Ti plasmid is very large, in the order of 200 kb, and therefore unwieldy to work with *in vitro*. It was soon discovered that all that is required for a gene to be introduced into a plant are the 25-bp repeat sequences at the borders of the *onc* region, known as the left and right borders (LB and RB), and the virulence genes (*vir*) of the Ti plasmid. It was possible, therefore, to separate these in a system of binary vectors. Genetic manipulation is done in *Escherichia coli* on a small plasmid carrying a multiple cloning site (MCS) downstream of a plant promoter, and a gene coding for resistance to a herbicide or antibiotic that is toxic to the plant of interest, situated between the LB and RB. This plasmid is then transformed into a strain of *A. tumefaciens* carrying a disarmed Ti plasmid, which essentially consists only of the *vir* region and an origin of replication (Fig. 14.2).

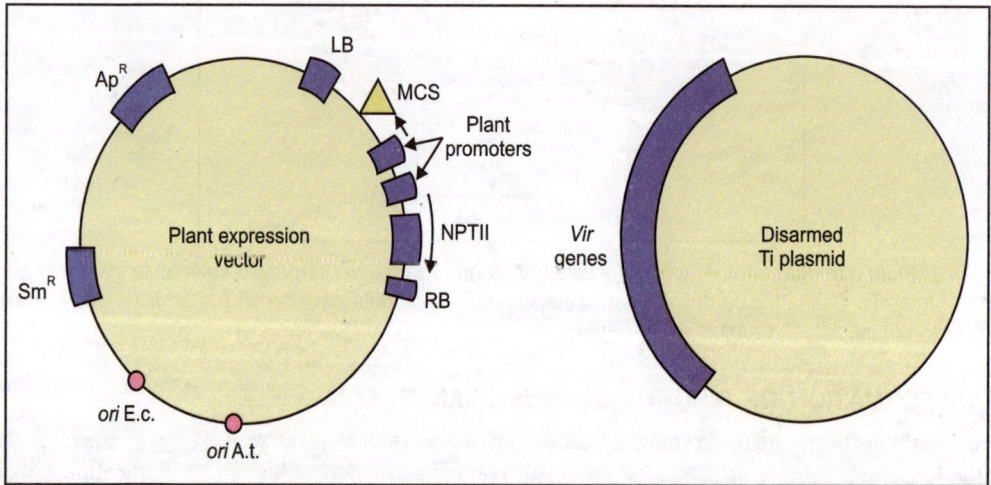

Fig. 14.2. Binary vectors. Ap^R, ampicillin resistance for selection in *E. coli*; Sm^R, streptomycin resistance for selection in *A. tumefaciens*; *ori* E.c, origin of replication for *E. coli*; *ori* A.t, origin of replication for *A. tumefaciens*; RB, right border; NPTII, kanamycin resistance for selection in plant cells; MCS, multiple cloning site; LB, left border.

This strain of *A. tumefaciens* is then used to transform plants. The earliest species to be transformed was tobacco, *Nicotiana tabacum*, which rapidly became the model dicot plant. However, more recently the workhorse has changed to *Arabidopsis thaliana* which has a very small genome of 120 Megabases and is easier to transform. In order to transform tobacco, and most other dicots, leaf disks are cut and placed in a Petri dish containing a liquid medium. The *A. tumefaciens* strain is placed on the surface of the disks and co-cultivation carried out for 2–3 days. The cutting of the leaf disks results in the plant producing wound-response compounds, such as acetosyringone, which induces the virulence genes. The leaf disks are then transferred to selection media containing the herbicide or antibiotic of choice. This is often kanamycin as many binary vectors carry the neomycin phosphotransferase gene (NPTII) which codes for kanamycin resistance. Transformation occurs along the cut edges of the disks, resulting in the formation of callus tissue which carries the DNA between the LB and RB integrated at random into the plant genome. The callus tissue is then transferred to regeneration medium also containing kanamycin, which only allows transgenic plants, expressing kanamycin resistance, to develop. The whole process takes about three to four months.

Agrobacterium as false positive results could be due to the expression of the T-DNA-carrying genes in the bacteria rather than in the plant. This is often found despite the fact that the genes are expressed from eukaryotic promoters. Antibiotics such as carbenicillin or cefotaxime can be used to eliminate the bacteria but they are not always sufficient. Another strategy is to introduce into the T-DNA a GUS gene, coding for β-glucuronidase, which carries a plant intron. The enzyme is very easy to detect histochemically and fluorometrically and will only be correctly spliced if it is expressed within the plant and not in *A. tumefaciens*.

Arabidopsis transformation is very simple and does not require tissue culture. This is advantageous because during the tissue culture process somatic mutations can occur which may adversely affect the plant of being very simple and not requiring any tissue culture. To transform *Arabidopsis* young flowering plants are inverted into a suspension of *A. tumefaciens* cells under a vacuum. This causes the bacteria to infiltrate into the flowers and transfer the T-DNA into the DNA of the developing seeds, which are collected and germinated on the selected antibiotic. Only transgenic seeds will germinate and although the frequency of transformation is only about 1 per cent, *Arabidopsis* produces such copious amounts of seed that transgenic plants are readily obtained. (Figure 14.3).

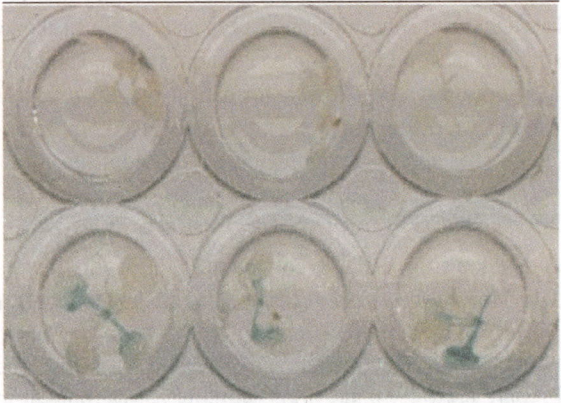

Fig. 14.3. Top row: untransformed *Arabidopsis* plants. Bottom row: transformed *Arabidopsis* plants stained blue due to expression of the β-glucuronidase gene.

Role of A. tumefaciens chromosomally encoded proteins and the Vir proteins

At least two loci on the *Agrobacterium* chromosome are required for the initial stage of binding the bacterium to the plant cell. The products of the genes *chv*A and *chv*B (chromosomal virulence) are responsible for the synthesis of a polysaccharide on the bacterial cell surface. ChvB is a membrane protein, which catalyses the conversion of UDP-glucose into cyclic glucans, which are transported into the periplasm by ChvA.

VirA and VirG make up a two-component signal transduction system. VirA is a periplasmic membrane protein, which senses the presence of wound-induced phenolic compounds, such as acetosyringone. VirA interacts with VirG, activating it by phosphorylation. In this state VirG acts as a transcriptional activator of the *vir* genes by binding to specific sequences, *vir* boxes, in their promoters. These Vir proteins have a number of functions. VirD1 and VirD2 nick the T-DNA within the RB, and VirD2 becomes covalently attached to the 5' end of the single-stranded T-DNA. It contains nuclear localising signals and will guide the DNA into the plant nucleus. When the nick is made it provides a priming end for the synthesis of a DNA single strand. This displaces the old strand, laying down a complementary strand in the Ti plasmid. The old strand is the one transferred. VirE2 proteins coat the single-stranded T-DNA, preventing it from degradation. VirB proteins form a pore in the bacterial membrane through which the coated T-DNA is transported (Fig. 14.4).

Little is known about the integration mechanism within the nucleus. The integrated DNA has a well-defined right junction with the plant DNA, retaining 1–2 bp of the RB. The left junction is variable, with the junction being at the LB or at one of a series of sites ~100 bp within the T-DNA.

This is because the LB is nicked with less precision, often resulting in the T-DNA extending further into the Ti plasmid. Sometimes multiple tandem copies of T-DNA are integrated at a single site.

Other Transformation Methods

For many years the only alternative to *A. tumefaciens*-mediated transformation was the direct uptake of naked DNA by plant protoplasts, achieved by electroporation or mediated by polyethylene glycol (PEG). This depends on the ability of plants to regenerate from protoplasts, which varies considerably between species. Early experiments focused on Solanaceae species which regenerate readily. Success has subsequently been obtained with *Arabidopsis*, rice, maize and forage grasses. Important parameters for successful PEG-mediated protoplast transformation include ion concentrations, the presence of inert carrier DNA, the molecular weight and concentration of PEG and the physical configuration of the nucleic acid. Linearised double-stranded plasmid DNA molecules are expressed and integrated most efficiently.

Now the most widely used alternative to transformation by *A. tumefaciens* is biolistics. Other techniques, which have been reported but not extensively used, include pollen co-cultivation, microinjection of somatic embryos and liposome fusion with protoplasts.

TRANSFORMATION OF MONOCOTYLEDONOUS PLANTS

Monocotyledonous plants develop from a single cotyledon in the seed. They can be recognised by the parallel veins in their leaves. Most of the world's crops belong to the monocots, including maize, wheat, rye and sorghum. Transformation of monocots with *A. tumefaciens* was not possible until relatively recently, and then only with certain plant varieties and bacterial strains. The exact reasons for the recalcitrance to this method are not fully understood. Initially it was thought that the triggering of the virulence process was impaired by the fact that monocots do not produce wound exudates such as acetosyringone. However, external addition of this compound did not facilitate the process. Resistance to *A. tumefaciens* is likely to be due to a number of factors, probably including integration into the chromosome, a process that is not well understood.

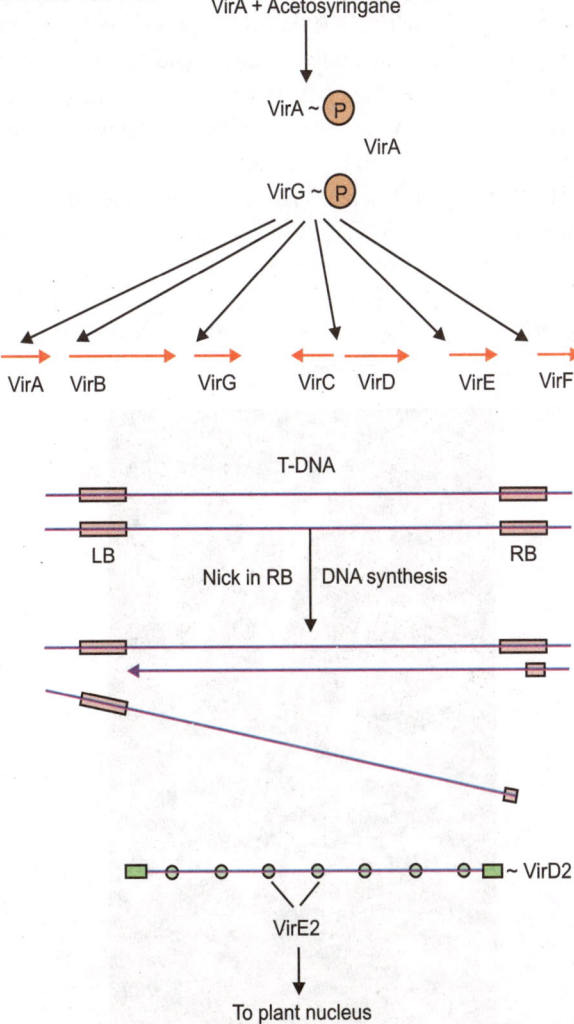

Fig. 14.4. VirA (sensor), a membrane-spanning protein in *A. tumefaciens*, reacts to the presence of acetosyringone, produced by wounded plant tissue. It autophosphorylates itself and then passes the phosphate group onto VirG. VirG in this activated state binds to the *vir* boxes in the promoters of the *vir* genes, inducing their expression. VirD1 and D2 nick the T- DNA in the RB and unwind the double helix. DNA synthesis lays down a complementary strand in the Ti plasmid. VirD2 becomes covalently attached to the leading edge of the T- DNA, guiding it to the plant nucleus, and VirE2 coats the single-stranded DNA, protecting it from nucleases.

Biolistic Transformation

Klein and others described a procedure in which high velocity microprojectiles were used to deliver nucleic acids into living cells. In their experiments they demonstrated transient expression of RNA or

DNA in epidermal cells of onion, *Allium cepa*. This technique of particle bombardment, or biolistics, is the most versatile and effective way of creating many transgenic plant species, including elite lines. Genes can be introduced into mitochondria and chloroplasts, present in many copies in a cell, as alternatives to delivery into the nucleus. This has the advantage of increasing the number of copies of the transgene. As these organelles are maternally inherited and therefore not transmitted by pollen, there is minimal chance of the transgene being transferred by cross-pollination, to plants in the field.

To transform plants biolistically, DNA is coated onto suitable metal particles, usually gold or tungsten, which are chemically inert. These are blasted into plant tissue using a biolistic device driven by a gas, usually helium. A series of baffles or mesh screens is used to reduce cell death. The type of plant tissue used can vary between different plant species, the most common being immature embryos, embryogenic callus and meristems. There are a number of instruments available for use in biolistics, based on various accelerating mechanisms. The most widely used is the one currently marketed by Bio-Rad, Inc (Biolistics®) but the Accell® device, based on a particle inflow mechanism, has been very useful in developing variety-independent gene transfer methods for recalcitrant monocots (Fig. 14.5).

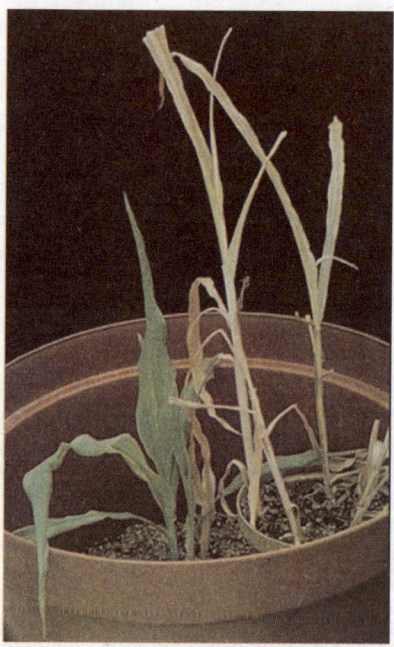

Fig. 14.5. A transgenic maize plant resistant to the herbicide bialaphos.

Gene silencing

Biolistic transformation is a useful transformation technique for plants not susceptible to transformation by *A. tumefaciens*. However there are negative features associated with this system such that multiple inserts are often obtained and there may also be genomic rearrangements. While naively this might be considered to be advantageous, in practice it is not so as the plant often responds by shutting off the expression of the transgene through a process referred to as gene silencing. Gene silencing is a natural defense pathway against viruses and transposons. Referred to as RNA interference in animals, post transcriptional (PTGS) in plants and quelling in fungi, the process of silencing is sequence specific and can be at the level of transcription, transcriptional gene silencing (TGS) or post transcriptional (PTGS). DNA methylation is involved in both TGS and PTGS. Transcriptional *cis*-inactivation is due to methylation when the transgene, in one or more copies, integrates in or next to hypermethlyated sequences. TGS involves the inhibition of transcription. However, silencing can also occur when transgenes integrate at hypomethylated regions. This can be due to differences between the DNA of the transgene and that of surrounding sequences, for instance when DNA from a dicot is transformed into a monocot, leading to specific methylation and silencing of foreign DNA. Methylation usually involves CG or CNG bases. Transcriptional *trans*-inactivation can also occur, probably by some sort of DNA-DNA pairing. This is in some cases correlated with inverted repeats, suggesting ectopic pairing between transgene copies or between transgenes and homologous host genes. This could lead to the synthesis of aberrant RNA that triggers specific degradation of all homologous RNA in the cytoplasm.

PTGS is associated with high transgene copy number and strength of the promoter. In PTGS, transgenes are transcribed at apparently normal rates in the nucleus but there is a strong reduction in the cytoplasm of steady-state mRNA levels. This is because when the transgene mRNA reaches a threshold level, the silencing mechanism is triggered and results in degradation of all homologous RNA in the cytoplasm. However, not all PTGS is consistent with the threshold model. Weakly or even untranscribed transgenes can also trigger silencing of homologous host genes. One explanation that has been proposed is that transgene RNA could be degraded if tagged by specific small complementary RNA molecules. A plant RNA dependent polymerase, using the transgene RNA as a template, could synthesise these. They can act with mRNA forming duplexes that act as targets for double stranded-RNAses. Viruses themselves are also able to trigger their own silencing on entry into a plant even in the absence of a transgene.

Plant viruses have however developed mechanisms to overcome being silenced by plants by expressing inhibitors that interfere with the PTGS pathway. These inhibitors are mainly proteins that interfere with one or more steps in the silencing pathway. Examples include the Cucumber mosaic virus 2b protein, p25 protein in Potexviruses, C2 gene in Tomato leaf curl virus and p19 protein from Tobamoviruses.

With a better understanding of gene silencing, however, design of vectors that minimise transgene silencing is being used to ensure that the transgene is not silenced upon entry into the plant cell. In addition, gene silencing can be harnessed to advantage to study gene function, for genetic improvement of crop plants and development of virus resistance.

Agrobacterium Transformation

Multiple inserts during *Agrobacterium* transformation are less frequent than with biolistics. Hence, if a plant can be transformed by this method it is usually the preferred technique. Although the host range of *A. tumefaciens* is broad, encompassing a large number of species of dicotyledonous plants and some monocots and Gymnosperms, a number of important monocot crops are recalcitrant to the method. These include maize, rice, wheat and other cereals. There has thus been considerable emphasis on the improvement of *A. tumefaciens* strains to transform these recalcitrant species. The greatest success to date has been with rice. Hiei and colleagues produced transformants with an efficiency similar to that of transformation in dicotyledons but using a 'super-binary' vector. Optimisation of the conditions of tissue culture and of the condition of co-cultivation was of critical importance and the choice of tissues as starting material was one of the most important factors. Callus cultures initiated from scutella were excellent materials for transformation whereas immature embryos and shoot apices were not. The DNA was randomly integrated into the rice genome and rearrangements, such as the deletion of part of the

T-DNA, was occasionally observed. However this is also the case in *Agrobacterium*-mediated transformation of dicotyledons. More recently successful transformation of maize by *Agrobacterium* has been achieved.

TRANSFORMATION OF ALGAE

Although this area of investigation is in its infancy there are reasons to be optimistic about the use of recombinant viruses as vectors of foreign DNA. There is growing interest in farming with marine microalgae in particular, and genetic modification could be used to develop strains, which can produce a variety of proteins, polysaccharides and high value secondary chemicals. The large brown algae, commonly known as kelps, can measure up to 50 m in length and weigh hundreds of kg. They are the basis of economically important industries worldwide. Viruses, or more often electron microscopic observations of viral like particles, have been described in a number of brown algae. Henry and Meints have isolated a strain of marine brown algae, which harbors a stable virus infection. The viral DNA appears to be stably integrated into the genome of the host and may have potential as a vehicle for the introduction of foreign genes into algae.

PROMOTER EFFICIENCY AND TISSUE SPECIFICITY

The 35S promoter of cauliflower mosaic virus (35S) was one of the earliest used in the transformation of dicots. It is still widely used but has been improved by duplicating a 250-bp up-stream enhancer. An A/T-rich positive regulatory region upstream of the translation start site of the pea plastocyanin gene can also enhance it. This enhancer acts as a quantitative element in all transgenic plant tissues.

In monocots the promoter of choice is from the maize ubiquitin gene, which consists of the promoter, the 5' untranslated exon and the first intron. Splicing out of the intron appears to increase gene expression by possibly increasing the stability of the mRNA or increasing the level of mature cytoplasmic RNA.

It is often advantageous to develop a transgenic plant in which the gene of interest is only expressed in certain tissues or under certain conditions. This could minimise the genetic load on a plant by ensuring the gene is only expressed in the targeted tissues or, for example, only after pathogen infection. Thus, for example, nematode resistance should be targeted to the roots, delayed fruit ripening to the fruit or stalk borer resistance to the stalk. This could also assist safety and regulatory aspects if, for example, nematode resistance is not expressed in edible fruits.

A recent example comes from work by Smith who introduced the snowdrop lectin into transgenic rice to confer resistance to rice brown planthopper. These insects feed by phloem abstraction and cause 'hopper burn' as well as transmitting an important virus. The snowdrop lectin has been shown to be toxic to the insects. The lectin gene was driven by a phloem-specific promoter from rice and was expressed only in the phloem. Transgenic plants were shown to have increased resistance to the brown planthopper, which showed decreased survival, lower fecundity and retarded development.

A tissue-specific promoter has also been used in rice. Rice (*Oryza sativa* L.), the major food staple for more than two billion people, contains neither β-carotene (provitamin A) nor precursors thereof in its kernel endosperm. To improve the nutritional value of rice, Burkhardt introduced the genes for β-carotene synthesis into rice behind an endosperm-specific promoter and showed accumulation of the provitamin in the kernels.

A useful way of detecting whether a particular promoter is able to target the desired tissue is to fuse it to a reporter gene that is readily visualised in a manner that is not destructive to the plant. One such gene is the luciferase gene, *lux*, which originates from the bacterium, *Vibrio harveyi* or from the firefly

(*Photinus pyralis*). Light emission can be monitored visually, photographically or electronically. It is rather pretty observing plants that glow in the dark! Another useful marker is the green fluorescent protein of the jellyfish, *Aequorea victoria*. In order to visualise the fluorescence in green tissues the mutant form of the gene with improved emission must be used and driven by a very strong promoter.

TARGETING GENES TO ORGANELLES

As mentioned above, targeting genes to chloroplasts and mitochondria can be beneficial. Recently, Kota and colleagues developed transgenic tobacco plants expressing a *Bacillus thuringiensis* toxin in their chloroplasts. Strains of *B. thuringiensis* (Bt) produce protein toxins specific to a variety of herbivorous insect pests. By expressing the gene in chloroplasts, which are present in cells in high numbers, the authors achieved toxin levels of between 2 per cent and 3 per cent of total soluble protein. This was so high that even Bt-resistant insects were killed when they were fed leaves from the transgenic plants. The added advantage is that the genes will be maternally inherited and therefore not spread by pollen, since there is concern that cross-pollination could spread transgenes in an uncontrolled fashion. This would be a particular problem if herbicide resistance were spread to potentially weedy relatives.

INTEGRATION AND STABILITY OF TRANSGENES

One of the first attributes of a transgenic plant to be determined is whether the transgenes are stably integrated, inherited in a Mendelian fashion and stably transferred to subsequent generations. This is usually the case when a few genes are integrated in one copy at one site. In many transgenic plants one or a few genes are transferred into a plant's genome along with the selectable marker. This has resulted in the production of transgenic crops expressing herbicide tolerance, resistance to viruses, fungi and bacteria, as well as to insect pests. Improved agricultural characteristics have also been achieved by overexpression of specific genes in a metabolic pathway or by inhibiting gene expression using antisense sequences. However, many agronomic characteristics are polygenic, requiring the engineering of multiple genes. This necessitates the integration of many transgenes, which must be stably inherited and expressed. Recently Chen and co-workers succeeded in tranforming rice with up to 11 transgenes. They co-bombarded the rice embryogenic tissue with 14 different plasmids and found that integration of the multiple transgenes occurred at either one or two genetic loci. Inheritance conformed to the 3:1 Mendelian ratio. Coexpression of four marker genes was followed until the R2 generation and found to be stable.

Although the mechanism of integration of transgenes into plant DNA is poorly understood, the integration of many genes at one or a few loci could not happen by chance. They may have been inserted individually at the same locus, or the plasmids might have become joined prior to integration. Experiments carried out by Collen and colleagues, also using biolistic transformation of rice, suggest a two-phase integration mechanism mediated by the establishment of integration hot spots. In the first stage, before integration, transforming plasmids appear to be spliced together. The cointegrate is then inserted into a site which subsequently acts as a hot spot, facilitating subsequent integration of successive transgenic molecules at the same locus.

A number of studies have been done on the mechanism of integration during *A. tumefaciens* transformation. De Neve and co-workers co-transformed plants with two *Agrobacterium* strains each carrying a different T-DNA and found that they were frequently integrated at the same locus. Out of 27 *Arabidopsis* transformants 12 contained the T-DNAs linked to each other in all possible configurations but with a preference for those with at least one RB involved. They also propose a model whereby separate T-DNAs are ligated prior to integration.

Hansen and Chilton have used a combination of biolistics and *Agrobacterium* transformation to develop transgenic plants carrying only the genes of interest without undesired vector sequences. They call this method 'agrolistic' transformation. The virulence proteins VirD1 and VirD2 from *A. tumefaciens* are required for the excision of T-DNA strands, and VirD2, covalently attached to the 5′ end of the strand, targets it to the plant nucleus. They cobombarded a plasmid carrying the *vir*D1 and *vir*D2 genes with one containing border sequences flanking their genes of interest. Agrolistic inserts were those which exhibited right junctions with plant DNA that corresponded precisely to the sequence expected for T-DNA.

PLANT TRANSFORMATION WITH Ti PLASMID OF *AGROBACTERIUM TUMEFACIENS*

Ti plasmid is a circular plasmid that often, but not always, is a part of the genetic equipment that *Agrobacterium tumefaciens* and *Agrobacterium rhizogenes* use to transduce its genetic material to plants. The Ti plasmid is lost when *Agrobacterium* is grown above 28°C. Such cured bacteria do not induce crown galls, i.e. they become avirulent. pTi and pRi share little sequence homology but are functionally rather similar. The Ti plasmids are classified into different types based on the type of opine produced by their genes. The different opines specified by pTi are octopine, nopaline, succinamopine and leucinopine.

The plasmid has 196 genes that code for 195 proteins. There is no one structural RNA. The plasmid is 206, 479 nucleotides long, the GC content is 56 per cent and 81 per cent of the material is coding genes. There are no pseudogenes. The modification of this plasmid is very important in the creation of transgenic plants, but only in dicotyledon plants.

Genes in the virulence region are grouped into the operons *vir*ABCDEFG, which code for the enzymes responsible for mediating transduction of T-DNA to plant cells.

Agrobacterium Tumefaciens

Agrobacterium tumefaciens is the causal agent of crown gall disease (the formation of tumours) in over 140 species of dicot. It is a rod shaped, Gram negative soil bacterium. Symptoms are caused by the insertion of a small segment of DNA (known as the T-DNA, for 'transfer DNA') into the plant cell, which is incorporated at a semi-random location into the plant genome.

Agrobacterium tumefaciens (or *A. tumefaciens*) is an alphaproteobacterium of the family Rhizobiaceae, which includes the nitrogen fixing legume symbionts. Unlike the nitrogen fixing symbionts, tumor producing *Agrobacterium* are pathogenic and do not benefit the plant. The wide variety of plants affected by *Agrobacterium* makes it of great concern to the agriculture industry.

Economically, *A. tumefaciens* is a serious pathogen of walnuts, grape vines, stone fruits, nut trees, sugar beets, horse radish and rhubarb.

In order to be virulent, the bacterium must contain a tumour-inducing plasmid (Ti plasmid or pTi), of 200 kb, which contains the T-DNA and all the genes necessary to transfer it to the plant cell. Many strains of *A. tumefaciens* do not contain a pTi.

Since the Ti plasmid is essential to cause disease, pre-penetration events in the rhizosphere occur to promote bacterial conjugation-exchange of plasmids amongst bacteria. In the presence of opines, *A. tumefaciens* produces a diffusible conjugation signal called 30C8HSL or the *Agrobacterium* autoinducer. This activates the transcription factor TraR, positively regulating the transcription of genes required for conjugation.

Method of infection

The *Agrobacterium tumefaciens* infects the plant through its Ti plasmid. The Ti plasmid integrates a segment of its DNA, known as T-DNA, into the chromosomal DNA of its host plant cells.

A. tumefaciens have flagella that allow them to swim through the soil towards photoassimilates that accumulate in the rhizosphere around roots. Chemotaxis: reaction of orientation and locomotion to chemical attractants. Without chemotaxis there will be no cell-cell contact. Some strains may chemotactically move towards chemical exudates coming out from wounded plant such as acetosyringone and sugars. Acetosyringone is recognised by the VirA protein, a transmembrane protein encoded in the virA gene on the Ti plasmid. Sugars are recognised by the chvE protein, a chromosomal gene-encoded protein located in the periplasmic space.

Induction of vir genes: At least 25 vir genes on Ti plasmid are necessary for tumor induction.In addition to their perception role, virA and chvE induce other vir genes. The VirA protein has a kinase activity, it phosphorylates itself on a histidine residue. Then the VirA protein phosphorylates the VirG protein on its aspartate residue.The VirG protein is a cytoplasmic protein produced from the virG Ti plasmid gene, it's a transcription factor. It induces the transcription of the vir operons.ChvE protein regulates the second mechanism of vir genes activation. It increases VirA protein sensibility to phenolic compounds.

Attachment is a two step process. Following an initial weak and reversible attachment, the bacteria synthesise cellulose fibrils that anchor them to the wounded plant cell. Four main genes are involved in this process: chvA, chvB, pscA and att. It appears that the products of the first three genes are involved in the actual synthesis of the cellulose fibrils. These fibrils also anchor the bacteria to each other, helping to form a microcolony.

After production of cellulose fibrils a Ca^{2+} dependent outer membrane protein called rhicadhesin is produced, which also aids in sticking the bacteria to the cell wall. Homologues of this protein can be found in other *Rhizobia* species.

Formation of the T-pilus

In order to transfer the T-DNA into the plant cell *A. tumefaciens* uses a Type IV secretion mechanism, involving the production of a T-pilus.

The VirA/VirG two component sensor system is able to detect phenolic signals released by wounded plant cells, in particular acetosyringone. This leads to a signal transduction event activating the expression of 11 genes within the VirB operon which are responsible for the formation of the T-pilus.

First, the VirB pro-pilin is formed. This is a polypeptide of 121 amino acids which requires processing by the removal of 47 residues to form a T-pilus subunit. The subunit is circularised by the formation of a peptide bond between the two ends of the polypeptide.

Products of the other VirB genes are used to transfer the subunits across the plasma membrane. Yeast two-hybrid studies provide evidence that VirB6, VirB7, VirB8, VirB9 and VirB10 may all encode components of the transporter. An ATPase for the active transport of the subunits would also be required.

Transfer of T-DNA into plant cell

The T-DNA must be cut out of the circular plasmid. A VirD1/D2 complex nicks the DNA at the left and right border sequences. The VirD2 protein is covalently attached to the 5′ end. VirD2 contains a motif that leads to the nucleoprotein complex being targeted to the type IV secretion system (T4SS).

In the cytoplasm of the recipient cell, the T-DNA complex becomes coated with VirE2 proteins, which are exported through the T4SS independently from the T-DNA complex. Nuclear localisation signals, or NLS, located on the VirE2 and VirD2 are recognised by the importin alpha protein, which then associates with importin beta and the nuclear pore complex to transfer the T-DNA into the nucleus.

VIP1 also appears to be an important protein in the process, possibly acting as an adapter to bring the VirE2 to the importin. Once inside the nucleus, VIP2 may target the T-DNA to areas of chromatin that are being actively transcribed, so that the T-DNA can integrate into the host genome.

Genes in the T-DNA

Hormones

In order to cause gall formation, the T-DNA encodes genes for the production of auxin or indole-3-acetic acid via the IAM pathway. This biosynthetic pathway is not used in many plants for the production of auxin, so it means the plant has no molecular means of regulating it and auxin will be produced constitutively. Genes for the production of cytokinins are also expressed. This stimulates cell proliferation and gall formation.

Opines

The T-DNA contains genes for encoding enzymes that cause the plant to create specialised amino acids which the bacteria can metabolise, called opines. Opines are a class of chemicals that serve as a source of nitrogen for *A. tumefaciens*, but not for most other organisms. The specific type of opine produced by *A. tumefaciens* C58 infected plants is nopaline.

Two nopaline type Ti plasmids, pTi-SAKURA and pTiC58, were fully sequenced. *A. tumefaciens* C58, the first fully sequenced pathovar, was first isolated from a cherry tree crown gall. The genome was simultaneously sequenced by Goodner and Wood in 2001. The genome of *A. tumefaciens* C58 consists of a circular chromosome, two plasmids, and a linear chromosome. The presence of a covalently bonded circular chromosome is common to bacteria, with few exceptions. However, the presence of both a single circular chromosome and single linear chromosome is unique to a group in this genus. The two plasmids are pTiC58, responsible for the processes involved in virulence, and pAtC58, coined the 'cryptic' plasmid.

The pAtC58 plasmid has been shown to be involved in the metabolism of opines and to conjugate with other bacteria in the absence of the pTiC58 plasmid. If the pTi plasmid is removed, the tumor growth that is the means of classifying this species of bacteria does not occur.

Beneficial uses

The DNA transmission capabilities of *Agrobacterium* have been extensively exploited in biotechnology as a means of inserting foreign genes into plants. Marc Van Montagu and Jeff Schell, discovered the gene transfer mechanism between *Agrobacterium* and plants, which resulted in the development of methods to alter *Agrobacterium* into an efficient delivery system for genetic engineering in plants. The plasmid T-DNA that is transferred to the plant is an ideal vehicle for genetic engineering. This is done by cloning a desired gene sequence into the T-DNA that will be inserted into the host DNA. This process has been performed using firefly luciferase gene to produce glowing plants. This luminescence has been a useful device in the study of plant *chloroplast* function and as a reporter gene. It is also possible to transform *Arabidopsis* by dipping their flowers into a broth of *Agrobacterium*, the seed produced will be transgenic. Under laboratory conditions the T-DNA has also been transferred to human cells, demonstrating the diversity of insertion application.

The mechanism by which *Agrobacterium* inserts materials into the host cell by a type IV secretion system, is very similar to mechanisms used by pathogens to insert materials (usually proteins) into human cells by type III secretion. It also employs a type of signaling conserved in many Gram-negative bacteria called quorum sensing. This makes *Agrobacterium* an important topic of medical research as well.

GENE TRANSFER METHODS IN PLANTS

To achieve genetic transformation in plants, we need the construction of a vector (genetic vehicle) which transports the genes of interest, flanked by the necessary controlling sequences, i.e. promoter and terminator, and deliver the genes into the host plant. The two kinds of gene transfer methods in plants are discussed below.

Vector-Mediated or Indirect Gene Transfer

Among the various vectors used in plant transformation, the Ti plasmid of *Agrobacterium tumefaciens* has been widely used. This bacteria is known as 'natural genetic engineer' of plants because these bacteria have natural ability to transfer T-DNA of their plasmids into plant genome upon infection of cells at the wound site and cause an unorganised growth of a cell mass known as crown gall. Ti plasmids are used as gene vectors for delivering useful foreign genes into target plant cells and tissues. The foreign gene is cloned in the T-DNA region of Ti-plasmid in place of unwanted sequences. To transform plants, leaf discs (in case of dicots) or embryogenic callus (in case of monocots) are collected and infected with *Agrobacterium* carrying recombinant disarmed Ti-plasmid vector. The infected tissue is then cultured (co-cultivation) on shoot regeneration medium for 2–3 days during which time the transfer of T-DNA along with foreign genes takes place. After this, the transformed tissues (leaf discs/calli) are transferred onto selection cum plant regeneration medium supplemented with usually lethal concentration of an antibiotic to selectively eliminate non-transformed tissues. After 3–5 weeks, the regenerated shoots (from leaf discs) are transferred to root-inducing medium, and after another 3–4 weeks, complete plants are transferred to soil following the hardening (acclimatisation) of regenerated plants. The molecular techniques like PCR and southern hybridisation are used to detect the presence of foreign genes in the transgenic plants.

Vectorless or Direct Gene Transfer

In the direct gene transfer methods, the foreign gene of interest is delivered into the host plant cell without the help of a vector. The methods used for direct gene transfer in plants are given below:

Chemical mediated gene transfer e.g. chemicals like polyethylene glycol (PEG) and dextran sulphate induce DNA uptake into plant protoplasts.Calcium phosphate is also used to transfer DNA into cultured cells.

Microinjection where the DNA is directly injected into plant protoplasts or cells (specifically into the nucleus or cytoplasm) using fine tipped (0.5–1.0 micrometerdiameter) glass needle or micropipette. This method of gene transfer is used to introduce DNA into large cells such as oocytes, eggs, and the cells of early embryo.

Electroporation involves a pulse of high voltage applied to protoplasts/cells/ tissues to make transient (temporary) pores in the plasma membrane which facilitates the uptake of foreign DNA. The cells are placed in a solution containing DNA and subjected to electrical shocks to cause holes in the membranes. The foreign DNA fragments enter through the holes into the cytoplasm and then to nucleus.

Particle gun/Particle bombardment in this method, the foreign DNA containing the genes to be transferred is coated onto the surface of minute gold or tungsten particles (1–3 micrometers) and bombarded onto the target tissue or cells using a particle gun (also called as gene gun/shot gun/microprojectile gun). The microprojectile bombardment method was initially named as biolistics by its inventor Sanford. Two types of plant tissue are commonly used for particle bombardment-Primary explants and the proliferating embryonic tissues.

Transformation this method is used for introducing foreign DNA into bacterial cells, e.g. *E. coli*. The transformation frequency (the fraction of cell population that can be transferred) is very good in this method, e.g. the uptake of plasmid DNA by *E. coli* is carried out in ice cold $CaCl_2$ (0–50C) followed by heat shock treatment at 37–450C for about 90 sec. The transformation efficiency refers to the number of transformants per microgram of added DNA. The $CaCl_2$ breaks the cell wall at certain regions and binds the DNA to the cell surface.

Conjuction it is a natural microbial recombination process and is used as a method for gene transfer. In conjuction, two live bacteria come together and the single stranded DNA is transferred via cytoplasmic bridges from the donor bacteria to the recipient bacteria.

Liposome mediated gene transfer or lipofection liposomes are circular lipid molecules with an aqueous interior that can carry nucleic acids. Liposomes encapsulate the DNA fragments and then adher to the cell membranes and fuse with them to transfer DNA fragments. Thus, the DNA enters the cell and then to the nucleus. Lipofection is a very efficient technique used to transfer genes in bacterial, animal and plant cells.

Selection of Transformed Cells from Untransformed Cells

The selection of transformed plant cells from untransformed cells is an important step in the plant genetic engineering. For this, a marker gene (e.g. for antibiotic resistance) is introduced into the plant along with the transgene followed by the selection of an appropriate selection medium (containing the antibiotic). The segregation and stability of the transgene integration and expression in the subsequent generations can be studied by genetic and molecular analyses.

REPORTER GENES

Some genes being transferred produce enzymes whose activities can be easily detected or used as a basis of selection for the transformed cells, e.g. genes for herbicide resistance.

However, most genes need to be tagged with another gene, called reporter gene, whose expression is easily detected either through highly sensitive enzyme assays (scorable reporter genes) or through expression of resistance to a toxin (selectable reporter genes). Some commonly used easily detectable enzyme producing genes are, *nos* (nopaline synthase, from *Agrobacterium*), lux (luciferase from bacteria or firefly), cat (chloramphenicol acetyltransferase from bacteria), and gus (β-glucuronidase from bacteria), etc.

Activities of the enzymes produced by scorable reporter genes are determined either *in situ*, i.e. in the transformed tissues, or by *in vitro* assays using plant tissue extracts. In addition, immunological methods may also be used to detect the protein products of marker genes either *in situ*, in plant extracts or by western blotting. The essential features of an ideal reporter gene are:

1. Lack of endogenous activity in plant cells of the concerned enzyme.
2. An efficient and easy detection.
3. A relatively rapid degradation of the enzyme.

Each reporter gene has some advantages and some disadvantages and none of them are ideally suited for all plant species. For example, there is little or no endogenous luciferase activity in plant cells, the enzyme serves as a visual marker, the assay is quite sensitive, but the enzyme is highly stable.

Similarly, the Gus enzyme serves as visual marker and the assay is highly sensitive so that expression in individual cells can be monitored, but the enzymes is highly stable and many plant species show variable endogenous Gus activity.

Reporter genes, more particularly, scorable reporter genes have been extensively used to assay the function of promoters and other regulatory sequences, and also to demonstrate the transformation of plant cells. A key step in gene transfer is the selection of few transformed cells from among the nontransformed ones. This is usually achieved by the use of selectable markers, which are genes that confer resistance to various compounds toxic to normal plant cells. The best selection agents are those that either inhibit growth or slowly kill the nontransformed cells so that the dying cells do not overwhelm the transformed ones.

The commonly used selectable marker genes include those conferring resistance to the antibiotics kanamycin (nptII, encoding neomycin phosphotransferase) and hygromycin (hptIV, encoding hygromycin phosphotransferase, isolated from *E. coli*); and broad range herbicides glyphosate (modified versions of the enzyme EPSPS, 5-enolpyruvate shikimate-3-phosphate synthase, isolated from *E. coli* or Salmonella typhimurium), phosphinothricin (bar, isolated from Streptomyces hygroscopicus, codes for phophinothricin acetyltransferase), etc. Each selectable marker presents some favourable and some unfavourable features. Therefore, the choice of a marker should be based on the plant species and other considerations in the study. The marker gene of choice is fused with a suitable plant promoter and is placed in a suitable vector along with the gene being transferred.

The bar gene confers resistance to the herbicide phosphinothricin, which inhibits the enzymes glutamine synthetase and, thereby, leads to an accumulation of ammonia to lethal levels. The bar product, phosphinothricin acetyl transferase, catalyses acetylation of phosphinothricin leading thereby to its inactivation. Transformed cells expressing bar gene almost normally grow on lethal concentrations of phosphinothricin, while nontransformed plant cells stop to grow, gradually become necrotic and die within 10–21 days. Phosphinothricin is used at 1–10 mg/l for selection of transformed cells.

The nptII gene from transposon Tn5 confers resistance to the aminoglycoside antibiotics kanamycin, neomycin and G418. The nptII gene product, neomycin phosphotransferase, inactivates these antibiotics through their phosphorylation. Kanamycin resistance due to nptII has been widely used as a selectable marker in many dicot plant species. But this gene is of limited value in monocots due to their tolerance to relatively high levels of kanamycin. The selection of transformed cells is done on a medium containing 50–350 mg/l of kanamycin sulphate in case of tobacco.

DEVELOPING VIRUS-RESISTANT PLANTS

Plant virus diseases cause severe constraints on the productivity of a wide range of economically important crops worldwide. In India the green revolution ushered in intensive agricultural practices and reduced varietal diversity, resulting in the emergence of viral diseases at an alarming pace in the cultivated crops. Some such diseases, which are especially relevant to India, along with their yield losses, are listed in Table 14.1.

Strategies for the management of viral diseases normally include control of vector population using insecticides, use of virus-free propagating material, appropriate cultural practices and use of resistant cultivars. However, each of the above methods has its own drawback. Rapid advances in the techniques of molecular biology have resulted in the cloning and sequence analysis of the genomic components of a number of plant viruses. A majority of plant viruses have a single-stranded positivesense RNA as the genome. However, some of the most important viruses in tropical countries like India have single-stranded and double-stranded DNA genomes and RNA genomes of ambisence polarity, i.e. genes oriented in both directions. Genome organisation, electron-microscopic structures and symptoms caused by some of the viruses, referred to in this review, are briefly illustrated in Fig. 14.6.

Table 14.1. Important viral diseases of crops in India

Crop	Disease	Yield loss (%)	Virus	Virus group
Cassava	Mosaic	18–25	Indian cassava mosaic virus	Begomovirus
Cotton	Leaf curl	68–71*	Cotton leaf curl virus	Begomovirus
Groundnut	Bud necrosis	> 80	Groundnut bud necrosis virus	Tospovirus
Mungbean Blackgram Soyabean	Yellow mosaic	21–70	Mungbean yellow mosaic virus	Begomovirus
Pigeonpea	Sterility Mosaic	> 80*	Pigeonpea sterility mosaic virus	Tenuivirus
Potato	Mosaic	85	Potato virus Y	Potyvirus
Rice	Rice tungro	10	Rice tungro badna and rice tungro spherical viruses	Badnavirus and waika virus
Sunflower	Necrosis	12–17	Sunflower necrosis virus	Ilarvirus
Tomato	Leaf curl	40–100	Tomato leaf curl virus	Begomovirus

*in epidemic years.

Concomitantly, tremendous advances have taken place in our understanding of plant–virus interaction in the process of pathogenesis and resistance. This, along with associated advances in the genetic transformation of a number of crop plants, have opened up the possibility of an entirely new approach of genetic engineering towards controlling plant virus diseases.

There are mainly two approaches for developing genetically engineered resistance depending on the source of the genes used. The genes can be either from the pathogenic virus itself or from any other source. The former approach is based on the concept of pathogen-derived resistance (PDR). For PDR, a part, or a complete viral gene is introduced into the plant, which, subsequently, interferes with one or more essential steps in the life cycle of the virus. This was first illustrated in tobacco by the group of Roger Beachy, who introduced the coat protein (CP) of tobacco mosaic virus (TMV) into tobacco and observed TMV resistance in the transgenic plants. The concept of PDR has generated lot of interest and today there are several host–virus systems in which it has been fully established. Non-pathogen-derived resistance, on the other hand, is based on utilising host resistance genes and other genes responsible for adaptive host processes, elicited in response to pathogen attack, to obtain transgenics resistant to the virus.

The use of non-PDR type of resistance, even though reported much less in the literature in comparison to PDR-based approaches, holds a better promise to achieve durable resistance. Various aspects of the above topics have been reviewed extensively.

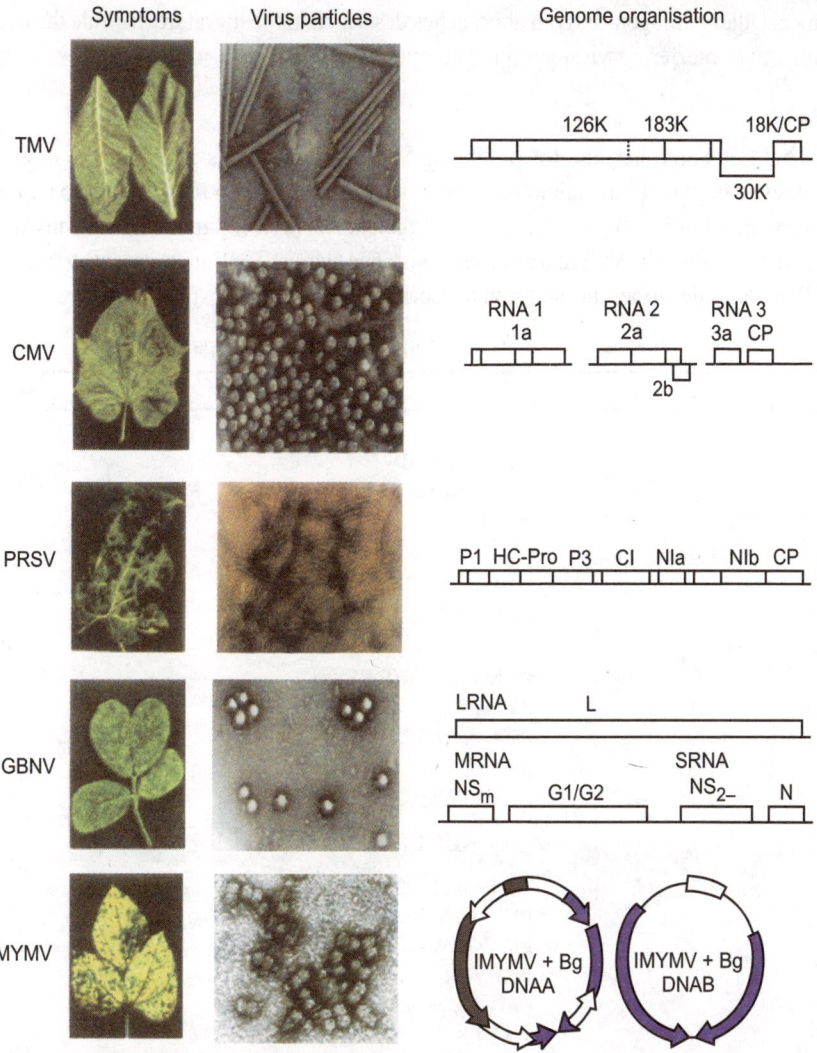

Fig. 14.6. Symptoms, particle morphology and genome organisation of some important viruses discussed in the text. Viral gene products and putative ORFs are indicated.

Transgenics with Pathogen-Derived Resistance

In a number of crops, transgenics resistant to an infective virus have been developed by introducing a sequence of the viral genome in the target crop by genetic transformation. Virus-resistant transgenics have been developed in many crops by introducing either viral CP or replicase gene encoding sequences. Resistance obtained by using CP is conventionally called CPMR. Replicasemediated resistance has been pursued in a number of laboratories and in most of these cases, resistance has been shown to be due to an inherent plant response, known as post-transcriptional gene silencing (PTGS), which is described in more detail later in this section. Because of the essential nature of the viral movement protein for intercellular movement of plant viruses, movement problem sequence has also been used for achieving viral resistance. Other pathogen-derived approaches described in the literature, include the use of satellite RNA and defective-interfering viral genomic components.

Coat protein

The use of viral CP as a transgene for producing virusresistant plants is one of the most spectacular successes achieved in plant biotechnology. Numerous crops have been transformed to express viral CP and have been reported to show high levels of resistance in comparison to untransformed plants (Table 14.2 and 14.3). Powell-Abel first reported resistance against TMV in transgenic tobacco expressing the TMV CP gene, as described in the previous section.

Table 14.2. Coat protein-mediated transgenic resistance to viruses in crops.

Crops	Viruses*	Field tested
Cereals		
Maize	MDMV, MCMV	–
Rice	RSV, RTSV	–
Wheat	WSMV	–
Fruits		
Apricot	PPV	–
Cantaloupe	ZYMV, WMV2, CMV	Yes
Citrus	CTV	–
Grape	GCMV, GFLV, ToRSV	–
Muskmelon	ZYMV	Yes
Papaya	PRV	Yes
Plum	PPV	–
Squash	ZYMV, WMV2	Yes
Vegetables		
Pepper	TSWV	–
Tomato	ToMV, YMV, CMV, TYLCV	Yes
Potato	PVX, PVY, PLRV	Yes
Lettuce	LMV, TSWV	–
Pea	PEMV	–
Cucumber	CMV	Yes
Sugarbeet	BNYVV	–
Legumes		
Peanut	TSWV	–
Soyabean	BPMV	–
Bean	BPMV	–

*MCMV, Maize chlorotic mottle virus; MDMV, Maize dwarf mosaic virus; RSV, Rice stripe virus; RTSV, Rice tungro spherical virus; WSMV, Wheat streak mosaic virus; CTV, Citrus tristeza virus; GCMV, Grapevine chrome mosaic virus; GFLV, Grapevine fanleaf virus; ToRSV, Tomato ringspot virus; YMV, Yellow mosaic virus; LMV, Lettuce mosaic virus; PEMV, Pea enation mosaic virus; BNYVV, Bean necrotic yellow vein virus; BPMV, Bean pod mottle virus; for rest of abbreviations, consult text.

The resistance was manifested as delayed appearance of symptoms as well as a reduced titre of virus in the infected transgenic plants, as compared to the controls. The resistance against TMV using TMV CP in tobacco was also reported to be effective against other tobamoviruses whose CP was closely related to that of TMV but not effective against viruses which were distantly related to TMV. Transgenic potato, expressing the CP of potato virus X (PVX) also showed resistance against PVX. However, in marked contrast to TMV, this resistance was not broken down when PVX RNA was used as the inoculum, thus indicating several possible mechanisms of CPMR.

Table 14.3. Comparative performance of transgenic virus resistant plants.

Host	Transgene	Yield increase (%)*
Tomato	TMV CP	40
Tomato	CMV satellite	14
Potato	PVX + PVY CP	38
Squash	CMV + ZYMV + WMV2 CP	97
Squash	ZYMV + WMV2 CP	90
Squash	ZYMV CP	77
Papaya	PRSV CP	90

*Yield increase over susceptible non-transgenic plants.

The stage of the viral life cycle at which the CPMR is effective has been shown to vary. In TMV, it is at the virus disassembly and in the long-distance transport stage. In the case of alfalfa mosaic virus (AMV), it is only at the disassembly stage, whereas in PVX, it is at multiple stages, including replication, cell-to-cell and systemic movement stages. In tospoviruses, the stage affected is believed to be replication.

Recently, considerable efforts have been made towards understanding the molecular basis of the CPMR especially in tobamoviruses. These studies may lead to more rational design of CP-derived transgenes. There is now enough evidence to suggest that CPMR results from the propensity of the transgenically expressed CP to form aggregates. For example, if the transgenically expressed CP was mutated such that there was an increase in inter—subunit interactions, the transgenic plant expressed higher levels of virus resistance. In the case of resistance to TMV, the transgenically expressed CP sub-units are believed to re-coat the nascent disassembled viral RNA which leads to a decreased pool of the available viral RNA for translation, resulting in resistance. However, in many other cases of CPMR, the mechanisms are unclear. Hence, further studies need to be conducted to investigate the existence of mechanisms underlying CPMR.

Substantial yield increase observed in field trials of transgenic papaya and squash (Table 14.3) has established CPMR as the most favoured strategy to engineer resistance against many viruses. The success of CPMR has prompted the production of transgenic plants expressing multiple CP genes from more than one virus. Several important crops have been engineered for virus resistance using CPMR approach and released for commercial cultivation. These include tomato resistant to TMV, tomato mosaic virus (ToMV) and cucumber mosaic virus (CMV); cucumber resistant to CMV, squash resistant to zucchini yellow mosaic virus (ZYMV) and watermelon mosaic virus (WMV2); cantaloupe resistant to ZYMV, WMV2 and CMV; potato resistant to PVX, potato virus Y (PVY) and potato leafroll virus (PLRV); papaya resistant to papaya ringspot virus, PRSV. In addition, transgenic tobacco containing the CP gene of three viruses has been shown to develop resistance to all of them, namely tomato spotted wilt virus (TSWV), tomato chlorotic spot virus and groundnut ringspot virus.

Since CP plays a major role in vector transmission, CPMR confers additional advantage of resistance to vector inoculation in a majority of cases. For example, potato, which express PVX and PVY CP and tobacco, tomato and cucumber expressing CMV CP were seen to be highly resistant to aphid transmissions.

Tomato plants, having TSWV CP transgene were resistant to thrips and plums transformed with PPV CP displayed resistance to *Sharka* virus transmission. Transgenic rice expressing high level of rice stripe virus CP gene expressed resistance to virus inoculation by plant-hopper. However, the mechanism of vector transmission is unclear in many viruses and thus remains a fertile field of research, having potential implications for further effective control of viral diseases.

The discussion on CPMR would not be complete without reference to the most successful story of resistance to PRSV in papaya. Papaya production in Hawaii, suffered due to high incidence of PRSV in 1950s. Transgenic papaya (var. sunset) with *CP* gene was grown from 1991 to 1993, and remained virus-free for 25 months. Subsequently, it was further crossed with other popular varieties. One such variety, called Rainbow, yielded 1,12,000 kg/ha marketable fruits in 1995, compared to 5600 kg/ha from non-transgenic lines. A remarkable increase in the yield clearly established the reliability of CPMR technology.

Replicase (Rep)

Replicase (Rep) protein-mediated resistance against a virus in transgenic plants was first shown in tobacco against TMV in plants containing the 54 kDa putative *Rep gene*. Similar resistances have been developed for several other viruses namely pea early browning virus, PVY and CMV.

Gene constructs of *Rep* genes that have been used for resistance include full-length, truncated or mutated genes. Many of the above resistance responses have now been shown not to require protein synthesis and to be mediated at the RNA level, which is described in more detail later under 'post-transcriptional gene silencing'. This type of resistance remains confined only to a narrow spectrum of viruses, the spectrum being narrower than that of CPMR. To make the resistance broad-based, it may be necessary to pyramid such genes from several dissimilar virussources into the test plant genome. However, the resistance generated by the use of Rep sequences is very tight; a high dosage of input virus can be resisted easily by the transgenic plant.

Movement protein

Movement proteins (MP) are essential for cell-to-cell movement of plant viruses. These proteins have been shown to modify the gating function of plasmodesmata, thereby allowing the virus particles or their nucleoprotein derivatives to spread to adjacent cells. This phenomenon was first used to engineer resistance against TMV in tobacco by producing modified MP which are partially active as a transgene. The conferred resistance is believed to be based on the competition between wild-type virusencoded MP and the preformed dysfunctional MP to bind to the plasmodesmatal sites. The above resistance was moreover seen to be effective against distantly related or unrelated viruses, for example resistance against TMV could be achieved in tobacco using the MP derived from brome mosaic virus, suggesting functional conservation of this protein among several viruses.

In contrast to the single MP gene in tobamoviruses, viral movement is mediated by a set of three overlapping genes, known as the triple-gene-block (TGB) in potex-, carla-and hordeiviruses. Expression of the modified central 12 kDa TGB gene of PVX, was shown to confer MP-derived resistance in potato to potexvirus PVX and carlaviruses potato virus M and potato virus S. However, resistance was overcome when inoculated with viruses lacking a TGB, like PVY. This indicated that the resistance depended upon the interaction of the viralderived and the transgene-derived MPs.

Satellite RNA

Besides using the genomic components of an infectious virus, a strategy exploiting the use of satellite RNA associated with certain viruses received great attention. Some strains of CMV encapsidate satellite RNA (sat RNA) in addition to the tripartite messenger sense, single-stranded RNA genome. CMV sat RNA depends on its helper virus (HV) CMV for replication, movement within the plant, encapsidation and transmission. The presence of sat-RNA modulates the symptoms induced by the HV and often depresses HV accumulation in different host species. Thus, transgenic tobacco plants expressing multiple or partial copies of CMV sat-RNA showed attenuated symptoms when challenged with CMV. In addition, tobacco plants transformed with anti-sense sat-RNA also showed delayed symptom development with the cognate virus.

Sat-RNA was tested as a bio-control agent in field trials in many countries with considerable success. Tomato, containing non-necrogenic sat-RNA sequences developed only faint symptoms following CMV infection. The timing of fruit set and fruit yield in transgenic plants was comparable with healthy plants. Thus, high-level of tolerance to CMV conferred by sat-RNA in tomato was demonstrated. This was further improved by combining sat-RNA and CMV CP. The mechanism behind sat-RNA-mediated resistance may be attributed to the reduction in accumulation of the HV and its long distance movement and down-regulation of replication. However, as sat-RNA spreads epidemically, sufficient caution will have to be exercised in adopting this technology.

Defective-interfering viral nucleic acids

In several viruses, truncated genomic components are often detectable in infected tissues, which interfere with the replication of the genomic components. These species of DNA are also called defective interfering (DI) DNA and expression of delayed disease symptoms and recovery, coupled with increased resistance upon repeated inoculation have been observed in plants engineered with (DI) DNA. For example, incorporation of subgenomic DNA B that interferes with the replication of full length genomic DNA A and B confers resistance to ACMV in *N. benthamiana*. Self-cleaving RNA (ribozymes), seen in viroids and some sat-RNA, were also used with high expectations. There are a few reports like targeting PLRV CP and replicase and 5' region of TMV RNA and citrus exocortis viroid. In most of the cases, ribozyme sequences were ineffective and the resistant phenotypes observed were duse to antisense RNA.

Transgenics with Non-Pathogen Derived Resistance

The following section describes the non-pathogen-derived strategies i.e. those utilising genes derived from either the host plant or any other non-pathogenic source. A new phenomenon called post-transcriptional gene silencing (PTGS) has recently been shown to be responsible for the inherent ability of many plants to specifically degrade nucleic acids in a sequence-specific manner, including those of viruses. Thus, this strategy can be very effective in engineering virus resistance. The other non-pathogen derived strategies are the utilisation of plant disease resistance genes, the ribosome-inactivating proteins, plant proteinase inhibitors, human interferon-like systems, antiviral antibodies expressed in plants, systemic acquired resistance and secondary metabolite engineering.

Post-transcriptional gene silencing

Post-transcriptional gene silencing (PTGS) is a specific RNA degradation mechanism of any organism that takes care of aberrant, unwanted excess or foreign RNA intracellularly in a homology-dependent manner. It is prevalent in various forms of life, namely plant, fungus and invertebrate animals. This activity could be present constitutively to help normal development or induced in response to cellular defense against pathogens. In this mechanism, the elicitor double-stranded RNA (ds RNA), commonly produced during viral infection, is degraded to 21–25 nucleotides, termed as small interfering RNA (siRNA), with the help of a variety of factors that have already been or are being identified. A complex of cellular factors, namely RNA-dependent RNA polymerase (RdRp), RNA-helicase, translation elongation factor, RNAse, etc. along with the small 21–25 nt RNA (of the elicitor RNA) acting as the guide RNA, supposedly degrade RNA molecules bearing homology with the elicitor RNA. This degradation process, initiating from a concerned cell having the elicitor RNA, spreads later within the entire organism in a systemic fashion. This process is generally regarded to have evolved as a plant defense mechanism against invading viruses containing either RNA or DNA genomes.

When the viral RNA is either the elicitor or target of PTGS, the degradation mechanism is known as virus-induced gene silencing (VIGS). VIGS comes into play when plants recover from initial viral infection (viral recovery) or plants resist superinfection of viruses with genomes bearing homology with those of the viruses used as primary inoculum. If tobacco rattle virus (TRV) infects *N. benthamiana*, the plant develops initial symptoms of viral infection at the inoculated region. But the plant shows signs of recovery later and newly emerging leaves are free of TRV. It was shown that viral replicative RNA forms are degraded during the process of recovery, thus indicating the presence of PTGS-related mechanisms.

In nepovirus-infected *Nicotiana* sp., there are severe viral symptoms on the inoculated and first systemic leaves. However, the upper leaves that develop after systemic infection are symptom-free and contain a lower concentration of virus than symptomatic leaves. Similarly, *N. clevelandii* inoculated with tomato black ring nepovirus (W-22 strain) initially shows symptoms and later recovers by PTGS mechanism. In addition, if a secondary inoculum of W22 is applied to the recovered leaves, no additional accumulation of W22 RNA above that resulting from the primary inoculation is seen and the plants remain symptom-free. This kind of resistance is not observed with secondary inoculation of viruses that are unrelated to the genomic sequence of W22. Thus, the resistance of the recovered leaves to subsequent viral challenge depends upon the homology-dependent process. A similar resistance involving PTGS applies not only to RNA viruses but also to DNA viruses.

Viruses can also induce silencing of host endogenes and transgenes that are similar in sequence to the inoculated virus. The applicability of this principle has been demonstrated by using a fused transgene containing TSWV–N gene and the PTGS-inducing turnip mosaic virus (TuMV) CP gene. The transgenic *N. benthamiana* showed resistance to both viruses by a PTGS-dependent phenomenon. Silencing can be achieved when the silenced gene is present in either sense or antisense orientation. During silencing, not only the target host gene transcripts but also the viral RNA forms are degraded. Thus it is easily conceivable that the infecting viruses could be inactivated by PTGS mechanisms if the host carries the transgene(s) of the same or similar virus. In fact, such phenomena of recovery/resistance can be explained using PTGS. In a majority of Rep-mediated resistance, mentioned earlier, resistance is now known to occur utilising the PTGS mechanisms, which provide the molecular basis of such phenomena. For the majority of the transgenic plants showing PDR phenotypes using antisense, untranslatable or non-coding regions of the virus, PTGS have been well documented and the level of resistance parallel the level of silencing. Direct correlation between the viral recovery or resistance and PTGS has been demonstrated using the mutant plants that are deficient in one or some of the components required for PTGS.

Resistance generated against PPV in *N. benthamiana* is a good example of application of this principle for virus control using PTGS. About 10-kb-long RNA genome of PPV is shown in Fig. 14.7. Isolated viral transgene(s) have been chosen from almost every segment of the genome and the transgenic plants are able to resist PPV. Since all the events of recovery or resistance were linked to the loss of viral replicative RNA and the transgenic RNA forms, PTGS must have played its part in conferring the resistance to PPV.

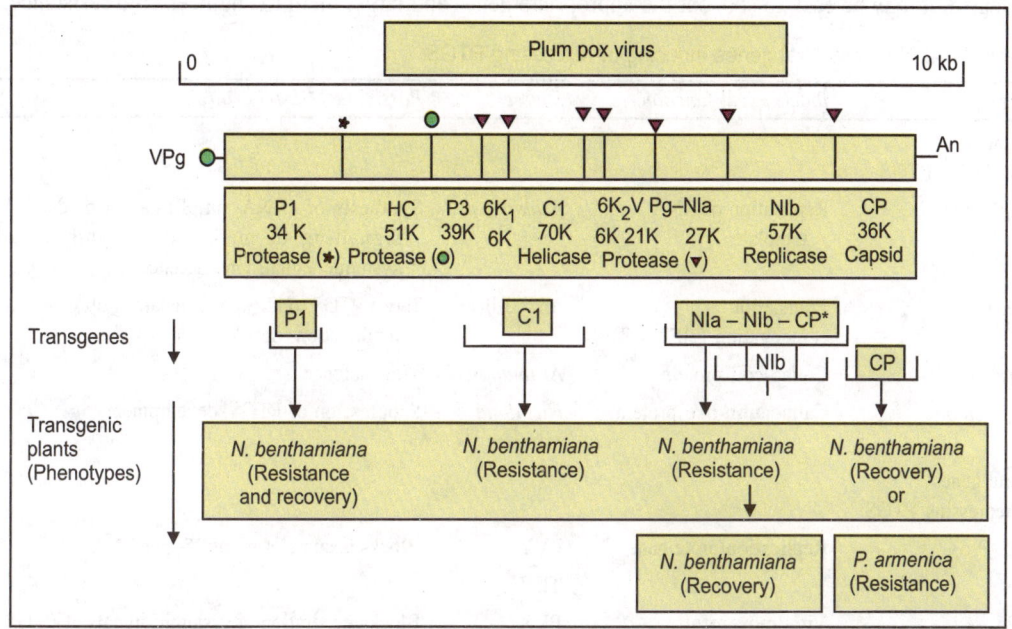

Fig. 14.7. Schematic diagram showing genetic map of PPV with the regions used for the production of transgenic plants for virus resistance. Gene products and the phenotype of the plants are indicated.

Antisense-mediated gene silencing (ASGS) and PTGS with sense transgenics are remarkably similar in mechanistic terms. Both forms of silencing are involved in production of 20–25 nt long degraded RNA (siRNA) and both forms are suppressible by the same viral proteins known to inhibit PTGS (as mentioned later). However PTGS works effectively only when both the sense and antisense RNAs are simultaneously present in the plant cell. Transgene constructs engineered to produce dsRNA as opposed to single stranded sense(s) or antisense (a/s) RNA cause higher incidence of RNA silencing. The pro-gene sequence of PVY was used to demonstrate this effect. Tobacco plants were generated using gene constructs encoding the 'Pro' sequence in the s, a/s or in both the orientations. The plants challenged with PVY were scored for symptoms and tested for PVY replication by ELISA. Results of progeny segregation analysis indicated that, unlike some of the simple s or a/s constructs, the s plus a/s constructs gave stable immunity to PVY, which was inherited in a Mendelian fashion. PVY immunity could also result when the sense and antisense Pro gene transcripts of the PVY-susceptible tobacco transformants were brought together by sexual crossing. Such findings confirm that the simultaneous expression of the sense and antisense RNA in the plant was responsible for enhanced PVY immunity.

Many viruses have evolved mechanisms to suppress host PTGS activity. The balance of the pro-PTGS and anti-PTGS activities probably determines the outcome of virus–plant interaction. Table 14.4 shows the known plant and viral genes inducing or repressing PTGS. PVX does not encode for any strong anti-PTGS activity by itself. Hence PVX-based recombinant viral vectors containing test genes from various viruses have been used for infecting silenced GFP-transgenic plants to screen for PTGS suppressing activity of the viruses. None of the genes shown in Table 14.4 has been used yet for plant transformation studies to develop or modulate viral resistance. Once the biochemical steps of PTGS are revealed, it may be easy to sort out the appropriate genes and target them to engineer viral resistance.

Table 14.4. Plant and viral genes inducing or repressing PTGS

Genes	Biochemical function	Source	Possible PTGS-related role
Plant genes inducing PTGS			
Sde1 or SgS2	Replication of RNA template	Arabidopsis	Synthesis of cRNA, amplification of dsRNA, signalling of methylation, synthesis of systemic signal, viral defence
Ago1	Translation elongation (eIF2C-like)	Arabidopsis	Target PTGS to ribosome, signalling of methylation, development
Sgs3	Coiled-coil protein	Arabidopsis	Viral defence
Rgs–CaM	Calmodulin-like protein	Nicotiana tabacum	Suppression of PTGS, development
Viral genes repressing PTGS			
HC–Pro	Replication/proteinase	PVY TEV	Blocks accumulation of 25-mer RNA
P25	Viral movement	PVX	Blocks generation of systemic signals of PTGS
2b	Viral movement	CMV	Blocks initiation of PTGS at the nuclear step
AC2	Virion-sense tran-scription enhancer	ACMV	PTGS inhibitor

Plant disease resistance genes

A number of disease resistance genes (R) have been reported against viruses of crop plants (Table 14.5). They encode products which respond to viral signals (avirulence (*avr*) gene products) culminating in a number of resistance responses in the plant. As shown in Table 14.5, many of the corresponding viral *avr* genes have also been identified. Some of the *R* genes have been shown to complement the disease susceptibility phenotype in the corresponding cultivars when used as transgenes, furnishing a direct proof of their action. The following section describes the current knowledge about *R* genes against viruses and their mechanisms of action. *R* genes in plants are defined by the classical gene-forgene hypothesis, which states that for every incompatible host pathogen interaction, there exist matching *R* genes in the host and *avr* genes in the pathogen. Resistance reaction against pathogen results generally by direct interaction between the products of *R* and *avr* genes. This interaction, in many cases, results in a resistance reaction, known as hypersensitive reaction (HR), which can be defined as a specific response of a host towards a pathogen. HR results in localised cell death, appearing as necrotic lesions at the site of pathogen entry. HR results in the arrest of pathogen spread, thereby effectively restricting it to the dead cells.

Table 14.5. *R* genes against viruses and corresponding *avr* gene products.

Resistance gene	Source plant	Avr product of the virus	Pathogen
HRT	*Arabidopsis thaliana* ecotype Dijon	Coat protein	TCV
I	*Phaseolus vulgaris*	–	BCMV
L2	*Capsicum* sp.	Coat protein	PMMV
L3	*Capsicum* sp.	Coat protein	PMMV
N	*N. tabacum* cultivar *Samsun*	Replicase	TMV
RRT	*Arabidopsis thaliana* ecotype Dijon	Coat protein	TCV
RTM	*Arabidopsis thaliana* ecotype *Columbia*-O	–	TCV
Rx, Nx, Nb	*Solanum tuberosum* cultivar *Cara*	Coat protein	PVX
Ry	*Solanum stoloniferum*	NIa protease	PVY
Tm1	*Lycopersicon esculentum*	Replicase	TMV
Tm2	*L. esculentum*	Movement protein	TMV
Tm2(2)	*L. esculentum*	Movement protein	TMV
TuRB01	*Brassica napus*	Cylindrical Inclusion protein	TuMV
Va	*Nicotiana tabacum* cultivar *Burley*	Covalently-linked viral genomic protein	TVMV

PMMV, Pepper mild mosaic virus; BCMV, Bean common mosaic virus; TVMV, Tobacco vein mottling virus; for rest of the viruses, consult Table 14.2 and text.

All known *R* genes encode products having two basic functions: to act as sensors for the corresponding *avr* factors/elicitors and to initiate signalling cascades for the expression of defence-related genes. A number of structural features are conserved across several *R* gene products. These include leucine-rich repeat (LRR), nucleotide-binding site (NBS), serine-threonine kinase, leucine zipper, toll-interleukin region (TIR), etc. These structural features are believed to have important roles to play in the execution of the above functions. The following sections describe different types of resistance responses initiated due to *R* genes against viruses and their mechanisms. One of the *R* genes against a viral pathogen (which has been analysed in great detail) is the *N* gene of tobacco and provides resistance against TMV. The *N* gene product has a prominent TIR (a signalling domain) at the amino-terminus and a LRR (a recognition domain) at the carboxyl-terminus of the polypeptide. The TIR domain exhibits a strong homology with the *Drosophila* toll receptor protein, which is a well-characterised signalling molecule. The *N* gene product recognises the TMV· replicase as the *avr* factor. Transposon mutagenesis was performed to obtain HR– lines of the tobacco cultivar Samsun, which were then used to clone the *N* gene adjacent to the sites of transposon insertion. The cloned *N* was shown to be sufficient for the production of a typical HR by complementation analysis. Transgenic tomato plants, expressing the cloned *N*, were also shown to develop resistance against the virus. The *N* gene was thus seen to retain its effectiveness for initiating a HR even in a heterologous system and was the first example of the use of a *R* gene in providing transgenic protection against virus in a useful crop plant.

Turnip crinkle virus (TCV) resistance in *A. thaliana* is mediated by an altogether different mechanism. The *RTM* gene, present in ecotype Columbia-O, brings about a HRindependent resistance against TCV by affecting its longdistance movement and is present as two alleles, *RTM1* and *RTM2*. Both the above allellic forms were cloned by map-based approach and shown to complement the TCVsusceptibility of the *rtm* mutant. The RTM protein is believed to interfere directly with an essential component of the long-distance movement of the virus. Thus, model plants like *Arabidopsis* can help us in looking for related *R* genes in crop plants.

Another type of resistance response is seen against PVX in certain varieties of potato carrying the *Rx* gene. This response, termed extreme resistance, is characterised by the rapid arrest of virus accumulation at the sites of infection and by the absence of HR. Gene *Rx* was cloned from potato cultivar Cara by a map-based cloning approach. The functionality of the gene was demonstrated by its ability to prevent the replication of a PVX-derived vector in tobacco *N. benthamiana* using a transient assay. The cloned DNA fragment was used to produce transgenic potato cultivar Maris Bard (*rx* genotype), which developed resistance against mechanically inoculated PVX. Moreover, the above resistance resembled that mediated by *Rx*. Similar results were also demonstrated in transgenic tobacco.

The other anti-viral *R* genes which have been identified are *Sw-5* and *Tsw* against TSWV from tomato and pepper respectively, *Ry* against PVY, from *Solanum stoloniferum*, *Va* against tobacco vein mottling virus (TVMV) from *N. tabacum* cultivar Burley, *TuRB01* from *Brassica napus* against TuMV, *I* against bean common mosaic virus (BCMV) from *Phaseolus vulgaris*, *L2* and *L3* against pepper mild mottle virus (PMMV) from *Capsicum* sp., *Nx* and *Nb* against PVX from *Solanum tuberosum* and *Tm1*, *Tm2* and *Tm2(2)* against TMV from *Lycopersicon esculentum*. There is, however, no report of use of the above resistance genes in engineering resistance against viruses in crop plants.

Many of the *R* genes studied so far are clustered in plant genomes and can induce resistance to diverse pathogens as exemplified by the *Rx* and the *Gpa2* genes, which are tightly linked, specifying resistance against PVX and nematode. Such a scenario can be expected to be more widespread, encompassing more than one viral pathogen. Thus, understanding the molecular interactions between the various *R* genes products and their elicitors would help in a better and more effective design for their use in providing resistance against a wide spectrum of pathogens at the field level.

Strategies to achieve broad-spectrum pathogen resistance utilising the *R* genes are also being developed and tested. Resistance in tomato to the bacterial pathogen *Pseudomonas syringae* pathovar tomato requires *Pto* and *Prf* genes. *Prf* belongs to the NBS-LRR superfamily of plant disease resistance genes. Overexpression of *Prf* in tomato cultivar lacking the gene leads to enhanced resistance to a number of pathogens, including TMV.

The most exciting approach towards engineering improved resistance to multiple diseases may be the development of new *R* genes having multiple specificities. The *Fen* (resistance to the insecticide Fenthion) and *Pto* genes are located in the same *R* gene cluster in the tomato genome and they are 86 per cent identical in nucleotide sequence. A functional gene was made by domain swapping of the two genes, thus raising the possibility of creating a hybrid gene containing multiple specificities. Another novel strategy, termed two-component approach, has been developed lately and holds lot of promise for introducing broad-spectrum resistance. This strategy involves generation of transgenic plants that express a pathogen *avr* gene under the control of a heterologous infection-inducible promoter. If the plant carries the matching *R* gene, it will respond with an HR at the site of infection thus limiting the pathogen. The key to this approach is the identification of suitable promoters that respond or are induced only following infection by broadrange pathogens. Such promoters have been described in the literature and the validity of this transgenic approach has also been demonstrated.

Ribosomal inactivating proteins

Several plants have been found to contain antiviral proteins, commonly termed as ribosome-inactivating proteins (RIPs). RIPs inhibit the translocation step of translation by catalytically removing a specific adenine base from 28S ribosomal RNA. They are synthesised either as pre-or pre-pro-proteins and targeted to vacuoles. Because of their specific intracellular localisation, RIPs do not affect the endogenous 28S RNA. It is supposed that RIPs enter cells together with the viruses and exert the damage to the host ribosome or possibly viral RNA.

The antiviral activity of several types of RIPs has been well-documented. When purified RIPs are mixed with viruses and applied on plants, virus multiplication and symptom development are dramatically suppressed. A broad range of viruses can be suppressed in this manner. Some RIPs not only inhibit local virus multiplication in RIP-treated leaves but also block viral multiplication systemically. Hence RIPs release a signal that induces systemic resistance to viruses. The development of systemic resistance was reported following studies on induction of a 34 kDa basic protein from the RIP (CA-SRI) treated *Cyamopsis tetragonoloba* plants.

The genes for RIPs have been isolated from a number of plant sources. The cDNAs for PAP (Pokeweed), MAP (*Mirabilis jalapa*), Trichoxanthin (*Trichoxanthes kirilowi*), Dianthin (*Dianthus caryophyllus*), Momorcharin (*Momordica charantia*), CA-SRI from *Clerodendrum aculeatum*, Ricin (*Ricinus communis*), etc. have been isolated and characterised. These cDNAs have also been used to transform plants and in many cases the transgenic plants have shown broad-range antiviral activities. Transgenic *N. benthamiana* plants expressing PAP have been shown to offer broad-spectrum virus resistance, to both mechanical and aphid transmission. In another experiment, the toxin gene, dianthin was placed downstream of a transactivatable geminivirus promoter from ACMV. When transgenic *N. benthamiana* plants were inoculated with ACMV, dianthin was synthesised only in the virusinfected tissues where it inhibited virus multiplication.

Protease inhibitors from plants

Many viruses, namely poty-, tymo-, nepo-, como-, and closteroviruses need cysteine protease activity to process their own polyproteins for their replication and propagation. Hence plants expressing cysteine protease inhibitors might resist the growth of viruses as mentioned above. This idea was tested by using cysteine protease inhibitors (oryzacystatin) of rice to successfully engineer resistance against potyviruses in transgenic tobacco plants. Tobacco lines expressing the rice cysteine proteaseinhibitor gene were examined for resistance against tobacco etch virus (TEV) and PVY infection. A clear, direct correlation between the level of oryzacystatin message, inhibition of papain (a cysteine protease) and resistance to TEV and PVY in all tested transgenic lines was observed. Expectedly, no protection has been found against the TMV infection because this virus does not require polyprotein-processing for its growth. These results indicate that plant proteinase inhibitors can be used against different potyviruses and potentially also against other viruses, where protein cleavage is an essential part of their life cycle.

Interferon-like systems

Higher vertebrates resist virus infections in part by catalysis of RNA decay using the interferon regulated 2–5A system. The 2–5A system consists of two enzymes, namely a 2–5A synthetase that makes 5′ phosphorylated, 2′–5′-linked oligoadenylates (2–5A) in response to doublestranded DNA, and the 2–5A dependent RNAse L. In plants, homologues of this system are not yet known but the inducers, i.e. interferon-like molecules have been reported. The above human enzymes have been co-expressed in transgenic tobacco plant. The transgenic tobacco produced low-level but functional 2–5A synthetase and activated RNAse L. These transgenic lines were tested positive for their proficiencies to resist at least three different types of viruses: TEV, TMV and AMV.

Anti-viral plantibodies

Another approach to control plant viruses is to express specific anti-viral antibodies in plants, commonly known as plantibodies. The efficacy of this approach has been demonstrated against Artichoke mottled crinkle virus in transgenic *N. benthamiana*. A panel of monoclonal antibodies was raised against AMCV and the gene for the most reactive of the above panel was cloned and expressed in *N. benthamiana*. The above transgenic plants and their progeny showed lower virus accumulation, reduced incidence of infection and delayed symptom appearance, compared to non-transgenic plants.

A similar approach was utilised to test *N. benthamiana* plants expressing single-chain antibody against the CP of beet necrotic yellow vein virus. A significant delay in symptom development in the above transgenic plants was reported, following mechanical inoculation and inoculation with the natural vector *Polymyxa betae*. Monoclonal antibodies against various gene products of TSWV have been introduced into tomato to generate continued resistance to both TSWV and root knot nematode.

Systemic acquired resistance

Following viral infections, plants develop an active resistance which is at first localised only at the site of infection, but spreads systemically in due course. This resistance, called systemic acquired resistance (SAR), is characterised by the coordinate activation of several genes in uninfected, distal parts of the inoculated plants. SAR is characteristically associated with accumulation of salicylic acid (SA), enhanced expression of pathogenesis-related (PR) proteins activation of phenylpropanoid pathway, leading to the synthesis of higher phenolic compounds, increase of active oxygen species and reinforcement of cell wall by the deposition of lignin and suberin. Involvement of SA in TMV resistance has been shown by expressing the bacterial salicylate hydroxylase (*NahG*) gene in tobacco plant, thus decreasing its endogenous salicylic acid, and causing susceptibility to TMV infection.

The discovery that SA-binding protein is a catalase, whose activity is blocked by SA led to the proposal that the mode of action of SA is to inhibit the hydrogen peroxide degrading enzyme catalase, resulting in elevation of hydrogen peroxide levels. Transgenic tobacco plants were developed that expressed catalase 1 (*Cat1*) or catalase 2 (*Cat2*) gene in an antisense orientation. Antisense catalase transgenic plants exhibiting severe reduction in catalase activity (approximately 90 per cent or more), developed chlorosis or necrosis on lower leaves. These plants also showed high level of SA and PR accumulation as well as enhanced resistance to TMV.

In another experiment, tobacco was transformed with two bacterial genes coding for enzymes that convert chorismate into SA by a two-step process. When the two enzymes were targeted to the chloroplast, the transgenic plants showed 500- to 1000-fold increased accumulation of SA and SA-glucoside, compared to control plants. The level of PR-proteins was enhanced and these plants showed resistance to viral and fungal infection, in a mode similar to SAR in nontransgenic plants.

Secondary metabolite pathways

Metabolic pathways which are important in viral pathogenesis are key targets for intervention against viral infection. One such step is mediated by *S*-adenosyl homocystein hydrolase (SAHH), which is a key enzyme in trans-methylation reactions that take place, using *S*adenosylmethionine as the methyl donor. It is suggested to play a role in 5′ capping of mRNA during replication. The antisense RNA for tobacco SAHH was expressed in transgenic tobacco plants. Though 50 per cent of the plants showed stunting, they were resistant to infection by various plant viruses. Analysis of the physiological changes in these plants showed that they contained excess level of cytokinin. Since cytokinin is known to induce acquired resistance, increased resistance observed might be attributed to increased level of cytokinin.

Another novel approach of interference with viral pathogenesis is to inhibit tetrapyrrole biosynthesis by expressing antisense RNA of uroporphyrinogen decarboxylase or coporphyrinogen oxidase in *N. tabacum*. The plants were characterised by accumulation of photosensitising tetrapyrrole intermediates, accumulation of highly fluorescent Coumarin scopolin, PR proteins and reduced levels of infecting viral RNA.

Essential Considerations for Developing Virus-Resistant Transgenics

Variability

Viral genes show high levels of variability. This may be due to lack of proof reading function of viral replicases and the high recombination rates of viral genomes during the progress of infection. Symptomatic variants or strains of viruses, as well as geographically distinct isolates, not showing such variations in symptoms, have been nevertheless, documented to contain significant variability in their genes. Under field conditions, most of the viruses are believed to exist as collection of variants, or 'quasispecies', as documented in cassava-infecting geminiviruses in Uganda and rice tungro bacilliform virus, a double-stranded DNA virus in southeast Asia.

As with naturally occurring virus resistance genes, when considering virus resistance under field conditions, strain specificity and breadth of protection are important questions. There is often a general correlation between the extent of protection and the relatedness between the challenge virus and virus from which the transgene was derived. It is clear from the case of transgenic papaya that the level of resistance is dependent upon the homology between the prevalent viral isolate and the transgene. It is imperative that in any viral transgene strategy, sequence of the aggressive prevalent strain of the virus in that region is used. Sufficient information on the degree of diversity amongst the biologically indistinguishable viral strains needs to be collected before designing the transgene. It is especially true of whitefly transmitted geminiviruses, where the evolution of the virus is rapid. A wide variety of virus genotypes may be present, either maintained in different cultivated hosts or on endogenous weed species. Depending upon change in the vector behaviour, e.g. feeding on to a new host more frequently than it was doing earlier and vector population build-up, viruses of different populations may start infecting new hosts leading to further changes in their genotype.

The success of any transgenic strategy is dependent upon the level of resistance to multiple inoculation of the same or related strains, by vector transmission. In recent years, efforts have been made to identify the variants and to assess the genetic relatedness between them. However, frequency distribution of these variants in a given virus population needs to be assessed to develop a transgenic strategy targeting any virus causing an economically important disease. The population structure of the virus is determined by evolutionary factors affecting its life cycle, the major factor being selection pressure on the gene products that interact with host and the vector. Variability may result due to host component as new host genotypes are introduced, or by vector component as they adapt to new host system or by the virus itself by mutation, complementation or recombination. A periodical assessment of population structure is mandatory if virus-derived transgenic resistance strategy is adopted for the control of the disease. It is especially true of India, where strain variability is observed and which would result in breakdown of resistance.

Biological risks

The concept of using pathogen-derived genes to induce transgenic resistance has no doubt raised a number of ecological concerns. Risk perceptions boil down to two major items, (i) recombination between viral-derived transgene and non target virus, and (ii) transmission/vector host range changes brought about by heteroencapsidation, i.e. encapsidation of the genome of non-target virus with the transgenically expressed CP. Field trials conducted so far with transgenics have not indicated that expression of viral transgenes leads to the emergence of new super strain or change in transmission behaviour of common viral pathogens. However, sufficient care should be taken to avoid any risks due to heteroencapsidation while designing the constructs.

The strong linkages shown by CP with insect transmission of viruses, have made possible heteroencapsidation, an important factor to be considered while designing CPbased transgenes. Coat protein genes have been designed from PPV, such that a 'DAG' motif in the CP, believed to play an important role in vector transmission, was deleted to prevent any further insect transmission of heteroencapsidated virions. The use of these constructs in producing transgenic plants has shown that heteroencapsidation of ZYMV was significantly reduced without compromising virus resistance of the plants. Similar results have also been reported recently in transgenic *N. benthamiana* expressing mutated PPV CP, which were not only resistant to PPV, but were also suppressed in heteroencapsidation, when infected with chilli vein mottle virus and PVY.

Comparison of anti-viral strategies

The success of transgenic approach varies for any specific host/virus combination. A range of phenotypes is observed amongst the virus-resistant transgenic plants. While CPMR confers broad-spectrum, less complete resistance, Rep-mediated resistance produces immunity against the virus, but to a limited spectrum of strains. Similarly, in RNA-mediated resistance, antisense RNA targeting mRNA of DNA viruses has more potential than against positive-stranded RNA virus. Any antisense RNA/ribozyme strategy should bear in mind the association/dissociation parameters of the molecules. Pyramiding of different transgenes or combination of transgenes with natural resistance targeting different events in viral life cycle will increase the confidence level in the management of viral diseases and will ensure stability of resistance at the field level. Durability, broad-spectrum character of the transgene-derived resistance coupled with enhanced crop yield of the transgenics *viv-à-vis* healthy, untransfomed plants, etc. are some of the essential parameters, which any important strategy must incorporate.

Economically Important Plant Viruses in India and Future Outlook

In India, the post-green revolution era saw an upsurge in agricultural operations all over the country. Practices like introduction of new genotypes, indiscriminate use of insecticides, change in cultivation practices, etc. tilted the balance in favour of vector-transmitted diseases in several crops. For example, cultivation of soyabean as an industrial crop in large areas, continued cropping of *moong* in summer months, without leaving any time lapse, introduction of susceptible germplasm of Nigerian cowpea, etc. led to the perpetuation of the vector whiteflies and to the availability of the viral inoculum throughout the year. The above reasons have been speculated to give rise to epidemics of yellow mosaic diseases of legumes. The scenario changes every year. In 1980s, the diseases caused by potyviruses and whitefly transmitted geminiviruses were the prominent ones resulting in considerable yield loss (Table 14.1). In the last five years, Ilarviruses causing severe necrosis and destruction of crop in sunflower and grain legumes and tospoviruses producing severe bud necrosis in groundnut, tomato, melons and grain legumes have emerged as serious pathogens. The host range of these viruses is spreading and in future, many more crops may get infected. We have listed ten most important viral diseases observed in crops extensively grown in India are already listed in (Table 14.1). Wide range in yield loss data given indicates the changes from year to year in the incidence and severity of the disease. The disparity is also due to diversity within particular virus and crop genotypes. Beside the viruses listed, viral diseases of horticultural crops like banana bunchy top disease in banana, tristeza virus disease in citrus, papaya ring spot viral diseases in papaya have also assumed serious and unmanageable proportions.

For most viral diseases, resistant lines have been developed by conventional breeding and along with judicious insecticide sprays to control the vector population, help in management of the disease. Some of the examples include cultivar Sree Vishakam in cassava against ICMV, LR5166 in cotton against CLCuV, K-134 in groundnut against bud necrosis virus, Kufri Chandramukhi in potato against PLRV and PVY and Vikramarya in rice against the tungro virus disease. However, when the source of resistance is not available, a biotechnological approach becomes necessary. For the whitefly-transmitted geminiviruses like ToLCV, CLCuV, ICMV and yellow mosaic virus in legumes, results obtained in many laboratories with transgenics containing replication initiation protein are encouraging and this approach could be adopted. CPMR for Ilarviruses, both CPMR and PTGS for potyviruses, have shown promising results, which could be adapted for viruses of India. The *NS* and *NM* genes, similarly, have been used for tospoviruses. Characterisation of *R* genes associated with the well-established resistant lines, if achieved, will lead to a long-lasting solution.

Efforts initiated in various research organisations in India towards the development of virus-resistant transgenics have been summarised in the following section.

Following the availability of molecular information on viruses, initiatives have been taken in some leading institutions in India towards the development of transgenic virus resistance in important crops. At the Indian Institute of Science, Bangalore, success has already been reported in controlling physalis mottle virus using pathogenderived resistance in tobacco and tomato. A similar approach has been recently shown to result in resistance to PVY in tobacco in a collaborative research programme between the Central Potato Research Institute, Shimla and the Bhabha Atomic Research Centre, Mumbai. Tobacco and tomato transformation using TLCV CP and replicase genes is being attempted at the National Botanical Research Institute, Lucknow. Similar approaches are also being used to generate resistance against viruses of important crops like cotton, rice, tomato and mungbean at the Indian Institute of Science, Bangalore, University of Delhi South Campus, New Delhi, the Indian Agricultural Research Institute, New Delhi, Madurai Kamaraj University, Madurai and Maharshi Dayanand University, Rohtak. Incorporation of PVY CP gene into tobacco and potato has been achieved by the Indian Agricultural Research Institute, New Delhi.

In conclusion, it can be said that genetic engineering of crop plants for virus resistance is undoubtedly a key biotechnological tool which can be used to minimise the losses to crop production incurred due to viral diseases in our country. Most of the important viruses have already been identified and the cloning and molecular characterisation of their genomic components is at advanced stages. However, to successfully develop and test a series of virus-resistant transgenic crops, the following bottlenecks need to be removed: (i) Absence of transformation and regeneration systems for all the major crops of the country, (ii) Insufficient variability studies of important viruses, and (iii) Lack of basic research on the functional genomics of pathogenesis.

Of all the major crop plants in our country, transformation systems are available for only a few cereals, vegetables, fibre crops and oilseed varieties. A major push needs to be given for transformation of pulses and legumes, which incur some of the heaviest losses due to viruses. The dominant and virulent strains of each important virus in the country need to be identified for obtaining genes for resistance engineering. Studies should also focus on the degree of variability and the recombination of viral genomes. This will help in the design of suitable constructs that will ensure durable resistance across the country. Emerging techniques of functional genomics need to be harnessed to understand the molecular interactions between the viral pathogen and the resistant and susceptible plants leading to resistance or pathogenesis. This is bound to result in novel insights at disease control. Insect-proof glasshouses and insectaries require to be modernised with facilities to provide ambient conditions for plant growth in our country. This needs to be looked into by funding agencies.

It is also clear that the effort for producing viral-resistant transgenic crop plants needs to be multidisciplinary, with a close cooperation among virologists, molecular biologists, tissue-culture specialists, agronomists and the government. Their combined effort is sure to deliver to the Indian farmers, a range of virus-resistant crops in the near future, which will help mitigate the losses in crop yields due to viruses in India.

GENETIC MANIPULATION OF FLOWER PIGMENTATION

As an alternative to traditional breeding techniques, uniquely coloured flowers can be developed by manipulating the genes for enzymes in the anthocyanin biosynthesis pathway. Anthocyanins, which are a class of flavonoids, are the most common type of flower pigment. They are synthesised from the amino acid phenylalanine by a series of enzyme-catalysed reactions. The colour of the flower is determined by the chemical side chain substitutions of different chemical structures, with the cynanidin derivatives producing more red and the delphinidin derivatives producing more.

While the petunia enzyme dihydroflavonol 4-reductase can convert colourless dihydroquercetin to red cyanidin-3-glucoside and colourless dihydromyricetin to blue delphinidin-3-glucoside, it cannot use colourless dihydrokaempferol as a substrate. However, when petunias were transformed with a dihydroflavonol 4-reductase gene from maize, the flowers of the transgenic plants was brick red — orange. This unique colour, which had never been seen before in petunias, was due to the production of pelargonidin-3-glucoside by the transgenic plants.

Four plants (roses, caranations, tulips, and chrysanthemums) account for approximately 70 per cent of the cut-flower industry worldwide. Moreover, since genetic transformation protocols have been worked out for these four plants, they should become the focus of efforts to develop plants with unique colours. For example, transgenic chrysanthemums with both sense and antisense constructs of the chrysanthemum chalcone synthase cDNA have been produced. Chalcone synthase catalyses the first step in anthocynanin biosyntheis. It is expected that both the sense and the antisense cDNA will suppress chalcone synthase gene expression in transgenic plants and produce white flowers instead of the normal pink. 'Sense suppression', which is also called 'cosuppression', occurs when an additional copy of an endogenous gene prevents the accumulation of the mRNA from the endogenous gene. On the other hand, the antisense chalcone synthase RNA should block translation of endogenous chalcone synthase mRNA.

The sense and antisense constructs were placed under the control of the cauliflower mosaic virus 35S promoter on a binary Ti plasmid vector and then introduced into plant cells. Three of the 133 sense transformants and three of the 83 antisense transformants produced white flowers, which indicated that endogenous chalcone synthase gene expression and, as a consequence, anthocyanin synthesis had been suppressed. The white-flowering plants were propagated vegetatively through cuttings, and approximately 90 to 98 per cent of the plants continued to produce white flowers when planted in the field. This work is an important step toward the development of commercial flower varieties with novel colours.

Manipulation of Carotenoids Astaxanthin

The carotenoids astaxanthin, which provides the characteristic pink colour to salmon, trout, and shrimp, is synthesised by marine bacteria and micro algae and then passed on to fish through the food chain.

More important, astaxanthin protects salmon and trout eggs from damage by UV radiation and improves the survival and growth rate of juveniles. Most likely, these properties of astaxanthin are related to its function as a powerful antioxidant. However, when fish are grown in aquaculture they are separated from the natural food chain and astaxanthin must be added to their feed in order to impart the typical pink colour to their flesh. Currently, astaxanthin is chemically synthesised and accounts for approximately 15 per cent of the total cost of salmon farming.

To produce astaxanthin biologically, one group of researchers first cloned a cDNA encoding the enzyme β-carotene Ketolase (β-C-4 oxygenase) from the unicellular green alga *Haematococcus pluvialis*. When this cDNA was expressed in an organism that contains β-carotene and the gene for β-carotene hydrolase, astaxanthin was synthesised. By appropriate genetic manipulation, astaxanthin has been synthesised in tobacco flowers. The cDNA for the algal β-carotene ketolase was fused to DNA encoding a chloroplast transit peptide and used to transform tobacco plants. To limit expression of astaxanthin to flowers and fruits, the cDNA for the algal β-carotene ketolase was fused to the promoter of the tomato *pds* gene, which encodes phytoene desaturase. To increase the expression of the cDNA for the algal β-carotene ketolase, the DNA fragment carrying the *pds* promoter was reduced in size and then fused to a β-glucuronidase gene. The construct, which had a 305-bp deletion from the 5′ terminus of the *pds* promoter, showed a decrease in β-glucuronidase activity in leaves, sepals, and petals and a very large increase in activity in flower ovaries (nectaries). To obtain maximal gene expression, 305 bp deleted *pds* promoter was placed upstream of the cDNA for the algal β-carotene ketolase. The net result of all these genetic manipulations was that, once the introduced T-DNA had been inserted into the plant genomic DNA, the algal β-carotene ketolase together with a transit peptide was inserted through the chromoplast membrane, with the transit peptide being removed in the process. Once inside the chromoplast, the algal β-carotene ketolase worked in concert with the endogenous β-carotene hydroxylase to convert the β-carotene to astaxanthin,which accumulated in the flower nectaries.The advantage to producing asataxanthin in plants can store large amounts of carotenoids inside cells in lipid vesicles within the plastids. Thus, plants can accumulate 10 to 50 fold greater concentrations of carotenoids than micro-organisms, whose membranes are damaged by high concentrations of carotenoids. These manipulations have the potiental to dramatically lower the cost of the astaxanthin that is used in salmon farming.

PLANT BIOREACTORS

The use of plants as bioreactors is a relatively new bioscience and a burgeoning new industry. It can be defined as the production of novel products in plants and, in the majority of instances, these products are products through the insertion and expression of new genes encoding the additional process(es) required by the plant to synthesise these products. Thus, 'molecular farming' involves the genetic modification of the 'host' plant.

Products that are currently being produced, either commercially or experimentally in plants, include human and animal therapeutics (including vaccines), proteins used in medical diagnostics, industrial proteins and other industrial products (such as bioplastics). The economic drivers for developing molecular farming as an industry include the capacity of crops to produce large amounts of desired products, safety issues (particularly microbiological safety) and most importantly, the cost benefits of plantbased production.

The tropical crops and biocommodities has the expertise and capacity to: (i) transform plants, (ii) express diagnostic/therapeutic proteins in those plants, and (iii) intellectual property access to molecular farming processes. The group have already generated an array of transgenic crops including tobacco, bananas, sugarcane and papaya. They have also developed and patented widely in the area of transgene expression in plants with particular emphasis on a platform technology known as INPACT (In plant ACTivation), which provides exquisite control over the time, place and level of proteins expression.

Bioreactors provide a rapid and efficient plant micropropagation system but as yet are not fully exploited commercially for agricultural crops and forest trees. The culture system was applied to herbaceous and woody plant species utilising liquid media to overcome intensive manual handling. Large-scale liquid cultures were used for propagation through organogenesis or somatic embryogenesis pathways depending on the species. Bioreactors have several advantages over agar cultures with a better control of the culture conditions. Direct contact of the plant tissue with the medium, optimal nutrient and growth regulators supply, continuous aeration and circulation, filtration of the medium for controlling exudates and contamination and the production of clusters of buds, meristems or protocorms for automated dispensing. The major issue imposed by liquid media in bioreactors is the phenomenon of hyperhydricity, morphogenic shoot and leaf malformation, due to the continuous immersion of the tissue in the medium. The malformations are manifested in glossy hyperhydrous leaves with distorted anatomy. The very nature of liquid tissue culture is an imposing stress to which the plants respond to the environmental signals in developmental aberration. The submerged tissue was found to exhibit oxidative stress symptoms, with elevated levels of reactive oxygen species that were associated with a change in anti-oxidant enzyme activity. These changes greatly affected the anatomy and physiology of the plants and their survival after transplanting. Two major solutions for malformation control were proposed: the use of growth retardants to control rapid proliferation and temporary immersion bioreactors. Growth retardants reduced water uptake during cell proliferation, decreased vacuolation and rapid growth, shortened stems and inhibited leaf expansion, inducing the formation of clusters. In tuber, bulb and corm producing plants growth retardants were found to enhance storage organs formation. Temporary immersion bioreactors were used to provide an improved aeration system to reduce hyperhydricity, by shortening plant duration in the liquid phase. The frequency of immersion and the medium composition improved plant development. Future prospects of micropropagation in bioreactors for optimal plant production will depend on both basic and applied studies. The former contributing to our understanding of plant responses to microenvironment signals to overcome the limitations of liquid cultures and the latter to provide specific culture manipulation to control the morphogenesis of plants *in vitro* improving survival *ex vitro*.

Chapter 15

Transgenic Animals

INTRODUCTION

Nowadays, breakthroughs in molecular biology are happening at an unprecedented rate. One of them is the ability to engineer transgenic animals. The term 'transgenics' refers to the science of inserting a foreign gene into an organism's genome. An animal is 'transgenic' once a scientist inserts DNA from another organism. This process allows scientists to transfer beneficial genes from a different animal, bacterium, or plant.

There are various definitions for the term transgenic animal. A transgenic animal is one whose genome has been changed to carry genes from other species.Transgenic animals are animals which have been genetically transformed by splicing and inserting foreign animal or human genes into their chromosomes. The term transgenic animal refers to an animal in which there has been a deliberate modification of the genome—the material responsible for inherited characteristics in contrast to spontaneous mutation.

A transgenic animal is one which has been genetically altered to have specific characteristics it otherwise would not have. In animals, transgenesis either means transferring DNA into the animal or altering DNA already in the animal. Transgenic animals contain elements of two different species—they are creatures that blur the barrier between species.

The Federation of European laboratory animal associations defines the term as an animal in which there has been a deliberate modification of its genome, the genetic makeup of an organism responsible for inherited characteristics.

The nucleus of all cells in every living organism contains genes made up of DNA. These genes store information that regulates how our bodies form and function. Genes can be altered artificially, so that some characteristics of an animal are changed. For example, an embryo can have an extra, functioning gene from another source artificially introduced into it, or a gene introduced which can knock out the functioning of another particular gene in the embryo. Animals that have their DNA manipulated in this way are knows as transgenic animals.

Transgenic animals are produced by inserting genes into embryos prior to birth. Each transferred gene is assimilated by the genetic material or chromosomes of the embryo and subsequently can be expressed in all tissues of the resulting animal. The objective is to produce animals which possess the transferred gene in their germ cells (sperm or ova). Such animals are able to act as 'founder' stock to produce many offspring that carry a desirable gene or genes. The animal that develops after receiving the transgene DNA is referred to as the founder (Fo) of a new transgenic lineage. If the germ cells of the founder (mosaic or not) transmit the transgene stably, then all descendants of this animal are members of a unique transgenic lineage.

A transgenic animal carries heterologous DNA stably integrated into its genome. A transgenic animal results from insertion of a foreign gene into an embryo. The foreign gene becomes a permanent part of the host animals' genetic material. As the embryo develops, the foreign gene may be present in many cells of the body, including the germ cells of the testis or the ovary. If the transgenic animal is fertile, the inserted foreign gene (transgene) will be inherited by future progeny. Thus, a transgenic animal, once created, can persist into future generations. Transgenic animals are different from animals in which foreign cells or foreign organs have been engrafted. The progeny of engrafted animals do not inherit the experimental change. The progeny of transgenic animals do.

In some cases over expression of human genes in bacteria (such as *E. coli*) does not yield a protein that is functionally active in humans. The reason for this is that some proteins need to be post-translationally modified (phosphorylated, glycosylated, etc.) before they are active. Bacteria generally lack the specific enzymes recognising the human protein sequences that need to be modified, and thus the bacterially produced gene product will differ from the native one. To counter this problem, certain human genes can be introduced into farm animals (usually yeast will do the job, too), and when these genes are expressed in the mammary glands of the animals, the post-translationally modified protein can be isolated from milk, tested whether its post-translationally modified product is identical or at least very similar to the native human one, and if so, be developed as a pharmaceutical. For example, the genes for two different human blood clotting factors (VIII and IX) have been hooked up to sheep and pig regulatory sequences that causes expression in mammary tissue; after transformation of sheep or pig embryos, genetically engineered animals have been selected that produce milk with a large percentage of human blood-clotting factor. This protein can be isolated from the milk, purified, and marketed. Similarly, transgenic rabbits have been created that produce human interleukin-2, which is a protein stimulating the proliferation of T-lymphocytes; the latter play an important role in fighting selected cancers.

The majority of transgenic animals produced so far are mice, the animal that pioneered the technology. Long life cycles of farm animals slow genetic analysis. That's why researchers use smaller, faster-breeding animals such as mice as model systems to test their ideas and their DNA constructs. The first successful transgenic animal was a mouse. Over 80 per cent of mouse genes function the same as those in humans. Mice also have a short reproduction cycle and their embryos are amenable to manipulation. Mice are therefore an ideal human surrogate in the study of most diseases. Currently over 95 per cent of transgenic animals used in biomedical research are mice. Other transgenic animals include rats, pigs and sheep. It is hoped that the refinement of transgenesis techniques in mice will ultimately allow for a corresponding reduction in the use of 'higher' animals, such as dogs and non-human primates, in biomedical research. A few years later; it was followed by rabbits, pigs, sheep, fish, poultry and cattle. Furthermore, the mouse is the only model system that combines homologous recombination with cloning to allow the study of modified genes in development of adult animals. Currently, in livestock homologous recombination is possible only with cells grown in tissue culture. This means a scientist can study the effect of knocked-out genes only on the physiology of the cell. The possible role of the gene in development from embryo to adult cannot be tested without a system of cloning: taking the original cell and growing an adult from it.

The insertion of a foreign gene (transgene) into an animal is successful only if the gene is inherited by offspring. The success rate for transgenesis is very low and successful transgenic animals need to be cloned or mated.

Since the early 1980s, methods have been developed and refined to generate transgenic animals or transgenic aquatic species. For example, transgenic livestock and transgenic aquatic species have been generated with increased growth rates, enhanced lean muscle mass, enhanced resistance to disease or improved use of dietary phosphorous to lessen the environmental impacts of animal manure. Transgenic poultry, swine, goats, and cattle also have been produced that generate large quantities of human proteins in eggs, milk, blood, or urine, with the goal of using these products as human pharmaceuticals. Examples of human pharmaceutical proteins include enzymes, clotting factors, albumin, and antibodies. The major factor limiting widespread use of transgenic animals in agricultural production systems is the relatively inefficient rate (success rate less than 10 per cent) of production of transgenic animals.

Scientists do this, creating a 'transgenic' organism, to study the function of the introduced gene and to identify genetic elements that determine which tissue and at what stage of an organism's development a gene is normally turned on. Transgenic animals have also been created to produce large quantities of useful proteins and to model human disease. Various human proteins that have been expressed in transgenic animals include: anti-thrombin III (to treat intravascular coagulation), collagen (to treat burns and bone fractures), fibrinogen (used for burns and after surgery), human fertility hormones, human haemoglobin, human serum albumin (for surgery, trauma, and burns), lactoferrin (found in mother milk), tissue plasminogen activator, and particular monoclonal antibodies (including one that is effective against a particular colon cancer). Animals mostly used for this work are pigs, cows, sheep, and goats.

Almost all the work on transgenic animals is still at the research level. But it enjoys inherent interest and the immense potential for future commercial applications. Scientists, farmers and business corporations hope that transgenic techniques will allow more precise and cost-effective animal and plant breeding programs. They also hope to use these new methods to produce animals with desirable characteristics that are not available using current breeding technology.

The technology has already produced transgenic animals such as mice, rats, rabbits, pigs, sheep, and cows. Although there are many ethical issues surrounding transgenesis, this chapter focuses on the basics of the technology and its applications in agriculture, medicine, and industry.

Scientists can now produce transgenic animals because, since Watson and Crick's discovery (in 1953), there have been breakthroughs in:

1. Recombinant DNA (artificially-produced DNA).
2. Genetic cloning.
3. Analysis of gene expression (the process by which a gene gives rise to a protein).
4. Genomic mapping.

PRODUCTION OF TRANSGENIC ANIMALS

The underlying principle in the production of transgenic animals is the introduction of a foreign gene or genes into an animal (the inserted genes are called transgenes). The foreign genes 'must be transmitted through the germ line, so that every cell, including germ cells, of the animal contains the same modified genetic material'. (Germ cells are cells whose function is to transmit genes to an organism's offspring).

This is a brief outline of the steps necessary to obtain transgenic mice or rats: DNA is prepared and microinjected into fertilised mouse or rat eggs. Potentially transgenic rodents are born. Transgenic founders are identified and bred to produce offspring for analysis. Core personnel are available for consultation on all aspects of transgenic research. Much genetic engineering goes into the choice of a foreign gene and building a construct. The construct must have promotes to turn on foreign gene expression at its new site within the host animal genome. By choosing a particular promoter and splicing it in front of the foreign gene, we can encourage expression of our transgene within a specific tissue.

A transgenic animal for pharmaceutical production should: (i) produce the desired drug at high levels without endangering its own health, and (ii) pass its ability to produce the drug at high levels to its offspring. The current strategy to achieve these objectives is to couple the DNA gene for the protein drug with a DNA signal directing production in the mammary gland. The new gene, while present in every cell of the animal, functions only in the mammary gland so the protein drug is made only in the milk. Since the mammary gland and milk are essentially 'outside' the main life support systems of the animal, there is virtually no danger of disease or harm to the animal in making the 'foreign' protein drug. After the DNA gene for the protein drug has been coupled with the mammary directing signal, this DNA is injected into fertilised cow, sheep, goat, or mouse embryos with the aid of a very fine needle, a tool called a micromanipulator, and a microscope. The injected embryos are then implanted into recipient surrogate mothers where, hopefully, they survive and are born normally.

MICROINJECTION OF DNA INTO FERTILISED EGGS

The production of transgenic mice and other higher animals by DNA microinjections is accomplished by essentially the same procedure that is widely used in *Drosophila*. There are two major differences. (i) P-element transformation in *Drosophila* utilises the transposase of the P-element for integration of the injected DNA molecules. Integration of microinjected DNA in fertilised mouse eggs depends on the recombination mechanisms of the mouse embryo itself, and (ii) DNA is usually injected into mouse eggs that are at an earlier stage of development than those used in Drosophila.

In microinjection, eggs are surgically removed from the female parent and are fertilised with sperm *in vitro*. The DNA (usually a plasmid vector carrying the gene of interest) is microinjected into the male pronucleus (the haploid nucleus contributed by the sperm, prior to nuclear fusion) of the fertilised egg through a very fine tipped glass needle. The injected DNA can be either linear or circular DNA molecules. However, linear DNA integrates with a higher efficiency (about fivefold higher) than circular DNA. Although the results for this difference is not known, it probably results from the recombinogenicity of ends of DNA molecules owing to their ability to invade homologous DNA molecules. Usually, several hundred to several thousand copies of the gene of interest are injected into each egg, and thus multiple integrations can occur. Surprisingly, when multiple copies do integrate into the genome, they usually do so as tandem, head-to-tail arrays at a single chromosomal site. These DNA molecules carrying multiple tandem copies of the transgene are believed to form by recombination events between injected DNA molecules prior to integration. The chromosomal sites of integration are apparently selected at random.

Because the DNA is injected so early during development, even before fusion of the haploid nuclei to form the diploid nucleus of the zygote, integration of the injected DNA molecules usually occurs early enough during embryogenesis so that some germ line cells do carry the transgene. As would be expected, the mice that develop from the injected eggs (called the G_0 generation) are almost always genetic mosaics with some somatic cells carrying the transgene and others not carrying the transgene. The initial (G_0) transgenic mice must be mated and G_1 progeny produced to obtain mice in which all cells carry the transgene.

In almost all the cases where progeny studies have been done, the transgenes were stably transmitted to progeny for as many generations as were examined. In a few cases, transgenes have undergone rearrangements in progeny generations. In mammals, transgenes do not seem to be maintained by autonomous replication (with a couple of exceptions). This is in contrast to the autonomous replication of transgenic DNAs observed after micro injection into eggs of other animals such as frogs, sea urchins, and *Caenorhabditis elegans*.

RETROVIRAL VECTORS

The ability of retroviral proviruses to integrate into host chromosomes and this capability of retroviruses to incorporate DNA copies of their genomes into the chromosomes of their hosts clearly suggests that one might be able to construct modified retroviral gene-transfer vectors that have properties analogous to the *P*-element vectors of *Drosophila*. The key to the development of such retroviral vectors is to modify the viral genome in some manner that will eliminate any chance of pathogenic effects of the vector when present in transgenic animals without changing its capacity to integrate into host chromosomes.

Several retroviral vectors have now been developed and shown to be effective vehicles for gene transfer. These retroviral vectors have proven especially useful in introducing genes into primary and established cell culture lines, although they have also been used to introduce genes into germ line cells by infecting eight-cell embryos. The use of retroviral vectors to introduce genes into primary cell lines may have major applications in somatic-cell 'gene therapy'. One promising approach is to initiate a primary cell line by tissue biopsy, to correct the enzyme deficiency in these primary cells by introducing a wild-type copy of the defective gene, and then to reimplant these transgenic cells back into the appropriate tissue of the affected individual. Whether or not this approach will prove to be effective in treating human diseases remains to be determined, but current work with mice has yielded very encouraging results. Although several different vectors have been developed, and several different gene-transfer strategies have been employed, a single example will suffice to illustrate the potential use of retroviral vectors as tools in future 'gene therapy' treatments of inherited diseases.

As already discussed phenylketonurea (PKU) is an inherited disease in humans caused by a deficiency of the enzyme phenylalanine hydroxylase (PAH). When untreated, individuals with PKU develop severe mental retardation as a result of the accumulation of toxic derivatives of phenylalanine. Current treatment of PKU involves limiting phenylalanine intake with a protein-restricted, carefully formulated diet. Somatic-cell 'gene therapy' might someday provide an alternative method of treatment of PKU.

Both the gene and a cDNA encoding human PAH have been cloned, thus setting the stage for PAH genetransfer experiments. One complication is that in human, PAH is synthesised only in the liver. Moreover, the PAH-catalysed, conversion of phenylalanine to tyrosine requires the cofactor tetrahydrobiopterin. This cofactor is present in Jiver cells, but is not present in most other tissues. Thus, corrective 'gene therapy' for PKU will probably require expression of the introduced PAH gene in liver cells. If so, this excludes the possibility of utilising the more common bonemarrow transplant technology to treat PKU. For that reason, Woo and colleagues have concentrated on the development of chimeric genes and vectors that could be used to express PAH in primary hepatocytes (liver cells). Their results to date are most promising; Woo and coworkers have demonstrated the expression of a chimeric human PAH transgene in primary mouse hepatocytes.

The chimeric human PAH gene was introduced into mouse hepatocytes by using a retroviral vector called N2 that was derived in part from the Moloney murine leukemia virus. The N2 vector contains the viral long terminal repeats (LTRs) that are required for integration of the provirus and additional viral sequences that are required for packaging of the vector into enveloped particles that are capable of adsorbing to and entering recipient cells. The coding sequences for the viral structural proteins have been deleted; thus, the vector is totally nonpathogenic. A chimeric selectable marker gene (a derivative of the neomycin-resistance gene of *E. coli* transposon Tn5) has been inserted to facilitate the identification of transgenic cells. Into this N2 vector, Woo and colleagues inserted a cassette that contained the human PAH cDNA clone and two key regulatory sequences: (i) the 5′ regulatory sequence of the human α_1-antitrypsin gene, and (ii) the promoter sequence from simian virus 40 (SV40). The human α_1-antitrypsin gene is known to be expressed at high levels in hepatocytes, and the 5′ sequence that controls this tissue-specific expression has been localised to the 5′ segment present in the PAH cassette. The structures of the chimeric human PAH 'gene' and the N2 vector are diagrammed in Fig. 15.1. Packaged vector is produced by transfection of a cell line that produces viral structural proteins, but no endogenous progeny viral genomes. Thus, only progeny RNA replicas of the vector genome are packaged, and these virions are purified for use in the gene-transfer experiments.

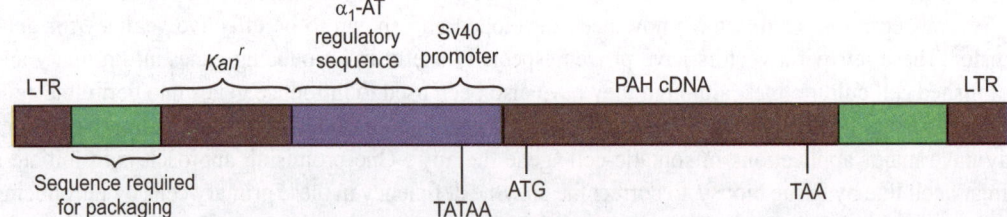

Fig. 15.1. Diagram of the structure of the retroviral phenylalanine hydroxylase expression vector pNASPAH (p, plasmid; N, N2 vector; A, α_1-antitrypsin gene tissue-specific regulatory sequence; S, SV40 promoter; PAR, phenylalanine hydroxylase cDNA). N2 vector sequences are shown in dark grey and light grey; components of the PAH expression cassette are shown in black. LTR, long terminal repeat sequences of the Moloney murine leukemia virus; packaging sequences are also those from the Moloney leukemia virus; Kan^r (often labelled NEO for neomycin resistance), a chimeric Kan^r gene containing the coding Sequence for neomycin phosphotransferase from the *E. coli* transposon Tn5; α_1-AT regulatory sequence, the 5′ regulatory region from the human α_1-antitrypsin gene that dictates the tissue-specific (hepatocyte specific) expression of this gene; SV40 promoter, the promoter from simian virus 40, but without the SV40 enhancer element; PAH cDNA, a cDNA encoding human phenylalanine hydroxylase; TATAA, position of the 'TATA box' of the SV40 promoter; ATG and TAA, translational-initiation and -termination codons, respectively, of the human PAH cDNA.

When primary mouse hepatocytes were infected with virions containing the retroviral vector carrying the chimeric human PAH 'gene,' transgenic cells were identified and were shown to express the chimeric 'gene.' Transcripts that contained the PAH coding sequence were found to have the predicted structure, and human PAH was shown to be synthesised in the transgenic mouse hepatocytes. Although considerable work remains to be done before somatic-cell 'gene therapy' is ready to be tried on PKU patients, these preliminary results with mice suggest that such 'gene therapy' will probably be feasible in the future.

Gene Expression in Transgenic Mice

As mentioned earlier in this chapter, transgenic mice are now routinely produced in laboratories throughout the world. These transgenic mice provide invaluable tools for the study of mammalian gene expression and provide a good model system with which to test the utility of various types of gene-transfer vectors and methodologies.

In excess of 50 different genes have been shown to exist as transgenes in mice, and, surprisingly, of these transgenes were found to exhibit their normal patterns of expression. This means that the adjacent regulatory sequences transferred with the transgenes were sufficient to produce normal patterns of transcription, processing, and translation in the new host.

The elastase-1 gene of the rat was one of the first genes to be studied in transgenic mice. The elastase gene is normally expressed only in the pancreas; elastase is a protease that is secreted into the upper intestine to aid digestion. When the rat elastase gene was cloned and micro injected into mouse eggs, the resulting transgenic mice expressed the fat elastase gene only in pancreatic secretory cells. Correct tissue-specific expression of the rat elastase gene was observed in transgenic mice that carried the gene integrated at different chromosomal sites and in their G_1 progeny that carried the gene in all somatic cells. When transgenic mice were produced with rat elastase genes that carried varying amounts of the adjacent 5′ sequence, it was demonstrated that only about 200 nucleotide pairs were necessary to obtain the normal tissue specific patterns of expression. Similar results have been obtained in studies of mammalian protamine genes and gamma-crystalin genes in transiliac mice. All of these genes contain compact promoters, and all the sequences required for the observed tissue-specific expression of these genes are located within a few hundred nucleotide-pairs 5′ to the coding sequences.

Similar studies of other genes in transgenic mice revealed more complex pictures of *cis*-acting regulatory elements, with tissue-specific enhancers located at considerable distances from the coding sequences. For example, the liver-specific expression of the mouse albumin gene is completely dependent on an enhancer element located about 10,000 nucleotidepairs upstream (5′ relative to the direction of transcription) from its promoter. Other genes exhibited even more complex regulatory circuits. The yolk sacspecific expression of the mouse alpha-fetoprotein gene was shown to be controlled by three different enhancer elements spread over a 7000-nucleotide-pair region upstream from the coding sequence. Transgenic mice have also been used to identify the sequences that regulate the expression of the embryonic, fetal, and adult hemoglobin genes during development. In short, transgenic mice have been used to study the expression of a large number of mammalian genes, far too many to discuss in detail here. Table 15.1 lists some of the genes that have been studied in transgenic mice.

Table 15.1. Expression of native genes in transgenic mice.

Gene	Species of gene donor	Tissue in which transgene is expressed
α-Actin	Rat	Muscle
Amylase-2.2	Mouse	Pancreas
Elastase-1	Rat	Pancreas
α-Fetoprotein	Mouse	Yolk sac and liver
β-Haemoglobin	Mouse	Erythrocytes
β-Haemoglobin	Rabbit	Erythrocytes
β-Haemoglobin	Human	Erythrocytes
Gonadotropin (alpha subunit)	Human	Pituitary
Immunoglobulin κ	Mouse	Lymphocytes
Immunoglobulin μ	Mouse	Lymphocytes
Immunoglobulin μ	Human	Lymphocytes
Insulin	Human	Pancreatic β-cells
α1(I)-Collagen	Human	Various tissues
Myosin (light chain-2)	Rat	Skeletal muscle
Protamine 1	Mouse	Testis
Transferrin	Chicken	Various tissues

The proper expression of genes from mammals as diverse as humans and rabbits in transgenic mice indicates that many of the regulatory sequences in mammals are quite highly conserved. This conservation of regulatory sequences will make the genetic engineering of animal species less difficult, since each gene of interest will not have to be provided with species-specific regulatory elements. Perhaps the most dramatic phenotypic effect of the expression of heterologous transgenes is the increased growth rate that occurs when rat, bovine, or human growth hormone is synthesised in transgenic mice.

As the preceding discussion indicates, the major use of transgenic mice to date has been in defining the *cis*-acting elements that regulate gene expression. Transgenic mice will obviously continue to be invaluable tools for use in dissecting the regulation of gene expression in the future. However, in addition, transgenic mice promise to provide tools for the study of animal development, of the immune response, and of the mode of action of oncogenes. Finally, there is the hope that appropriately manipulated transgenic mice may provide valuable animal models for the study of inherited human diseases such as PKU and of infectious diseases such as AIDS.

DNA MICROINJECTION METHOD

In this method, DNA solution is injected directly into the nucleus of a cell or into the male pronucleus of a fertilised one - to two-cell ovum. Typically, a microinjection assembly consists of a low power sterioscopic dissecting microscope (to view the ovum and the entire process) and two micromanipulators, one for a glass micropipette to hold the ovum by partial suction and the other for a glass injection needle to introduce the DNA into the male pronucleus. The male pronucleus is much larger than the female pronucleus of fertilised mammalian ova. However, in fish ova, the DNA is injected into the egg cytoplasm.

The general procedure for microinjection is as follows (Fig. 15.2). Donor females are induced to superovulate using appropriate hormone treatments. Female mice are subjected to a regime of pregnant mare serum gonadotrophin (PMSG) which stimulates growth and development of follicles which contain the developing oocytes. The release of these oocytes or ovulation is induced by the subsequent treatment with human chorionic gonadotrophin (hCG). The superovulated females are then mated with fertile males, and large numbers of fertilised one- to two-cell ova/embryos are collected surgically. Alternatively, unfertilised ova are collected from superovulated females; the ova are then fertilised *in vitro*.

The transgene construct is prepared in a buffer solution and is injected into the male pronuclei of fertilised eggs using a microinjection assembly. Typically, 2 pl (picolitre = 10^{-12} 1 = 10^{-9} ml) of the DNA solution is injected in a pronucleus. But in case of fish, 20 nl (nanolitre = 10^{-9} 1 = 10^{-6} ml) DNA solution, containing 10^6–10^8 linearised transgene constructs, is injected into the cytoplasm of a single ovum. In mice, the microinjected embryos are cultured *in vitro* upto the morula or blastocyst stage. The surviving embryos are then transferred into the uterus of surrogate mothers, i.e. females which have been made receptive or synchronised by hormone treatments; these embryos develop to full term and give rise to normal mice (Fig. 15.2). A proportion of the progeny so produced will be transgenic in that all their cells will contain the transgene stably integrated into their genomes. But in case of fish, the microinjected embryos are incubated in water until hatching.

In mice, an average of about 3–6 per cent of the progeny derived from microinjected embryos are transgenic; the frequency is much lower in other animals, e.g. <1 per cent in sheep and pigs. In case of fish about 35–80 per cent of the embryos survive microinjection, of which 10–70 per cent may be transgenic. The transgenic animals contain the transgene in their germ cells and, as a consequennce, pass it on to their progeny; transgenes show typical mendelian inheritance.

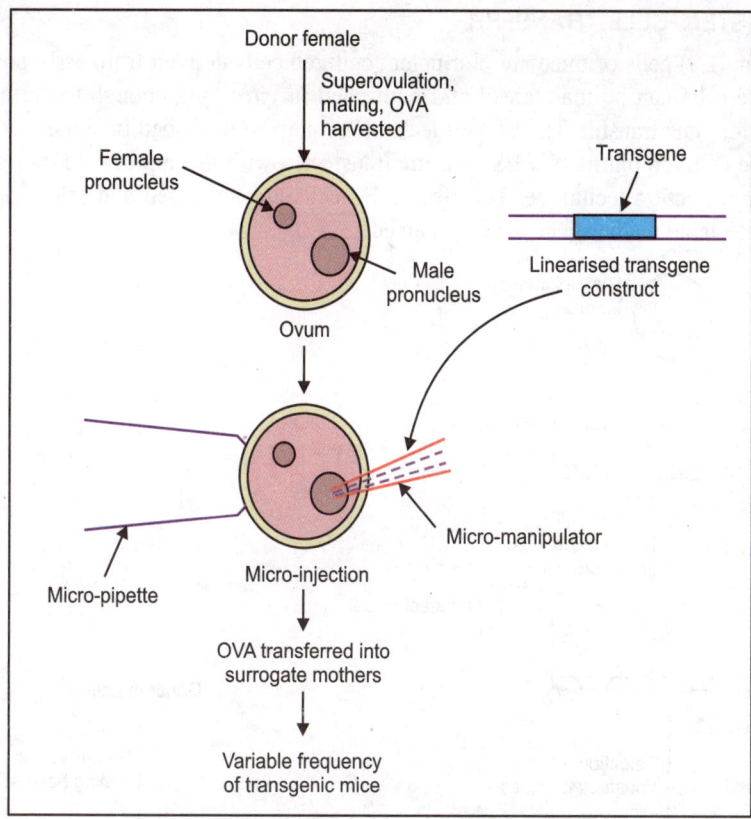

Fig. 15.2. A schematic representation of the microinjection technique of transfection for producing transgenic mice.

The transgene integration occurs at random sites in the genome, but in a given cell or embryo usually only a single chromosomal site is involved. However, there is generally a wide variation in the number of copies integrated ranging from the common one copy to several hundred copies. The multiple copies are integrated at a single site in a head-to-tail arrangement. Consequently, the site of integration of a transgene indifferent transgenic animals differs greatly and may involve different locations of the same chromosome or different chromosomes. The transgene integration occurs at an early stage of embryo development following microinjection, and ordinarily all the cells of an embryo are involved. But often the integration may be delayed, and the transgene remains in the extrachromosomal state during this period. Subsequently, transgene integration occurs only in some cells of the embryo; this results in chimeric progeny. Pure transgenic individuals can be recovered through suitable breeding schemes from such chimeric animals in whose germ cells the transgene has become suitably integrated.

All the transfection techniques are applicable to cultured animal cells, but microinjection is ordinarily not used due to the tediousness of the technique and the limited number of cells that can be handled. For transfection of mice embryos, the preferred techniques are microinjection, retroviral infection and embryonic stem cell technology, microinjection being the most commonly used. Embryos of other animals are generally, transfected by microinjection technique only. In case of fish embryos, microinjection and electroporation are routinely employed.

EMBRYONIC STEM CELL TRANSFER

Embryonic stem (ES) cells of mice are pluripotent cultured cells derived from early pre-implantation embryos. These cells can be maintained and multiplied *in vitro* long enough to permit the various manipulations for gene transfer. The ES cell technology may be described in simple terms as follows (Fig. 15.3). The cultured pluripotent ES cells are transfected with the appropriate transgene construct by a suitable transfection technique. Transfected ES cells are identified and selected, generally by employing a selectable marker gene, and are cloned.

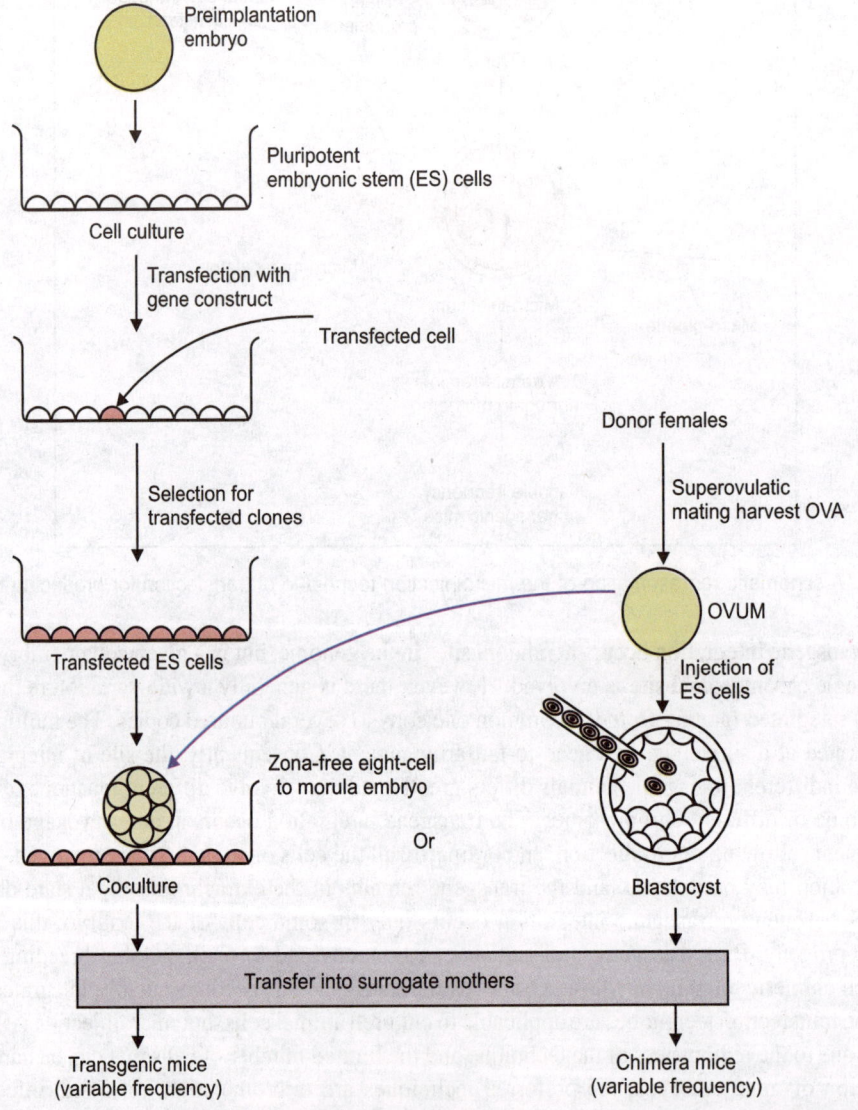

Fig. 15.3. A summary of the steps in embryonic stem (ES) cell transfer technology. When ES cells are injected into blastocoel embryos, chimera mice are obtained. But when 8-cell to morula stage embryos are co-cultured with ES cells non-chimeric transgenic mice are recovered.

The production of transgenic animals using transfected ES cell clones may be achieved in one of the following two ways: (i) injection, and (ii) coculture. The cloned ES cells are injected into the blastocoel of blastocyst stage embryos; the blastocysts are obtained from donor females in a similar manner as that for microinjection. Alternatively, the zona-pellucida of 8-cell to morula stage embryos is removed, and the morulae are co-cultured with the ES cells; the ES cells are preferentially incorporated into the inner cell mass of the developing embryo. It is also possible to transplant the ES cell nucleus into an enucleated fertilised ovum (an ovum whose nuclei have been removed), but this technique is not commonly employed as it is quite tedious although all the progeny obtained by this technique are transgenic.

The embryos cocultured or injected with transfected ES cells are transferred into surrogate mothers where they complete their development. About 30 per cent of the progeny derived from such embryos contain tissues derived from the ES cells, i.e. they are chimeric. The pluripotent ES cells can give rise to germ cells as well. Therefore, pure transgenic mice can be recovered from the chimeric mice using a suitable breeding scheme.

Since DNA integration in genome is random, the frequency of targetted gene transfer, i.e. integration of transgene at a specified site, is discouragingly low. Therefore, transfection techniques like microinjection are not suited to the targetted gene transfer. ES cell line technology, on the other hand, permits the selection of clones(s) having targetted gene transfers from among several clones showing stable transfection. The desired clone can then be used to produce transgenic animals having targetted gene transfer.

ES cell technology is at present confined to mice because embryos of most other mammals do not survive *in vitro* so that it is extremely difficult to produce and maintain their ES cell lines. Even in case of mice, ES cell lines rarely give rise to germ cells in individuals of some strains making it is virtually impossible to produce transgenic animals of these strains using this technology. Recently, ES cell lines have been developed in some mammalian species other than mice, but so far chemeric individuals have not been produced using them. It may be hoped that in the near future it may become possible to apply this technology in some more mammalian species.

DETECTION OF TRANSGENIC ANIMALS AND OF TRANSGENE FUNCTION

It is essential to identify the transgenic animals and to establish that they have stably integrated transgenes which are transcribed and the protein encoded by them is produced. A variety of techniques have been utilised for this purpose.

Identification of Transgenic Animals

Transgenic individuals are the most easily identified when the transgene produces a distinct phenotypic effect, but such cases are only occasional. A more general approach utilises either dot-blot technique or PCR amplification using genomic DNAs extracted from tail biopsies from 6–7 week old mice (produced by one or the other technique for transgenic production). In case of fish, genomic DNA is usually extracted from pectoral fin tissue. PCR amplification can be used if the transgene has unique sequences, not found in the host genome, that can be used as primers. This allows very small amounts of DNA from presumptive transgenic individuals to be suitably amplified for a reliable detection of the transgene. The PCR approach is briefly described below (Fig. 15.4).

1. The test DNA is amplified using unique transgene sequences as primers in a PCR.
2. The amplified DNA is subjected to agarose gel electrophoresis; the transgene construct also run as a control.

3. DNA from the gel is blotted onto a solid support following the protocol for Southern blotting.
4. A radioactive probe specific for the transgene is used for hybridisation and the hybridising samples are detected by autoradiography in the same manner as for Southern hybridisation.

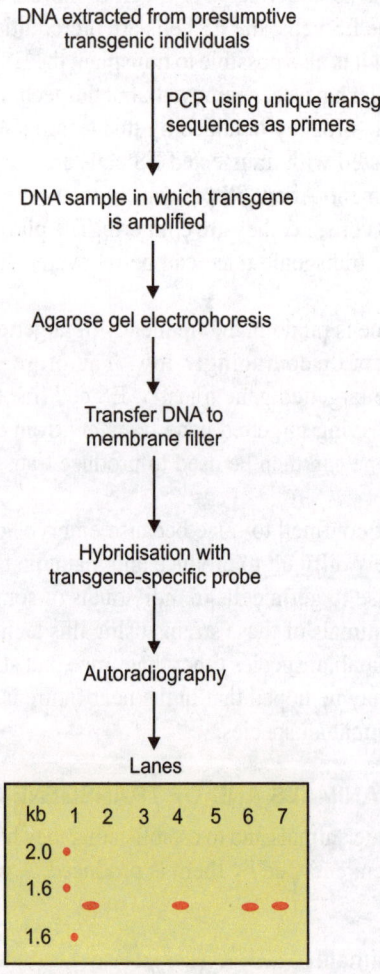

Fig. 15.4. A schematic representation of use of PCR for identification of transgenic animals. Kb, Kilobase (size is determined by running in the gel DNAs of known size); Lane 1, transgene construct used for transfection (control); Lanes 2–7, PCR amplified DNAs from presumptive transgenic animals (lanes 4, 6, 7 test positive for the transgene).

The samples that test positive for hybridisation with the probe are from putative or suspected transgenic individuals. It should be kept in mind that both dot blot and PCR techniques detect the transgene irrespective of whether it is integrated in the genome or is present in an extrachromosomal state. Therefore, dot blot or PCR assay positive individuals are subjected to further assays, such as, Southern hybridisation, etc. for confirmation of transgene integration, etc. The DNA amplified by PCR can be utilised for dot blot and Southern hybridisation as well. In many laboratories, PCR is routinely used as a first screen for transgenics from thousands of presumptive transgenic individuals.

Analysis of Transgene Integration

The integration of transgene into the genome is confirmed by Southern hybridisation of genomic DNA extracted from putative transgenic individuals; the DNA is digested with a suitable restriction enzyme prior to electrophoresis. By choosing appropriate restriction enzymes for DNA digestion, not only the integration of transgene can be established beyond doubt, but information on the number of copies per cell, the orientations of tandemly arranged copies and the presence of single or multiple integration sites is also obtained from Southern hybridisation. All the individuals that give positive result with Southern hybridisation are regarded as confirmed transgenics.

Detection of mRNA Expression

The mRNA produced by transgenes is the most readily detected if they produce mRNAs with unique sequences, i.e. which have no counterparts among those produced by the host genome. A high purity RNA preparation is obtained from the appropriate tissue of transgenic individuals, and is subjected to RNA dot blot hybridisation with a radioactive probe specific for the transgene. Alternatively, the RNA preparation may be used for northern blot hybridisation, which provides additional information on transcript size as well.

Techniques like nuclease protection assay, reverse transcription PCR and *in situ* hybridisation can be used to obtain information on the relative levels of mRNA present in the tissues of different transgenic individuals.

Assays for Protein Expression

Detection of the proteins produced by transgenes are either based on antibodies specific for or on the enzymatic properties of the concerned proteins. Specific antibodies can be employed for a variety of immunological assays of which ELISA is the most rapid and convenient; some other assays are immunoblotting, radioimmunoprecipitation and immunohistochemical staining of tissue sections. Assays of enzyme activities are usually applicable to scorable marker genes (Table 15.2) which produce unique enzyme activities not found in the host, and are efficiently detected by using relatively simple procedures.

Expression of a transgene must be assayed in two or more unrelated transgenic lines of the given animal. This is necessary because the level of expression in different individuals may vary widely due to the site of integration of the transgene.

TRANSGENIC ANIMALS PRODUCED

The ease with which transgenic animals can be produced and the transfection techniques to be employed depend chiefly on the reproductive biology, husbandry requirements and responses to various experimental procedures of the concerned animal. The following features greatly facilitate gene transfer efforts.

1. Production of larger number of eggs either naturally, e.g. in fish, or in response to hormone regimens used for superovulation, e.g. in mice, pigs, etc.
2. Short breeding cycle, i.e. time taken from birth to reaching the reproductive age, greatly facilitates analysis of the transgenic individuals produced.
3. It is desirable that ovulation occurs throughout the year so that ova are readily available for experimentation. For example, fish like rainbow trust, salmon, common carp spawn only once a year which is not desirable.

4. The size and the structure of eggs should be amenable to microinjection, the only transfection technique successful with almost all animal species. For example, tough chorions of fertilised eggs of some fish, e.g. rainbow trout, Atlantic salmon, etc. make microinjection difficult and treatments to remove the chorion may often become necessary.

5. In many animal species, e.g. fish, body size may be an important factor to allow sufficient tissue samples to be taken for the detection of transgene integration and function without sacrificing the individual.

6. In case of mammals where transfected ova/embryos must be transferred into surrogate mothers, the following features are critical: (i) synchronisation of females used for superovulation and as surrogate mother by hormone administration, (ii) *in vitro* fertilisation and culture, at least for some time, of the transfected ova/young embryos, and (iii) transfer of the embryos into surrogate mothers and completion of embryo development in them. These steps are essential for the production of transgenic mammals, and difficulty in any of them will seriously hamper the success of efforts.

7. Production and maintenance of embryonic stem (ES) cell lines capable of giving rise to germ cells is essential for the application of ES cell transfer technology. So far this is possible only in mice.

Transgenics have been produced in a variety of animal species, e.g. mice (including rats), rabbits, swine, sheep, goat, cattle, poultry, fish, amphibians, insects land nematodes. However, these activities are so far limited to experimental stages, and production technologies or transgenic animals have not yet reached commercial applications. This is highlighted by the fact that upto the beginning of 1995, patents had been taken in USA only on transgenic mice. It may be emphasised that much work and uncertainty lies between taking a patent and its commercial exploitation.

Transgenic Mice

Mouse is the most preferred mammal for studies on gene transfers due to its many favourable features like short oestrous cycle and gestation period, relatively short generation time, production of several offspring per pregnancy (i.e. litter), convenient *in vitro* fertilisation, successful culture of embryos *in vitro* at least for a period of time, production and maintenance of ES cell lines, availability of a diverse array of genetic stocks, etc. As a result, the techniques for gene transfer and transgenic production have been developed using mice as models; subsequently these approaches have been modified to adapt them to other animal species. More recently, rats and rabbits are being increasingly used for research work on gene transfer.

Transgenic Rabbits

Rabbits are quite promising for gene farming or molecular farming which aims at the production of recoverable quantities of pharmaceutically or biologically important proteins encoded by the transgenes. Transgenic animals used for this purpose are popularly called bioreactors. Generally, the transgenes are designed to be expressed in mammary tissue so that their protein products are secreted in milk. Consequently, the protein product is easily harvested with milk from which it is conveniently purified.

The following human genes encoding valuable proteins have been separately transferred into rabbits; interleukin 2, growth hormone, tissue plasminogen activator, α_1 antitrypsin, etc. In addition, bovine α-lactalbumin has also been expressed. These genes were expressed in the mammory tissues and their proteins were harvested from milk (Table 15.2).

Table 15.2. Some notable gene transfers and their consequences in animals of economic importance.

Gene transferred	Objective	Achievements	Remarks
Cattle, goat, sheep and swine			
Human genes α₁ antitrypsin, tissue plasminogen activator, blood clotting factor IX, and protein C.	Gene farming	Genes expressed in mammary tissue; proteins secreted in milk in functional form	Experimental stages
Sheep			
Bacterial genes *cysE* and *cysM* (genes concerned with cysteine biosynthesis)	Improved wool production/quality	Genes expressed in transgenic animals	
Mice and Swine			
Human haemoglobin and specific circulating immunoglobulins (antibodies)	Proteins from blood serum for blood transfusion and disease diagnosis	Genes expressed; proteins released in blood serum	Experimental stages
Swine and Sheep	Increased and desirable growth	Improvements in body weight gain, feed efficiency, lean/fat ratio, fat composition, etc.	Produces joint pathology, skeletal defects, ulcers, infertility, etc.
Human growth hormone			
Rabbits			
Human genes: Interleukin 2, growth hormone, tissue plasminogen activator, α₁-antitrypsin, etc. Bovine gene: α-lactoglobulin	Molecular farming or gene farming	Genes expressed in mammary tissue; proteins harvested from milk	Experimental stage
Fish			
Salmon or rainbow trout growth hormone	Increased body growth	Upto 60% increase in size	Transgenes stably inherited; growth improved by selection
Anti-freeze protein gene, α-globin gene, chicken δ-crystalline protein gene, etc.	Variable	Genes expressed in transgenic individuals	Transgenes are stably inherited

Transgenic Cattle

The only successful transfection technique in cattle is microinjection of fertilised ova which may either be recovered surgically or may be obtained from ovaries extracted from slaughtered cows and cultured *in vitro*. The two chief objectives of transgenic production are as follows: (i) increased milk or meat production, and (ii) molecular farming. Several human genes have been successfully transferred in cows and expressed in the mammary tissue. The transgenic protein is secreted in milk from where it is easily harvested (Table 15.2). Other objectives for transgenic cattle are: improved properties and proportions of caseins, contents of lactose and butterfat in milk, and enhanced resistance to viral and bacterial pathogens, including the development of constitutive immunity due to germ line transmission of rearranged antibody genes specific to selected pathogens.

Transgenic Goat

Goats are being evaluated as bioreactors. Some human genes have been introduced in goats and their expression achieved in mammary tissues (Table 15.2). The initial results have been quite encouraging and, in the near future, commercial production may become feasible.

Transgenic Sheep

Transgenic sheep have been produced to achieve better growth and meat production as well as to serve as bioreactors. For example, human genes for blood clotting factor IX and for α_1 antitryspin have been transferred in sheep and expressed in mammary tissue (Table 15.2); this was achieved by fusing the genes with the mammary tissue-specific promoter of the bovine β-lactoglobulin gene. Human growth hormone gene has also been introduced in sheep in order to promote growth and meat production. The transgenic animals showed improvements in body weight gain, feed efficiency, lean meat/fat ratio, fat composition, etc. However, they also showed several undesirable effects like joint pathology, skeletal defects, gastric ulcers, infertility, etc. (Table 15.2). These problems have been attributed to chronic overexpression of the growth hormone transgene. This gains support from the fact that in many cases long term administration of elevated levels of growth hormones produces similar abnormalities.

Increased wool production and improved wool quality are important objectives of transgenic sheep research efforts. Towards this end, genes involved in the biosynthesis of amino acids important in keratin biosynthesis are being identified and cloned. Keratin proteins are found in wool. For example, two bacterial genes involved in cystein biosynthesis, viz. cysE (serine acetyltransferase) and cysM (O-acetylserine sulphhydrolase) have been cloned and introduced in sheep. The transgenic sheep do express these genes, but much further work is needed to improve wool production and/or quality of transgenic sheep.

Transgenic Pigs

The rate of transgenic production in pigs, sheep, cattle and goats is much lower (usually <1 per cent) than that in mice (usually between 3–6 per cent). In addition, swine ova contain a large amount of lipids which makes the visualisation of male pronuclei very difficult. When DNA was injected into the ova cytoplasm, no transgenics could be recovered; this is in contrast to fish. It was found that centrifugation of pig ova facilitates visualisation of the pronuclei, which enables, microinjection of DNA into the male pronuclei.

The objectives in transgenic swine production are: (i) increased growth and meat production, and (ii) to serve as bioreactors (Table 15.2). Transgenic pigs expressing human growth hormone do show improved growth and meat production, but they also show several health problems most likely due to the chronic overproduction of growth hormone. Several human genes have been expressed ill swine with a view to harvest their protein products; these proteins were either secreted in milk or in blood serum from where they are easily recoverable. The human proteins expressed in blood serum are: haemoglobin and specific circulating immunoglobulins; these proteins can be used in blood transfusion (haemoglobin) and disease diagnosis (antibodies).

Transgenic Fish

Gene transfers have been successful in several fish, e.g. common carp, rainbow trout, Atlantic salmon, catfish, goldfish, loach, medaka, tilapia, zebra-fish, etc. The genes transferred into fish include salmon or rainbow trout growth hormone, chicken δ-crystalline protein, winter flounder antifreese protein, E. coli β-galactosidase and E. coli hygromycin resistance gene. Transfection is achieved either by microinjection of the DNA construct into egg cyptoplasm (typically 20 nl DNA solution per ovum; it would contain 10^6–10^8 copies of linearised gene construct) or by electroporation. Microinjection is performed within few hours after fertilisation. Transfected ova are cultured in water where they hatch.

The rate of survival of microinjected embryos varies from 35 to 80 per cent of which 10–70 per cent may be transgenic. Electroportation is much less tedious than microinjection and can be used to transfect a very large number of eggs within a limited period of time. About 20 per cent or more of the embryos surviving electroporation give rise to transgenic fish.

Improved growth was sought to be achieved by transferring salmon or rainbow trout growth hormone (GH) gene in channel catfish, common carp, goldfish, loach, medaka, rainbow trout, salmon and tilapia. Transgenic families of a fish differ in the level of expression of GH as well their body growth; this is most likely the consequence of positional effects due to random integration of the transgene. Some transgenic families show upto 60 per cent increase in body growth. A combination of family selection with mass selection among the transgenic individuals has yielded the fastest growing fish lines. Generally, the transgene is stably inherited.

In addition, many other genes have been successfully introduced and expressed in fish; these genes include, antifreeze protein gene, hygromycin resistance gene, neomycin resistance gene, α-globin gene, β-galactosidase gene, chicken δ-crystalline protein gene, bacterial or insect luciferase gene. In most of the studies, gene transfers were successful, the trans genes were expressed and inherited stably.

APPLICATIONS OF TRANSGENIC ANIMAL TECHNOLOGY

Introduction of growth hormone genes into animal species has been carried out, notably in pigs, but in many cases there are undesirable side effects. Pigs with the bovine growth hormone gene show greater feed efficiency and have lower levels of subcutaneous fat than normal pigs. However, problems such as enlarged heart, high incidence of stomach ulcers, dermatitis, kidney disease and arthritis have demonstrated that the production of healthy transgenic farm animals is a difficult undertaking. Although progress is being made, it is clear that much more work is required before genetic engineering has a major impact on animal husbandry. The study of development is one area of transgenic research that is currently yielding much useful information. By implanting genes into embryos, features of development such as tissue-specific gene expression can be investigated. The cloning of genes from the fruit fly *Drosophila melanogaster*, coupled with the isolation and characterisation of transposable elements (*P*-elements) that can be used as vectors, has enabled the production of stable transgenic *Drosophila* lines. Thus the fruit fly, which has been a major contributor to the field of classical genetic analysis, is now being studied at the molecular level by employing the full range of gene manipulation techniques.

In mammals, the mouse is proving to be one of the most useful model systems for investigating embryological development, and the expression of many transgenes has been studied in this organism. One such application which demonstrates the use of the *lacZ* gene as a means of detecting tissue-specific gene expression. In this example the *lacZ* gene was placed under the control of the weak thymidine kinase (TK) promoter from herpes simplex virus (HSV), generating an HSV-TK–*lacZ* construct. This was used to probe for active chromosomal domains in the developing embryos, with one of the transgenic lines showing the brain-specific expression seen.

Although the use of transgenic organisms is providing many insights into developmental processes, inserted genes may not always be expressed in exactly the same way as would be the case in normal embryos. Thus a good deal of caution is often required when interpreting results. Despite this potential problem, transgenesis is proving to be a powerful tool for the developmental biologist. Mice have also been used widely as animal models for disease states. One celebrated example is the oncomouse, generated by Philip Leder and his colleagues at Harvard University. Mice were produced in which the *c-myc* oncogene and sections of the mouse mammary tumour (MMT) virus gave rise to breast cancer. The oncomouse has a place in history as the first complex animal to be granted a patent in the USA. Other transgenic mice with disease characteristics include the prostate mouse (prostate cancer), mice with severe combined immunodeficiency syndrome (SCIDS), and mice that show symptoms of Alzheimer disease.

Many new variants of transgenic mice have been produced, and have become an essential part of research into many aspects of human disease. Increased knowledge of molecular genetics, and the continued development of the techniques of transgenic animal production, have enabled mice to be generated in which specific genes can be either activated or inactivated. Where a gene is inactivated or replaced with a mutated version, a knockout mouse is produced. If an additional gene function is established, this is sometimes called a knockout mouse. The use of knockout mice in cystic fibrosis (CF) research is one example of the technology being used in both basic research and in developing gene therapy procedures. Mice have been engineered to express mutant CF alleles, including the prevalent ΔF508 mutation that is responsible for most serious CF presentations. Having a mouse model enables researchers to carry out experiments that would not be possible in humans, although (as with developmental studies) results may not be exactly the same as would be the case in a human subject.

In 1995 a database was established to collate details of knockout mice. This is known as MKMD and can be found at URL [http://research.bmn.com/mkmd/]. This demonstrates that the mouse is proving to be one of the mainstays of modern transgenic research.

Early examples of protein production in transgenic animals include expression of human tissue plasminogen activator (tPA) in transgenic mice, and of human blood coagulation factor IX (FIX) in transgenic sheep. In both cases the transgene protein product was secreted into the milk of lactating organisms by virtue of being placed under the control of a milk-protein gene promoter. In the mouse example the construct consisted of the regulatory sequences of the whey acid protein (WAP) gene, giving a WAP–tPA construct. Control sequences from the β-lactoglobulin (BLG) gene were used to generate a BLG–FIX construct for expression in the transgenic sheep. Other examples of transgenic animals acting as bioreactors include pigs that express human haemoglobin, and cows that produce human lactoferrin.

Producing a therapeutic protein in milk provides an ideal way of ensuring a reliable supply from lactating animals, and downstream processing to obtain purified protein is relatively straightforward. This approach was used by scientists from the Roslin Institute near Edinburgh, working in conjunction with the biotechnology company PPL Therapeutics. In 1991 PPL's first transgenic sheep (called Tracy) was born. Yields of human proteins of around 40 g l^{-1} were produced from milk, demonstrating the great potential for this technology. PPL continues to develop a range of products, such as at-antitrypsin (for treating cystic fibrosis), fibrinogen (for use in medical procedures) and human factor IX (for haemophilia B).

Using animals as bioreactors offers an alternative to the fermentation of bacteria or yeast that contain the target gene. The technology is now becoming well established, with many biotechnology companies involved. As we have already seen, this area is sometimes called pharming, with the transgenic animals referred to as pharm animals. Given the problems in achieving correct expression and processing of some mammalian proteins in non-mammalian hosts, this is proving to be an important development of transgenic animal technology.

Transgenic animals also offer the potential to develop organs for xenotransplantation. The pig is the target species for this application, as the organs are of similar size to human organs. In developing this technology the key target is to alter the cell surface recognition properties of the donor organs, so that the transplant is not rejected by the human immune system. In addition to whole organs from mature animals, there is the possibility of growing tissue replacements as an additional part of a transgenic animal. Both these aspects of xenotransplantation are currently being investigated, with a lot of scientific and ethical problems still to be solved. Given the shortfall in organ donors, and the consequent loss of life or quality of life that results, many people feel that the objections to xenotransplantation must be discussed openly, and overcome, to enable the technology to be implemented when fully developed.

In January 2001 the birth of the first transgenic non-human primate, a rhesus monkey, was announced. This was developed by scientists in Portland, Oregon. He was named ANDi, which stands for inserted DNA (written backwards). A marker gene from jellyfish, which produces green fluorescent protein (GFP) was used to confirm the transgenic status of a variety of ANDi's cells. ANDi is particularly significant in that he opens up the possibility of a near-human model organism for the evaluation of disease and therapy. He also brings the ethical questions surrounding transgenic research a little closer to the human situation, which some people are finding a little uncomfortable. It will certainly be interesting to follow the developments in transgenic technology over the next few years.

ETHICAL ISSUES RELATED TO TRANSGENIC ANIMALS

The social opinion on transgenic animal research is divided almost in the middle. Opinion surveys in USA, Japan and New Zealand reveal that only 42, 54 and 58 per cent, respectively, of the people participating in the survey favour such research. The main reasons for opposition of people may be summarised as follows:

1. Use of animals in biotechnological research causes greater suffering to the animals. But most people seem to accept some animal suffering to serve the basic interest and welfare of mankind; this attitude has been termed as interest-sensitive speciesism. European Patent convention recognises this position in form of a provision of rejection of patent applications on the basis of the balance between human welfare and animal suffering. The patent application for a transgenic mouse designed to screen hair growth stimulants was rejected on this ground, but that for Onco-mouse was allowed.

2. It is felt that by using animals for the production of pharmaceutical proteins we reduce them to mere factories. This seems not to recognise that animals also are living beings which feel pleasure and pain just as we do.

3. Some people feel that animals should be regarded as equal to humans in that they have the same basic rights as human beings. However, in most societies animals are relegated to a position several steps below that of man.

4. An argument attempts to focus on integrity of species in that each biological species has a right to exist as a separate identifiable entity. But biologists do not regard a species as a fixed, clearly delineated, water-tight entity; rather they are regarded as dynamic, constantly evolving groups. Further, genetic modification of a small fraction (usually <1 per cent) of the individuals of given species can hardly be expected to change the definition of that species.

5. Finally, the introduction of human genes into animals, and vice versa, may be seen by many as clouding the definition of 'humanness'. But it may be pointed out that the known human genes are not unique, and comparable genes do occur in animals. In addition, many retroviruses, the lowest form of life imaginable, have integrated into the human genome without any recognisable devaluation of our humanness.

Chapter 16

Isolation of Human Genes

INTRODUCTION

The human genome is the genome of *Homo sapiens*, which is stored on 23 chromosome pairs. Twenty-two of these are autosomal chromosome pairs, while the remaining pair is sex-determining. The haploid human genome occupies a total of just over 3 billion DNA base pairs. The Human Genome Project (HGP) produced a reference sequence of the euchromatic human genome, which is used worldwide in biomedical sciences.

There are estimated to be between 20,000 and 25,000 human protein-coding genes. The estimate of the number of human genes has been repeatedly revised down from initial predictions of 1,00,000 or more as genome sequence quality and gene finding methods have improved. Surprisingly, the number of human genes seems to be less than a factor of two greater than that of many much simpler organisms, such as the roundworm and the fruit fly. However, human cells make extensive use of alternative splicing to produce several different proteins from a single gene, and the human proteome is thought to be much larger than those of the aforementioned organisms. Besides, most human genes have multiple exons, and human introns are frequently much longer than the flanking exons. Human genes are distributed unevenly across the chromosomes. Each chromosome contains various gene-rich and gene-poor regions, which seem to be correlated with chromosome bands and GC-content. The significance of these nonrandom patterns of gene density is not well understood. In addition to protein coding genes, the human genome contains thousands of RNA genes, including tRNA, ribosomal RNA, microRNA, and other noncoding RNA genes.

The human genome has many different regulatory sequences which are crucial to controlling gene expression. These are typically short sequences that appear near or within genes. A systematic understanding of these regulatory sequences and how they together act as a gene regulatory network is only beginning to emerge from computational, high-throughput expression and comparative genomics studies. Some types of noncoding DNA are genetic 'switches' that do not encode proteins, but do regulate when and where genes are expressed.

Most studies of human genetic variation have focused on single-nucleotide polymorphisms (SNPs), which are substitutions in individual bases along a chromosome. Most analyses estimate that SNPs occur on average somewhere between every 1 in 100 and 1 in 300 base pairs in the euchromatic human genome, although they do not occur at a uniform density. Thus follows the popular statement that 'we are all, regardless of race, genetically 99.9 per cent the same', although this would be somewhat qualified by most geneticists.

Most aspects of human biology involve both genetic (inherited) and non-genetic (environmental) factors. Some inherited variation influences aspects of our biology that are not medical in nature (height, eye colour, ability to taste or smell certain compounds, etc.). Moreover, some genetic disorders only cause disease in combination with the appropriate environmental factors (such as diet). With these caveats, genetic disorders may be described as clinically defined diseases caused by genomic DNA sequence variation. In the most straightforward cases, the disorder can be associated with variation in a single gene.

Comparative genomics studies of mammalian genomes suggest that approximately 5 per cent of the human genome has been conserved by evolution since the divergence of extant lineages approximately 200 million years ago, containing the vast majority of genes. Intriguingly, since genes and known regulatory sequences probably comprise less than 2 per cent of the genome, this suggests that there may be more unknown functional sequence than known functional sequence.

The human mitochondrial genome, while usually not included when referring to the 'human genome', is of tremendous interest to geneticists, since it undoubtedly plays a role in mitochondrial disease. It also sheds light on human evolution; for example, analysis of variation in the human mitochondrial genome has led to the postulation of a recent common ancestor for all humans on the maternal line of descent. Due to the lack of a system for checking for copying errors, mitochondrial DNA (mtDNA) has a more rapid rate of variation than nuclear DNA. This 20-fold increase in the mutation rate allows mtDNA to be used for more accurate tracing of maternal ancestry.

Epigenetics are a variety of features of the human genome that transcend its primary DNA sequence, such as chromatin packaging, histone modifications and DNA methylation, and which are important in regulating gene expression, genome replication and other cellular processes. Basically they are marks on DNA that are influenced within an individual's own life.

TARGETING THE HUMAN GENOME TO MAKE GENE ISOLATION EASY

The human genome project has made great strides in the decade since its inception including the cloning of most of the chromosomal DNA, the identification of unique sequences (sequence tags sites, STS's) approximately every 150 kb and the sequencing of short regions of almost all the expressed genes (expressed sequence tags, EST's). In addition to understanding chromosome organisation, this vast amount of information is leading to the isolation of genes that correspond to specific diseases, particularly through positional cloning. Furthermore, the genetic make-up of humans is better understood because of sequence relatedness between species.

Until now there has been little opportunity to utilise the information being generated to isolate specific large regions (i.e. greater than 10 to 20 kb) or genes directly from total genomic material. Virtually all cloning of chromosomal DNA from humans, or any organism, has involved the isolation of random DNA fragments into vectors through several steps of enzymatic treatment plus ligation and the subsequent transfer into the desired bacterial or yeast host. The isolation of specific DNAs would provide a variety of opportunities, including studies of human polymorphisms, clinical diagnosis, gene therapy and the filling-in of gaps in sequenced regions. However, the only available enrichment procedure has been the physical isolation of entire chromosomes. Even then, the subsequent cloning of human DNAs has involved random DNA fragments.

Over the past year a new approach has emerged that is providing for the specific isolation of genes and regions directly from total human DNA. The approach draws upon several features of the yeast *Saccharomyces cerevisiae*. The first is that during transformation, yeast can take up several small and large molecules. Secondly, intermolecular, as well as intramolecular, recombination is highly efficient during transformation between homologous, as well diverged DNAs. This includes double-strand break recombination between broken molecules. Thirdly, human DNA contains sequences (about 1 per 20–30 kb) that can function as origins of replication (ARS-autonomously replicating sequence) in yeast.

These features have provided for the development of a novel method based on transformation-associated recombination (TAR) to target the isolation of specific DNAs from total human DNAs. As described in Fig. 16.1, genomic DNA is presented to yeast along with a molar excess of vector containing a selectable marker, a centromere (CEN) to assure production of a single copy of the cloned material and targeting sequence *hooks* A and B (the original circular plasmid is linearised at a site between A and B). [The TAR procedure simply involves the presentation of gently prepared human DNA, originally isolated in low-melt agarose plugs, to competent yeast spheroplasts along with vector DNA.]

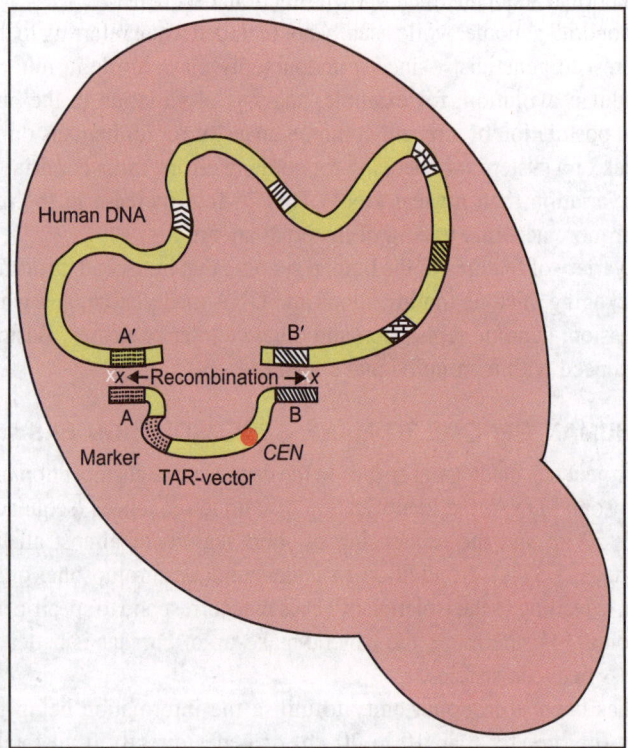

Fig. 16.1. Model of TAR cloning to generate circular YACs. Human DNA is taken up by a yeast cell along with linearised vector DNA. The vector contains a centromere and a marker for selection. If the human DNA contains segments corresponding to the segments—*hooks*—A and B on the plasmid, recombination will lead to the establishment of a circular YAC. Propagation of the YAC depends on the presence of a yeast ARS-like sequence in the human DNA. The various blocks could be diverged repeats, such as *Alu's* or LINES.

The minimum size of the hooks required for TAR cloning appears to be less than 150 bp. If a human fragment containing a sequence A′ and B′ winds up in the same cell as the vector, recombination between the cut plasmid and the fragment will generate a circular yeast artificial chromosome (YAC) which can be selected using the plasmid marker. Because the plasmid has no yeast replication origin, sequences in human DNAs capable of functioning as ARS's in yeast provide for the propagation of the YAC. Thus, the isolation of human DNA is essentially accomplished by marker rescue through recombination. The generation of YACs with large human segments was proposed to be due to preferential double-strand break repair at or near ends of molecules rather than internal regions. [The original model for double-strand break repair has now had many applications and refinements that extend from the repair of radiation-induced breaks, natural breaks and gap repair of incoming molecules to gene replacement in mammalian cells and the development of knockout mice and now TAR cloning.]

The opportunity to TAR clone human DNA was suggested from experiments in which it was shown that during transformation there was efficient recombination between an incoming plasmid with an *Alu* and an incoming human yeast artificial chromosome (YAC) that contained several *Alu's*. With this in mind, transformation-associated recombination was explored as an alternative means of generating linear YAC libraries containing large fragments of chromosomal DNA. Subsequently, the original scheme—which does not involve restricting or ligating DNA—was modified to yield circular YACs as described in Fig. 16.1.

The efficiency and selectivity of TAR cloning was initially demonstrated by the specific isolation of human DNA from a radiation hybrid rodent cell line containing a 5 Mb human chromosome fragment that had the Ku80 gene. A circularising TAR vector was used that had the same human *Alu* for the targeting A and B hooks (Fig. 16.1 and Table 16.1). Approximately 25 per cent of the transformants for the vector marker had YACs containing human DNA and most were greater than 150 kb. Based on the relative number of YACs isolated containing rodent DNA, this corresponded to a nearly 5000-fold enrichment over the 0.1 per cent human DNA present in the hybrid cells.

These results led to the demonstration that TAR cloning could be used to isolate a specific human gene, the breast cancer gene BRCA2. Although it had been sequenced, no complete BRCA2 gene had been isolated either as a YAC or a BAC (a bacterial artificial chromosome in *E. coli*). To do this, the TAR vector with hooks of approximately 500 bp each of the promoter sequence and the noncoding region of the last exon (Fig. 16.1) was presented to yeast cells along with total DNA isolated from human fibroblasts. About 1 in 300 transformants selected for the vector marker also contained the BRCA2 gene and these could be easily identified by PCR analysis (Table 16.1). Further physical analysis established that several independent copies of the complete gene had indeed been isolated.

Table 16.1. Specific isolation of human DNA by TAR cloning.

DNA cloned and source	Hook A	Hook B
100 Mb Chromosome 16 in a monochromosomal hybrid	Consensus *Alu*	BLUR13 *Alu*
5 Mb Ku80 in a radiation hybrid	Consensus *Alu*	BLUR13 *Alu*
43 kb rDNA unit in total human DNA	Nontranscribed spacer	BLUR13 *Alu*
90 kb BRCA2 in total human DNA*	5′ Upstream sequence	3′ Downstream sequence
82 kb BRCA1 in total human DNA*	5′ Upstream sequence	3′ Downstream sequence
70–350 kb HPRT in total human DNA*	BLUR13 *Alu*	3′ Downstream sequence

*Up to 1 per cent of the yeast transformants had the gene of interest. The genes were identified through pooling of transformants, PCR analysis, followed by isolation of clones.

The utility of TAR cloning for the specific isolation of human genes has now been demonstrated further for the BRCA1 and the HPRT genes (unpublished) and the human ribosomal RNA gene family. As shown in Table 16.1, specific isolation can be accomplished with one hook that is unique to the gene(s) being isolated and the other hook being a common repeat. The numbers of unique genes isolated per mg of total DNA presented to yeast were comparable for the BRCA1 and the HPRT genes. Thus, direct gene isolation is now possible using information derived from only a small portion of a gene. Because only a few weeks are required once the vectors are built, TAR cloning provides new opportunities for investigating genes and chromosomal regions directly from individuals. Previously, isolation of specific chromosomal regions would have required the development of a library for each person studied followed by extensive analysis to find the region of interest. These features suggest that TAR cloning can open the way to clinical investigations of whole genes or large chromosomal regions since, for example, only 10 to 20 ml of blood would be needed for the isolation of a specific gene. Another novel utility—referred to as radial TAR cloning—derives from the isolation of the rDNA and the HPRT genes with a vector that has a unique sequence hook and an *Alu* repeat hook (A and B, respectively, in Fig. 16.1 and Table 16.1). YACs are generated that extend from the unique position to various *Alu's*. By changing the orientation of the unique hook, a radial series of YACs is developed that surround the unique sequence. There are many applications that include isolating a unique region surrounding a particular STS or EST site. In addition chromosomal changes such as amplifications and translocations in individuals become directly accessible with TAR cloning once a chromosomal sequence is identified. Radial TAR cloning also provides the opportunity to clone a region lacking an ARS-like sequence since the hook with the common repeat enables the isolation of chromosome fragments that are sufficiently large that they are likely to contain such a sequence.

The TAR cloning can be used in a cycle that provides for specific human DNA isolation and reintroduction, as described in Fig. 16.2. Once DNA is isolated as a circular molecule it can be modified and even retrofitted with bacterial artificial chromosome sequences and mammalian selectable markers such as neomycin (NEO) or hygromycin resistance (or alternatively the original TAR vector could contain these sequences) using recombination methods standard to yeast.

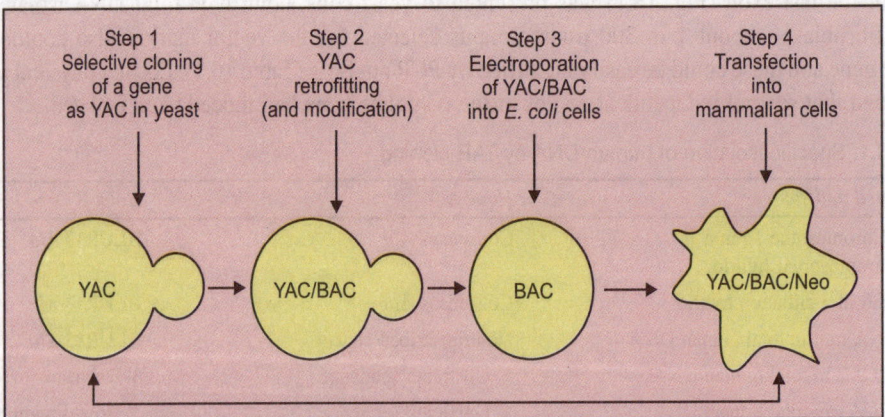

Fig. 16.2. A TAR cloning cycle for the specific isolation of human DNA and its reintroduction into mammalian cells. Human DNA can be specifically isolated in yeast by TAR cloning, modified for transfer to bacteria and then transferred to mammalian cells. Alternatively, the TAR vector can contain sequences that would enable selection in mammalian cells enabling direct transfer from yeast.

The YAC/BAC can than be transferred into *E. coli* in order to obtain large amounts of this DNA and it could subsequently be introduced into human cells. (Large circular molecules may be isolated directly from yeast, so that the step involving transfer to *E. coli* could be eliminated.) This approach is being applied to the BRCA2, BRCA1 and HPRT genes initially isolated as YACs. The subsequent YAC/BACs are reintroduced into mammalian cells using the NEO marker for selection. Since, as recently shown for HPRT, most of the isolated genes are functional when transferred to mammalian cells (in preparation), the cycle of human DNA isolation and reintroduction can be accomplished with high fidelity. The tremendous success of the human genome project has relied on the development of new approaches. The information generated can be applied to many areas including functional genomics, investigations of genetic diseases, gene manipulation and gene therapy. TAR cloning is one of the new tools that will make our chromosomes more accessible.

GENETIC LINKAGE AND GENE MAPPING

Genetic Linkage

Genetic linkage is a term which describes the tendency of certain *loci* or alleles to be inherited together. Genetic *loci* on the same chromosome are physically close to one another and tend to stay together during meiosis, and are thus genetically linked. At the beginning of normal meiosis, a chromosome pair (made up of a chromosome from the mother and a chromosome from the father) intertwine and exchange sections or fragments of chromosome. The pair then breaks apart to form two chromosomes with a new combination of genes that differs from the combination supplied by the parents. Through this process of recombining genes, organisms can produce offspring with new combinations of maternal and paternal traits that may contribute to or enhance survival. This crossing over of DNA can cause alleles previously on the same chromosome to be separated and end up in different daughter cells. The further the two alleles are apart, the greater the chance that a crossover event may occur between them, possibly separating the alleles. The relative distance between two genes can be calculated using the offspring of an organism showing two linked genetic traits, and finding the percentage of the offspring where the two traits do not run together.

The higher the percentage of descendants that does not show both traits, the farther apart on the chromosome the two genes are. Among individuals of an experimental population or species, some phenotypes or traits occur randomly with respect to one another in a manner known as independent assortment. Today scientists understand that independent assortment occurs when the genes affecting the phenotypes are found on different chromosomes or separated by a great enough distance on the same chromosome that recombination occurs at least half of the time.

An exception to independent assortment develops when genes appear near one another on the same chromosome. When genes occur on the same chromosome, they are usually inherited as a single unit.

Linkage map

A linkage map is a genetic map of a species or experimental population that shows the position of its known genes or genetic markers relative to each other in terms of recombination frequency, rather than as specific physical distance along each chromosome. Linkage mapping is critical for identifying the location of genes that cause genetic diseases. A genetic map is a map based on the frequencies of recombination between markers during crossover of homologous chromosomes. The greater the frequency of recombination (segregation) between two genetic markers, the farther apart they are assumed to be. Conversely, the lower the frequency of recombination between the markers, the smaller the physical distance between them.

Gene Mapping

Gene mapping, also called genome mapping, is the creation of a genetic map assigning DNA fragments to chromosomes. When a genome is first investigated, this map is nonexistent. The map improves with the scientific progress and is perfect when the genomic DNA sequencing of the species has been completed. During this process, and for the investigation of differences in strain, the fragments are identified by small tags. These may be genetic markers (PCR products) or the unique sequence-dependent pattern of DNA-cutting enzymes. The ordering is derived from genetic observations (recombinant frequency) for these markers or in the second case from a computational integration of the fingerprinting data. The term 'mapping' is used in two different but related contexts. Two different ways of mapping are distinguished.

Genetic mapping uses classical genetic techniques (e.g. pedigree analysis or breeding experiments) to determine sequence features within a genome. Using modern molecular biology techniques for the same purpose is usually referred to as physical mapping. In physical mapping, the DNA is cut by a restriction enzyme. Once cut, the DNA fragments are separated by electrophoresis. The resulting pattern of DNA migration (i.e. its genetic fingerprint) is used to identify what stretch of DNA is in the clone. By analysing the fingerprints, contigs are assembled by automated (FPC) or manual means (Pathfinders) into overlapping DNA stretches.

Now a good choice of clones can be made to efficiently sequence the clones to determine the DNA sequence of the organism under study. Macrorestriction is a type of physical mapping wherein the high molecular weight DNA is digested with a restriction enzyme having a low number of restriction sites. The ultimate goal of gene mapping is to clone genes, especially disease genes. Once a gene is cloned, we can determine its DNA sequence and study its protein product.

Linkage analysis

The genetic mapping is based on the linkage between 'loci' (locations of genes). If two loci are usually inherited together, they are said to be 'linked'. Two loci on different chromosomes are not linked, because they are usually separated by independent assortment. A locus (singular of loci) may have different sequences, referred to as alleles. Consider two loci A and B, each having two alleles (one from mother, another from father). A_1 and A_2 are the two alleles of locus A ; B_1 and B_2 are the two alleles of locus B. Initially, A_1 and B_1 are located on the same chromosome. A_2 and B_2 are located on a different chromosome (Fig. 16.3).

The DNA crossover may cause recombination of *loci* A and B. Namely, A_1 and B_2 (or A_2 and B_1) are located on the same chromosome. The recombination frequency depends on the distance between the two *loci* and the position of crossover (the chiasma). The closer they are, the less likely the recombination will occur, because recombination occurs only when the chiasma is located between the two loci.

To apply this basic principle to map a disease gene, we need to analyse the pedigree and estimate recombination frequency.

Disease-association

The process to identify a genetic element that signs responsible for a disease is also referred to as 'mapping'. If the locus in which the search is performed is already considerably constrained, the search is called the 'fine-mapping' of a gene. This information is derived from the investigation of disease-manifestations in large families (genetic linkage) or from populations-based genetic association studies.

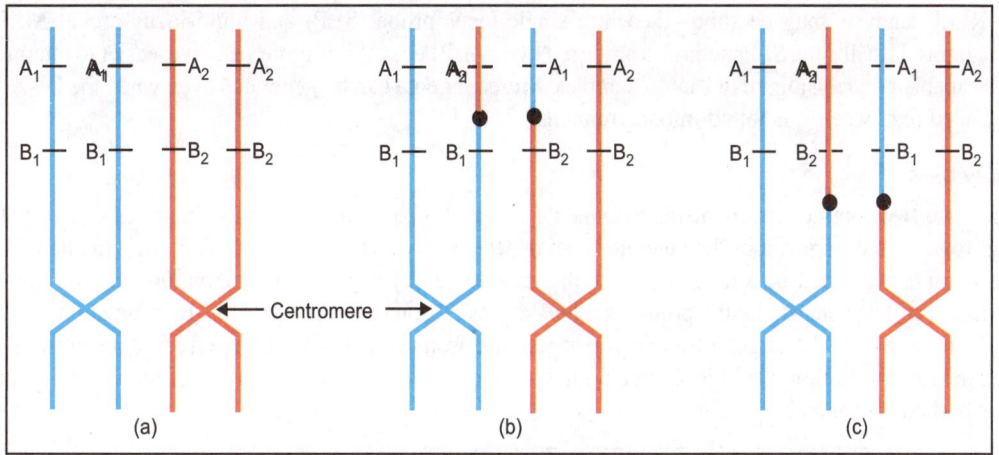

Fig. 16.3. Illustration of recombination between two loci A and B. (a) Two pairs of sister chromatids align during meiosis. A_1 and B_1 are located on the same chromosome. A_2 and B_2 are located on a different chromosome. (b) DNA crossover leads to recombination if the chiasma is located between the two loci. (c) DNA crossover does not lead to recombination if the chiasma is not located between the two loci.

RESTRICTION FRAGMENT LENGTH POLYMORPHISM

In molecular biology, the term restriction fragment length polymorphism, or RFLP, (commonly pronounced 'rif-lip') refers to a difference between two or more samples of homologous DNA molecules arising from differing locations of restriction sites, and to a related laboratory technique by which these segments can be distinguished. In RFLP analysis the DNA sample is broken into pieces (digested) by restriction enzymes and the resulting restriction fragments are separated according to their lengths by gel electrophoresis. Restriction fragment length polymorphism or RFLP analysis is used to identify a change in the genetic sequence that occurs at a site where a restriction enzyme cuts. RFLPs can be used to trace inhertitance patterns, identify specific mutations, and for other molecular genetic techniques. Restriction enzymes are proteins isolated from bacteria that recognise specific short sequences of DNA and cut the DNA at those sites. The normal function of these enzymes in bacteria is to protect the organism by attacking foreign DNA, such as viruses.

The restriction enzyme is added to the DNA being analysed and incubated for several hours, allowing the restriction enzyme to cut at its recognition sites. The DNA is then run through a gel, which separates the DNA fragments according to size. We can then visualise the size of the DNA fragments and assess whether or not the DNA was cut by the enzyme.

Analysis Technique

The basic technique for detecting RFLPs involves fragmenting a sample of DNA by a restriction enzyme, which can recognise and cut DNA wherever a specific short sequence occurs, in a process known as a restriction digest. The resulting DNA fragments are then separated by length through a process known as agarose gel electrophoresis, and transferred to a membrane via the Southern blot procedure. Hybridisation of the membrane to a labelled DNA probe then determines the length of the fragments which are complementary to the probe. A RFLP occurs when the length of a detected fragment varies between individuals. Each fragment length is considered an allele, and can be used in genetic analysis.

RFLP analysis may be subdivided into single-locus probe (SLP) and multi-locus probe (MLP) paradigms. Usually, the SLP method is preferred over MLP because it is more sensitive, easier to interpret and capable of analysing mixed-DNA samples. Moreover data can be generated even when the DNA is degraded (e.g. when it is found in bone remains.)

Examples

There are two common mechanisms by which the size of a particular restriction fragment can vary. In Fig. 16.4, a small segment of the genome is being detected by a DNA probe (thicker line). In allele 'A', the genome is cleaved by a restriction enzyme at three nearby sites (triangles), but only the rightmost fragment will be detected by the probe. In allele 'a', restriction site 2 has been lost by a mutation, so the probe now detects the larger fused fragment running from sites 1 to 3. Figure 16.5 shows how this fragment size variation would look on a Southern blot, and how each allele (two per individual) might be inherited in members of a family.

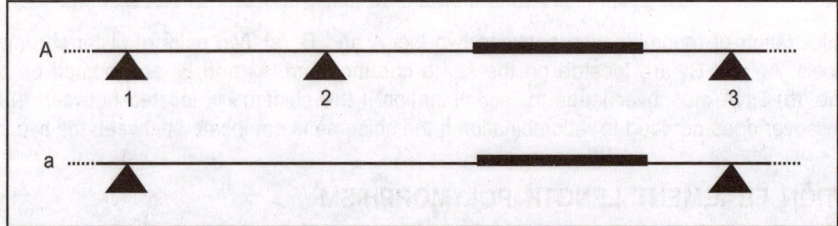

Fig. 16.4. Schematic for RFLP by cleavage site loss.

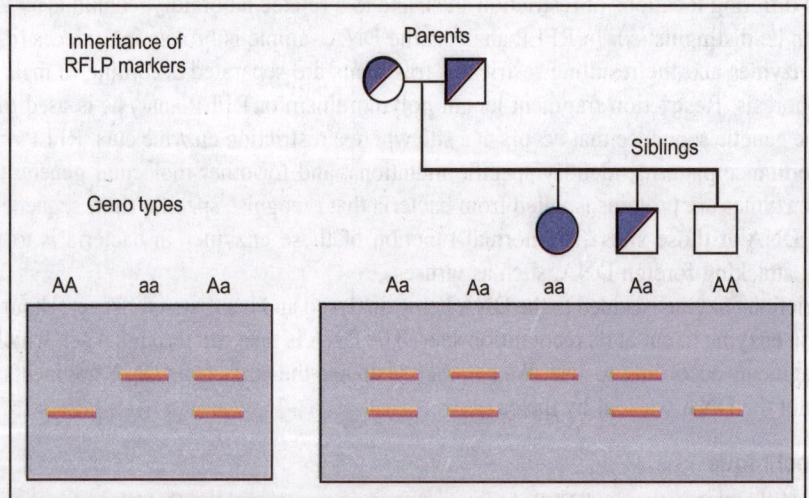

Fig. 16.5. Analysis and inheritance of allelic RFLP fragments (NIH).

In Fig. 16.6, the probe and restriction enzyme are chosen to detect a region of the genome that includes a variable VNTR segment (boxes). In allele 'c' there are five repeats in the VNTR, and the probe detects a longer fragment between the two restriction sites. In allele 'd' there are only two repeats in the VNTR, so the probe detects a shorter fragment between the same two restriction sites. Other genetic processes, such as insertions, deletions, translocations, and inversions, can also lead to RFLPs.

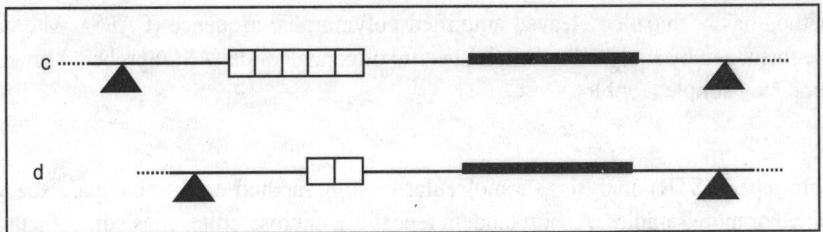

Fig. 16.6. Schematic for RFLP by VNTR length variation.

Applications

Analysis of RFLP variation in genomes was a vital tool in genome mapping and genetic disease analysis. If researchers were trying to initially determine the chromosomal location of a particular disease gene, they would analyse the DNA of members of a family afflicted by the disease, and look for RFLP alleles that show a similar pattern of inheritance as that of the disease (see Genetic linkage). Once a disease gene was localised, RFLP analysis of other families could reveal who was at risk for the disease, or who was likely to be carriers of the mutant genes.

RFLP analysis was also the basis for early methods of Genetic fingerprinting, useful in the identification of samples retrieved from crime scenes, in the determination of paternity, and in the characterisation of genetic diversity or breeding patterns in animal populations.

Alternatives

The technique for RFLP analysis is, however, slow and cumbersome. It requires a large amount of sample DNA, and the combined process of probe labelling, DNA fragmentation, electrophoresis, blotting, hybridisation, washing, and autoradiography could take up to a month to complete. A limited version of the RFLP method that used oligonucleotide probes was reported in 1985. Fortunately, the results of the Human Genome project have largely replaced the need for RFLP mapping, and the identification of many single-nucleotide polymorphisms (SNPs) in that project (as well as the direct identification of many disease genes and mutations) has replaced the need for RFLP disease linkage analysis. The analysis of VNTR alleles continues, but is now usually performed by polymerase chain reaction (PCR) methods. For example, the standard protocols for DNA fingerprinting involve PCR analysis of panels of more than a dozen VNTRs.

RFLP is still a technique used in marker assisted selection. Terminal restriction fragment length polymorphism (TRFLP or sometimes T-RFLP) is a molecular biology technique initially developed for characterising bacterial communities in mixed-species samples. The technique has also been applied to other groups including soil fungi. TRFLP works by PCR amplification of DNA using primer pairs that have been labelled with fluorescent tags. The PCR products are then digested using RFLP enzymes and the resulting patterns visualised using a DNA sequencer. The results are analysed either by simply counting and comparing bands or peaks in the TRFLP profile, or by matching bands from one or more TRFLP runs to a database of known species. The technique is similar in some aspects to DGGE or TGGE. The sequence changes directly involved with an RFLP can also be analysed more quickly by PCR. Amplification can be directed across the altered restriction site, and the products digested with the restriction enzyme.

This method has been called cleaved amplified polymorphic sequence (CAPS). Alternatively, the amplified segment can by analysed by Allele specific oligonucleotide (ASO) probes, a process that can often be done by a simple Dot blot.

STR Analysis

Short tandem repeat (STR) analysis is a molecular biology method used to compare specific loci on DNA from two or more samples. A short tandem repeat is a microsatellite, consisting of a unit of two to thirteen nucleotides repeated hundreds of times in a row on the DNA strand. STR analysis measures the exact number of repeating units. This method differs from restriction fragment length polymorphism analysis since STR analysis does not cut the DNA with restriction enzymes. Instead, probes are attached to desired regions on the DNA, and a polymerase chain reaction is employed to discover the lengths of the short tandem repeats.

Forensic uses

STR analysis is a tool in forensic analysis that evaluates specific STR regions found on nuclear DNA. The variable (polymorphic) nature of the STR regions that are analysed for forensic testing intensifies the discrimination between one DNA profile and another. Forensic science takes advantage of the population's variability in STR lengths, enabling scientists to distinguish one DNA sample from another. For example, the likelihood that any two individuals (except identical twins) will have the same 13-loci DNA profile can be as high as 1 in 1 billion or greater.

AFLP may refer to:

1. Amplified fragment length polymorphism, a highly sensitive tool used in molecular biology to detect DNA polymorphisms.
2. Acute fatty liver of pregnancy, a life-threatening liver condition that may occur during pregnancy.

MAPPING AND SEQUENCING THE HUMAN GENOME

A primary goal of the Human genome project is to make a series of descriptive diagrams maps of each human chromosome at increasingly finer resolutions. Mapping involves: (i) dividing the chromosomes into smaller fragments that can be propagated and characterised, and (ii) ordering (mapping) them to correspond to their respective locations on the chromosomes. After mapping is completed, the next step is to determine the base sequence of each of the ordered DNA fragments. The ultimate goal of genome research is to find all the genes in the DNA sequence and to develop tools for using this information in the study of human biology and medicine. Improving the instrumentation and techniques required for mapping and sequencing a major focus of the genome project will increase efficiency and cost-effectiveness. Goals include automating methods and optimising techniques to extract the maximum useful information from maps and sequences. A genome map describes the order of genes or other markers and the spacing between them on each chromosome. Human genome maps are constructed on several different scales or levels of resolution. At the coarsest resolution are genetic linkage maps, which depict the relative chromosomal locations of DNA markers (genes and other identifiable DNA sequences) by their patterns of inheritance. Physical maps describe the chemical characteristics of the DNA molecule itself. Geneticists have already charted the approximate positions of over 2300 genes, and a start has been made in establishing high- resolution maps of the genome (Fig. 16.7). More precise maps are needed to organise systematic sequencing efforts and plan new research directions. Human genome project goals and resolution are given in Table 16.2.

Table 16.2. Human genome project goals and resolution.

Human genome project goals	Resolution
Complete a detailed human genetic map	2 Mb
Complete a physical map	0.1 Mb
Acquire the genome as clones	5 kb
Determine the complete sequence	1 bp
Find all the genes	

With the data generated by the project, investigators will determine the functions of the genes and develop tools for biological and medical applications.

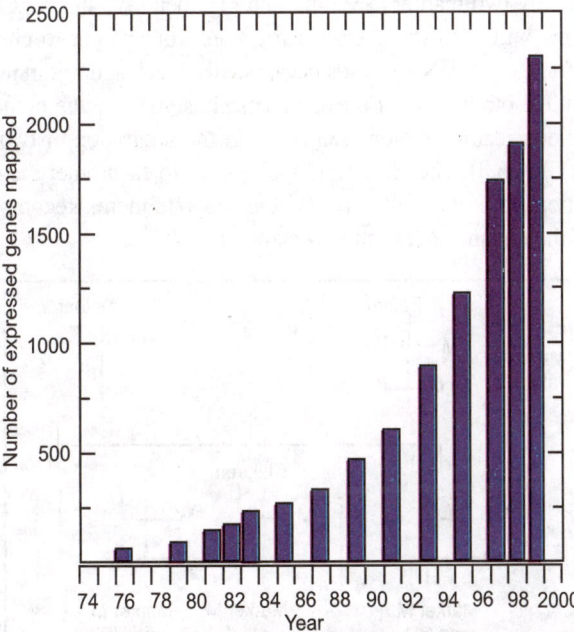

Fig. 16.7. Assignment of genes to specific chromosomes. The number of genes assigned (mapped) to specific chromosomes has greatly increased since the first autosomal (i.e. not on the X or Y chromosome) marker was mapped in 1974. Most of these genes have been mapped to specific bands on chromosomes. The acceleration of chromosome assignments is due to: (i) a combination of improved and new techniques in chromosome sorting and band analysis, (ii) data from family studies, and (iii) the introduction of recombinant DNA technology.

Mapping Strategies

Genetic linkage maps

A genetic linkage map shows the relative locations of specific DNA markers along the chromosome. Any inherited physical or molecular characteristic that differs among individuals and is easily detectable in the laboratory is a potential genetic marker. Markers can be expressed DNA regions (genes) or DNA segments that have no known coding function but whose inheritance pattern can be followed. DNA sequence differences are especially useful markers because they are plentiful and easy to characterise precisely.

Markers must be polymorphic to be useful in mapping; that is, alternative forms must exist among individuals so that they are detectable among different members in family studies. Polymorphisms are variations in DNA sequence that occur on average once every 300 to 500 bp. Variations within exon sequences can lead to observable changes, such as differences in eye colour, blood type, and disease susceptibility. Most variations occur within introns and have little or no effect on an organisms appearance or function, yet they are detectable at the DNA level and can be used as markers. Examples of these types of markers include: (i) restriction fragment length polymorphisms (RFLPs), which reflect sequence variations in DNA sites that can be cleaved by DNA restriction enzymes, and (ii) variable number of tandem repeat sequences, which are short repeated sequences that vary in the number of repeated units and, therefore, in length (a characteristic easily measured). The human genetic linkage map is constructed by observing how frequently two markers are inherited together. Two markers located near each other on the same chromosome will tend to be passed together from parent to child. During the normal production of sperm and egg cells, DNA strands occasionally break and rejoin in different places on the same chromosome or on the other copy of the same chromosome (i.e. the homologous chromosome). This process (called meiotic recombination) can result in the separation of two markers originally on the same chromosome (Fig. 16.8). The closer the markers are to each other the more tightly linked the less likely a recombination event will fall between and separate them. Recombination frequency thus provides an estimate of the distance between two markers.

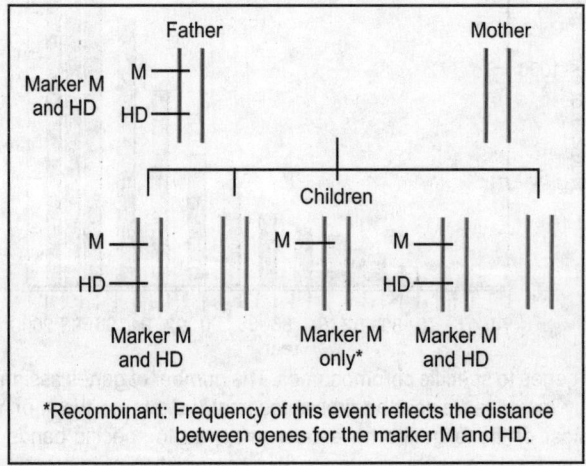

Fig. 16.8. Constructing a genetic linkage map. Genetic linkage maps of each chromosome are made by determining how frequently two markers are passed together from parent to child. Because genetic material is sometimes exchanged during the production of sperm and egg cells, groups of traits (or markers) originally together on one chromosome may not be inherited together. Closely linked markers are less likely to be separated by spontaneous chromosome rearrangements. In this diagram, the vertical lines represent chromosome 4 pairs for each individual in a family. The father has two traits that can be detected in any child who inherits them: a short known DNA sequence used as a genetic marker (M) and Huntingtons disease (HD). The fact that one child received only a single trait (M) from that particular chromosome indicates that the fathers genetic material recombined during the process of sperm production. The frequency of this event helps determine the distance between the two DNA sequences on a genetic map .

On the genetic map, distances between markers are measured in terms of centimorgans (cM), named after the American geneticist Thomas Hunt Morgan. Two markers are said to be 1 cM apart if they are separated by recombination 1 per cent of the time. A genetic distance of 1 cM is roughly equal to a physical distance of 1 million bp (1 Mb). The current resolution of most human genetic map regions is about 10 Mb. The value of the genetic map is that an inherited disease can be located on the map by following the inheritance of a DNA marker present in affected individuals (but absent in unaffected individuals), even though the molecular basis of the disease may not yet be understood nor the responsible gene identified. Genetic maps have been used to find the exact chromosomal location of several important disease genes, including cystic fibrosis, sickle cell disease, Tay-Sachs disease, fragile X syndrome, and myotonic dystrophy. One short-term goal of the genome project is to develop a high- resolution genetic map (2 to 5 cM); recent consensus maps of some chromosomes have averaged 7 to 10 cM between genetic markers. Genetic mapping resolution has been increased through the application of recombinant DNA technology, including *in vitro* radiation-induced chromosome fragmentation and cell fusions (joining human cells with those of other species to form hybrid cells) to create panels of cells with specific and varied human chromosomal components. Assessing the frequency of marker sites remaining together after radiation- induced DNA fragmentation can establish the order and distance between the markers. Because only a single copy of a chromosome is required for analysis, even nonpolymorphic markers are useful in radiation hybrid mapping. [In meiotic mapping (described already), two copies of a chromosome must be distinguished from each other by polymorphic markers.]

Restriction enzymes: microscopic scalpels

Isolated from various bacteria, restriction enzymes recognise short DNA sequences and cut the DNA molecules at those specific sites. (A natural biological function of these enzymes is to protect bacteria by attacking viral and other foreign DNA.) Some restriction enzymes (rare- cutters) cut the DNA very infrequently, generating a small number of very large fragments (several thousand to a million bp). Most enzymes cut DNA more frequently, thus generating a large number of small fragments (less than a hundred to more than a thousand bp). On average, restriction enzymes with:

1. 4-Base recognition sites will yield pieces 256 bases long.
2. 6-Base recognition sites will yield pieces 4000 bases long.
3. 8-Base recognition sites will yield pieces 64,000 bases long.

Since hundreds of different restriction enzymes have been characterised, DNA can be cut into many different small fragments.

Physical maps

Different types of physical maps vary in their degree of resolution. The lowest- resolution physical map is the chromosomal (sometimes called cytogenetic) map, which is based on the distinctive banding patterns observed by light microscopy of stained chromosomes. A cDNA map shows the locations of expressed DNA regions (exons) on the chromosomal map. The more detailed cosmid contig map depicts the order of overlapping DNA fragments spanning the genome. A macrorestriction map describes the order and distance between enzyme cutting (cleavage) sites. The highest- resolution physical map is the complete elucidation of the DNA base-pair sequence of each chromosome in the human genome. Physical maps are described in greater detail below.

Low-resolution physical mapping

Chromosomal map

In a chromosomal map, genes or other identifiable DNA fragments are assigned to their respective chromosomes, with distances measured in base pairs. These markers can be physically associated with particular bands (identified by cytogenetic staining) primarily by *in situ* hybridisation, a technique that involves tagging the DNA marker with an observable label (e.g. one that fluoresces or is radioactive). The location of the labelled probe can be detected after it binds to its complementary DNA strand in an intact chromosome.

As with genetic linkage mapping, chromosomal mapping can be used to locate genetic markers defined by traits observable only in whole organisms. Because chromosomal maps are based on estimates of physical distance, they are considered to be physical maps. The number of base pairs within a band can only be estimated. Until recently, even the best chromosomal maps could be used to locate a DNA fragment only to a region of about 10 Mb, the size of a typical band seen on a chromosome. Improvements in fluorescence *in situ* hybridisation (FISH) methods allow orientation of DNA sequences that lie as close as 2 to 5 Mb. Modifications to *in situ* hybridisation methods, using chromosomes at a stage in cell division (interphase) when they are less compact, increase map resolution to around 1,00,000 bp. Further banding refinement might allow chromosomal bands to be associated with specific amplified DNA fragments, an improvement that could be useful in analysing observable physical traits associated with chromosomal abnormalities.

cDNA map

A cDNA map shows the positions of expressed DNA regions (exons) relative to particular chromosomal regions or bands. (Expressed DNA regions are those transcribed into mRNA). cDNA is synthesised in the laboratory using the mRNA molecule as a template; base-pairing rules are followed (i.e. an A on the mRNA molecule will pair with a T on the new DNA strand). This cDNA can then be mapped to genomic regions.

Because they represent expressed genomic regions, cDNAs are thought to identify the parts of the genome with the most biological and medical significance. A cDNA map can provide the chromosomal location for genes whose functions are currently unknown. For disease-gene hunters, the map can also suggest a set of candidate genes to test when the approximate location of a disease gene has been mapped by genetic linkage techniques.

High-resolution physical mapping

The two current approaches to high-resolution physical mapping are termed top-down and bottom-up. With either strategy the maps represent ordered sets of DNA fragments that are generated by cutting genomic DNA with restriction enzymes (see previously discussed Restriction enzymes). The fragments are then amplified by cloning or by polymerase chain reaction (PCR) methods. Electrophoretic techniques are used to separate the fragments according to size into different bands, which can be visualised by direct DNA staining or by hybridisation with DNA probes of interest. The use of purified chromosomes separated either by flow sorting from human cell lines or in hybrid cell lines allows a single chromosome to be mapped.

A number of strategies can be used to reconstruct the original order of the DNA fragments in the genome. Many approaches make use of the ability of single strands of DNA and/or RNA to hybridise to form double-stranded segments by hydrogen bonding between complementary bases. The extent of sequence homology between the two strands can be inferred from the length of the double-stranded segment. Finger printing uses restriction map data to determine which fragments have a specific sequence (fingerprint) in common and therefore overlap. Another approach uses linking clones as probes for hybridisation to chromosomal DNA cut with the same restriction enzyme.

Macrorestriction maps: Top-down mapping

In top-down mapping, a single chromosome is cut (with rare-cutter restriction enzymes) into large pieces, which are ordered and subdivided; the smaller pieces are then mapped further. The resulting macro-restriction maps depict the order of and distance between sites at which rare-cutter enzymes cleave [Fig. 16.9(a)]. This approach yields maps with more continuity and fewer gaps between fragments than contig maps, but map resolution is lower and may not be useful in finding particular genes; in addition, this strategy generally does not produce long stretches of mapped sites. Currently, this approach allows DNA pieces to be located in regions measuring about 1,00,000 bp to 1 Mb.

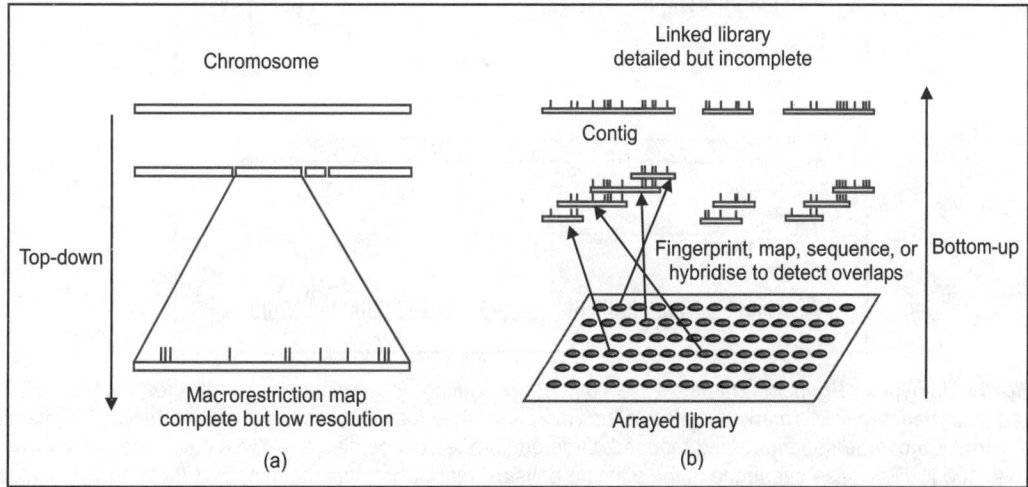

Fig. 16.9. Physical mapping strategies. Top-down physical mapping (a) produces maps with few gaps, but map resolution may not allow location of specific genes. Bottom-up strategies (b) generate extremely detailed maps of small areas but leave many gaps. A combination of both approaches is being used.

The development of pulsed-field gel (PFG) electrophoretic methods has improved the mapping and cloning of large DNA molecules. While conventional gel electrophoretic methods separate pieces less than 40 kb (1 kb = 1000 bases) in size, PFG separates molecules up to 10 Mb, allowing the application of both conventional and new mapping methods to larger genomic regions.

Contig maps: Bottom-up mapping

The bottom-up approach involves cutting the chromosome into small pieces, each of which is cloned and ordered. The ordered fragments form contiguous DNA blocks (contigs). Currently, the resulting library of clones varies in size from 10,000 bp to 1 Mb [Fig. 16.9(b)]. An advantage of this approach is the accessibility of these stable clones to other researchers. Contig construction can be verified by FISH, which localises cosmids to specific regions within chromosomal bands.

Contig maps thus consist of a linked library of small overlapping clones representing a complete chromosomal segment. While useful for finding genes localised to a small area (under 2 Mb), contig maps are difficult to extend over large stretches of a chromosome because all regions are not clonable. DNA probe techniques can be used to fill in the gaps, but they are time consuming. Figure 16.10 is a diagram relating the different types of maps.

Technological improvements now make possible the cloning of large DNA pieces, using artificially constructed chromosome vectors that carry human DNA fragments as large as 1 Mb. These vectors are maintained in yeast cells as artificial chromosomes (YACs). Before YACs were developed, the largest cloning vectors (cosmids) carried inserts of only 20 to 40 kb. YAC methodology drastically reduces the number of clones to be ordered; many YACs span entire human genes. A more detailed map of a large YAC insert can be produced by subcloning, a process in which fragments of the original insert are cloned into smaller-insert vectors. Because some YAC regions are unstable, large-capacity bacterial vectors (i.e. those that can accommodate large inserts) are also being developed.

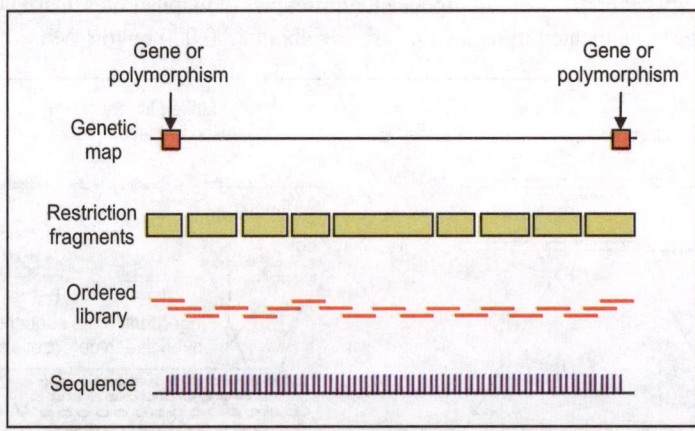

Fig. 16.10. Types of genome maps. At the coarsest resolution, the genetic map measures recombination frequency between linked markers (genes or polymorphisms). At the next resolution level, restriction fragments of 1 to 2 Mb can be separated and mapped. Ordered libraries of cosmids and YACs have insert sizes from 40 to 400 kb. The base sequence is the ultimate physical map. Chromosomal mapping (not shown) locates genetic sites in relation to bands on chromosomes (estimated resolution of 5 Mb); new *in situ* hybridisation techniques can place *loci* 100 kb apart. This direct strategy links the other four mapping approaches.

Separating chromosomes

Flow sorting

Flow sorting employs flow cytometry to separate, according to size, chromosomes isolated from cells during cell division when they are condensed and stable. As the chromosomes flow singly past a laser beam, they are differentiated by analysing the amount of DNA present, and individual chromosomes are directed to specific collection tubes.

Somatic cell hybridisation

In somatic cell hybridisation, human cells and rodent tumour cells are fused (hybridised); over time, after the chromosomes mix, human chromosomes are preferentially lost from the hybrid cell until only one or a few remain. Those individual hybrid cells are then propagated and maintained as cell lines containing specific human chromosomes. Improvements to this technique have generated a number of hybrid cell lines, each with a specific single human chromosome.

Sequencing Technologies

The ultimate physical map of the human genome is the complete DNA sequence the determination of all base pairs on each chromosome. The completed map will provide biologists with a Rosetta stone for studying human biology and enable medical researchers to begin to unravel the mechanisms of inherited diseases. Much effort continues to be spent locating genes; if the full sequence were known, emphasis could shift to determining gene function. The Human Genome Project is creating research tools for 21st-century biology, when the goal will be to understand the sequence and functions of the genes residing therein. Achieving the goals of the Human Genome Project will require substantial improvements in the rate, efficiency, and reliability of standard sequencing procedures. While technological advances are leading to the automation of standard DNA purification, separation, and detection steps, efforts are also focusing on the development of entirely new sequencing methods that may eliminate some of these steps. Sequencing procedures currently involve first subcloning DNA fragments from a cosmid or bacteriophage library into special sequencing vectors that carry shorter pieces of the original cosmid fragments (Fig. 16.11).

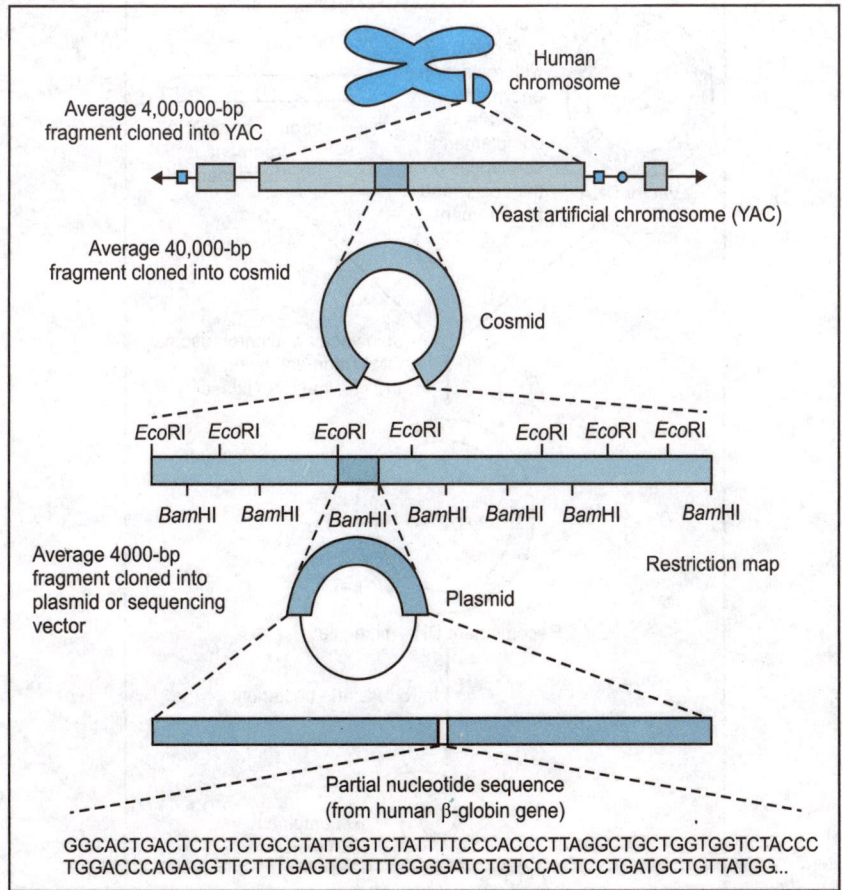

Fig. 16.11. Constructing clones for sequencing. Cloned DNA molecules must be made progressively smaller and the fragments subcloned into new vectors to obtain fragments small enough for use with current sequencing technology. Sequencing results are compiled to provide longer stretches of sequence across a chromosome.

The next step is to make the subcloned fragments into sets of nested fragments differing in length by one nucleotide, so that the specific base at the end of each successive fragment is detectable after the fragments have been separated by gel electrophoresis.

DNA amplification: cloning and polymerase chain reaction

Cloning (in vivo DNA amplification)

Cloning involves the use of recombinant DNA technology to propagate DNA fragments inside a foreign host. The fragments are usually isolated from chromosomes using restriction enzymes and then united with a carrier (a vector). Following introduction into suitable host cells, the DNA fragments can then be reproduced along with the host cell DNA. Vectors are DNA molecules originating from viruses, bacteria, and yeast cells. They accommodate various sizes of foreign DNA fragments ranging from 12,000 bp for bacterial vectors (plasmids and cosmids) to 1 Mb for yeast vectors (yeast artificial chromosomes). Bacteria are most often the hosts for these inserts, but yeast and mammalian cells are also used (Fig. 16.11a).

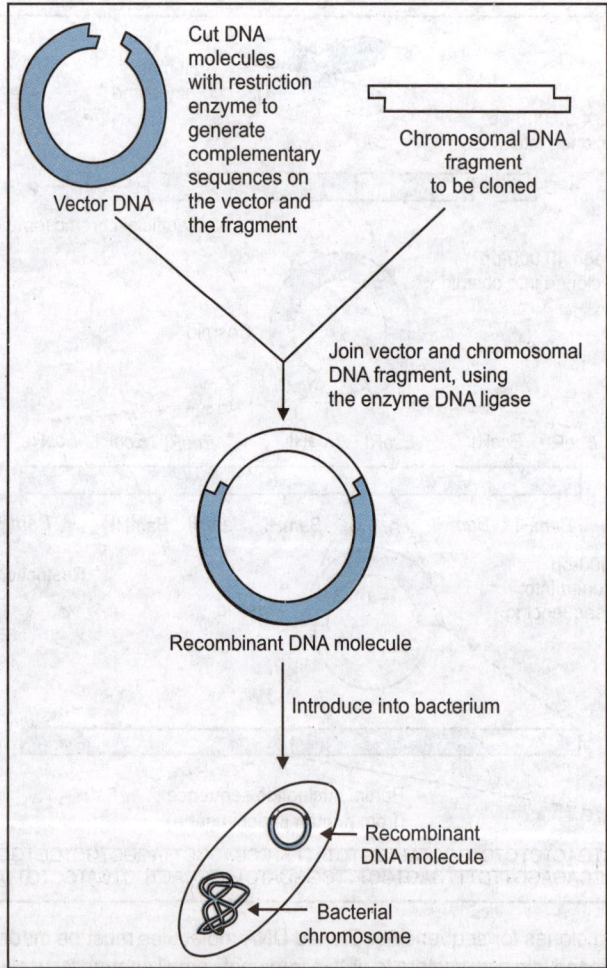

Fig. 16.11a. Cloning DNA in plasmids. By fragmenting DNA of any origin (human, animal, or plant) and inserting it in the DNA of rapidly reproducing foreign cells, billions of copies of a single gene or DNA segment can be produced in a very short time. DNA to be cloned is inserted into a plasmid (a small, self- replicating circular molecule of DNA) that is separate from chromosomal DNA. When the recombinant plasmid is introduced into bacteria, the newly inserted segment will be replicated along with the rest of the plasmid.

Cloning procedures provide unlimited material for experimental study. A random (unordered) set of cloned DNA fragments is called a library. Genomic libraries are sets of overlapping fragments encompassing an entire genome (Fig. 16.11b). Also available are chromosome-specific libraries, which consist of fragments derived from source DNA enriched for a particular chromosome.

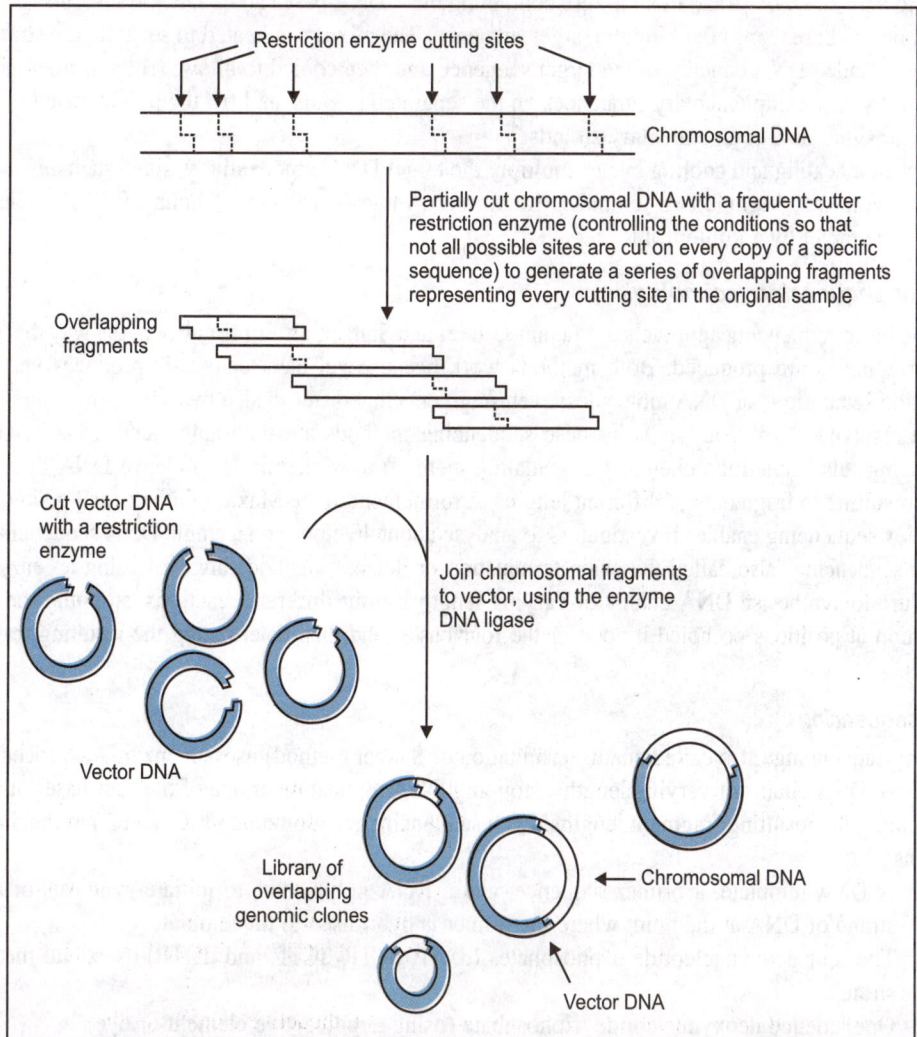

Fig. 16.11b. Constructing an overlapping clone library. A collection of clones of chromosomal DNA, called a library, has no obvious order indicating the original positions of the cloned pieces on the uncut chromosome. To establish that two particular clones are adjacent to each other in the genome, libraries of clones containing partly overlapping regions must be constructed. These clone libraries are ordered by dividing the inserts into smaller fragments and determining which clones share common DNA sequences.

PCR (in vitro DNA amplification)

PCR can amplify a desired DNA sequence of any origin (virus, bacteria, plant, or human) hundreds of millions of times in a matter of hours, a task that would have required several days with recombinant technology. PCR is especially valuable because the reaction is highly specific, easily automated, and capable of amplifying minute amounts of sample. For these reasons, PCR has also had a major impact on clinical medicine, genetic disease diagnostics, forensic science, and evolutionary biology.

PCR is a process based on a specialised polymerase enzyme, which can synthesise a complementary strand to a given DNA strand in a mixture containing the 4 DNA bases and 2 DNA fragments (primers, each about 20 bases long) flanking the target sequence. The mixture is heated to separate the strands of double- stranded DNA containing the target sequence and then cooled to allow: (i) the primers to find and bind to their complementary sequences on the separated strands, and (ii) the polymerase to extend the primers into new complementary strands.

Repeated heating and cooling cycles multiply the target DNA exponentially, since each new double strand separates to become two templates for further synthesis. In about 1 hour, 20 PCR cycles can amplify the target by a millionfold.

Current sequencing technologies

The two basic sequencing approaches, Maxam-Gilbert and Sanger, differ primarily in the way the nested DNA fragments are produced. Both methods work because gel electrophoresis produces very high resolution separations of DNA molecules; even fragments that differ in size by only a single nucleotide can be resolved. Almost all steps in these sequencing methods are now automated. Maxam-Gilbert sequencing (also called the chemical degradation method) uses chemicals to cleave DNA at specific bases, resulting in fragments of different lengths. A refinement to the Maxam-Gilbert method known as multiplex sequencing enables investigators to analyse about 40 clones on a single DNA sequencing gel. Sanger sequencing (also called the chain termination or dideoxy method) involves using an enzymatic procedure to synthesise DNA chains of varying length in four different reactions, stopping the DNA replication at positions occupied by one of the four bases, and then determining the resulting fragment lengths.

DNA sequencing

Dideoxy sequencing (also called chain- termination or Sanger method) uses an enzymatic procedure to synthesise DNA chains of varying lengths, stopping DNA replication at one of the four bases and then determining the resulting fragment lengths. Each sequencing reaction tube (T, C, and A) in the diagram contains

1. A DNA template, a primer sequence, and a DNA polymerase to initiate synthesis of a new strand of DNA at the point where the primer is hybridised to the template.
2. The four deoxynucleotide triphosphates (dATP, dTTP, dCTP, and dGTP) to extend the DNA strand.
3. One labelled deoxynucleotide triphosphate (using a radioactive element or dye).
4. One dideoxynucleotide triphosphate, which terminates the growing chain wherever it is incorporated. Tube A has didATP, tube C has didCTP, etc.

For example, in the A reaction tube the ratio of the dATP to didATP is adjusted so that each tube will have a collection of DNA fragments with a didATP incorporated for each adenine position on the template DNA fragments. The fragments of varying length are then separated by electrophoresis (a) and the positions of the nucleotides analysed to determine sequence. The fragments are separated on the basis of size, with the shorter fragments moving faster and appearing at the bottom of the gel. Sequence is read from bottom to top (b) (Fig. 16.12). These first-generation gel-based sequencing technologies are now being used to sequence small regions of interest in the human genome. Although investigators could use existing technology to sequence whole chromosomes, time and cost considerations make large-scale sequencing projects of this nature impractical. The smallest human chromosome (Y) contains 50 Mb; the largest (chromosome 1) has 250 Mb.

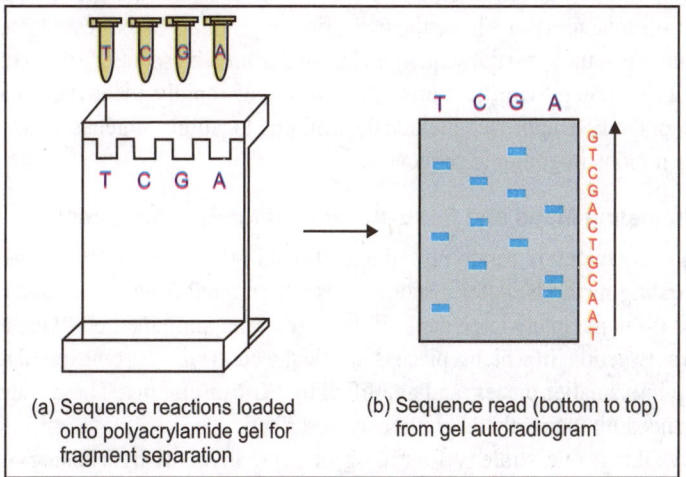

(a) Sequence reactions loaded onto polyacrylamide gel for fragment separation

(b) Sequence read (bottom to top) from gel autoradiogram

Fig. 16.12. DNA sequencing.

Sequencing technologies under development

A major focus of the Human Genome Project is the development of automated sequencing technology that can accurately sequence 1,00,000 or more bases per day at a cost of less than $0.50 per base. Specific goals include the development of sequencing and detection schemes that are faster and more sensitive, accurate, and economical. Many novel sequencing technologies are now being explored, and the most promising ones will eventually be optimised for widespread use.

Second-generation (interim) sequencing technologies will enable speed and accuracy to increase by an order of magnitude (i.e. 10 times greater) while lowering the cost per base. Some important disease genes will be sequenced with such technologies as: (i) high-voltage capillary and ultrathin electrophoresis to increase fragment separation rate, and (ii) use of resonance ionisation spectroscopy to detect stable isotope labels. Third-generation gel-less sequencing technologies, which aim to increase efficiency by several orders of magnitude, are expected to be used for sequencing most of the human genome. These developing technologies include: (i) enhanced fluorescence detection of individual labelled bases in flow cytometry, (ii) direct reading of the base sequence on a DNA strand with the use of scanning tunnelling or atomic force microscopies, (iii) enhanced mass spectrometric analysis of DNA sequence, and (iv) sequencing by hybridisation to short panels of nucleotides of known sequence. Pilot large-scale sequencing projects will provide opportunities to improve current technologies and will reveal challenges investigators may encounter in larger-scale efforts.

Partial sequencing to facilitate mapping, gene identification

Correlating mapping data from different laboratories has been a problem because of differences in generating, isolating, and mapping DNA fragments. A common reference system designed to meet these challenges uses partially sequenced unique regions (200 to 500 bp) to identify clones, contigs, and long stretches of sequence. Called sequence tagged sites (STSs), these short sequences have become standard markers for physical mapping. Because coding sequences of genes represent most of the potentially useful information content of the genome (but are only a fraction of the total DNA), some investigators have begun partial sequencing of cDNAs instead of random genomic DNA. (cDNAs are derived from mRNA sequences, which are the transcription products of expressed genes.) In addition to providing unique markers, these partial sequences [termed expressed sequence tags (ESTs)] also identify expressed genes. This strategy can thus provide a means of rapidly identifying most human genes. Other applications of the EST approach include determining locations of genes along chromosomes and identifying coding regions in genomic sequences.

End Games: Completing Maps and Sequences; Finding Specific Genes

Starting maps and sequences is relatively simple; finishing them will require new strategies or a combination of existing methods. After a sequence is determined using the methods described above, the task remains to fill in the many large gaps left by current mapping methods. One approach is single-chromosome microdissection, in which a piece is physically cut from a chromosomal region of particular interest, broken up into smaller pieces, and amplified by PCR or cloning. These fragments can then be mapped and sequenced by the methods previously described.

Chromosome walking, one strategy for filling in gaps, involves hybridising a primer of known sequence to a clone from an unordered genomic library and synthesising a short complementary strand. The complementary strand is then sequenced and its end used as the next primer for further walking; in this way the adjacent, previously unknown, region is identified and sequenced. The chromosome is thus systematically sequenced from one end to the other. Because primers must be synthesised chemically, a disadvantage of this technique is the large number of different primers needed to walk a long distance. Chromosome walking is also used to locate specific genes by sequencing the chromosomal segments between markers that flank the gene of interest (Fig. 16.13).

The current human genetic map has about 1000 markers, or 1 marker spaced every 3 million bp; an estimated 100 genes lie between each pair of markers. Higher-resolution genetic maps have been made in regions of particular interest. New genes can be located by combining genetic and physical map information for a region. The genetic map basically describes gene order. Rough information about gene location is sometimes available also, but these data must be used with caution because recombination is not equally likely at all places on the chromosome. Thus the genetic map, compared to the physical map, stretches in some places and compresses in others, as though it were drawn on a rubber band.

The degree of difficulty in finding a disease gene of interest depends largely on what information is already known about the gene and, especially, on what kind of DNA alterations cause the disease. Spotting the disease gene is very difficult when disease results from a single altered DNA base; sickle cell anemia is an example of such a case, as are probably most major human inherited diseases. When disease results from a large DNA rearrangement, this anomaly can usually be detected as alterations in the physical map of the region or even by direct microscopic examination of the chromosome. The location of these alterations pinpoints the site of the gene.

Identifying the gene responsible for a specific disease without a map is analogous to finding a needle in a haystack. Actually, finding the gene is even more difficult, because even close up, the gene still looks like just another piece of hay. However, maps give clues on where to look; the finer the maps resolution, the fewer pieces of hay to be tested.

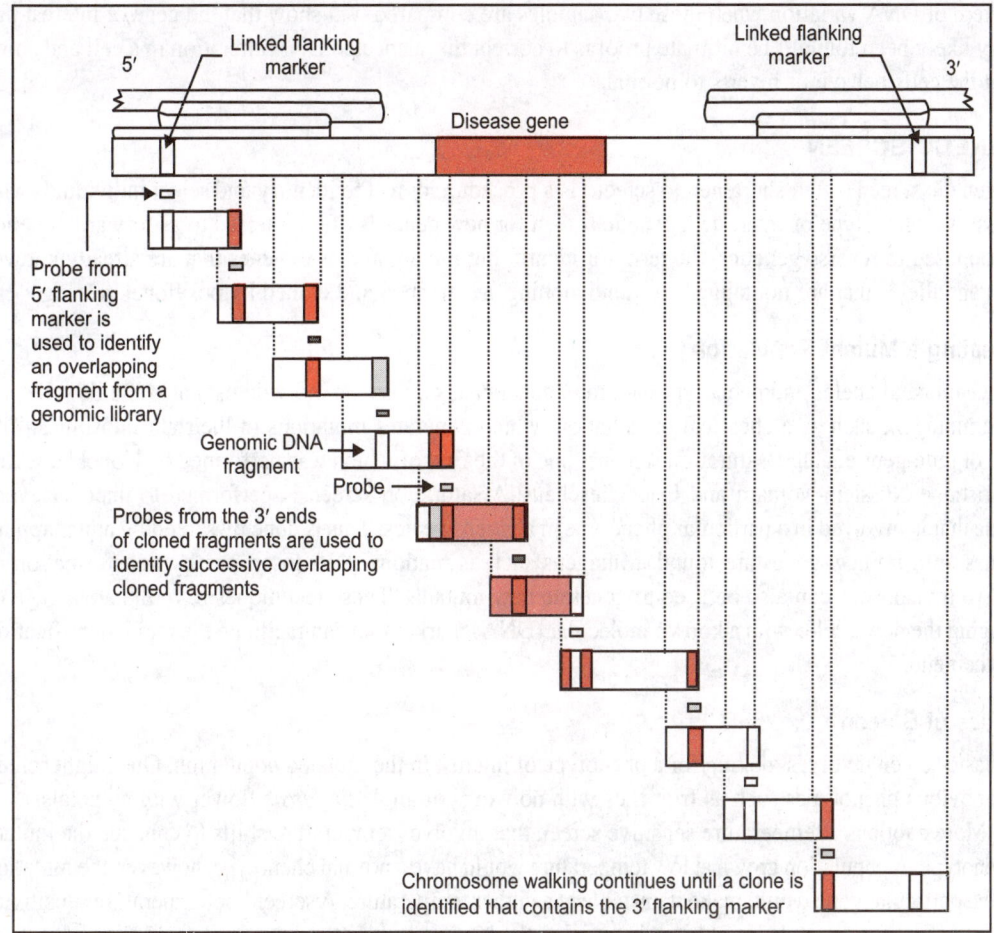

Fig. 16.13. Cloning a disease gene by chromosome walking. After a marker is linked to within 1 cM of a disease gene, chromosome walking can be used to clone the disease gene itself. A probe is first constructed from a genomic fragment identified from a library as being the closest linked marker to the gene. A restriction fragment isolated from the end of the clone near the disease locus is used to reprobe the genomic library for an overlapping clone. This process is repeated several times to walk across the chromosome and reach the flanking marker on the other side of the disease- gene locus

Once the neighbourhood of a gene of interest has been identified, several strategies can be used to find the gene itself. An ordered library of the gene neighbourhood can be constructed if one is not already available.

This library provides DNA fragments that can be screened for additional polymorphisms, improving the genetic map of the region and further restricting the possible gene location. In addition, DNA fragments from the region can be used as probes to search for DNA sequences that are expressed (transcribed to RNA) or conserved among individuals. Most genes will have such sequences. Then individual gene candidates must be examined. For example, a gene responsible for liver disease is likely to be expressed in the liver and less likely in other tissues or organs. This type of evidence can further limit the search. Finally, a suspected gene may need to be sequenced in both healthy and affected individuals. A consistent pattern of DNA variation when these two samples are compared will show that the gene of interest has very likely been found. The ultimate proof is to correct the suspected DNA alteration in a cell and show that the cells behaviour reverts to normal.

GENETIC SCREEN

A genetic screen (often shortened to screen) is a procedure or test to identify and select individuals who possess a phenotype of interest. A genetic screen for new genes is often referred to as forward genetics as opposed to reverse genetics, the term for identifying mutant alleles in genes that are already known. Mutant alleles that are not tagged for rapid cloning are mapped and cloned by positional cloning.

Creating a Mutant Population

Since unusual alleles and phenotypes are rare, geneticists expose the individuals that are to be screened to a mutagen, such as a chemical or radiation, which generates mutations in their chromosomes. The use of mutagens enables 'saturation screens' one of the first of which was performed by Nobel laureates Christiane Nüsslein-Volhard and Eric Wieschaus. A saturation screen is performed to uncover every gene that is involved in a particular phenotype in a given species. This is done by screening and mapping genes until no new genes are found. Mutagens such as random DNA insertions by transformation or active transposons can also be used to generate new mutants. These techniques have the advantage of tagging the new alleles with a known molecular (DNA) marker that can facilitate the rapid identification of the gene.

Types of Screen

A basic screen involves looking for a phenotype of interest in the mutated population. One might screen for obvious phenotypes such as fruit flies with no wings or an *Arabidopsis* flower with no petals.

More subtle is a temperature sensitive screen that involves temperature shifts to enhance the mutant phenotype. A population grown at low temperature would have a normal phenotype, however, the mutation in the particular gene would make it unstable at a higher temperature. A screen for temperature sensitivity in fruit flies, for example, might involve raising the temperature in the cage until some flies faint, then opening a portal to let the others escape. Individuals selected in a screen are liable to carry an unusual version of a gene involved in the phenotype of interest. An advantage of alleles found in this type of screen is that the mutant phenotype is conditional and can be activated by simply raising the temperature. A null mutation in such a gene may be lethal to the embryo and such mutants would be missed in a basic screen. An enhancer/suppressor screen is the most sophisticated type of genetic screen. In this case a mutagenised population has an allele of a gene that leads to a weak mutant phenotype in the biological process of interest.

For example, with regard to fruit fly wing development, a weak allele may have small abnormal wings whereas a strong/null allele would have no wings. In this sensitised background it is possible to discover new mutants that either enhance the phenotype (small wings to no wings) or suppress the phenotype (small wings to normal wings). Such a screen has two advantages. First, new genes identified in the screen are often involved in the same biological process as the weak allele in the genetic background, in this case wing formation. Second, due to genetic redundancy, the mutant genes discovered may not have a visible phenotype of their own. In a more basic screen these would not be discovered, however, in the sensitised genetic background a visible phenotype is clear.

Mapping Mutants

By the classical genetics approach, a researcher would then locate (map) the gene on its chromosome by crossbreeding with individuals that carry other unusual traits and collecting statistics on how frequently the two traits are inherited together. Classical geneticists would have used phenotypic traits to map the new mutant alleles.

With the advent of genomic sequences for model systems such as *Drosophila, Arabidopsis* and *C. elegans* many SNPs have now been identified that can be used as traits for mapping. SNPs are the preferred traits for mapping since they are very frequent, on the order of one difference per 1000 base pairs, between different varieties of organism.

Positional Cloning

Positional cloning is a method of gene identification in which a gene for a specific phenotype is identified, with only its approximate chromosomal location (but not the function) known, also known as the candidate region. Initially, the candidate region can be defined using techniques such as linkage analysis, and positional cloning is then used to narrow the candidate region until the gene and its mutations are found. Positional cloning typically involves the isolation of partially overlapping DNA segments from genomic libraries to progress along the chromosome toward a specific gene. During the course of positional cloning, one needs to determine whether the DNA segment currently under consideration is part of the gene. Tests used for this purpose include cross-species hybridisation, identification of unmethylated CpG islands, exon trapping, direct cDNA selection, computer analysis of DNA sequence, mutation screening in affected individuals, and tests of gene expression. For genomes in which the regions of genetic polymorphisms are known, positional cloning involves identifying polymorphisms that flank the mutation. This process requires that DNA fragments from the closest known genetic marker are progressively cloned and sequenced, getting closer to the mutant allele with each new clone. This process produces a contig map of the locus and is known as chromosome walking. With the completion of genome sequencing projects such as the Human Genome Project, modern positional cloning can use ready-made contigs from the genome sequence databases directly.

For each new DNA clone a polymorphism is identified and tested in the mapping population for its recombination frequency compared to the mutant phenotype. When the DNA clone is at or close to the mutant allele the recombination frequency should be close to zero. If the chromosome walk proceeds through the mutant allele the new polymorphisms will start to show increase in recombination frequency compared to the mutant phenotype. Depending on the size of the mapping population, the mutant allele can be narrowed down to a small region (<30 Kb). Sequence comparison between wild type and mutant DNA in that region is then required to locate the DNA mutation that causes the phenotypic difference.

Modern positional cloning can more directly extract information from genomic sequencing projects and existing data by analysing the genes in the candidate region. Potential disease genes from the candidate region can then be prioritised, potentially reducing the amount of work involved. Genes with expression patterns consistent with the disease phenotype, showing a (putative) function related to the phenotype, or homologous to another gene linked to the phenotype are all priority candidates. Generalisation of positional cloning techniques in this manner is also known as positional gene discovery.

Positional cloning is an effective method to isolate disease genes in an unbiased manner, and has been used to identify disease genes for Duchenne Muscular Dystrophy, Huntington's and Cystic Fibrosis. However, complications in the analysis arise if the disease exhibits locus heterogeneity.

Exon

An exon is a nucleic acid sequence that is represented in the mature form of an RNA molecule after either portions of a precursor RNA (introns) have been removed by *cis*-splicing or when two or more precursor RNA molecules have been ligated by *trans*-splicing. The mature RNA molecule can be a messenger RNA or a functional form of a noncoding RNA such as rRNA or tRNA. Depending on the context, exon can refer to the sequence in the DNA or its RNA transcript.

Function

In many genes, each exon contains part of the open reading frame (ORF) that codes for a specific portion of the complete protein. However, the term exon is often misused to refer only to coding sequences for the final protein. This is incorrect, since many noncoding exons are known in human genes.

Figure 16.14 of a heterogeneous nuclear RNA (hnRNA), which is an unedited mRNA transcript, or pre-mRNAs. Exons can include both sequences that code for amino acids (red) and untranslated sequences (grey). Stretches of unused sequence called introns (blue) are removed, and the exons are joined together to form the final functional mRNA. The notation 5′ and 3′ refer to the direction of the DNA template in the chromosome and is used to distinguish between the two untranslated regions (grey).

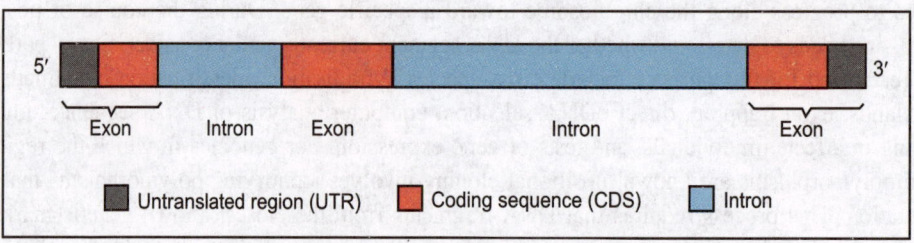

Fig. 16.14. Diagram of a heterogeneous nuclear RNA (hnRNA).

Some of the exons will be wholly or part of the 5′ untranslated region (5′ UTR) or the 3′ untranslated region (3′ UTR) of each transcript. The untranslated regions are important for efficient translation of the transcript and for controlling the rate of translation and half life of the transcript. Furthermore, transcripts made from the same gene may not have the same exon structure since parts of the mRNA could be removed by the process of alternative splicing. Some mRNA transcripts have exons with no ORF's and thus are sometimes referred to as noncoding RNA. Exonisation is the creation of a new exon, as result of mutations in intronic sequences. Polycistronic messages have multiple ORF's in one transcript and also have small regions of untranslated sequence between each ORF.

Experimental approaches that utilise exons

Exon trapping or 'gene trapping' is a molecular biology technique that exploits the existence of the intron-exon splicing to find new genes. The first exon of a 'trapped' gene splices into the exon that is contained in the insertional DNA. This new exon contains the ORF for a reporter gene that can now be expressed using the enhancers that control the target gene. A scientist knows that a new gene has been trapped when the reporter gene is expressed.

Splicing can be experimentally modified so that targeted exons are excluded from mature mRNA transcripts by blocking the access of splice-directing small nuclear ribonucleoprotein particles (snRNPs) to pre-mRNA using Morpholino antisense oligos. This has become a standard technique in developmental biology. Morpholino oligos can also be targeted to prevent molecules that regulate splicing (e.g. splice enhancers, splice suppressors) from binding to pre-mRNA, altering patterns of splicing.

A tendency for exons to correspond to discrete units of protein structure in protein-coding genes of ancient origin would provide clear evidence in favour of the exon theory of genes, which proposes that split genes arose not by insertion of introns into unsplit genes, but from combinations of primordial mini-genes (exons) separated by spacers (introns). Although putative examples of such correspondence have strongly influenced previous debate on the origin of introns, a general correspondence has not been rigorously proved.

Chapter 17

Human Somatic Cell Gene Therapy

INTRODUCTION

The prelude to successful human somatic gene therapy, i.e. the efficient transfer and expression of a variety of human genes into target cells, has already been accomplished in several systems. Safe methods have been devised to do this using nonviral and viral vectors. Potentially therapeutic genes have been transferred into many accessible cell types, including haematopoietic cells, hepatocytes and cancer cells, in several different approaches to *ex vivo* gene therapy. Successful *in vivo* gene therapy requires improvements in tissue-targeting and new vector design, which are already being sought. Gene-transfer protocols have been approved for human use in inherited diseases, cancer and acquired disorders. Human somatic cell gene therapy promises to be an effective addition to the arsenal of approaches to the therapy of many human diseases in the 21st century if not sooner.

Somatic gene therapy of human disease with retrovirus vectors is a new technology with potentially important medical benefits. Although it involves recombinant DNA technologies and modified retroviruses, proper design of the vectors and delivery systems removes most potential foreseen risks. Furthermore, even in the very remote possibility that there is a nontherapeutic biological effect of the treatment, it is unlikely to be a harmful one.

Thus, once very safe retrovirus vector–helper cell systems are constructed and in use, safety considerations should not hold up further human trials of retrovirus vectors. There are many techniques of gene therapy, all of them still in experimental stages. The two basic methods are called *in vivo* and *ex vivo* gene therapy. The *in vivo* method inserts genetically altered genes directly into the patient; the *ex vivo* method removes tissue from the patient, extracts the cells in question, and genetically alters them before returning them to the patient.

The challenge of gene therapy lies in development of a means to deliver the genetic material into the nuclei of the appropriate cells, so that it will be reproduced in the normal course of cell division and have a lasting effect. One technique involves removing cells from a patient, fortifying them with healthy copies of the defective gene, and reinjecting them into the patient. Another involves inserting a gene into an inactivated or nonvirulent virus and using the virus's infective capabilities to carry the desired gene into the patient's cells.

A liposome, a tiny fat-encased pouch that can traverse cell membranes, is also sometimes used to transport a gene into a body cell. Another approach employing liposomes, called chimeraplasty, involves the insertion of manufactured nucleic acid molecules (chimeraplasts) instead of entire genes to correct disease-causing gene mutations. Once inserted, the gene may produce an essential chemical that the patient's body cannot, remove or render harmless a substance or gene causing disease, or expose certain cells, especially cancerous cells, to attack by conventional drugs.

Gene therapy was first used in humans in 1990 to treat a child with adenosine deaminase deficiency (ADA), a rare hereditary immune disorder. It is hoped that gene therapy can be used to treat cancer, genetic diseases, and AIDS, but there are concerns that the immune system may attack cells treated by gene therapy, that the viral vectors could mutate and become virulent or that altered genes might be passed to succeeding generations. In the United States, gene therapy techniques must be approved by the federal government.

The Recombinant DNA Advisory Committee of the National Institutes of Health oversees gene therapy experiments. Like drugs, products must pass the requirements of the Food and Drug Administration. Gene therapy is a competitive and potentially lucrative field, and patents have been awarded for certain techniques.

Today, most gene therapy studies are aimed at cancer and hereditary diseases linked to a genetic defect. Antisense therapy is not strictly a form of gene therapy, but is a related, genetically-mediated therapy (Fig. 17.1).

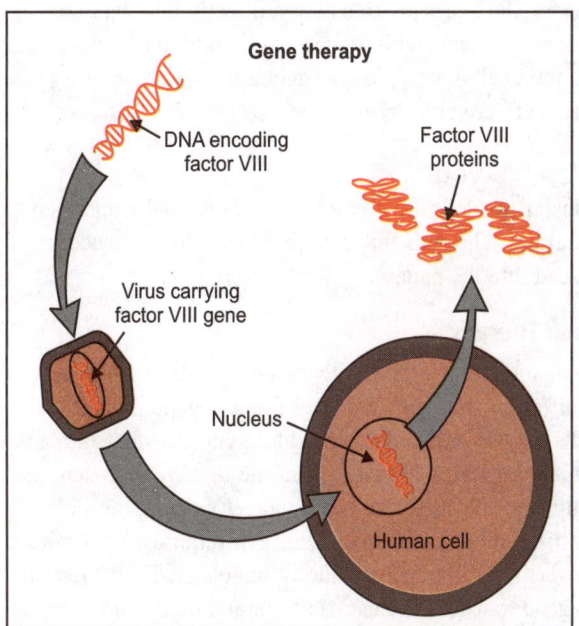

Fig. 17.1. Human gene therapy.

The biology of human gene therapy remains complex and many techniques need further development. Many diseases and their strict genetic link need to be understood more fully before gene therapy can be used appropriately. The public policy debate surrounding the possible use of genetically engineered material in human subjects has been equally complex. Major participants in the debate have come from the fields of biology, government, law, medicine, philosophy, politics, and religion, each bringing different views to the discussion.

TYPES OF GENE THERAPY

Gene therapy may be classified into the two following types:

Germ Line Gene Therapy

In the case of germ line gene therapy, germ cells, i.e. sperm or eggs, are modified by the introduction of functional genes, which are ordinarily integrated into their genomes. Therefore, the change due to therapy would be heritable and would be passed on to later generations. This new approach, theoretically, should be highly effective in counteracting genetic disorders and hereditary diseases. However, many jurisdictions prohibit this for application in human beings, at least for the present, for a variety of technical and ethical reasons.

Somatic Gene Therapy

In the case of somatic gene therapy, the therapeutic genes are transferred into the somatic cells of a patient. Any modifications and effects will be restricted to the individual patient only, and will not be inherited by the patient's offspring or later generations.

In vivo gene transfer

During *in vivo* gene transfer, the genes are transferred directly into the tissue of the patient and this can be the only possible option in patients with tissues where individual cells cannot be cultured *in vitro* in sufficient numbers (e.g. brain cells). Also, *in vivo* gene transfer is necessary when cultured cells cannot be re-implanted in patients effectively.

Ex vivo gene transfer

During *ex vivo* gene transfer the cells are cultured outside the body and then the genes are transferred into the cells grown in culture. The cells that have been transformed successfully are expanded by cell culture and then introduced into the patient.

Ex vivo vs In vivo Gene Therapy

In gene therapy, recombinant vector with the therapeutic gene is used for gene delivery to specified cells and tissues. Two different strategies are used for this gene delivery, i.e. *ex vivo* and *in vivo*. In *ex vivo* approach the cells may be cultured and used for gene transfer, so that these transfected cells are then introduced in a targeted tissue. Alternatively in the *in vivo* approach, the gene may be delivered through a vector directly into the target cell or tissue. *Ex vivo* gene delivery is common and more certain, but at the same time more problematic, since it requires: (i) a mitotic cell population, (ii) a tissue culture method, and (iii) a cell transplantation technology. There are also following advantages of an *ex vivo* approach: (i) gene transfer efficiency is generally high and retroviral vectors are particularly effective, (ii) the transduced cells can be enriched if the vector has a selectable marker gene, and (iii) transduction efficiency can be assessed before re-implantation.

Bone marrow cells, can be multiplied and modified and are the common candidates for *ex vivo* gene delivery, but for other types of cells, *ex vivo* modification may be difficult. However, the use of embryonic stem (ES) cells may be really useful. For this purpose, although earlier ES cells were available only from mouse, rat, pig, rabbit, etc. but human ES cells have also become available recently (1998–2002).

Despite some advantage of *ex vivo* gene delivery, *in vivo* gene delivery would be preferred, if feasible. However, one major precaution required during *in vivo* gene delivery is that the gene be delivered only to the targeted cells and no other cells, and in no case to the gene line cells. Retrovirus delivers the gene only to dividing cells and therefore is safe for delivery of gene to cancer cells. But in other cases receptor mediated endocytosis (RME) may have to be used, so that the vector will have to carry a ligand for the receptor available on the target cells. Sometimes, instead of targeting specific cell types, selective expression of a transferred gene can also be achieved by the use of tissue specific enhancers/promoters. However, the disadvantages of *in vivo* gene delivery include the following: (i) specificity and low efficiency of stable gene transfer, (ii) for clinically useful therapeutic application, repeated treatments may be needed raising the problem of a host immune response (Fig. 17.2).

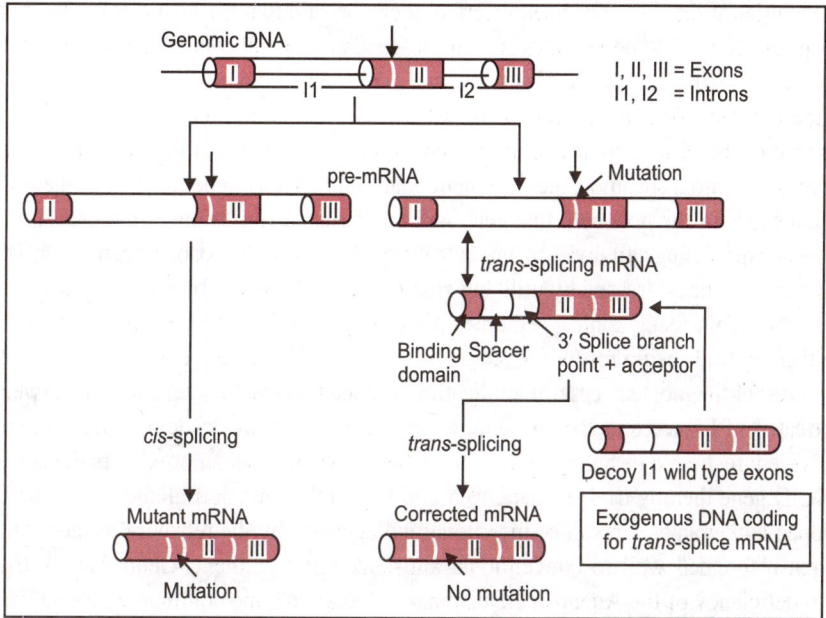

Fig. 17.2. *Ex vivo* vs. *in vivo* gene therapy.

In view of the above advantages and disadvantages of *ex vivo* and *in vivo* approaches, the choice will depend on the relative ease of *in vitro* culture (*ex vivo* approach) and the gene transfer efficiency of the target tissue (*in vivo* approach).

VECTORS IN GENE THERAPY

Viruses

All viruses bind to their hosts and introduce their genetic material into the host cell as part of their replication cycle. This genetic material contains basic 'instructions' of how to produce more copies of these viruses, hijacking the body's normal production machinery to serve the needs of the virus. The host cell will carry out these instructions and produce additional copies of the virus, leading to more and more cells becoming infected. Some types of viruses physically insert their genes into the host's genome.

Retroviruses

The genetic material in retroviruses is in the form of RNA molecules, while the genetic material of their hosts is in the form of DNA. When a retrovirus infects a host cell, it will introduce its RNA together with some enzymes, namely reverse transcriptase and integrase, into the cell. This RNA molecule from the retrovirus must produce a DNA copy from its RNA molecule before it can be integrated into the genetic material of the host cell. The process of producing a DNA copy from an RNA molecule is termed reverse transcription. It is carried out by one of the enzymes carried in the virus, called reverse transcriptase.

After this DNA copy is produced and is free in the nucleus of the host cell, it must be incorporated into the genome of the host cell. That is, it must be inserted into the large DNA molecules in the cell (the chromosomes). This process is done by another enzyme carried in the virus called integrase. Now that the genetic material of the virus has been inserted, it can be said that the host cell has been modified to contain new genes. If this host cell divides later, its descendants will all contain the new genes. Sometimes the genes of the retrovirus do not express their information immediately.

One of the problems of gene therapy using retroviruses is that the integrase enzyme can insert the genetic material of the virus into any arbitrary position in the genome of the host; it randomly shoves the genetic material into a chromosome. If genetic material happens to be inserted in the middle of one of the original genes of the host cell, this gene will be disrupted (insertional mutagenesis). If the gene happens to be one regulating cell division, uncontrolled cell division (i.e. cancer) can occur. This problem has recently begun to be addressed by utilising zinc finger nucleases or by including certain sequences such as the beta-globin locus control region to direct the site of integration to specific chromosomal sites. Gene therapy trials using retroviral vectors to treat X-linked severe combined immunodeficiency (X-SCID) represent the most successful application of gene therapy to date. More than twenty patients have been treated in France and Britain, with a high rate of immune system reconstitution observed. Similar trials were restricted or halted in the USA when leukemia was reported in patients treated in the French X-SCID gene therapy trial. To date, four children in the French trial and one in the British trial have developed leukemia as a result of insertional mutagenesis by the retroviral vector. All but one of these children responded well to conventional anti-leukemia treatment. Gene therapy trials to treat SCID due to deficiency of the Adenosine Deaminase (ADA) enzyme continue with relative success in the USA, Britain, Italy and Japan.

Adenoviruses

Adenoviruses are viruses that carry their genetic material in the form of double-stranded DNA. They cause respiratory, intestinal, and eye infections in humans (especially the common cold). When these viruses infect a host cell, they introduce their DNA molecule into the host. The genetic material of the adenoviruses is not incorporated (transient) into the host cell's genetic material. The DNA molecule is left free in the nucleus of the host cell, and the instructions in this extra DNA molecule are transcribed just like any other gene.

The only difference is that these extra genes are not replicated when the cell is about to undergo cell division so the descendants of that cell will not have the extra gene. As a result, treatment with the adenovirus will require readministration in a growing cell population although the absence of integration into the host cell's genome should prevent the type of cancer seen in the SCID trials. This vector system has been promoted for treating cancer and indeed the first gene therapy product to be licensed to treat cancer, Gendicine, is an adenovirus. Gendicine, an adenoviral p53-based gene therapy was approved by the Chinese FDA in 2003 for treatment of head and neck cancer.

Adeno-associated viruses

Adeno-associated viruses, from the parvovirus family, are small viruses with a genome of single-stranded DNA. The wild type AAV can insert genetic material at a specific site on chromosome 19 with near 100 per cent certainty.

Envelope protein pseudotyping of viral vectors

The viral vectors described above have natural host cell populations that they infect most efficiently. Retroviruses have limited natural host cell ranges, and although adenovirus and adeno-associated virus are able to infect a relatively broader range of cells efficiently, some cell types are refractory to infection by these viruses as well. Attachment to and entry into a susceptible cell is mediated by the protein envelope on the surface of a virus. Retroviruses and adeno-associated viruses have a single protein coating their membrane, while adenoviruses are coated with both an envelope protein and fibres that extend away from the surface of the virus. The envelope proteins on each of these viruses bind to cell-surface molecules such as heparin sulphate, which localises them upon the surface of the potential host, as well as with the specific protein receptor that either induces entry-promoting structural changes in the viral protein, or localises the virus in endosomes wherein acidification of the lumen induces this refolding of the viral coat. In either case, entry into potential host cells requires a favourable interaction between a protein on the surface of the virus and a protein on the surface of the cell. For the purposes of gene therapy, one might either want to limit or expand the range of cells susceptible to transduction by a gene therapy vector.

To this end, many vectors have been developed in which the endogenous viral envelope proteins have been replaced by either envelope proteins from other viruses or by chimeric proteins. Such chimera would consist of those parts of the viral protein necessary for incorporation into the virion as well as sequences meant to interact with specific host cell proteins. Viruses in which the envelope proteins have been replaced as described are referred to as pseudotyped viruses. For example, the most popular retroviral vector for use in gene therapy trials has been the lentivirus Simian immunodeficiency virus coated with the envelope proteins, G-protein, from Vesicular stomatitis virus. This vector is referred to as VSV G-pseudotyped lentivirus, and infects an almost universal set of cells. This tropism is characteristic of the VSV G-protein with which this vector is coated. Many attempts have been made to limit the tropism of viral vectors to one or a few host cell populations. This advance would allow for the systemic administration of a relatively small amount of vector. The potential for off-target cell modification would be limited, and many concerns from the medical community would be alleviated. Most attempts to limit tropism have used chimeric envelope proteins bearing antibody fragments. These vectors show great promise for the development of 'magic bullet' gene therapies.

Replication-competent vectors

A replication-competent vector called ONYX-015 is used in replicating tumour cells. A replication-defective vector deletes some essential genes. These deleted genes are still necessary in the body so they are replaced with either a helper virus or a DNA molecule.

Cis and trans-acting elements

Replication-defective vectors always contain a 'transfer construct'. The transfer construct carries the gene to be transduced or 'transgene'. The transfer construct also carries the sequences which are necessary for the general functioning of the viral genome: packaging sequence, repeats for replication and, when needed, priming of reverse transcription. These are denominated *cis*-acting elements, because they need to be on the same piece of DNA as the viral genome and the gene of interest. Transacting elements are viral elements, which can be encoded on a different DNA molecule. For example, the viral structural proteins can be expressed from a different genetic element than the viral genome.

Herpes simplex virus

Herpes Simplex Virus is a human neurotropic virus. This is mostly examined for gene transfer in the nervous system. The wild type HSV-1 virus is able to infect neurons. Infected neurones are not rejected by the immune system. Though the latent virus is not transcriptionally apparent, it does possess neurone specific promoters that can continue to function normally. Antibodies to HSV-1 are common in humans, however complications due to herpes infection are somewhat rare.

Nonviral Methods

Nonviral methods present certain advantages over viral methods, with simple large scale production and low host immunogenicity being just two. Previously, low levels of transfection and expression of the gene held non-viral methods at a disadvantage; however, recent advances in vector technology have yielded molecules and techniques with transfection efficiencies similar to those of viruses.

Naked DNA

This is the simplest method of nonviral transfection. Clinical trials carried out of intramuscular injection of a naked DNA plasmid have occurred with some success; however, the expression has been very low in comparison to other methods of transfection. In addition to trials with plasmids, there have been trials with naked PCR product, which have had similar or greater success.

Oligonucleotides

The use of synthetic oligonucleotides in gene therapy is to inactivate the genes involved in the disease process. There are several methods by which this is achieved. One strategy uses antisense specific to the target gene to disrupt the transcription of the faulty gene. Another uses small molecules of RNA called siRNA to signal the cell to cleave specific unique sequences in the mRNA transcript of the faulty gene, disrupting translation of the faulty mRNA, and therefore expression of the gene. A further strategy uses double stranded oligodeoxynucleotides as a decoy for the transcription factors that are required to activate the transcription of the target gene. The transcription factors bind to the decoys instead of the promoter of the faulty gene, which reduces the transcription of the target gene, lowering expression. Additionally, single stranded DNA oligonucleotides have been used to direct a single base change within a mutant gene. The oligonucleotide is designed to anneal with complementarity to the target gene with the exception of a central base, the target base, which serves as the template base for repair. This technique is referred to as oligonucleotide mediated gene repair, targeted gene repair, or targeted nucleotide alteration.

Lipoplexes and polyplexes

To improve the delivery of the new DNA into the cell, the DNA must be protected from damage and its entry into the cell must be facilitated. To this end new molecules, lipoplexes and polyplexes, have been created that have the ability to protect the DNA from undesirable degradation during the transfection process. Plasmid DNA can be covered with lipids in an organised structure like a micelle or a liposome. When the organised structure is complexed with DNA it is called a lipoplex. There are three types of lipids, anionic (negatively charged), neutral, or cationic (positively charged). Initially, anionic and neutral lipids were used for the construction of lipoplexes for synthetic vectors. However, inspite of the facts that there is little toxicity associated with them, that they are compatible with body fluids and that there was a possibility of adapting them to be tissue specific; they are complicated and time consuming to produce so attention was turned to the cationic versions.

Cationic lipids, due to their positive charge, were first used to condense negatively charged DNA molecules so as to facilitate the encapsulation of DNA into liposomes. Later it was found that the use of cationic lipids significantly enhanced the stability of lipoplexes. Also as a result of their charge, cationic liposomes interact with the cell membrane, endocytosis was widely believed as the major route by which cells uptake lipoplexes. Endosomes are formed as the results of endocytosis, however, if genes cannot be released into cytoplasm by breaking the membrane of endosome, they will be sent to lysosomes where all DNA will be destroyed before they could achieve their functions. It was also found that although cationic lipids themselves could condense and encapsulate DNA into liposomes, the transfection efficiency is very low due to the lack of ability in terms of 'endosomal escaping'. However, when helper lipids (usually electroneutral lipids, such as DOPE) were added to form lipoplexes, much higher transfection efficiency was observed. Later on, it was figured out that certain lipids have the ability to destabilise endosomal membranes so as to facilitate the escape of DNA from endosome, therefore those lipids are called fusogenic lipids. Although cationic liposomes have been widely used as an alternative for gene delivery vectors, a dose dependent toxicity of cationic lipids were also observed which could limit their therapeutic usages.

The most common use of lipoplexes has been in gene transfer into cancer cells, where the supplied genes have activated tumour suppressor control genes in the cell and decrease the activity of oncogenes. Recent studies have shown lipoplexes to be useful in transfecting respiratory epithelial cells, so they may be used for treatment of genetic respiratory diseases such as cystic fibrosis.

Complexes of polymers with DNA are called polyplexes. Most polyplexes consist of cationic polymers and their production is regulated by ionic interactions. One large difference between the methods of action of polyplexes and lipoplexes is that polyplexes cannot release their DNA load into the cytoplasm, so to this end, co-transfection with endosome-lytic agents (to lyse the endosome that is made during endocytosis, the process by which the polyplex enters the cell) such as inactivated adenovirus must occur. However, this isn't always the case, polymers such as polyethylenimine have their own method of endosome disruption as does chitosan and trimethylchitosan.

Hybrid Methods

Due to every method of gene transfer having shortcomings, there have been some hybrid methods developed that combine two or more techniques. Virosomes are one example; they combine liposomes with an inactivated HIV or influenza virus. This has been shown to have more efficient gene transfer in respiratory epithelial cells than either viral or liposomal methods alone. Other methods involve mixing other viral vectors with cationic lipids or hybridising viruses.

Dendrimers

A dendrimer is a highly branched macromolecule with a spherical shape. The surface of the particle may be functionalised in many ways and many of the properties of the resulting construct are determined by its surface. In particular it is possible to construct a cationic dendrimer, i.e. one with a positive surface charge. When in the presence of genetic material such as DNA or RNA, charge complimentarity leads to a temporary association of the nucleic acid with the cationic dendrimer. On reaching its destination the dendrimer-nucleic acid complex is then taken into the cell via endocytosis.

In recent years the benchmark for transfection agents has been cationic lipids. Limitations of these competing reagents have been reported to include: the lack of ability to transfect a number of cell types, the lack of robust active targeting capabilities, incompatibility with animal models, and toxicity. Dendrimers offer robust covalent construction and extreme control over molecule structure, and therefore size. Together these give compelling advantages compared to existing approaches.

PROSPECTS FOR HUMAN GENE THERAPY

Gene therapy the insertion into an organism of a normal gene which then corrects a genetic defect has been carried out in fruit flies: (i) *Drosophila melanogaster*, and (ii) mice. How soon gene therapy might be available for the treatment of human genetic diseases and what criteria should be used in determining when clinical trials should begin are issues examined in this section. Several investigators are now preparing protocols for clinical trials of gene therapy in seriously ill patients. Since most of these protocols will be based on the use of retroviral vectors as a delivery system, these structures will be emphasised. It may well be, however, that one of the other delivery systems described below, or a new one not yet developed, will be the procedure of choice in the future.

Gene Therapy in Lower Species

The most elegant system thus far demonstrating successful gene therapy is the work in *Drosophila*. The transposable genetic element, the P factor, has been used to transfer a normal gene coding for the enzyme that produces the wild-type red eve colour in *Drosophila* embryos which have a genetically defective gene. The result is that the treated flies acquire normal eye colour. Similar transfer experiments under way use other genes. Despite considerable searching, transposon-like elements have not been identified in vertebrates. Retroviruses, however, are structurally and functionally similar in many ways to the mobile genetic elements found in lower organisms, and retroviral vectors have now been used to transfer functioning genes into mouse bone marrow cells.

Gene Therapy in Humans

Human disease candidates for gene therapy. Pituitary dwarfism in humans is not a reasonable initial candidate. Genes making hormones that circulate in the bloodstream are probably not appropriate for early attempts at gene therapy in humans. First the normal feedback controls in DNA that regulate the expression of hormone genes in the body are not now known. Therefore, physiologically correct levels of hormone production would probably not be possible. Second, it would be easier and safer to use recombinant DNA manufacturing techniques to produce sufficiently large quantities of hormone so that the active polypeptide itself could be given to the patient. Hormone levels could then be titrated precisely.

At first, clinical investigators thought that the human genetic diseases most likely to be the initial ones successfully treated by gene therapy would be the haemoglobin abnormalities (specifically, β-thalassemia) because these disorders are the most obvious ones carried by blood cells, and bone marrow is the easiest tissue to manipulate *in vitro*. Regulation of globin synthesis, however, is unusually complicated. Not only are the embryonic, fetal and adult globin chains carefully regulated during development, but also the α- and β-globin-like chains are always maintained in a 1 to 1 ratio despite the fact that the α- and β-globin loci are on different chromosomes. To understand the regulatory signals that control such a complicated system and to develop means for obtaining controlled expression of an exogenous β-globin gene will take considerably more research effort. The recent development of a mouse model for β-thalassemia should aid these investigations.

Gene therapy should be beneficial primarily for the replacement of a defective or missing enzyme or protein that must function inside the cell that makes it, or of a deficient circulating protein whose level does not need to be exactly regulated. Early attempts at gene therapy will almost certainly be done with genes for enzymes that have a simple 'always-on' type of regulation. Three genes are the initial prime candidates: hypoxanthine-guanine phosphoribosyl transferase (HPRT), the absence of which results in Lesch-Nyhan disease: purine nucleoside phosphorylase (PNP), the absence of which results in a severe immunodeficiency disease: and adenosine deaminase (ADA), the absence of which results in severe combined immunodeficiency disease. For all three the clinical syndrome is profoundly debilitating.

The defect in each is found in the patient's bone marrow (although the severe central nervous system manifestations of Lesch-Nyhan disease are due to absence of HPRT in brain cells and probably cannot be corrected with current techniques). In all three there is no or minimal detectable enzyme in marrow cells from patients homozygous (or hemizygous) for the defect and the production of a small fraction of the normal enzyme level should be beneficial. Furthermore a mild over production of enzyme should not be harmful to the cell. In addition in all three the gene has been cloned and a complementary DNA is available.

Since combined immunodeficiency due to a defect in the ADA gene in Tlymphocytes can be corrected by infusion of normal bone marrow cells from a histocompatible donor selective replication of the normal T cells appears to take place. This observation offers hope that defective bone marrow can be removed from a patient, the normal ADA gene inserted into a number of cells through gene therapy and the treated marrow reimplanted into the patient where it may have a selective growth advantage. There is also evidence that marrow cells containing HPRT (HPRT-) may have a selective advantage (in both mice and humans) over cells that do not (HPRT-). If selective growth occurs no ablation of the patient's own marrow would be necessary. If however, corrected stem cells have no growth advantage over endogenous ones, then partial or complete marrow destruction (either by irradiation or by other means) may be required in order to allow the corrected marrow cells an environment favourable for expansion.

Ethics: Essentially all observers have stated that they believe that it would be ethical to insert genetic material into a human being for the sole purpose of medically correcting a severe genetic defect in that patient that is somatic cell gene therapy. Attempts to correct germ cells (that is to permit the new gene to be passed on to the patient's children) or to enhance or improve a 'normal' person by gene manipulation do not have societal acceptance at this time. However, somatic cell gene therapy for a patient suffering a serious genetic disorder would be ethically acceptable if carried out under the same strict criteria that cover other new and experimental medical procedures. The techniques that are now being developed for human application are for somatic cell, not germ line gene therapy. The question examined here is: What criteria should be used in evaluating gene therapy protocols? Three general requirements first presented in 1980 are that it should be shown in animal studies that (I) the new gene can be put into the correct target cells and will remain there long enough to be effective (II) the new gene will be expressed in the cell at an appropriate level and (III) the new gene will not harm the cell or by extension, the animal. These three requisites summarised as delivery expression and safety will each be examined in turn.

Delivery

At present the only human tissues that can be used for gene transfer are bone marrow and skin cells. No other cells can be extracted from the body grown in culture to allow manipulation and then successfully reimplanted into the patient from whom the tissue was taken. In the future as more is learned on how to package the injected DNA and to make it tissue or even cell type specific the intravenous route would be the simplest and most desirable. Attempting to give a foreign gene by injection directly into the bloodstream is not advisable with our present state of knowledge, since the procedure would be enormously inefficient and there would be little control over the DNA's fate.

Studies are considerably more advanced with bone marrow than skin cells as a recipient tissue for gene transfer. Bone marrow consists of a heterogeneous population of cells, most of which are committed to differentiation into erythrocytes, lymphocytes, megakaryocytes and so on. Only a small proportion (0.1 to 0.5 per cent) of nucleated bone marrow cells are stem cells (that is cells that have not yet differentiated into specific cell types and which divide as needed to maintain the marrow population. In gene therapy, stem cells would be the primary target. Because they are low in number and are not recognisable a delivery system for transferring a gene into stem cells must be efficient.

Techniques for transferring cloned genes into cells can be grouped in four categories: (i) viral both RNA viruses (or retroviruses) and DNA viruses (for example SV40 adenovirus and bovine papilloma), (ii) chemical such as calcium phosphate-mediated DNA uptake, (iii) fusion, that is fusion of DNA-loaded membranous vesicles, such as liposomes, red blood cell ghosts or protoplasts to cells, and (iv) physical, that is, microinjection or electroporation. Each technique is valuable for certain types of experiments but none can yet be used to insert a gene into a specific chromosomal site in a target cell. Fusion techniques are the least well characterised and will not be discussed. As noted retroviral-based vectors appear to be the most promising approach at present for use in humans.

Viral Techniques

RNA viruses (retroviruses): There are a number of advantages of vectors derived from retroviruses as a gene delivery system. First up to 100 per cent of cells can be infected and can express the integrated viral (and exogenous) genes: this is in contrast to chemical methods where although most cells take in the DNA as shown by positive assays after 48 hours only one cell in 10^{-3} to 10^{-7} stably expresses the exogenous gene. Second as many cells as desired can be infected simultaneously: 10^{-6} to 10^{-7} is a convenient number for a Simple protocol. Third under appropriate conditions the DNA can integrate as a single copy at a single albeit random site, whereas the chemical and physical techniques often result in the insertion of multiple copies of the transferred gene all linked head-to-tail in tandem repeats. Fourth although integration is random with respect to the host genome it is precise with respect to the viral genome-that is the structure of the integrated DNA is known. Fifth the infection and long-term harbouring of the retroviral vector usually does not harm cells. Finally a wide and controllable host range is available. A number of retroviral vector systems have been developed. Here we concentrate on vectors based on Maloney murine leukemia virus (MoMLV).

Life cycle and structure: The details of the life cycle of retroviruses have been reviewed recently. In brief the retrovirus composed of an RNA-protein core and a glycoprotein envelope enters a cell where the RNA acts as a template for the reverse transcription of the genetic information into a double strand of DNA. This DNA can precisely integrate as a single copy called a provirus at a random location in the genome of the host. Although much has been learned about the regulatory features of retroviruses uncertainties remain. Those features of the proviral structure that are thought to be necessary for transcription and transmission of the viral genome are (Fig. 17.3): a long terminal repeat (LTR) sequence on each end containing regulatory signals for initiating and terminating transcription sequences required for reverse transcription and others for PF (viral integration: short sequences (called here for short,

r^- and r') immediately adjacent to each LTR and necessary for reverse transcription: the packaging sequence called/in MoMLV necessary for the viral RNA to be packaged into an infectious viral particle and the donor (D) and acceptor (A) splice sites. Retroviral RNA is synthesised from the proviral DNA by the host cell's own RNA polymerase. A portion of this RNA is used in the cell's translational machinery to synthesise the viral proteins that go into the final viral particles along with the genomic RNA. These viral particles bud off from the cell and can then infect other cells.

From experimental studies as well as the existence of a number of naturally occurring defective viruses, it is known that almost all of the regions coding for viral proteins (*gag*, *pol* and *env* in Fig. 17.3) can be deleted and some or all of these sequences replaced with other DNA. Once the viral genes are deleted the retroviral vector becomes defective. In order to obtain infectious viral particles a cell harbouring a defective provirus must be infected with a 'helper' virus which carries all the viral functions needed that is, the genes for *gag*, *pol*, and *env*.

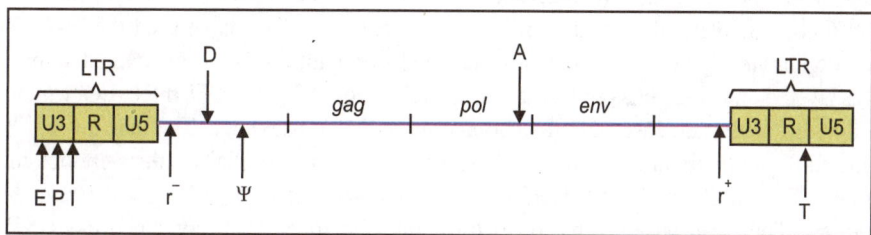

Fig. 17.3. Simplified structure of MoMLV retroviral provirus DNA. Abbreviations: E, enhancer; P, promoter; I, initiation (Cap) site for viral RNA synthesis; r^-, replication initiation site for minus DNA strand (transfer RNA binding site); D, donor splice site: Ψ packaging sequence; A, the major acceptor splice site; r^+, replication initiation site for plus DNA strand (purine-rich site); T, terminal [poly(A) addition] site for viral RNA synthesis; LTR, long terminal repeat; U3, R, and U5 are portions of the LTR; *gag*, group-specific (that is viral core) antigens: pl5, p12, p30, and p10; *pol*, RNA dependent DNA polymerase (reverse transcriptase); and *env*, envelope proteins: gp70, pl5E and R (Not drawn to scale).

Use as gene delivery system: The proviral DNA for the desired retrovirus [commonly either MoMLV or murine sarcoma virus (MSV)] is isolated and inserted into a convenient plasmid. The viral genes can then be replaced with the exogenous genes of choice by standard recombinant DNA techniques. This construct is used to transfect tissue culture cells (for example NIH 3T3 cells) by a convenient gene transfer procedure (for example, calcium phosphate). After infecting the cells with a helper virus (such as intact MoMLV) infectious viral particles, possessing both the retroviral vector and the helper virus bud off from the cells into the surrounding medium. This particle-containing supernatant is collected and used to infect bone marrow cells in culture or more simply freshly extracted bone marrow is incubated directly with the cells budding the viral particles. The marrow cells are removed and injected intravenously into a mouse whose bone marrow has been killed by X-rays (lethally irradiated). The animal is then studied to determine if the transferred marrow cells express the desired gene from the vector.

Successful gene transfer into adult mice: Joyner have successfully used this procedure to transfer a functional gene for neomycin resistance (*neo'*) into mouse haematopoietic progenitor cells by use of a MoMLV retroviral vector. The presence and expression of this gene in granulocytic progenitor cells rendered these cells resistant to the neomycin-like antibiotic G418 as determined by *in vitro* colony assays. Treated cells were injected into lethally irradiated mice. Southern blot analysis, and colony assays showed that the *neo'* gene is present and functional in the spleens of the recipient animals.

An improvement on this procedure would be to treat bone marrow cells with a retroviral particle that could deliver the vector but which would not itself produce a spreading infection. Mann and others have developed a technique for accomplishing this goal. The regulatory signal Ψ (Fig. 17.3) contains a sequence, the exact size and structure of which are not yet known. That must be present in the viral RNA for it to be packaged into a viral particle. A helper virus was constructed with this sequence deleted (Ψ-) by making use of convenient restriction endonuclease sites (Bal I and Pst I) flanking the Ψ sequence in MoMLV. The Ψ-helper is able to produce all the viral proteins required to make a particle but the particle does not package its own RNA. Since the retroviral vector has a Ψ sequence it is packaged. Consequently, the particle can just infect once: it is only a delivery system for the vector, not an infectious agent.

In order to use the Ψ-helper virus conveniently, a line of NIH 3T3 cells was established with the helper provirat DNA permanently integrated: Ψ-helper viral RNA is produced constitutively. The transfection of this cell line (called Ψ-2) with the retroviral vector DNA results 48 hours later in a supernatant that contains viral particles with only the vector. William have used the Ψ-2 cell line to place a functioning *neo'* gene into the hematopoietic cells of adult mice. Freshly extracted murine bone marrow was layered onto Ψ-2 cells producing a retroviral vector called MSV DHFR-NEO, which contains genes for dihydrofolate reductase (DHFR) and *neo'* in an MSV backbone. The marrow and Ψ-2 cells were incubated for 48 hours under standard incubation conditions. Similar results were obtained when bone marrow cells with the Ψ-2 MSV DHFR-NEO cell layer were incubated for 6 days under Dexter-type conditions. The viral particles that budded off into the supernatant contained the MSV DHFR. NEO vector but to the extent that could be determined, no Ψ-helper viral RNA. Ten days after lethally irradiated mice were injected with the treated bone marrow cells analysis of the regenerating spleens showed that the mice carried the MSV DHFR-NEO proviral DNA in their hematopoietic cells. Individual spleen colonies each arising from a single stem cell were generated by injecting an estimated one to ten stem cells into another group of lethally irradiated mice. Cells from individual colonies were able to produce spleen colonies in a secondary group of lethally irradiated animals. These mice also were shown to carry MSV DHFR-NEO DNA in their total spleen DNA and in each case to have the same integration site restriction pattern as the colony from the primary mouse. These data show that the delivery system is effective at least for mouse bone marrow cells. Preliminary evidence indicates that the *neo'* gene is expressed.

Southern blot analysis of total spleen DNA with a number of restriction enzymes revealed in some cases a small number of proviral integration sites. This result suggests that only a few infected stem cells were proliferating to repopulate the irradiated spleen. Secondary transfers of individual colonies showed that only 7 of 48 colonies (15 per cent) contained the *neo'* gene. This is a lower limit since an occasional colony might have been formed from endogenous stem cells that survived the irradiation. These data suggest that the present bone marrow procedure might still be made more efficient as a delivery system.

A similar retroviral vector system based primarily on MoMLV has been developed by Smith and his co-workers. In their Ψ-helper virus they substituted an amphotrophic (that is wide host ange) *env* gene for the MoMLV env gene which produces a particle coat with a narrow host range. This helper viral construct is called *p*SAM. Miller built a retroviral vector containing a full-length complementary DNA for the human enzyme HPRT. This vector called PLPL was cotransfected along with the Ψ-helper, pSAM, into HPRT-BALB/3T3 cells. One clone (c7cl) was obtained, that produced high levels of viral particles containing the HPRT vector. Injection of these cells into lethally irradiated mice resulted in animals that continued to produce HPRT-vector particles for at least 6 months. The infectious particles resulted from the presence of low levels (<0.l per cent of the HPRT-vector virus) of packageable helper virus along with the injection of MoMLV as additional helper which led to multiple rounds of replication in the host. In addition human HPRT enzyme was detected in spleen cells.

Shortcomings of retroviral delivery systems: The evidence indicates that retroviruses can be used as a reasonably efficient delivery system. A gene therapy procedure however, also requires a reliable system. In most of the work reported to date a number of cells are found to contain altered proviral DNA. The biggest problem appears to be that retroviruses have a strong propensity for deleting sequences during virus replication. Many vectors have been ineffective because the foreign DNA is partially or totally removed from the construct or is rearranged. For example Joyner and Bernstein have used the Friend spleen focus-forming virus as a potential vector system for hematopoietic cells. Constructs containing a thymidine kinase (TK) gene in the *gag* region and an intact *env* gene (gp55) were used along with MoMLV as helper to obtain viral particles. The particles were injected into lethally irradiated mice and also layered onto rat TK-(LTA) cells. Southern blot analysis of the integrated proviral DNA in erythroleukemic spleens demonstrated vector constructs with intact gp55 genes but deleted TK sequences, whereas TK-LTA clones possessed intact TK genes but deleted or rearranged gp55 sequences . In other words in no case could a provirus be found that still contained both the TK and gp55 genes. Even the successful MSV DHFRNEO vector which produces *neo'* expression in mice has lost a portion of its DHFR gene during production of the viral particles. Several approaches are being tried to circumvent this problem of instability.

Properties still needed for an optimal delivery system. An ideal delivery system not only would be stable but also would be tissue-specific. When a genetic disorder is in the hematopoietic system, then the isolated bone marrow can be treated. But no other tissue, except skin cells can be removed, treated and replaced at present. Since many viruses are known to infect only specific tissues (that is to bind to receptors that are present only on certain cell types) a retroviral particle containing a coat glycoprotein that recognises only human hematopoietic stem cells would permit the retroviral vector to be given intravenously with little danger that cells other than those in the marrow would be infected. Such specificity could permit the liver and brain for example to be treated individually. In addition, the danger of inadvertently infecting germ cells could be eliminated. One problem however, is that cell replication appears to be necessary for integration. It would not be possible to infect nondividing brain cells for example as far as we now know.

The optimal system not only would deliver the vector specifically into the cell type of choice but would also direct the vector to a predetermined chromosomal site. Specific insertion into a selected site of a chromosome by means of homologous recombination can be readily achieved in lower organisms but appears to be a formidable task in mammals, whether retroviral vectors or plasmid based vectors are used. Present evidence suggests that homologous site- specific integration occurs at a very low level, when it occurs at all in mammals.

DNA viruses: Viruses such as SV40 with DNA as the nucleic acid in their core have been employed for several years as gene transfer vectors. A conditionally nonreplicating adenoviral vector has recently been developed that will efficiently infect animal and human cells (including hematopoietic cells) with the result that one or a few copies of the recombinant virus are integrated into the host cell's genome. Whether adenoviral vectors will be as efficient as retroviral vectors or will offer other advantages as a gene transfer delivery system remains to be determined. One subcategory of DNA viruses should be mentioned: bovine papilloma virus (BPV). This viral DNA replicates extra-chromosomally so that BPV-based vectors may prove to be useful for maintaining genes in cells in a nonintegrated manner. Transfection of hematopoietic cells with BPV-vectors has not yet been reported.

Expression

The second criterion for evaluating a human gene therapy protocol is that there is appropriate expression of the new gene in the target cells. Even when a delivery system can transport an exogenous gene into the DNA of the correct cells of an organism it has been a major problem to get the integrated DNA to function. A vast array of cloned genes have been introduced into a wide range of cells by the several gene transfer techniques discussed above. 'Normal' expression of exogenous genes is the exception rather than the rule.

Active exogenous promoters in tansgenic mice: Microinjection of fertilised eggs with exogenous DNA to obtain transgenic mice carrying an expressing gene has resulted in several spectacular successes but also in a considerable number of unpublished failures. Thus far only four genomic promoters have been reported to show significant activity: metallothionein, transferrin, immunoglobulin and elastase. However essentially any complementary DNA can be attached to an active promoter such as metallothionein and the coding sequence will usually be expressed in a transgenic mouse under the control of that promoter. Why are most promoters inactive after microinjection into mouse oocytcs? Al least one promoter has been examined in this regard: mouse B-ma) globin. The sequences are found to be heavily methylated in mouse tissues where they are inactive but relatively unmethylated in tissue culture cells where they are active. Therefore, the mouse zygote appears to respond to this foreign DNA by covering it with methyl groups, which remain on the DNA throughout the lifetime of the animal. Attempts to decrease the methylation of the genomic DNA by treating adult mice carrying an exogenous β-globin promoter with the hypomethylating drug 5-azacytidine have been essentially unsuccessful. The metallothionein promoter, however, even if methylated can remain active. Why some promoters are inactivated by methylation or other mechanisms while others are not is not known.

Expression from retroviral vectors: If a retroviral vector is used for gene transfer the transcriptional signals in the retrovirus's own LTR's can be used (Fig. 17.3). Expression of exogenous genes carried by retroviral vectors into bone marrow cells has been reported by three laboratories. The two studies in which a *neo'* gene was expressed in mouse bone marrow were described above. The most extensive data, however, are from Willis. A homozygous Lesch-Nyhan (LN) lymphoblast cell line was used to determine whether an HPRT-human hematopoietic cell could be corrected by a retroviral vector containing a functional HPRT gene. The LN cells have all the characteristics of a cell line totally defective in HPRT, specifically a disruption in their inosinate cycle that leads to a high purine production and a number of other metabolic abnormalities. LN cells infected with viral particles containing the HPRT-vector could be rescued in selective medium. Seventeen HPRT-clones were isolated and studied. These cell lines had HPRT levels ranging from 4 to 23 per cent of the normal level and the abnormalities associated with a deranged inosinate cycle were partially to nearly completely corrected. In a corollary study viral particles containing the HPRT-vector ere used to infect mouse bone marrow cells that were then injected into lethally irradiated mice. Both human HPRT proteins and chronic production of HPRT-vector particles were detected in the hematopoietic tissue of the mice.

A problem must still be overcome, however. Even though expression of HPRT and *neo'* genes has been obtained in the hematopoietic tissue of irradiated mice, the efficiency of the combined delivery-expression system is poor. If 15 per cent of stem cells can be infected and if 4 to 23 per cent of normal expression can be obtained in them, can sufficient enzyme be synthesised to be of benefit to a patient?

The issue, once again is whether or not the treated cells will have a selective growth advantage in the patient's body. If they do not, then, either the patient's own bone marrow must be partially or totally eliminated before re-implantation of the treated cells or the gene therapy protocol must demonstrate at least some expression in nonirradiated animals. It must be recognised, however, that in the absence of a true animal model for a given genetic disease, it might be difficult or impossible to demonstrate selective growth advantage except in human patients.

Use of enhancers to increase expression: How can the level of expression be increased and properly regulated? One key element may be the enhancers. These are DNA sequences usually 50 to 150 base pairs in length that increase the expression of the adjacent gene 10 to 1000 times. A retrovirus has its own enhancer immediately upstream from its promoter in the LTR (Fig. 17.3). Enhancers are known to be species-specific. A primate enhancer (for example, the 72 base pair repeat from SV40) is several times more active in primate tissue culture cells than in rodent cells. Likewise, a mouse enhancer (for example, the 73 base pair repeat from MSV) is more active in rodent cells than in primate cells. The promoter acted upon does not influence the species specificity (a mouse β-globin promoter and a primate SV40 promoter are both activated more by a primate enhancer in primate cells than in rodent cells), although different promoters can be enhanced to different extents. Retroviral vectors designed for therapeutic application in humans may need primate, or even human, enhancing sequences rather than the mouse ones that are now used. Some enhancers may even be tissue-specific. With a tissue-specific enhancer it may not be necessary to develop a cell-specific delivery system. The DNA could be integrated into all cells but only be expressed significantly in that tissue in which the enhancer is active. Even more precision may be achieved if one could place a tissue- specific coat on a retroviral particle that would direct the virus into the target cell, along with a tissue-specific (and possibly even a developmental-time-period-specific) enhancer in the construct itself.

Systems like globin undoubtedly have other regulatory regions in addition to enhancers which recognise cellular factors that are involved in control. Much information still needs to be learned about the regulatory signals in these multigene families.

Expression from plasmid-based expression vector: If a chemical gene transfer technique is used as a delivery system, then the gene must be inserted into an appropriate expression vector. An expression vector is a plasmid (usually pBR322) in which the complementary DNA (or genomic gene) of interest is inserted together with regulatory signals. A typical expression vector would be composed of a promoter (for example, from the mouse metallothionein gene), the complementary DNA of choice, a splice site and polyadenylation site (necessary for correct processing of the transcribed RNA), and an enhancer.

Plasmid-based expression vectors containing an enhancer have not yet been used to transfect bone marrow cells. Therefore, how effective expression might be is unknown. The inefficiency of the presently available delivery systems for these vectors was discussed above. One additional complication is that calcium phosphate-directed transfection, as well as microinjection does not usually result in the integration of a single copy of the expression vector. The plasmid DNA vector appears to be ligated or replicated, or both, inside the cell to form a long head-to-tail structure called a tandem repeat. This tandem repeat, which can be a few or up to hundreds of copies in length, is randomly inserted usually in one site in the genome. The tandem repeats may produce problems for genes requiring intricate regulation because of the uncertainty as to how many of the copies are active.

Regulation by genomic control signals: Can either plasmid-based expression vectors or retroviral vectors be used to transfer genes that are controlled by the gene's own genomic regulatory sequences? Plasmid-based expression vectors in transgenic mice do respond to normal physiological control signals in some cases. Metallothionein-promoted genes express primarily in the liver, the normal tissue for metallothionein synthesis, and can be induced by cadmium, as occurs *in vivo* for the endogenous gene: however, they do not respond to steroids, which are another physiologic inducer *in vivo*. An immunoglobulin gene is expressed in the spleen, the correct *in vivo* tissue, and not in liver. A mouse-human β-globin fusion gene expresses in haematropoietic tissue. In tissue culture cells, a number of plasmid-based expression vectors have demonstrated at least a degree of normal regulation. For example, the human β-globin gene with approximately 1 kilobase of genomic 5' flanking sequence can be induced (along with endogenous mouse globin) in a transfected MEL cell. The level of expression is not as high as that of the normal endogenous β-globin gene, suggesting that other regulatory signals are needed. However, transfection of MEL cells with cosmids carrying 30 to 40 kilobases of human genomic DNA containing the human β-globin gene does not result in higher expression of human β-globin messenger RNA. Miller and others obtained encouraging results when they placed a rat growth hormone complementary DNA together with 237 bases of genomic 5' flanking sequence into the *env*, region of the HPRT-vector already described above. This growth hormone gene was regulated in rescued HPRT-fibroblast cells by its own genomic promoter and regulatory sequences as shown by: (i) stimulation by glucocorticoid and thyroid hormones, which are normal *in vivo* regulators, and (ii) equal activity whether the fragment was placed in the same direction or opposite to the vector's LTR's. Expression of the vector in an animal has not yet been studied. These data provide hope that vectors can be built with all the genomic regulatory signals necessary to produce correctly controlled expression in target cells. In the future, one might use only selected portions of a retrovirus in order to construct a delivery and integration system that would place one copy of the vector DNA into the target cell's genome. Expression would be controlled by the exogenous gene's own genomic regulatory signals. One possible problem is size: it appears that MoMLV constructs must not be over 9 to 12 kilobases in order to be packaged. Since 2 or 3 kilobases are necessary for essential function, only 6 to 9 kilobases are available for insert. This amount may be adequate, but further studies are needed to determine the answer.

Importance of chromosomal location: A major question that remains is. How important is chromosome location? Integration of a proviral structure can in some cases activate a downstream gene, as can occur with oncogenes. This problem could be eliminated by deleting the enhancer and promoter regions from the 3' (right-hand) LTR in the retroviral vector. One round of reverse transcription could then occur which would result in double-stranded retroviral DNA with both LTR's defective. The retroviral vector DNA would then integrate with no transcription initiation signals. Therefore, expression would have to be controlled by exogenous signals in the inserted gene, and no downstream activation of other genes could take place. Certainly an integration site that disrupts an important gene or regulatory sequence would normally be detrimental. How often this would occur must be determined by experiment. It is probable though that in most such cases the insertional event would diminish the fitness of the recipient cell so that it would be outgrown by normal cells. Are there only certain active chromatin regions that can allow expression of a gene? Or could an expression vector take its own-active domain with it so that essentially any location would be acceptable? The answers to these questions are still not known.

Safety

The third and final criterion for evaluating a human gene therapy protocol is that the delivery-expression system be safe.

Retroviral vectors: Although retroviruses have many advantages for gene transfer, they also have disadvantages. One problem is that they can rearrange their own structure as well as exchange sequences with other retroviruses. In the future it might be possible to modify retroviral vectors in such a way that they become less unstable. At present, however, there is the possibility that a retroviral vector might recombine with an endogenous viral sequence to produce packageable, infectious recombinant virus. Properties that such a recombinant would have are unknown, but the potential homology between retroviral vectors and as-yet unknown primate cancer retroviruses or human T-cell leukemia viruses might be sufficiently close so that possible recombinants should be sought. There is, however, a built-in safety feature with the mouse retroviral vectors now in use.

These mouse structures have a very different sequence from known primate retroviruses, and there appears to be little or no homology between the two. Therefore, a potentially 'safe' proviral vector construct might be one composed of mouse LTR's with their enhancer and promoter regions deleted and a human gene controlled by the appropriate human genomic regulatory signals. With the present constructs, three types of experiments ought to be carried out before any retrovirus-treated bone marrow is injected into a patient. These protocols, designed to test the safety of the delivery-expression system are necessary since once treated bone marrow is reinserted into a patient, it and all retroviruses that it contains are irretrievable. First studies *in vitro* with human bone marrow are needed. Marrow cultures infected with the therapeutic vector should be tested for a period of time for the production of recombinant viruses. Any infectious virus isolated should be studied for possible pathogenicity. Second studies *in vivo* with mice are needed. Since many retroviral vectors are constructed from mouse retroviruses, and expression studied in mouse bone marrow transplanted into lethally irradiated (or nonirradiated) mice, these animals should be followed to determine if genomic rearrangement or the site of chromosomal integration has resulted in any pathologic manifestations or the production of any infectious viruses.

Third studies *in vivo* with primates are needed. A protocol similar to the one planned for human application should be carried out in primates, not just mice, because the endogenous proviral sequences in primate, including human. DNA are different from those in mouse DNA. Therefore, the nature of any viral recombinants would be different. Treated bone marrow should be reimplanted into primates, the successful transfer of intact vector DNA into haematopoietic cells demonstrated, the expression of at least small amounts of gene product verified, and the existence of infectious recombinant viruses sought and, if found, analysed.

Plasmid-based expression vectors: The calcium-phosphate procedure for transferring a plasmid-based expression vector into human bone marrow has not yet been demonstrated to be an effective delivery system. However, the procedure itself does not appear to represent a significant risk of harm. In theory, of course, a stem cell could be altered to make it carcinogenic so that it would still be necessary to follow treated mice over time to determine the likelihood of pathology. Primate studies, however, would appear not to be necessary. The initial clinical protocols designed to carry out gene therapy in patients will probably be evaluated in the following way. Under current Department of Health and Human Services regulations for the protection of human research subjects, a human gene therapy protocol must be reviewed by the Institutional Review Board at the investigator's home institution. In addition, because of the widespread public interest and concern in this area, the National Institutes of Health has announced that any federally funded gene therapy experiment involving recombinant DNA must first be approved by the NIH after review by the Recombinant DNA Advisory Committee (RAC). Prior to review by RAC, proposals will be examined by a special RAC working group on human gene therapy. In addition, the Food and Drug Administration could regulate the DNA used in a human trial as a biological drug, analogous to polynucleotide interferon inducers, interferons, and vaccines. The Food and Drug Administration is currently exploring its regulatory responsibilities in this area.

Representative Albert Gore's proposal for a President's Commission on the Human Applications of Genetic Engineering has just passed both houses of Congress in a modified form. This commission, if signed into law, would probably concern itself primarily with matters of policy and procedure rather than the review of individual recombinant DNA research proposals: the initial protocols, however, might be of particular interest to the commission in helping it to define the scope of its efforts.

Thus, it now appears that effective delivery expression systems are becoming available that will allow reasonable attempts at human gene therapy. These systems are based on treatment of bone marrow cells with retroviral-vectors carrying a normal gene. The safety of the procedures is the remaining major issue. Patients severely debilitated by being homozygous for a defect in the gene for one of the enzymes HPRT, PNP, or ADA are the most likely first candidates for gene therapy. It is unrealistic to expect a complete cure from the initial attempts at gene therapy. Many patients, who suffer from severe genetic diseases, as well as their families, are eager to participate in early clinical trials even if the likelihood is low that the original experiments will alleviate symptoms. However, for the protection of the patients, particularly since those with the most severe diseases and therefore, the most ethically justifiable first candidates are children.

Gene therapy trials should not be attempted until there are good animal data to suggest that some amelioration of the biochemical defect is likely. Then it would be necessary to weigh the potential risks to the patient, including the possibility of producing a pathologic virus or a malignancy against the anticipated benefits to be gained from the functional gene. This risk to benefit determination, a standard procedure for all clinical research protocols, would need to be carried out for each patient. In summary, institutional review boards should carefully evaluate therapeutic protocols to ensure that the delivery system is effective. That sufficient expression can be obtained in bone marrow cultures, and in laboratory animals to predict probable benefit, even if small, for the patient, and that safety protocols have demonstrated that the probability is low for the production of either a malignant cell or a harmful infectious retrovirus.

Once these criteria are met, we believe that it would be unethical to delay human trials. Patients with serious genetic diseases have little other hope at present for alleviation of their medical problems. The issues of germ line therapy and enhancement engineering need to be debated widely in society; but arguments that genetic engineering might someday be misused do not justify the needless perpetuation of human suffering that would result from an unnecessary delay in the clinical application of this potentially powerful therapeutic procedure.

IN VIVO GENE THERAPY INTO CAROTID ARTERY BY ELECTROPORATION

There are tremendous interests in the scientific and clinical community on introduction of DNA into cells using with gene therapy. Several modes of gene therapy have been pursued. The common ones are virus based, ultrasound and electroporation. The virus based method, might cause side effects and complications, such as immune reactions. Ultrasound is a possible method for gene therapy, however, efficacy of the transfection was above seven times greater with electroporation than ultrasound treatment. Electroporation is a physical process of inducing transient pores in the cell membrane by the application of short electric pulses. Electroporation has been successfully applied to gene therapy with various types of cells using *in vitro* and *in vivo*. Experiments with muscle, liver, cardiac tissue and solid tumours, using specially designed electrodes have been reported. *In vivo* electroporation of artery has yet to be studied intensively. Scientists have successfully conducted *in vivo* experimental studies on electroporation induced gene transfer in rabbit carotid artery with specific parameters.

Methods

Electroporation

Electroporation is a physical process of inducing nanometer-sized transient pores in the cell membrane by the application of short duration, high intensity electric field pulses to cells or tissues. In this permeabilised state, the membrane can allow passage of DNA, enzymes, antibodies and other macromolecules into the cells. The most important parameters for effective electroporation are the voltage [V], the length of time the field is applied (pulse duration), plasmid concentration and electrodes.

Electrode

Plate electrode model consists of two 5 mm × 10 mm stainless steel plates (Fig. 17.4). Artery is placed between those plate electrodes.

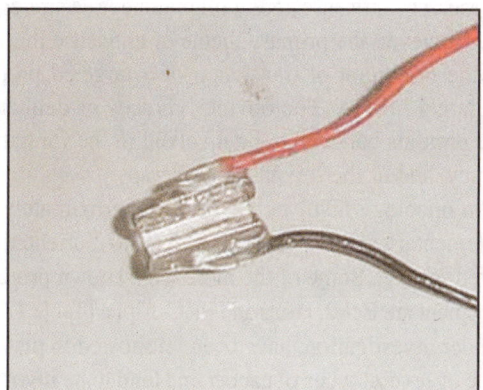 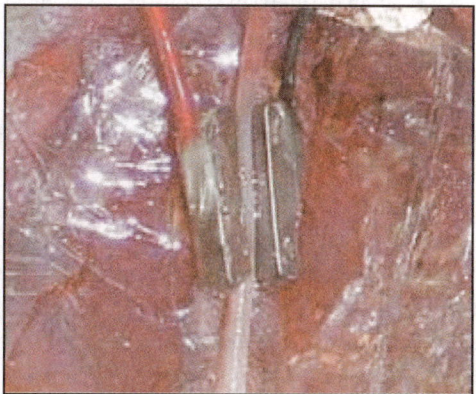

Fig. 17.4. Plate electrode model consists of two stainless steel plates.

Plasmid

Plasmid (*p*CAGGS-Lac-Z plasmid DNA and pCAGGS-Luc plasmid DNA) was used as carrier to carry the gene into the cell.

Result

Scientists have been carried out *in vivo* experiments on rabbits using different voltages, different number of pulses and pulse duration. Scientists have successfully transferred the plasmid with LacZ as a marker into the rabbits' carotid artery. Microscopic examination of the artery demonstrated frequent blue staining in endothelial layers with and 30V, 10 times of 20 ms of pulses with plasmid DNA (LacZ). These result is the appropriate setting in transferring the plasmid into artery tissue with minimum damages and high volume transferred.

ANTISENSE THERAPY

Antisense therapy is a form of treatment for genetic disorders or infections. When the genetic sequence of a particular gene is known to be causative of a particular disease, it is possible to synthesise a strand of nucleic acid (DNA, RNA or a chemical analogue) that will bind to the messenger RNA (mRNA) produced by that gene and inactivate it, effectively turning that gene 'off'. This is because mRNA has to be single stranded for it to be translated. Alternatively, the strand might be targeted to bind a splicing site on pre-mRNA and modify the exon content of an mRNA. This synthesised nucleic acid is termed an 'antisense' oligonucleotide because its base sequence is complementary to the gene's messenger RNA (mRNA), which is called the 'sense' sequence (so that a sense segment of mRNA '5'-AAGGUC-3'' would be blocked by the antisense mRNA segment '3'-UUCCAG-5'').

Antisense drugs are being researched to treat cancers (including lung cancer, colorectal carcinoma, pancreatic carcinoma, malignant glioma and malignant melanoma), diabetes, ALS, Duchenne muscular dystrophy and diseases such as asthma and arthritis with an inflammatory component. Most potential therapies have not yet produced significant clinical results, though one antisense drug, fomivirsen (marketed as Vitravene), has been approved by the US Food and Drug Administration (FDA) as a treatment for cytomegalovirus retinitis. As the aim of cancer therapeutics is becoming streamlined to target more specific biological pathways, genetic components, and/or cellular proteins, the role of antisense therapy utilising oligonucleotides is evolving as a potential treatment strategy in the fight against cancer. In the arena of scientific and medical research, antisense and/or oligonucleotide strategies may involve several strategic mechanisms of action. However, the primary theme of antisense therapy currently being explored for oncology purposes is the inhibition of translation of a targeted protein through complementary oligonucleotide binding to target mRNA. The obvious choices of deliberate inhibition through antisense therapy include specific proteins believed to be involved in the formation of malignancy, the continued expression of malignancy, and/or the resistance to therapy.

At present, the main focus of antisense therapy in oncology involves the use of approximately 20 nucleotides (oligonucleotide) synthesised to be complementary to the specific 'sense' (5' to 3' orientation) mRNA sequence responsible for coding of the targeted protein. Some of the more well-known proteins currently being targeted with antisense agents in development are Bcl-2, H-ras and PKC-Alpha (Table 17.1). These proteins, as well as several others presently under investigation, have been implicated in playing a role in the development, growth, and/or maintenance of several types of cancer and tend to be involved in messaging systems involving anti-apoptotic signalling and/or unregulated cellular proliferation.

Table 17.1. Antisense agents and their targets.

Agent	Target
Genasense (oblimersen)	Bcl-2
Affinitak (ISIS 3521)	PKC-alpha
ISIS 112989 (OGX 011)	Secretory protein clusterin
ISIS 23722	Survivin
AP 12009	TGF-beta2
GEM 231	Protein kinase A
GEM 240	MDM2
IGF-1R/AS ODN	Insulin-like growth factor
MG98	DNA methyltransferase
LErafAON	C-raf-1
Ki-67 antisense oligonucleotide	Ki-67
GTI-2040	Ribonucleotide reductase
ISIS 2503	H-ras
AP11014	TGF-Beta1

Once introduced into a cell, the 'antisense' oligonucleotide hybridises to the corresponding mRNA sequence through Watson-Crick binding, forming a heteroduplex. Once the duplex is formed, translation of the protein coded by the sequence of bound mRNA is inhibited. There are several mechanisms through which the oligonucleotide/mRNA duplex may hinder subsequent translation. The most widely accepted explanation for several different antisense agents involves the degradation of the mRNA in the heteroduplex by the ubiquitous enzyme Rnase H. Rnase H is attracted to the heteroduplex and cleaves the bound mRNA, while leaving the oligonucleotide sequence intact, allowing the oligonucleotide to continue seeking and binding to corresponding mRNA sequences. Some other accepted explanations of translation inhibition through antisense therapy which may occur separately or in conjunction with Rnase H activity include, but are not limited to, the blocking of appropriate ribosome assembly that disables the ribosomal complexes' ability to translate, blocking of RNA splicing and/or impeding appropriate exportation of mRNA.

Potential Advantages

There are several aspects of antisense therapy utilising oligonucleotides that are potentially advantageous over traditional drug mechanisms.

1. Oligonucleotides may be manufactured quickly, some within one week, and the sequence of a gene is all that is needed.
2. Potential sensitivity to therapy may be easily measured, as the target is often one-dimensional versus multiple-dimensional domains often targeted within proteins. Sensitivity can be measured through database scanning or Northern/Southern blotting for unknown genes.
3. Potential to produce longer lasting responses, as clonal expansion may require more time to produce clinical disease once mRNA is inhibited, versus just inhibition of protein typical with conventional therapies.
4. Potential for enhanced binding affinity to target, as hydrogen bonding between oligonucleotide and target appears to exceed, by several orders of magnitude, van der Waals and other forces used by standard agents to bind to protein targets.

Structure

The concept of synthesising a short strand of nucleotides complementary to a desired mRNA sequence appears fundamentally simple. However, several obstacles were recognised as this technique progressed through experimentation. One important hurdle that had to be addressed was the intrinsic nature of ubiquitous nucleases existent in living tissues and serum to degrade single-stranded nucleotide chains (i.e. the oligonucleotide). To overcome this initial impediment, a sulphur atom was substituted for the non-bridging oxygen in the nucleotide linkages of the synthesised chain. This chemical modification gives rise to a phosphorothioate backbone of the oligonucleotide that eludes immediate nuclease degradation while maintaining the ability to attract Rnase H. The phosphorothioate modification is considered to be a first-generation antisense oligonucleotide, and is currently the most commonly seen modification in chemical structure in antisense therapy involved in clinical trials for oncology. In addition, oligonucleotides used for antisense therapy in oncology tend to be around 20 bases in length, as much longer oligonucleotides demonstrated poor permeation into cells and required involved carrier systems, and those much shorter in length are theoretically poor at recognising a very specific RNA sequence, resulting in the potential binding of untargeted mRNA.

Future Directions

Currently, research efforts in antisense strategies are aimed at understanding the degree of involvement of single genes, or combinations of genes, in the course of disease. The purpose of this important area of research is to isolate the most critical targets and identify the feasibility of using genes as targets for therapeutic purposes. Other issues being actively pursued include altering chemical structures of the oligonucleotides to provide greater resistance against degradation, enhance binding affinity to target, and improving pharmacokinetics. Improving these properties will, in theory, reduce possible side effects, increase efficacy, enable lower dosing, and provide an opportunity for oral dosing. Future generation compounds include modifications to address these issues, such as composition of more RNA-like nucleotides versus DNA nucleotides, alkyl modifications at the 2' position of the ribose, polyamide linkages replacing deoxyribose phosphate backbones, and 3' amino groups to replace the 3'-hydroxyl group of the 2'-deoxyribose ring, to name a few. The ever-present issue of optimal drug delivery persists with antisense therapy, and research continues to refine delivery systems in order to achieve the goal of directing active treatment only to the target while sparing untargeted molecules, and maintaining active levels of the compound through the delivery process.

Chapter 18

Regulating the Use of Biotechnology

INTRODUCTION

Molecular biotechnology can potentially affect many aspects of modern society—including agricultural production and medical treatment—there are significant ethical, legal, economic, and social issues that need to be considered. For example, since its inception in 1973, serious doubts have been voiced by some individuals about the safety of recombinant DNA technology. These concerns promoted scientists to declare a self-imposed moratorium on certain types of recombinant DNA experiments until the adoption of official regulatory guidelines designed to ensure that recombinant micro-organisms were unable to proliferate outside of the laboratory and that laboratory workers were protected from any potential hazard. Moreover, there has been much discussion about the ethics of genetic manipulation of humans. The objective of these discussions has been to distinguish between inappropriate and acceptable procedures. There are no easy answers to the ethical, legal, and social questions raised by the various applications of molecular biotechnology. However, because the stakes are so high, many of these issues have been examined extensively.

REGULATING RECOMBINANT DNA TECHNOLOGY

Regulation of recombinant DNA is perhaps the ideal case study in science and public policy, and for several reasons. First, it offers an unparalleled sweep of new opportunity. Those who are practicing the technology, let alone the investors, see exciting prospects of new medications, new agricultural crops, new means of remediating environmental problems. It is, in short, the source of stupendous possibilities.

But second, each opportunity affords an array of potential problems: unwanted side effects, unanticipated social costs, unforeseen public health and environmental risks. But these, not in themselves unusual because they often accompany newly introduced technology, are compounded by a very special kind of drama—the specter of genetic monsters running amuck, and some feel, furthermore, that in undertaking this kind of work we have begun to interfere with a process so fundamental in nature that we may be guilty of the sin of hubris. And that reservation—so deep, that at times in the history of this business, it has seemed almost theological—has been of profound significance in the politics of recombinant DNA regulation.

Moreover, this is one of the very few instances in which scientists themselves, the very developers of the technology, were the first to recognise its potential risks and to call public attention to the need for evaluating them. Perhaps partly as a result, scientists were given more than the usual amount of responsibility for the early development of regulation in this area. In the view of some, that's made the process more sensible, more appropriately suited to the nature of the risk, and in the view of others, it has removed critical issues from public scrutiny and thereby reduced accountability.

So there's lots to argue about. It is a fascinating exercise, and partly because it illuminates a special part of the American character. On the one hand, we are a creative people bursting with entrepreneurial zeal, fearless about risk, and on the other we are full of suspicion and concerned about what others may do to us—in particular, what our own government may do to us. On the one hand, we believe that our leaders owe us a measure of protection against hazards, but on the other hand, we deeply resent any intrusions on personal freedom, even when those intrusions are for exactly that kind of protection.

Scientist Paul Berg, had recognised the hazards of working with animal viruses like SV40 well before the issue of recombinant DNA technology itself came to the fore, and he organised a conference to deal with those issues.

So there was a precedent when Paul and other colleagues assembled a group of scientists, first to co-sign a moratorium letter that temporarily halted their research and was published in Science Magazine. And then he organised the now-famous Asilomar Conference, at which the issue of recombinant DNA regulation was first considered in 1975. That meeting, and the cloud of controversy that developed around it and lingered long afterward, set the tone for much of what followed.

The first obstacles came up when it was necessary to take the work out of the laboratory and start field trials. In the first instance, this came not with transgenic plants but when recombinant DNA technologies were used to move useful genes from one kind of bacterium to another. We already heard about *Bt*, the insecticidal protein from *Bacillus theringiensis*. Bear in mind, *Bacillus theringiensis*, the bacterium, has been used in absolutely unregulated or almost unregulated fashion by farmers for years. They mix up vats of it in the barn and spray it on. It is sprayed by air frequently. It is a microbial insecticide that is of proven effectiveness.

REGULATING FOOD AND FOOD INGREDIENTS

Food products designed and marketed for children are regulated under the Food, Drug, and Cosmetic (FD&C) Act administrated by the Food and Drug Administration (FDA), Department of Health and Human Services (DHHS) and/or the Meat and Poultry Inspection Act administered by the Food Safety and Inspection Service (FSIS), US Department of Agriculture. Foods that contain 3 per cent or more of red meat or 2 per cent or more of poultry are subject to the provisions of the Meat and Poultry Inspection Acts, whereas all other foods are only subject to the provisions of the FD&C Act. The differences between how the two groups of products are regulated have more to do with compliance procedures than with requirements. The FSIS, relying on continuous inspection by FSIS inspectors who are assigned to each meat processing plant for compliance, reviews and approves labels prior to marketing of meat and poultry products. The FDA relies on quality assurance procedures, inspections of food processors, sample analyses, and review of product labelling.

The major difference is that, for FDA-regulated products, quality assurance of food products resides completely with the manufacturer and the government role is entirely enforcement, whereas FSIS takes on significant responsibility for quality assurance by inspecting and approving all products under its jurisdiction. In the even of problems with product safety, quality, or misrepresentation, the manufacturer is totally responsible for FDA-regulated products, but both the government and the manufacturer share responsibility for FSIS-regulated products. If these were infant formulas made from meat or poultry, as there were at one time such products would be subject to the additional requirements of the Infant Formula Act, a part of the FD&C Act, and additional FDA jurisdiction. This difference in the way products are regulated dates back to the origins of each law. The present FD&C Act has its origins in the Pure Food and Drug Act passed by Congress in 1906. This law covered a larger number of products and production facilities, and premarket approval of product composition and labels was considered impractical. The Federal Meat Inspection Act, which was passed one year later, covered a fewer number of products and production establishments, and continuous inspection and premarket approval were considered essential for meat.

Chymosin

Chymosin or rennin is an aspartic acid protease enzyme found in rennet. It is produced by cows in the lining of the abomasum (the fourth and final, chamber of the stomach). Chymosin is produced by gastric chief cells in infants to curdle the milk they ingest, allowing a longer residence in the bowels and better absorption. Bovine chymosin is now produced recombinantly in *E. coli*, *Aspergillus niger* var *awamori*, and *K. lactis* as alternative resource. The gene is found in humans (on chromosome 1), but it is not expressed.

Enzymatic reaction

Chymosin causes cleavage of a specific linkage—the peptide bond between phenylalanine and methionine in the K-casein. If this reaction applies to milk, the specific linkage between the hydrophobic (para-casein) and hydrophilic (acidic glycopeptide) group of casein inside milk would be broken, since they are joined by phenylalanine and methionine. The hydrophobic group would unite together and would form a 3-D network to trap the aqueous phase of the milk. The resultant product is calcium phosphocaseinate. Due to this reaction, rennin is used to bring about the extensive precipitation and curd formation in cheese making.

Tryptophan

Tryptophan (IUPAC-IUBMB abbreviation: Trp or W; IUPAC abbreviation: L-trp or D-trp; sold for medical use as Tryptan) is one of the 20 standard amino acids, as well as an essential amino acid in the human diet. It is encoded in the standard genetic code as the codon UGG. Only the L-stereoisomer of tryptophan is used in structural or enzyme proteins, but the D-stereoisomer is occasionally found in naturally produced peptides (for example, the marine venom peptide contryphan). The distinguishing structural characteristic of tryptophan is that it contains an indole functional group. It is an essential amino acid as defined by its growth effects on rats.

L-Tryptophan

Isolation

The isolation of tryptophan was first reported by Frederick Hopkins in 1901 through hydrolysis of casein. From 600 grams of crude casein one obtains 4–8 grams of tryptophan.

Biosynthesis and industrial production

Plants and micro-organisms commonly synthesise tryptophan from shikimic acid or anthranilate. The latter condenses with phosphoribosylpyrophosphate (PRPP), generating pyrophosphate as a by-product. After ring opening of the ribose moiety and following reductive decarboxylation, indole-3-glycerinephosphate is produced, which in turn is transformed into indole. In the last step, tryptophan synthase catalyses the formation of tryptophan from indole and the amino acid serine.

The industrial production of tryptophan is also biosynthetic and is based on the fermentation of serine and indole using either wild-type or genetically modified bacteria such as *Corynebacterium glutamicum*, *Bacillus subtilis*, *Bacillus amyloliquefaciens* or *E. coli*. These strains carry either mutations that prevent the reuptake of aromatic amino acids or multiple/overexpressed trp operons. The conversion is catalysed by the enzyme tryptophan synthase.

Bovine Somatotropin

Bovine somatotropin (abbreviated bST and BST), also known as bovine growth hormone, or BGH, is a protein hormone produced in cattle. Since 1994 it has been possible to synthesise the hormone using recombinant DNA technology to create recombinant bovine somatotropin (rBST), recombinant bovine growth hormone (rBGH), or artificial growth hormone. Monsanto was the first to develop the technology and marketed it as 'Posilac' — a brand now owned by Elanco Animal Health, a division of Eli Lilly and Company. Posilac was banned from use in Canada, Australia, New Zealand and most of Europe, by 2000 or earlier. In the United States, concern about potential side-effects from drinking milk produced by cows injected with artificial growth hormone has slowly grown, with a number of products and retailers now becoming rBST-free.

Use of BST is controversial primarily due to concerns over potential effects on animal and human health. The past and present business practices of Monsanto as they relate to Posilac and its other products is also debated. Some, for instance, are suspicious concerning the company's ethics and how it is regulated by government given that it produced such chemicals as Agent orange, DDT, and produces a number of pesticides and genetically modified organisms.

Animal health

Two meta-analyses have been published on rBST's effects on bovine health. Findings indicated an average increase in milk output ranging from 11–16 per cent, a nearly 25 per cent increase in the risk of clinical mastitis, a 40 per cent reduction in fertility and 55 per cent increased risk of developing clinical signs of lameness. However, the study did not show if using 'natural' growth hormones had the same or worse effects (the study in fact notes that synthetic BST can be made to be identical to natural BST). The same study reported a decrease in body condition score for cows treated with rBST even though there was an increase in their dry matter intake.

Human health

According to the Food and Drug Administration, food products made from rBST treated cows are safe for human consumption, and no significant difference exists between milk derived from rBST-treated and non-rBST-treated cows. The FDA found BGH to be biologically inactive when consumed by humans and found no biological distinction between rBST and BST. In 1990, an independent panel convened by the National Institute of Health supported the FDA opinion that milk and meat from cows supplemented with rBST is safe for human consumption.

DIRECTIVE ON THE RELEASE OF GENETICALLY MODIFIED ORGANISMS (GMOs)

In accordance with the precautionary principle and in view of the potential risk to the environment and human health of the release of genetically modified organisms (GMOs), the Directive strengthens the legislative framework on the deliberate release of GMOs into the environment and the placing of GMOs on the market. In particular, the Directive improves the efficiency and transparency of the authorisation procedures for such deliberate release and placing on the market, establishes a common methodology for risk assessment and a safety mechanism. It also introduces mandatory public consultation and GMO labelling.

Ice-minus Bacteria

Ice-minus bacteria is a nickname given to a variant of the common bacterium *Pseudomonas syringae* (*P. syringae*). This strain of *P. syringae* lacks the ability to produce a certain surface protein, usually found on wild-type *P. syringae*. The 'ice-plus' protein (Ina protein, 'ice nucleation-active' protein) found on the outer bacterial cell wall acts as the nucleating centers for ice crystals. This facilitates ice formation, hence the designation 'ice-plus'. The ice-minus variant of *P. syringae* is a mutant, lacking the gene responsible for ice-nucleating surface protein production. This lack of surface protein provides a less favourable environment for ice formation. Both strains of *P. syringae* occur naturally, but recombinant DNA technology has allowed for the synthetic removal or alteration of specific genes, enabling the creation of the ice-minus strain. Modifying *P. syringae* may have unexpected consequences for climate. A study has shown that its ice nucleating proteins may play an important part in causing ice crystals to form in clouds. If humans increase the frequency of bacteria lacking these proteins then it may affect rainfall (Fig. 18.1).

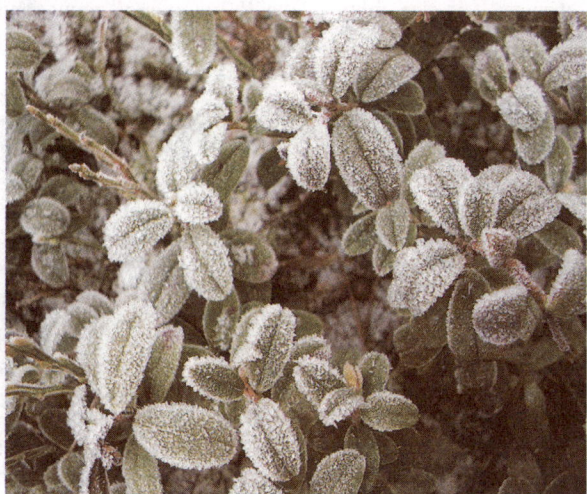

Fig. 18.1. Icy Lingoberry.

Production

To systematically create the ice-minus strain of *P. syringae*, its ice-forming gene must be isolated, amplified, deactivated and reintroduced into *P. syringae* bacterium.

The following steps are often used to isolate and generate ice-minus strains of *P. syringae*:

1. Digest *P. syringae*'s DNA with restriction enzymes.

2. Insert the individual DNA pieces into a plasmid. Pieces will insert randomly, allowing for different variations of recombinant DNA to be produced.

3. Transform the bacterium *Escherichia coli* (*E. coli*) with the recombinant plasmid. The plasmid will be taken in by the bacteria, rendering it part of the organism's DNA.

4. Identify the ice-gene from the numerous newly developed *E. coli* recombinants. Recombinant *E. coli* with the ice-gene will possess the ice-nucleating phenotype, these will be 'ice-plus'.

5. With the ice nucleating recombinant identified, amplify the ice gene with techniques such as polymerase chain reactions (PCR).

6. Create mutant clones of the ice gene through the introduction of mutagenic agents such as UV radiation to inactivate the ice gene, creating the 'ice-minus' gene.

7. Repeat previous steps (insert gene into plasmid, transform *E. coli*, identify recombinants) with the newly created mutant clones to identify the bacteria with the ice-minus gene. They will possess the desired ice-minus phenotype.

8. Insert the ice-minus gene into normal, ice-plus *P. syringae* bacterium.

9. Allow recombination to take place, rendering both ice-minus and ice-plus strains of *P. syringae*.

Pseudomonas syringae

Pseudomonas syringae is a rod shaped, Gram-negative bacterium with polar flagella. It is a plant pathogen which can infect a wide range of plant species, and exists as over 50 different pathovars, all of which are available to legitimate researches via international culture collections such as the NCPPB, ICMP, and others. Many of these pathovars were once considered to be individual species within the *Pseudomonas* genus, but molecular biology techniques such as DNA hybridisation have shown these to in fact all be part of the *P. syringae* species. It is a member of the *Pseudomonas* genus, and based on 16S rRNA analysis, *P. syringae* has been placed in the *P. syringae* group. It is named after the lilac tree (*Syringa vulgaris*), from which it was first isolated (Fig. 18.2).

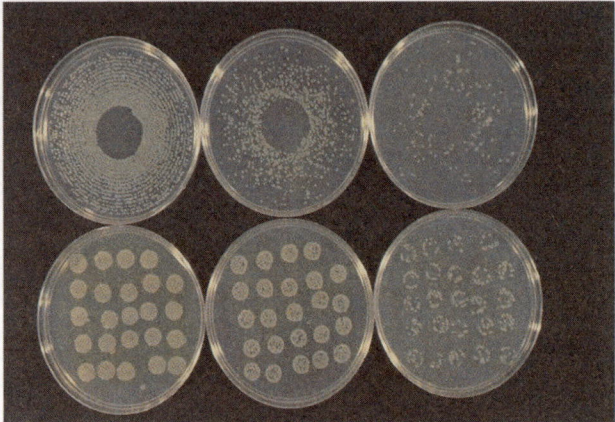

Fig. 18.2. *Pseudomonas syringae.*

P. syringae tests negative for arginine dihydrolase and oxidase activity, and forms the polymer levan on sucrose nutrient agar. It is known to secrete the lipodepsinonapeptide plant toxin syringomycin, and it owes its yellow fluorescent appearance when cultured *in vitro* on King's B medium to production of the siderophore pyoverdin. *P. syringae* also produce Ina proteins which cause water to freeze at fairly high temperatures, resulting in injury to plants. Since the 1970s, *P. syringae* has been implicated as an atmospheric 'biological ice nucleator', with airborne bacteria serving as cloud condensation nuclei. Recent evidence has suggested that the species plays a larger role than previously thought in producing rain and snow. These Ina proteins are also used in making artificial snow. *P. syringae*, more than any mineral or other organism, is responsible for the surface frost damage in plants, exposed to the environment. *P. syringae* can cause water to freeze at temperatures as high as –1.8°C, but strains causing ice nucleation at lower temperatures (down to –8°C) are more common. The freezing causes injuries in the epithelia and makes the nutrients in the underlying plant tissues available to the bacteria. Figure 18.3 shows Canker on an Ash tree.

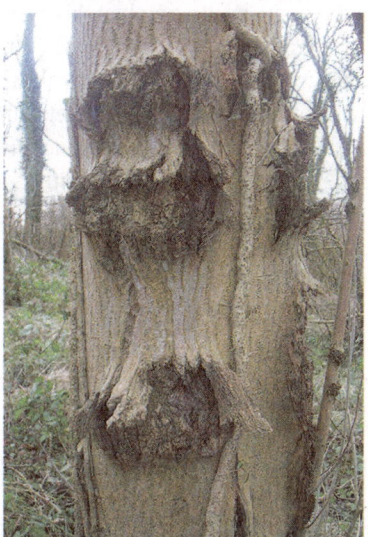

Fig. 18.3. Canker on an Ash tree.

P. syringae have *ina* (ice nucleation-active) genes that make Ina proteins which translocate to the outer bacterial cell wall on the surface of the bacteria where the Ina proteins act as nuclei for ice formation. Artificial strains of *P. syringae* known as ice-minus bacteria have been created to reduce frost damage.

SOMATIC CELL THERAPY AND GENE THERAPY

Recently, various innovative therapies involving the *ex vivo* manipulation and subsequent reintroduction of somatic cells into humans have been used or proposed. Somatic cell therapy is the administration to humans of autologous, allogeneic, or xenogeneic living cells which have been manipulated or processed *ex vivo*. Manufacture of products for somatic cell therapy involves the *ex vivo* propagation, expansion, selection, or pharmacologic treatment of cells, or other alteration of their biological characteristics. Such cellular products might also be used for diagnostic or preventive purposes. Manufacturers should review policy and regulations to determine how a particular somatic cell therapy or gene therapy product is regulated.

Recently, various innovative therapies involving the introduction of somatic cells into humans have been used or proposed. For the purpose of this Guidance, the term somatic cell therapy refers to the administration to humans of autologous, allogeneic, or xenogeneic living non-germline cells, other than transfusable blood products, for therapeutic, diagnostic, or preventive purposes. Gene therapy is a medical intervention based on modification of the genetic material of living cells. Cells may be modified *ex vivo* for subsequent administration to humans, or may be altered *in vivo* by gene therapy given directly to the subject. When the genetic manipulation is performed *ex vivo* on cells which are then administered to the patient, this is also a form of somatic cell therapy. The genetic manipulation may be intended to have a therapeutic or prophylactic effect, or may provide a way of marking cells for later identification. Recombinant DNA materials used to transfer genetic material for such therapy are considered components of gene therapy and as such are subject to regulatory oversight.

Examples of somatic cell therapies include implantation of cells as an *in vivo* source of a molecular species such as an enzyme, cytokine or coagulation factor; infusion of activated lymphoid cells such as lymphokine activated killer cells and tumour-infiltrating lymphocytes; and implantation of manipulated cell populations, such as hepatocytes, myoblasts, or pancreatic islet cells, intended to perform a complex biological function. Initial approaches to gene therapy have involved the alteration and administration of somatic cells. However, additional approaches such as the direct administration to patients of retroviral vectors or other forms of genetic material have been used. The concerns described below apply regardless of the method used, though the applicable tests may be different.

Cells for therapeutic purposes may be delivered in various ways. For example, they may be infused, injected at various sites or surgically implanted in aggregated form or along with solid supports or encapsulating materials. Any matrices, fibres, beads, or other materials which are used in addition to the cells may be categorised as excipients, additional active components, or medical devices.

Because of the complexities of potential interactions with the cells and other constituents, additional components should be considered as part of the final biological product for purposes of preclinical evaluation.

GENE THERAPY

Gene therapy is the insertion of genes into an individual's cell and biological tissues to treat disease, such as cancer where deleterious mutant alleles are replaced with functional ones. Although the technology is still in its infancy, it has been used with some success. Scientific breakthroughs continue to move gene therapy toward mainstream medicine. Scientists have taken the logical step of trying to introduce genes directly into human cells, focusing on diseases caused by single-gene defects, such as cystic fibrosis, haemophilia, muscular dystrophy and sickle cell anemia. However, this has proven more difficult than modifying bacteria, primarily because of the problems involved in carrying large sections of DNA and delivering them to the correct site on the comparatively large genome. Today, most gene therapy studies are aimed at cancer and hereditary diseases linked to a genetic defect. Antisense therapy is not strictly a form of gene therapy, but is a related, genetically-mediated therapy.

The biology of human gene therapy remains complex and many techniques need further development. Many diseases and their strict genetic link need to be understood more fully before gene therapy can be used appropriately. The public policy debate surrounding the possible use of genetically engineered material in human subjects has been equally complex. Major participants in the debate have come from the fields of biology, government, law, medicine, philosophy, politics, and religion, each bringing different views to the discussion.

Defective Genes

Genetic disorders are caused by missing or abnormal genes. Sometimes only these defective genes are responsible for disorders, but more often than not, they are compounded by environmental factors. Our genes play a role in most of the illnesses that affect us. Some of these illnesses can be attributed to an anomaly in one gene. They are called monogenic. This is the case with cystic fibrosis. Other diseases such as cancer, or conditions like dyslexia, are the result of several genes interacting with environmental factors, including diet and lifestyle. These genes are called susceptibility genes. Researchers say we all carry several such genes.

Future of Gene Therapy

Delivery of genes into cells

Gene delivery can be used in cells that have been removed from the body (*ex vivo* gene therapy) or in cells that are still in the body (*in vivo* gene therapy). Genes can be delivered into cells in different ways. The selection of a gene delivery system depends on the target cell, the duration of gene expression required for therapeutic effect, and the size of the piece of DNA to be used in the gene therapy.

Genes can be carried into cells by viruses. Viral vectors or carriers take advantage of the natural ability of a virus to enter a cell and deliver genetic material to the nucleus of the cell that contains its DNA. In developing virus carriers, the DNA coding for some or all of the normal genes of the virus to be used as a carrier are removed and replaced with a treatment gene. Most of these virus carriers are engineered so that they are able to enter cells, but they cannot reproduce themselves and so are innocuous.

Genes can also be delivered within tiny synthetic 'envelopes' of fat molecules. Cell membranes contain a very high concentration of fat molecules. The fat molecule 'envelope' can carry the therapeutic gene into the cell by being admitted through the cell membrane as if it were one of its own molecules.

Genes can also gain entrance into cells when an electrical charge is applied to the cell to create tiny openings in the membrane that surrounds a cells. This technique is called electroporation.

A 'bionic chip'

A new 'bionic chip' has been developed to help gene therapists using electroporation to slip fragments of DNA into cells. Electroporation was originally a hit-or-miss technique because there was no way to determine how much of an electrical jolt it took to open the cell membrane.

The 'bionic chip' solves this problem. It contains a single living cell embedded in a tiny silicon circuit. The cell acts as a diode, or electrical gate. When it is hit with just the right charge, the cell membrane opens, allowing the electricity to pass from the top to the bottom of the bionic chip. By recording what voltage caused this phenomenon to occur, it is now possible to determine precisely how much electricity it takes to pry open different types of cells.

Route of administration of gene therapy

The choice of route for gene therapy depends on the tissue to be treated and the mechanism by which the therapeutic gene exerts its effect. Gene therapy for cystic fibrosis, a disease which effects cells within the lung and airway, may be inhaled. Most genes designed to treat cancer are injected directly into the tumour. Proteins such as factor VIII or IX for haemophilia are also being introduced directly into target tissue (the liver).

Potential power of gene therapy

Most gene therapy for diseases such as cystic fibrosis and haemophilia has been designed only to ease, not to cure, the disease. However, the delivery of functional copies of genes provides a potential method to correct a disease at its most basic level. Gene therapy also holds the potential to provide 'patient-friendly' treatment regimens for a variety of diseases. Today, many patients with haemophilia and diabetes must have repeated injections in order to manage their disease because proteins exist in the blood stream for a limited period of time before they are degraded or eliminated. Since DNA is more stable and functions inside the cell, the delivery of genes may result in longer-term expression of the necessary proteins. Because of its accuracy, gene therapy has the potential to eliminate cancer cells without damaging normal, healthy tissue. Furthermore, cancer gene therapies may provide alternatives when a disease does not respond to other older treatments.

The potential of gene therapy is great but, compared to its promise, the results to date are still quite limited. However, the benefits of gene therapy are believed to be on the near horizon. Gene therapy is one of the hottest areas of medical research today.

The remarkable advances in genetics, including the human genome project, have opened new doors for the exploration of gene therapy. New technologies are needed to speed the progress of gene therapy. As these new technologies such as the 'bionic chip' arrive, we believe that, without a doubt, gene therapy will play an increasingly important and prominent part in medicine in the decades to come.

Chapter 19

Biotechnology Patents and Intellectual Property Rights

INTRODUCTION

A patent portfolio is often the most important asset for a biotechnology company. US patents are granted for useful, new and non-obvious products or processes. While this appears to be a pretty big hurdle even improvements to current inventions or technologies may be patentable. In fact, a complex system may result in multiple US patents. While many inventors have a tremendous scientific ability, a patent is a legal document and should be prepared by a licensed patent attorney.

Patents are granted by the government for the commercial exploitation of an invention for a specific period of time in consideration of the disclosure of the invention so that expiry of the terms of the patent, the information can benefit the public at large. The patents system provides a solid benefit as it bestows monetary reward for revealing technological innovation along with accolades for the inventor. Patent is an award for the inventor and a reward for the investor.

The grant of patent for an invention attracts investment because the commercial exploitation of the invention is possible to its fullest extent during the term of patent. Another major advantage of the patent system is that it promotes; invent around concept. Patent is granted only when the invention and its operation or use and the method by which it is to be performed are fully disclosed. When the patentee launches the product (in which the invention is incorporated) in the market, his competitors may lose the market if the product is technically advanced and cheap as compared to the existing one.

The patentee can prevent others from manufacturing the same product without his authorisation and can resort to legal means to enforce his right. But the competitors have an option to 'invent around' the patented product by conducting further research around to bring out a better invention, which may result in cheaper and better product.

It paves the way for healthy competition among manufactures that results in day-to-day improvement of technology. Ultimately, it contributes to the economic growth of the country, thereby enhancing living standard of the people. By virtue of the grant, patentee gets the exclusive right to prevent the third parties (not having his consent) from the act of making, using, offering for sale, selling or importing the patented product or process within the territory of grant.

The granting of special exclusive rights (for trading new articles) has been a practice to encourage innovations. As an example, monopoly rights (only to inventors) were granted in some countries like Europe, as an incentive to develop new articles that would be of benefit to the society.

Under the USA law, a patent means grant of 'right to exclude others from making, using or selling' an invention for a 17-years period. Patents are usually allowed for a specified period. Before 1970, when the discovery of an oil-eating bacterium (*Pseudomonas*) by a nonresident Indian (Dr. Chakrabarty), was patented in the USA by a multinational corporation, the life forms could not be patented. A latter patent issued for 'oncomouse' was another milestone in patenting of life forms. In patents for food, chemicals, drug and pharmaceuticals, the duration of the patent in India is five years from the date of grant of patent or seven years from the date of filing the application, whichever is less.

How can biotechnology products and processes be protected and the due financial profits returned to the rightful inventors and industrial developers? Inventors in the area of biotechnology can be protected by way of different titles of protection including patents for inventions, plant breeder's rights and trade secrets. In the context of biotechnology, inventions can be in the form of product or processes.

Products These can be considered either as: (i) living entities of natural or artificial origin such as animals, plants and micro-organism, cell lines, organelles, plasmids and DNA sequences, and (ii) naturally occurring substances, primary or secondary, derived from living system.

Processes These can include those of isolation, cultivation, multiplication, purification and bioconversion. Such processes can be involved in the isolation or the creation of the above products, e.g. antibiotic production; the production of substances through bioconversion of products, e.g. enzymatic conversion of sugar to alcohol; the used of the products for many purposes, e.g. monoclonal antibodies for analysis or diagnosis; and the use of microbes for biocontrol of pathogens.

INTELLECTUAL PROPERTY RIGHTS FOR BIOTECHNOLOGY

Intellectual Property is the term used to describe the branch of law which protects the application of thoughts, ideas and information which are of commercial value. It thus covers the law relating to patents, copyrights, trademarks, trade secrets and other similar rights.

The development of the genetic resources of biodiversity is known as biotechnology. Broadly defined, biotechnology includes any technique that uses living organisms or parts of organisms to make or modify products, to improve plants or animals, or to develop micro-organisms for specific uses. Mankind has used forms of biotechnology since the dawn of civilisation. However, it has been the recent development of new biological techniques (e.g., recombinant DNA, cell fusion, and monoclonal antibody technology) which has raised fundamental social and moral questions and created problems in intellectual property rights.

Intellectual property protection for biotechnology is currently in a state of flux. Whilst it used to be the case that living organisms were largely excluded from protection, attitudes are now changing and increasingly biotechnology is receiving some form of protection. These changes have largely taken place in the USA and other industrialised countries, but as other countries wish to compete in the new biotechnological markets, they are likely to change their national laws in order to protect and encourage investment in biotechnology.

There is at the moment no clear international consensus on how biotechnology should be treated. Although bodies such as the World Intellectual Property Organisation (WIPO, the United Nations permanent body primarily responsible for international cooperation in intellectual property), and the Organisation for Economic Cooperation and Development (OECD) have conducted separate studies and produced various reports, these have only sought to make governments more aware of the potential problems and to offer some suggested solutions. In view of the highly controversial nature of providing intellectual property protection for biotechnology, it is likely that in the short term developments will be at a national and regional level.

Intellectual Property Protection Currently Available

There are currently two main systems of protection for biotechnology: rights in plant varieties, and patents. Both systems provide exclusive, time-limited rights of exploitation and are described in more detail below.

Keeping biotechnology 'secret' can also be a valuable form of protection. National treatment of trade secrets is diverse, and all attempts to harmonise trade secret laws in Europe, for example, have failed. Most jurisdictions do provide some form of protection against those who steal or use others' trade secrets unfairly. However, the problem with this form of protection is that the secret generally becomes public once the biotechnology is used commercially and thus the protection is lost.

It is conceivable that the law of copyright could afford some protection for biotechnology. Lines of genetic code are analogous to some extent with computer program code, which has now been incorporated into the copyright systems of most industrialised countries. However, this route to protection is fraught with practical and conceptual difficulties and is generally thought to be unsuitable. There is as yet no recorded case of biotechnologists claiming copyright in their inventions.

Trademarks are also unlikely to be of much use in protecting biotechnology, though they may of course prove important later in regard to marketing products, processes or services. An attempt to register the name of a plant or an animal as a trade mark is unlikely to be successful as public policy would prevent it (in England, registrations for names of varieties of roses have been removed from the Trade Mark Register for lack of distinctiveness and because of the likelihood of confusion).

Rights in Plant Varieties

Prior to the mid-1960s only a few countries (e.g. Germany, USA) gave any intellectual property protection to plant varieties. Because of pressure from their plant breeding industries, 10 western European countries entered into a diplomatic process in the early-1960s which eventually culminated in the formation of an International Union for the Protection of New Varieties of plants (UPOV) and the signing of a Convention (the UPOV Convention 1961). Since that time a number of other countries have become parties to the UPOV Convention. Amendments were made to the UPOV Convention in 1978, principally to facilitate the entry of the USA.

The UPOV Convention requires that each member country must adopt national legislation to give at least 24 genera or species protection, in accordance with the provisions of the convention, within eight years of signing. A plant variety is protectable (a protectable variety) under the UPOV system if it is distinct, uniform, stable (DUS) and satisfies a novelty requirement. Novelty and distinctiveness equate broadly to novelty under patent law, but are more leniently applied in comparison to the patent rule. Satisfaction of the DUS criteria is conducted by the national authority responsible, usually by growing the variety over at least two seasons. There is also an important requirement that the variety be maintained throughout the duration of protection. A country may apply the system to all genera or species, but there is no obligation to do so and thus the system has been extended only gradually. In addition, the UPOV Convention allows national legislation to discriminate against foreigners (including nationals of a UPOV Convention country) under the principle of reciprocity. Thus amongst the UPOV members there is still some disparity in protection.

Duration of protection depends on national legislation and on the plant species to which the variety belongs, but is generally for 20–30 years. Grant of plant variety rights confers certain exclusive rights on the holder, including the exclusive right to sell the reproductive material (e.g. seed, cuttings, whole plants) of the protected variety. However the rights do not extend to consumption material (e.g. fruit, wheat seed grown for milling flour). Essentially the exclusive rights define what others may or may not do in relation to the protected varieties.

Plant breeders were for some time dissatisfied with the protection provided by the UPOV system. This eventually resulted in a major diplomatic conference in March 1991, at which the UPOV Convention was substantially revised. The new 1991 text will provide far greater protection than is afforded at present, most notably by requiring that all member countries apply the convention to all genera and species, by extending the exclusive rights to include harvested material (e.g. fruit, wheat grown for milling into flour) and, most controversially, by allowing enforcement against farm-saved seed (where a farmer produces further seed of the protected variety from the previous year's crop). However, until the national governments ratify the new convention the system will continue to be based on the 1978 text. There will be considerable national opposition to the strengthening of plant variety rights and thus these changes may take years before they are implemented and may even be superseded by greater availability of patent protection in the meantime.

Patents for Biotechnology

A patent is a grant of exclusive rights for a limited time in respect of a new and useful invention. The exact requirements for grant of a patent, the scope of protection it provides and its duration differs depending on national legislation. However, generally the invention must be of patentable subject matter, novel (new), non-obvious (inventive), of industrial application and sufficiently disclosed. A patent will provide a wide range of legal rights, including the right to possess, use, transfer by sale or gift, and to exclude others from similar rights. Duration will be for around 20 years (although for only 17 years in the USA). These rights are generally restricted to the territorial jurisdiction of the country granting the patent and thus an inventor wishing to protect his/her invention in a number of countries will need to seek separate patents in each of those countries. Whilst the majority of countries provide some form of patent protection, only a few provide patent protection for biotechnology (these include: Australia, Bulgaria, Canada, Czechoslovakia, Hungary, Romania, Japan, the Soviet Union and the parties to the European Patent Convention). The reasons for this may differ, but generally it has been because biotechnology has been thought inappropriate for patent protection, either because the system was originally designed for mechanical inventions, or for technical or practical reasons, or for one or more ethical, religious or social concerns. In all the National Patent Offices where patents are granted for biotechnology there is a considerable backlog of pending applications. Even in those countries where patent protection is provided, the type and extent of that protection is different in nearly every national system.

It has largely been the USA which has broken new ground in providing the possibility of patent protection for 'anything under the sun that is made by man'. Patents have been granted for plants since 1930 in the USA, under The Plant Patent Act. However, prior to 1980, the US Patent Office would not grant utility patents (separate from The Plant Patent Act) living matter because it deemed products of nature not to be within the terms of the utility patent statute. That was until the landmark decision of the US Supreme Court in Diamond v Chakrabarty (from which the above quote is taken), which held that a particular genetically engineered bacterium was statutory subject matter for a utility patent. This decision has been the basis upon which patents have been granted for higher life forms. Subsequently it has been held that a utility patent may be granted for plants and a patent has been granted for an animal. Polyploid oysters, not naturally occurring, were held to be patentable subject matter and US Patent no. 3,736,866, was issued in respect of a 'transgenic nonhuman mammal all of whose germ cells and somatic cells contain a recombinant activated oncogene sequence introduced into the said mammal, or an ancestor of said animal, at an embryonic stage' popularly known as the 'oncomouse'.

Elsewhere, the treatment of applications for patents for living matter is far from certain. Whilst patents are granted in many countries for plants and micro-organisms, it has been the issue of patents for animals which has been most controversial. Whilst it is not possible to summarise succinctly the position in the rest of the world, it is possible to describe the present approach of those countries which are party to the European Patent Convention (the EPC). The EPC is a regional arrangement entered into by 14 European countries for the purpose of making multiple applications for any of the member countries a great deal easier and to introduce a common system for patent protection. An application under the EPC is for a European patent, or Europatent, for short. If a Europatent is granted by the European Patent Office (EPO) it has the same effect, and is subject to the same conditions, as a national patent in each of the member countries designated in the application. In other words, through a single application a bundle of national patents can be obtained. The EPC provides that 'plant or animal varieties or essentially biological processes for the production of plants or animals' are excluded from patent protection (although the exclusion is expressly stated not to apply to microbiological processes and products). These exclusions would appear to place unequivocal prohibition on Europatents for macrobiotechnology. However, the EPO has been taking an increasingly narrow view of these exclusions, and has held that they do not exclude all plants and animals *per se*, but only claims for varieties of plants or animals and that a process is not 'essentially biological' if there has been substantial interference by man.

It is also important to note that there is currently before the European Parliament of the European Community (EC) a proposal for a Council Directive for harmonisation of the legal protection provided for biotechnology in the EC. This does not propose to amend the EPC, but the present draft proposal would make even more opportunities available for patenting biotechnology and thus make the EC more attractive in terms of investment in biotechnology research.

Attempts to harmonise patent law and practice internationally have not yet fully succeeded. For example, at present the US allows a one-year grace period between an inventor's publication and the deadline for filing a US patent application. In contrast, any public disclosure of an invention before filing any application is usually fatal to the prospects of protection in European countries. Again, the US settles disputes over priority as between rival claimants for the same invention by comparing actual dates of invention, whereas, in other countries, whoever has the earlier effective patent application date will usually prevail. Therefore patents encourage secrecy up to the point of filing but ensure publication of the information after the granting of a patent, and thus making it available for research purposes.

Another difference is that in US patent law the term 'invention' means invention or discovery. In European law 'discovery' is distinguished from 'invention' and is unpatentable. The distinction is not easy to define. A discovery involves new knowledge whereas an invention is a practical application of knowledge. For example: the elucidation by Crick and Watson of the double helix structure of DNA was an unpatentable discovery whereas later exploitation of this to produce DNA artificially and to produce new forms of DNA have given rise to many patents.

Naturally occurring substances, present as components of complex mixtures of natural origin, can in principle be patented where they are isolated from their natural surrounding, identified, and made available for the first time and a process is developed for producing them so that they can be put to a useful purpose. This applies to inanimate substances as well as to living materials. In appropriate circumstances such substances are not ruled out as mere discoveries but are considered as invention by the EPO and other legal authorities.

Micro-organism patents are now routinely granted by the US, European and Japanese Patent offices. Although a US patent had been granted in 1873 to Pasteur for 'yeast free from germs of disease as an article of manufacture', the US courts later held that the 'discovery of some of the handiwork of nature' was unpatentable. In the Chakrabarty case in 1980 the US Supreme Court decided that a micro-organism was not precluded from patentability solely because it was alive. Thus a Pseudomonas bacterium manipulated to contain more than one plasmid controlling the breakdown of hydrocarbons (therefore more useful in dispersing oil slicks than the natural organism containing only one such plasmid) was 'a new bacterium with markedly different characteristics from any found in nature' and hence not nature's handiwork but that of the inventor. The 'product of nature' objection therefore failed and the modified organism was held patentable. This decision was influential in most other industrially developed countries and the issue is now settled in law.

Plant patents are also obtainable in US, Europe and Japan. The US Plant Patent Act of 1930 is restricted to asexually propagated plants and over 6500 of such plant patents have been granted (mostly for rose and fruit trees). In the Hibberd case, following the principle established in the Chakrabarty case, it was decided that normal US 'utility' patents could be granted for other types of plant, e.g. genetically modified plants.

In Europe, patent law was originally considered unsuitable for protecting new plant varieties developed by traditional breeding methods. Special national laws of plant breeder's rights, which are also called Plant Variety Rights (PVR), were therefore established in the 1960s in some countries as well as the International Union for the Protection of New Varieties of Plants (UPOV, 1961). To avoid legal confusion, patent law in Europe subsequently excluded plant varieties from patentability, e.g. EPC Article 53(b) which excludes patents for 'plant and animal varieties' as such and 'essentially biological processes for the production' of plants and animals. The UPOV Convention was revised in 1991 and now does not prevent dual protection by PVR or patents. This revision awaits ratification by Member States and is therefore not yet in force.

Plant breeder's rights have been highly successful in their own sphere. However, legal experts now generally recognise that patent law is better suited to the protection of recombinant methods for producing transgenic plants and the resulting products. Patents of this type, claiming methods and products *per se*, have been granted by the EPO.

Animal breeds produced by traditional methods have no legal system for their protection comparable to plant breeder's rights. Based on the micro-organism and plant patent precedents, the US Commissioner of Patents declared in 1987 that US patents would be granted for 'non-naturally occurring nonhuman multicellular living organisms including animals'. The first transgenic animal patent was issued in 1988 to Harvard University with claims covering the 'oncomouse', one in which an oncogene has been introduced to make the animal more susceptible to cancer and therefore more sensitive in testing possible carcinogens. After initial reluctance by the EPO to grant the corresponding European patent (and a successful appeal to the Appeal Board) the European patent was issued. This is now under formal opposition by anti-vivisection and animal rights groups. More than 300 patent applications for transgenic animals have been filed but so far few have been granted (3 in the EPO, 6 in the US Patent Office).

Gene patents are available in all fields of biotechnology. For recombinant DNA inventions, the patent will claim the nucleotide sequence coding for the protein expression product, vectors, e.g. plasmids containing this sequence, micro-organisms or higher organisms transformed with the sequence, and in appropriate cases the expression product itself (normally only if the product is new *per se*). Corresponding process technology will also be claimed. The patentability of DNA sequences of unknown function is dubious and controversial. The Human Genome Organisation accepts that patents should be granted for full length genes but is against patenting fragmentary cDNA sequences having no established utility.

Debate About Patents in Biotechnology

The industries that utilise biotechnology are convinced that intellectual property protection should be obtainable for the inventions that stem from research and which have commercial potential. Biotechnology research workers in academic institutions increasingly share this view because of their need for research funding which is in part conditional on patentability. A serious challenge to this assumption has come from a number of interest groups concerned variously with matters of ecology, animal welfare and rights, moral issues and the interests of small farmers and the developing countries.

Some of these groups have formally opposed specific European patents and demanded their revocation. For many such groups 'patenting life' is considered unethical in principle. The opposition extends also to possible structural change in the agricultural industry which might stem from biotechnology and especially from the acquisition by the larger corporations of legal rights on the advances that are being made.

Legal and moral issues: A legally permissible ground of objection is that genes are naturally occurring entities and that the methods for transferring them to plants or animals are well-known and straightforward. This is a challenge to the inventiveness content of the particular patent at issue; it is an argument that industrial competitors will sometimes use against each other's patents but so far it has not achieved a high success rate. The argument also lies at the heart of the moral objections many with religious beliefs have to patenting genes. They regard claims of invention, instead of discovery, tantamount to claiming to be God.

Some feel that patenting living things change the relationship between humanity and the rest of nature. This is particularly sensitive as regards animals, where patents are seen as conferring 'ownership', thereby undermining the animal's right to independence of being and relegating it to the status of a mere object. However, plants and animals are owned by the farmers who produce them and use them as agricultural commodities. All such owners, whether of patented or unpatented organisms, are bound to respect animal welfare legislation. The opposers can raise the morality issue where the patent law allows, as in Europe under EPC Article 53(a) which forbids patents for inventions 'the publication or exploitation of which is contrary to order public (public order) or to morality'. The morality objection is being currently used against the European oncomouse patent. To programme an animal genetically for certain death in laboratory experiments is morally repugnant to these opposing groups and they feel in conscience bound to protest. Animals have, however, long been used as disease models. The response of the patent authorities may depend on whether, in the light of general public acceptance of the use of test animals in research to find cures for serious human diseases, the use of the oncomouse would be generally condemned.

The objection to animal suffering may also apply to the genetic modification of farm animals. One early experiment to insert a growth hormone gene into a pig in order to increase growth rate succeeded but caused severe unforeseen side effects including arthritis. Animal welfare groups argue that patents will encourage more research on animal genetic modification, which they oppose on grounds of possible suffering and of principle. Intended to prevent undue suffering, legislation requires the granting of animal experimentation licenses and full disclosure of the experimentation.

Freedoms for breeders and farmers are seen by some groups as threatened by patents on transgenic plants and animals. Under PVR breeders previously enjoyed the so-called 'breeder's privilege' or 'research exemption' which gave them the freedom not only to use protected plant varieties in their breeding programmes but also to commercialise the further varieties developed therefrom (often only 'cosmetically' different from the original) without any royalty payment to the owner of the initial variety. The UPOV Convention as revised in 1991 now expands the scope of the right of the initial variety breeder to include what are termed 'essentially derived varieties' (both the terms 'essentially derived' and 'variety' are defined). This expansion of the right is not automatic but depends on Member States amending their national PVR legislation in conformity with UPOV 1991.

Freedom to research and to commercialise: The freedom to research is safeguarded equally under both patent law and PVR law. But the freedom to commercialise the resulting products of research depends on whether or not they infringe the patent claims or are 'essentially derived' under PVR law. A strengthened UPOV-type protection would therefore go part of the way towards the strong protection given by patents. Neither system is a threat to the free use of existing germ plasm since these rights can in no sense monopolise known material as such. Again, until the UPOV revision is taken up in national laws, farmers legitimately sowing seed of a protected variety are legally free to save part of the seed from the first crop of plants for sowing on their own farms to produce a second and subsequent crops (the 'farmer's privilege').

Recognising that the current scale of use of farm-saved seed thus deprives the breeder of significant royalty income, the strengthened right under the 1991 version of UPOV would make this subject to authorisation of the breeder. However, Contracting States can 'reintroduce' this freedom under their national legislation 'within reasonable limits and subject to the safeguarding of the legitimate interests of the breeder'.

INTERNATIONAL TREATIES

There are three international intellectual property treaties which are of particular importance for the protection of biotechnology: the Paris Convention for the Protection of Industrial Property (the Paris Convention); the Budapest Treaty on the International Recognition of the Deposit of micro-organisms for the Purposes of Patent Procedure (the Deposit Treaty) and the Patent Cooperation Treaty (PCT).

The Paris Convention was originally signed in 1883 by just 11 countries, but now the majority of countries who have any form of intellectual property law are parties to it. The keystone to the convention is the principle of national treatment: an applicant from one convention country shall have the same rights in a second convention country as a national of that second country. The convention covers patents and defines them so broadly that it permits application to any of the forms of industrial patents granted under the laws of the convention countries. The most important practical result of the convention is that it is possible to claim priority from an application made in a convention country for all subsequent convention countries within 12 months of the original filing.

The Deposit Treaty, as the full title suggests, is concerned with the deposit of examples of micro-organisms for the purposes of patent applications. Applications for patents for biotechnology often face considerable difficulties in describing the nature of the invention sufficiently. The Deposit Treaty is a vehicle for solving these problems, primarily through the setting up of a series of International Depository Authorities (IDA) and through the recognition by all member countries of a deposit in a single IDA.

The PCT simplifies the process of filing patent applications simultaneously in a number of countries. Under the PCT a single application may be filed in one of the official receiving offices, designating any number of PCT member countries, which can eventually result in a national patent being granted in each of the designated states (and/or a Europatent). A prior-art search is performed by the receiving office and a report sent to the applicant. The application and report are published and the application will then move on either to an international preliminary examination followed by national examination, or alternatively straight to the national examination stage. Unfortunately, the eventual outcome is not a 'world patent' and there is no harmonisation patent law under the PCT apart from the procedural aspects.

ETHICAL ISSUES IN BIOTECHNOLOGY

New ethical questions have arisen from our ability to intervene in the structure of the genome. Responsible use of this technique requires ethical evaluation in which experts, potential beneficiaries and the general public should all participate. The examples of genetically modified food and of human genetics help to illustrate the issues involved.

From the time when the earliest pioneers of medicine took the Hippocratic oath, the importance of ethical considerations in relation to actions affecting living entities has been recognised by professionals. The general principles are still of fundamental importance: respect for life and the need for a balance of benefit over harm resulting from any intervention.

Contemporary Features

There are three particular contemporary features that account for the heightened public concern on the threshold of the 21st century. First, much of the current development in biotechnology results from a greatly enhanced understanding of the nature of genetics and the consequent ability to perform manipulations in the genomes of plants and animals. This power to intervene in what might be thought of as 'the fabric of life' raises the question of whether or not this, in itself, is an ethically questionable activity. Some feel that 'respect for life' implies that there should be no interference with it in this basic way. Conversely, the issue of the integrity of nature is itself complex and open to interpretation in an evolutionary world in which there is natural genomic plasticity. Moreover, the ethical does not simply equate with the natural. Heart transplants are as radically unnatural as gene transplants, but most people consider them to be ethically acceptable.

Second, the pace of discovery in genetics-based biotechnology is very rapid and there is anxiety that a kind of technological compulsion ('if we can do it, let's do it') will drive developments ahead of proper ethical consideration of their propriety. Not everything that can be done should be done but, once technology is 'on the shelf', it is hard not to take it off. The moratorium on human germ-line therapy is an example of the recognition that there must be ethical restraints on the use of what is technically feasible. Part of the reason for this restriction is uncertainty about the long-term effects of such interventions. There is also considerable uncertainty about the environmental consequences of the genetic manipulation of plants. These issues are scientific questions that need to be answered before we have an adequate basis of knowledge for reaching final ethical decisions.

Third, advanced technology involves processes that are only well understood by the experts who develop and use them. This places considerable power in the hands of the companies that employ these experts. Currently, there is much public suspicion about the reliability and independence of this 'expert' advice. Some of this suspicion derives from a difficulty in understanding that absolutely certain answers often cannot be given to complex questions and that every element of risk can seldom be eliminated. It is also exacerbated by memories of unfortunate incidents, such as the bovine spongiform encephalopathy (BSE) crisis in the UK.

There is also much suspicion of transnational corporations, which are perceived by many as wanting to maximise their profits by making users dependent on their products and then controlling availability.

The ethical use of biotechnology clearly includes it being provided on a fair and just basis, neither denying reasonable reward to those who have undertaken the considerable expense and risk of R&D nor putting small-scale users in thrall to large-scale suppliers.

Genetically Modified Foods

These general considerations can be illustrated by the current controversy about the development and use of genetically modified (GM) organisms in the food chain.

Selectivity

Selective breeding has been used since agriculture began, with the development of cultivated crops from wild species and of domestic herds from wild animals. However, it is now possible to carry out gene transfers that could not occur in nature, even gene transfers from the animal kingdom to the plant kingdom.

Some people have characterised this as 'playing God', with the implication that it is ethically unacceptable to interfere with nature. However, human beings are themselves part of nature and many religious people would see the responsible exercise of scientific skills as being the employment of God-given abilities. We have already seen that the natural-unnatural division is not in itself of intrinsic ethical significance, otherwise much of medicine, for instance, would be morally outlawed. Three particular points are notable.

1. The genetic code is only significant when operating in the context of a living cell. In isolation, genes are simply complex chemicals. This has led some people to believe — to take the most ethically sensitive example — that if a human gene were transferred to a pig cell, it would, in that context, become simply a pig gene, although admittedly one of human origin. Other people do not accept this, but believe that the gene would continue to have the ethical status of a human gene.
2. Current gene transfers involve single genes or, at most, small gene clusters. They represent a highly accurate and targeted form of crossing. The creation of chimeras with substantial interspecies mingling would raise different and difficult ethical issues, including questions of animal welfare.
3. There is a widely recognised obligation to use this new technology for serious and valuable means, not for speculative or trivial purposes. Obvious examples of responsible projects to choose include the generation of therapeutic proteins from transgenic animals and the modification of crops so that they can grow in and or saline environments.

Environmental effects

One of the major concerns about GM crops is their possible environmental effects. Insect-resistant strains may reduce the use of insecticides, but will genes spread from herbicide-resistant strains to produce 'superweeds'? All interventions in nature run the risk of unanticipated upsets to its balance and, from the time that humans with stone axes began felling trees, agriculture has had significant environmental consequences. Even in the next millennium, our intellectual ability to foresee environmental effects is unlikely to be perfect. Some form of precautionary principle is ethically required, but it should not induce total paralysis. Because consequences are difficult to predict accurately, it is important that carefully controlled and monitored trials are used to gain the detailed knowledge on which ethically responsible decisions can be based.

Moral duties

It is predicted that the world population, currently approximately six billion, will rise to approximately eight billion by the year 2020. Present agricultural resources, if their produce was fairly distributed, could sustain approximately 6.4 billion people. Biotechnology offers considerable possibilities to help eliminate the anticipated shortfall. However, there is also considerable concern that small-scale farmers should not be exploited by large international companies.

Moral perplexities often arise when there is a clash between two different ethically desirable goals. The possible use of 'terminator' genes (that make seeds sterile) illustrates this point. On the one hand, they would help to reduce the hazards of environmental dispersal; on the other, farmers in developing countries traditionally save seed from one season to the next and cannot afford to buy new supplies each year. If these problems are to be solved, there must be recognition of the common good, understood on a worldwide basis and calling for fairness in the policies of big corporations and in the international regulation of biotechnological trading.

To these considerations must be added the universal ethical obligation to respect the duty of safety. With regard to food safety, GM products do not seem to raise issues or demand the monitoring of techniques, different to those employed to assess the effects of ordinary foods.

Human Genetics

The use of biotechnology in relation to human beings is governed by the Hippocratic principle that interventions must be for the benefit of the individual person concerned. Controversy in this area is not generated by dissent from this principle but by disagreement about what constitutes a human person, with all the moral rights appertaining to that status.

Some believe that this status is established at the moment of conception. If that is the case then no manipulation of the early embryo, other than for its own direct benefit, could be ethically justified. Others, however, take a more developmental view of the way in which a human foetus grows into a person, with the dawning of sentience and eventually of mentality. This latter view forms the basis of the legal restriction in the UK on research using embryos to the 14-day period before the development of the primitive streak. Currently, that research is also limited to projects investigating aspects of human fertility. However, it has recently been suggested that the scope of possible investigation should be extended to include the use of cell-nuclear-replacement (CNR) techniques to generate immunologically compatible tissue for therapeutic purposes and for the treatment of mitochondrial disease. At present, there has been no decision by the UK Government on whether or not to accept this recommendation.

In the UK, GM embryos may not legally be implanted, so there is an absolute embargo on the use of CNR to generate cloned human beings. There is extensive ethical support for this legal position. The moral necessity to use new technology for acceptable means plays a determinative role in forming this view. Although the repair of damaged tissues in the ill or injured is seen as being highly desirable, the creation of a 'replacement person' is not so acceptable. Respect for the human person forbids this—not because there is an intrinsic human right to possess a unique genome (identical twins do not, but each is a human person) but because a human being is to be valued for their self and not used as a surrogate for another. The same moral intuition leads to an abhorrence of the idea of using genetic manipulation to produce 'designer babies' with qualities according to parental specification. Persons are never to be commodified: ethically, they are never means but always ends.

The example of the regulation of human genetics in the UK provides an answer to the so-called 'slippery slope' argument. It is sometimes argued that to allow CNR for therapeutic purposes would soon lead to it being used for reproductive purposes. The ban on exceeding the 14-day limit and on implanting GM embryos shows that there are effective barriers in place to prevent this happening.

Public Debate

Debates on the ethical issues raised by biotechnology will certainly continue into the 21st century. Science, by gaining knowledge, confers power; if that power is to be used to choose the good and refuse the bad then wisdom must be added to knowledge. This quest for judicious decisions will involve the participation of at least three parties:

1. The experts.
2. The community of possible beneficiaries.
3. The general public.

Participation of the experts is essential, as only they can assess the potential risks and benefits of new developments. They have an ethical obligation to do this in as fair and as balanced a way as possible. Final decisions cannot be left to them alone, however, because their monopoly of expertise does not confer a monopoly of wisdom. They cannot be judges in their own cause, because the excitement of the research may cloud their judgement. The interest of the community of possible beneficiaries, whether it be sufferers from a particular disease or farmers on a marginal kind of land, is obvious but, again, they cannot be judges in their own cause.

The general public has an indispensable ethical stake in what is decided. If this general influence is to be exercised well, it will call for the development of informed and ethically sensitive public opinion. However, there are obstacles in the path to this happening. Much contemporary ethical debate takes the form of the confrontation of opposing single-issue pressure groups. One side claims that X is the best thing ever and we cannot have too much of it; the other, that X is the worst thing ever and we must avoid it at all costs. Whatever X may be, it is unlikely that either of these extreme positions is justified. It is important that society should seek to create forums in which ethical issues can be discussed in a truth-seeking and nonconfrontational manner. The issues that face us are too complex to be dealt with in slogan form.

If this prospect of a rational debate about biotechnology is to be realised, a considerable educational programme will be required. It is clear that many people still lack the rudimentary degree of scientific understanding that is indispensable as the basis for reaching informed, ethical conclusions on these issues. A saddening but instructive example is provided by the case of irradiated food. Because 'radiation' is, in many minds, a sinister word, conjuring up the image of an invisible hazard, this effective way of improving food safety was rejected by the public, who simply refused to buy food so labelled. We must hope that the debates of the 21st century will be both scientifically better informed, and also ethically more subtle, than those of the past decade of the 20th century have often proved to be.

Glossary

Abundance class	:	Refers to the relative abundance of different mRNA molecules in a cell at any given time.
ADA	:	Adenosine deaminase, deficiency results in SCIDS.
Adaptor	:	A synthetic single-stranded non self-complementary oligonucleotide used in conjunction with a linker to add cohesive ends to DNA molecules.
Adenine (A)	:	Nitrogenous base found in DNA and RNA
Adeno-associated virus	:	Virus used in gene therapy delivery methods.
Adenovirus	:	Virus that can infect through nasal passages, used in gene therapy delivery methods.
Aetiology	:	Of disease; relating to the causes of the disease.
Agrobacterium tumefaciens	:	Bacterium that infects plants arid causes crown gall disease. Carries a plasmid (the Ti plasmid) used for gene manipulation in plants.
Agarose	:	Jellylike matrix, extracted from seaweed, used as a support in the separation of nucleic acids by gel electrophoresis.
Alkaline phosphatase	:	An enzyme that removes 5′ phosphate groups from the ends of DNA molecules, leaving 5′ hydroxyl groups.
Allele	:	One of two or more variants of a particular gene.
Allele-specific oligonucleotide	:	Oligonucleotide with a sequence that can be matched precisely to a particular allele by using stringent hybridisation conditions.
Alpha-peptide	:	Part of the β-galactosidase protein, encoded by the *lacZ′* gene fragment.
Ampicillin (Ap)	:	A semisynthetic β-lactam antibiotic.
Aneuploidy	:	Variation in chromosome 'number where single chromosomes are affected, thus the chromosome complement is not an exact multiple of the haploid chromosome number.
Animal model	:	Usually a transgenic mouse in which a disease state has been engineered.
Antibody	:	An immunoglobulin that specifically recognises and binds to an antigenic determinant on an antigen.
Anticodon	:	The three bases on a tRNA molecule that are complementary to the codon on the mRNA.
Antigen	:	A molecule that is bound by an antibody. Also used to describe molecules that can induce an immune response, although these are more properly described as immunogens.
Antiparallel	:	The arrangement of complementary DNA strands, which run in different directions with respect to their 5′–3′ polarity.
Antisense RNA	:	Produced from a gene sequence inserted in the opposite orientation, so that the transcript is complementary to the normal mRNA and can therefore bind to it and prevent translation.

Arabidopsis thaliana	:	Small plant favoured as a research organism for plant molecular biologists.
Autoradiograph	:	Image produced on X-ray film in response to the emission of radio active particles.
Autosome	:	A chromosome that is not a sex chromosome.
Auxotroph	:	A cell that requires nutritional supplements for growth.
Bacillus thuringiensis	:	Bacterium used in crop protection, and in the generation of *Bt* plants that are resistant to insect attack. The bacterium produces a toxin that affects the insect.
Bacteriophage	:	A bacterial virus.
Baculovirus	:	A particular type of virus that infects insect cells, producing large inclusions in the infected cells.
Bal 31 nuclease	:	An exonuclease that degrades both strands of a DNA molecule at the same time.
Bioinformatics	:	The emerging discipline of collating and analysing biological information, especially genome sequence information.
Biolistic	:	Refers to a method of introducing DNA into cells by bombarding them with microprojectiles, which carry the DNA.
Blunt ends	:	DNA termini without overhanging 3′ or 5′ ends. Also known as flush ends.
Bovine somatotropin (BST)	:	Bovine growth hormone, produced as rBST for use in dairy cattle to increase milk production.
Bt plants	:	Plants which carry the toxin-producing gene from *Bacillus thuringiensis* as a means to protect the plant from insect attack.
Callus	:	A mass of relatively unspecialised tissue used in plant tissue culture as the starting material for the propagation of plant clones.
Carboxyl (C) terminus	:	Carboxyl terminus, defined by the –COOH group of an amino acid or protein.
CAAT box	:	A sequence located approximately 75 base-pairs upstream from eukaryotic transcription start sites. This sequence is one of those that enhance binding of RNA polymerase.
Caenorhabditis elegans	:	A nematode worm used as a model organism in developmental and molecular studies.
Cap	:	A chemical modification that is added to the 5′ end of a eukaryotic mRNA molecule during post-transcriptional processing of the primary transcript.
Capsid	:	The protein coat of a virus.
cDNA	:	DNA that is made by copying mRNA using the enzyme reverse transcriptase.
cDNA library	:	A collection of clones prepared from the mRNA of a given cell or tissue type, representing the genetic information expressed by such cells.
Central dogma	:	Statement regarding the unidirectional transfer of information from DNA to RNA to protein.
CFTR gene (protein)	:	Cystic fibrosis transmembrane conductance regulator, the gene and protein involved in defective ion transport that causes cystic fibrosis.
Chimaera	:	An organism (usually transgenic) composed of cells with different genotypes.
Chromosome	:	A DNA molecule carrying a set of genes. There may be a single chromosome, as in bacteria, or multiple chromosomes, as in eukaryotic organisms.
Chromosome jumping	:	Technique used to isolate non-contiguous regions of DNA by 'jumping' across gaps that may appear as a consequence of uncloned regions of DNA in a gene library.
Chromosome walking	:	Technique used to isolate contiguous cloned DNA fragments by using each fragment as a probe to isolate adjacent cloned regions.
Chymosin (chymase)	:	Enzyme used in cheese production, available as recombinant product.

Cis-acting element	:	A DNA sequence that exerts its effect only when on the same DNA molecule as the sequence it acts on. For example, the CAAT box is a *cis*-acting element for transcription in eukaryotes.
Cistron	:	A sequence of bases in DNA that specifies one polypeptide.
Clone	:	(1) A colony of identical organisms; often used to describe a cell carrying a recombinant DNA fragment. (2) Used as a verb to describe the generation of recombinants. (3) A complex organism (e.g. sheep) generated from a totipotent cell nucleus by nuclear transfer into an enucleated ovum.
Codon	:	The three bases in mRNA that specify a particular amino acid during translation.
Cohesive ends	:	Those ends (termini) of DNA molecules that have short complementary sequences that can stick together to join two DNA molecules. Often generated by restriction ˙enzymes.
Competent	:	Refers to bacterial cells that are able to take up exogenous DNA.
Competitor RT-PCR	:	Technique used to quantify the amount of PCR product by spiking samples with known amounts of a competitor sequence.
Complementation	:	Process by which genes on different DNA molecules interact. Usually a protein product is involved, as this is a diffusible molecule that can exert its effect away from the DNA itself. For example, a *lacZ*⁺ gene on a plasmid can complement a mutant (*lacZ*⁻) gene on the chromosome by enabling the synthesis of β-galactosidase.
Concatemer	:	A DNA molecule composed of a number of individual pieces joined together via cohesive ends.
Congenital	:	Present at birth, usually used to describe genetically derived abnormalities.
Conjugation	:	Plasmid-mediated transfer of genetic material from a 'male' donor bacterium to a 'female' recipient.
Consensus sequence	:	A sequence that is found in most examples of a particular genetic element, and which shows a high degree of conservation. An example is the CAAT box.
Copy number	:	(1) The number of plasmid molecules in a bacterial cell. (2) The number of copies of a gene in the genome of an organism.
cos site	:	The region generated when the cohesive ends of λ DNA join together.
Cosmid	:	A hybrid vector made up of plasmid sequences and the cohesive ends (*cos* sites) of bacteriophage lambda.
Crown gall disease	:	Plant disease caused by the Ti plasmid of *Agrobacterium tumefaciens*, in which a 'crown gall' of tissue is produced after infection.
Cyanogen bromide	:	Chemical used to cleave a fusion protein product from the N-terminal vector-encoded sequence after synthesis.
Cystic fibrosis	:	Disease affecting lungs and other tissues, caused by ion transport defects in the cm gene.
Cytosine (C)	:	Nitrogenous base found in DNA and RNA.
Deletion	:	Change to the genetic material caused by removal of part of the sequence of bases in DNA.
Deoxynucleoside triphosphate (dNTP)	:	Triphosphorylated (high energy) precursor required for synthesis of DNA, where N refers to one of the four bases (A,G,T or C).
Deoxyribonucleic acid (DNA)	:	A condensation heteropolymer composed of nucleotides. DNA is the primary genetic material in all organisms apart from some RNA viruses. Usually double-stranded.
Deoxyribose	:	The sugar found in DNA.

Deoxyribonuclease (*DNase*)	:	An nuclease enzyme that hydrolyses (degrades) single- and double-stranded DNA.
Dicotyledonous plant	:	Plant which develops from two cotyledons in the seed.
Dideoxynucleoside triphosphate (ddNTP)	:	A modified form of dNTP used as a chain terminator in DNA sequencing.
Diploid	:	Having two sets of chromosomes.
Disarmed vector	:	A vector in which some characteristic (e.g. conjugation) has been disabled.
DNA chip	:	A DNA microarray used in the analysis of gene structure and expression. Consists of oligonucleotide sequences immobilised on a 'chip' array.
DNA footprinting	:	Method of identifying regions of DNA to which regulatory proteins will bind.
DNA ligase	:	Enzyme used for joining DNA molecules by the formation of a phosphodiester bond between a 5′ phosphate and a 3′ OH group.
DNA polymerase	:	An enzyme that synthesises a copy of a DNA template.
DNA profiling	:	Term used to describe the various methods for analysing DNA to establish identity of an individual.
Dominant	:	An allele that is expressed and appears in the phenotype in heterozygous individuals.
Dot-blot	:	Technique in which small spots, or dots, of nucleic acid are immobilised on a nitrocellulose or nylon membrane for hybridisation.
Downstream processing	:	Refers to the procedures used to purify products (usually proteins) after they have been expressed in bacterial, fungal or mammalian cells.
Drosophila melanogaster	:	Fruit fly used as a model organism in genetic, developmental and molecular studies.
Duchenne muscular dystrophy	:	X-linked muscle-wasting disease caused by defects in the gene for the protein dystrophin.
Dystrophin	:	Large protein linking the cytoskeleton to the muscle cell membrane, defects in which cause muscular dystrophy.
Ectopic	:	Occurring in an unusual place or in an unusual form or manner.
Electroporation	:	Technique for introducing DNA into cells by giving a transient electric pulse.
ELSI	:	Sometimes used as shorthand to describe the ethical, legal and social implications of genetic engineering.
Embryo splitting	:	Technique used to clone organisms by separating cells in the early embryo, which then go on to direct development and produce identical copies of the organism.
End labelling	:	Adding a radioactive molecule onto the end(s) of a polynucleotide.
Endonuclease	:	An enzyme that cuts within a nucleic acid molecule, as opposed to an exonucleas, which digests DNA from one or both ends.
Enhancer	:	A sequence that enhances transcription from the promoter of a eukaryotic gene. May be several thousand base-pairs away from the promoter.
Enzyme	:	A protein that catalyses a specific reaction.
Enzyme replacement therapy	:	Therapeutic procedure in which a defective enzyme function is restored by replacing the enzyme itself.
Epigenesis	:	Theory of development that regards the process as an iterative series of steps, in which various signals and control events interact to regulate development.
Escherichia coli	:	The most commonly used bacterium in molecular biology.
Ethidium bromide	:	A molecule that binds to DNA and fluoresces when viewed under ultraviolet light. Used as a stain for DNA.
Eukaryotic	:	The property of having a membrane-bound nucleus.

Exon	:	Region of a eukaryotic gene that is expressed via mRNA.
Exonuclease	:	An enzyme that digests a nucleic acid molecule from one or both ends.
Explant	:	A piece of living tissue taken from its normal situation to a culture medium
Expressivity	:	The degree to which a particular genotype generates its effect in the phenotype.
Extrachromosomal element	:	A DNA molecule that is not part of the host cell chromosome.
Ex vivo	:	Outside the body. Usually used to describe gene therapy procedure in which the manipulations are performed outside the body, and the altered cells returned after processing.
Flavr Savr (sic)	:	Transgenic tomato in which polygalacturonase synthesis is restricted using antisense technology.
Foldback DNA	:	Class of DNA which has palindromic or inverted repeat regions that reanneal rapidly when duplex DNA is denatured.
Fusion protein	:	A hybrid recombinant protein that contains vector-encoded amino acid residues at the N terminus.
β-Galactosidase	:	An enzyme encoded by the *lacZ* gene. Splits lactose into glucose and galactose.
Gamete	:	Refers to the haploid male (sperm) and female (egg) cells that fuse to produce the diploid zygote (q.v.) during sexual reproduction.
Gel electrophoresis	:	Technique for separating nucleic acid molecules on the basis of their movement through a gel matrix under the influence of an electric field.
Gel retardation	:	Method of determining protein-binding sites on DNA fragments on the basis of their reduced mobility, relative to unbound DNA, in gel electrophoresis experiments.
Gene	:	The unit of inheritance, located on a chromosome. In molecular terms, usually taken to mean a region of DNA that encodes one function. Broadly, therefore, one gene encodes one protein.
Gene cloning	:	The isolation of individual genes by generating recombinant DNA molecules, which are then propagated in a host cell which produces a clone that contains a single fragment of the target DNA.
Gene protection technology	:	Range of techniques used to ensure that particular commercially derived recombinant constructs cannot be used without some sort of control or process, usually supplied by the company marketing the recombinant. Also known as genetic use restriction technology and genetic trait control technology.
Gene therapy	:	The use of cloned genes in the treatment of genetically-derived malfunctions. May be delivered *in vivo* or *ex vivo*. May be offered as gene addition or gene replacement versions.
Genetic code	:	The triplet codons that determine the types of amino acid that are inserted into a polypeptide during translation. There are 61 codons for 20 amino acids (plus three stop codons), and the code is therefore referred to as degenerate.
Genetic fingerprinting	:	A method which uses radioactive probes to identify bands derived from hypervariable regions of DNA. The band pattern is unique for an individual, and can be used to establish identity or family relationships.
Genetic mapping	:	Low-resolution method to assign gene locations (loci) to their position on the chromosome.
Genetic marker	:	A phenotypic characteristic that can be ascribed to a particular gene.

Genetic trait control technology	:	Version of gene protection technology, sometimes called 'traitor technology'.
Genetically modified organism (GMO)	:	An organism in which a genetic change has been engineered. Usually used to describe transgenic plants and animals.
Genome	:	Used to describe the complete genetic complement of a virus, cell or organism.
Genomics	:	The study of genomes, particularly genome sequencing.
Genomic library	:	A collection of clones which together represent the entire genome of an organism.
Genotype	:	The genetic constitution of an organism.
Germ line	:	Gamete producing (reproductive) cells that give rise to eggs and sperm.
Guanine (G)	:	Nitrogenous base found in DNA and RNA.
Haploid	:	Having one set of chromosomes.
Heterologous	:	Refers to gene sequences that are not identical, but show variable degrees of similarity.
Heteropolymer	:	A polymer composed of different types of monomer. Most protein and nucleic acid molecules are heteropolymers.
Heterozygous	:	Refers to a diploid organism (cell or nucleus) which has two different alleles at a particular locus.
Homologous	:	(1) Refers to paired chromosomes in diploid organisms. (2) Used to strictly describe DNA sequences that are identical; however, the percentage homology between related sequences is sometimes quoted.
Homopolymer	:	A polymer composed of only one type of monomer, such as polyphenylalanine (protein) or polyadenine (nucleic acid).
Homozygous	:	Refers to a diploid organism (cell or nucleus) which has identical alleles at a particular locus.
Host	:	A cell used to propagate recombinant DNA molecules.
Hybrid-arrest translation	:	Techniques used to identify the protein product of a cloned gene, in which translation of its mRNA is prevented by the formation of a DNA·mRNA hybrid.
Hybrid-release translation	:	Technique in which a particular mRNA is selected by hybridisation with its homologous cloned DNA sequence, and is then translated to give a protein product that can be identified.
Hybridisation	:	The joining together of artificially separated nucleic acid molecules via hydrogen bonding between complementary bases.
Hyperchromic effect	:	Change in absorbance of nucleic acids, depending on the relative amounts of single-stranded and double-stranded forms. Used as a measurement in denaturation/renaturation studies.
Hypervariable region (HVR)	:	A region in a genome that is composed of a variable number of repeated sequences and is diagnostic for the individual.
Ice-minus bacteria	:	Bacteria engineered to disrupt the normal ice-forming process, used to protect plants from frost damage.
Insertion vector	:	A bacteriophage vector that has a single cloning site into which DNA is inserted.
Insulin-like growth factor (IGF-1)	:	Polypeptide hormone, synthesis of which is stimulated by growth hormone. Implicated in some concerns about the safety of using recombinant bovine growth hormone in cattle to increase milk yields.
Intervening sequence	:	Region in a eukaryotic gene that is not expressed via the processed mRNA.
Inverted repeat	:	A short sequence of DNA that is repeated, usually at the ends of a longer sequence, in a reverse orientation.
In vitro	:	Literally 'in glass', meaning in the test-tube, rather than in the cell or organism.

In vivo	:	Literally 'in life', meaning the natural situation, within a cell or organism.
IPTG	:	*iso*-Propyl-thiogalactoside, a gratuitous inducer which de-represses transcription of the lac operon.
Kilobase (kb)	:	10^3 bases or base-pairs, used as a unit for measuring or specifying the length of DNA or RNA molecules.
Klenow fragment	:	A fragment of DNA polymerase I that lacks the 5'–3' exonuclease activity.
Knockin mouse	:	A transgenic mouse in which a gene function has been added or 'knocked in'. Used primarily to generate animal models for the study of human disease.
Knockout mouse	:	A transgenic mouse in which a gene function has beep disrupted or 'knocked out'. Used primarily to generate animal models for the study of human disease, e.g. cystic fibrosis.
Linkage mapping	:	Genetic mapping technique used to establish the degree of linkage between genes.
Linker	:	A synthetic self-complementary oligonucleotide that contains a restriction enzyme recognition site. Used to add cohesive ends to DNA molecules that have blunt ends.
Lipase	:	Enzyme that hydrolyses fats (lipids).
Liposome (lipoplex)	:	Lipid-based method for delivering gene therapy.
Locus	:	The site at which a gene is located on a chromosome.
Lysogenic	:	Refers to bacteriophage infection that does not cause lysis of the host cell.
Lytic	:	Refers to bacteriophage infection that causes lysis of the host cell.
Maternal inheritance	:	Pattern of inheritance from female cytoplasm. Mitochondrial genes are inherited in this way, as the mitochondria are inherited with the ovum.
Mega (M)	:	SI prefix, 10^6.
Messenger RNA (mRNA)	:	The ribonucleic acid molecule transcribed from DNA that carries the codons specifying the sequence of amino acids in a protein.
Micro (μ)	:	SI prefix, 10^{-6}.
Microinjection	:	Introduction of DNA into the nucleus or cytoplasm of a cell by insertion of a microcapillary and direct injection.
Microsatellite DNA	:	Type of sequence repeated many times in the genome. Based on dinucleotide repeats, microsatellites are highly variable and can be used in mapping and profiling studies.
Milli (m)	:	SI prefix, 10^{-3}.
Minisatellite DNA	:	Type of sequence based on variable number tandem repeats (VNTRs). Used in genetic mapping and profiling studies.
Molecular cloning	:	Alternative term for gene cloning.
Molecular ecology	:	Use of molecular biology and recombinant DNA techniques in studying ecological topics.
Molecular paleontology	:	Use of molecular techniques to investigate the past, as in DNA profiling from mummified or fossilised samples.
Monocistronic	:	Refers to a RNA molecule encoding one function.
Monogenic	:	Trait caused by a single gene.
Monocotyledonous plant	:	Plant which develops from a single cotyledon in the seed.
Monomer	:	The unit that makes up a polymer. Nucleotides and amino acids are the monomers for nucleic acids and proteins, respectively.

Monosomic	:	Diploid cells in which one of a homologous pair of chromosomes has been lost.
Monozygotic	:	Refers to identical twins, generated from the splitting of a single embryo at an early stage.
Mosaic	:	An embryo or organism in which not all the cells carry identical genomes.
mRNA	:	Messenger RNA transcribed from DNA in the nucleus, exported into the cytoplasm and translated into protein.
Multifactorial	:	Caused by many factors, e.g. genetic trait in which many genes and environmental influences may be involved.
Multi-locus probe	:	DNA probe used to identify several bands in a DNA fingerprint or profile. Generates the 'bar code' pattern in a genetic fingerprint.
Multiple cloning site (MCS)	:	A short region of DNA in a vector that has recognition sites for several restriction enzymes.
Multipotent	:	Cell which can give rise to a range of differentiated cells.
Mutagenesis	:	The process of inducing mutations in DNA.
Mutant	:	An organism (or gene) carrying a genetic mutation.
Mutation	:	An alteration to the sequence of bases in DNA. May be caused by insertion, deletion or modification of bases.
Nano (n)	:	SI prefix, 10^{-9}.
Native protein	:	A recombinant protein that is synthesised from its own N terminus, rather than from an N terminus supplied by the cloning vector.
Nested fragments	:	A series of nucleic acid fragments that differ from each other (in terms of length) by one or only a few nucleotides. Nick translation Method for labelling DNA with radioactive dNTPs.
Northern blotting	:	Transfer of RNA molecules onto membranes for the detection of specific sequences by hybridisation.
N terminus	:	Amino terminus, defined by the $-NH_2$ group of an amino acid or protein.
Nuclear transfer	:	Method for cloning organisms in which a donor nucleus is taken from a somatic cell and transferred to the recipient ovum.
Nuclease	:	An enzyme that hydrolyses phosphodiester bonds.
Nucleoside	:	A nitrogenous base bound to a sugar.
Nucleotide	:	A nucleoside bound to a phosphate group.
Nucleoid	:	Region of a bacterial cell in which the genetic material is located.
Nucleus	:	Membrane-bound region in a eukaryotic cell that contains the genetic material.
Oligo	:	Prefix meaning few, as in oligonucleotide or oligopeptide.
Oligo(dT)-cellulose	:	Short sequence of deoxythymidine residues linked to a cellulose matrix, used in the purification of eukaryotic mRNA.
Oligomer	:	General term for a short sequence of monomers.
Oligonucleotide	:	A short sequence of nucleotides.
Oligonucleotide-directed mutagenesis	:	Process by which a defined alteration is made to DNA using a synthetic oligonucleotide.
Oncogene	:	Gene involved in the formation of cancerous tissue.
Oncomouse	:	Transgenic mouse engineered to be susceptible to cancer.
Oocyte	:	Stage in development of the female gamete or ovum (egg). Often the terms oocyte and ovum are used interchangeably.
Operator	:	Region of an operon, close to the promoter, to which a repressor protein binds.
Operon	:	A cluster of bacterial genes under the control of a single regulatory region.

Organelle	:	Any discrete structure in an individual cell of a multicellular organism that is adapted and/or specialised for the performance of one or more vital functions.
Organismal cloning	:	The production of an identical copy of an individual organism by techniques such as embryo splitting or nuclear transfer. Used to distinguish the process from molecular cloning.
Ovum	:	The mature female gamete or egg cell, derived from the oocyte. Often the terms ovum and oocyte are used interchangeably.
Palindrome	:	A DNA sequence that reads the same on both strands when read in the same (e.g. 5′–3′) direction. Examples include many restriction enzyme recognition sites.
Pedigree analysis	:	Determination of the transmission characteristics of a particular gene by examination of family histories.
Penetrance	:	The proportion of individuals with a particular genotype that show the genotypic characteristic in the phenotype.
Phagemid	:	A vector containing plasmid and phage sequences.
Pharm animal	:	Transgenic animal used for the production of pharmaceuticals.
Phenotype	:	The observable characteristics of an organism, determined both by its genotype and its environment.
Phosphodiester bond	:	A bond formed between the 5′ phosphate and the 3′ hydroxyl groups of two nucleotides.
Physical mapping	:	Mapping genes with reference to their physical location on the chromosome. Generates the next level of detail compared to genetic mapping.
Physical marker	:	A sequence-based tag that labels a region of the genome. There are several such tags that can be used in mapping studies.
Pico (p)	:	SI prefix, 10^{-12}.
Plaque	:	A cleared area on a bacterial lawn caused by infection by a lytic bacteriophage.
Plasmid	:	A circular extrachromosomal element found naturally in bacteria and some other organisms. Engineered plasmids are used extensively as vectors for cloning.
Ploidy number	:	Refers to the number of sets of chromosomes, e.g. haploid, diploid, triploid, etc.
Pluripotent	:	Cell which can give rise to a range of differentiated cells.
Polyacrylamide	:	A cross-linked matrix for gel electrophoresis of small fragments of nucleic acids, primarily used for electrophoresis of DNA. Also used for electrophoresis of proteins.
Polyadenylic acid	:	A string of adenine residues. Poly(A) tails are found at the 3′ ends of most eukaryotic mRNA molecules.
Polycistronic	:	Refers to an RNA molecule encoding more that one function. Many bacterial operons are expressed via polycistronic mRNAs.
Polygalacturonase	:	Enzyme involved in pectin degradation. Target for antisense control in the Flavr Savr tomato.
Polygenic trait	:	A trait determined by the interaction of more than one gene, e.g. eye colour in humans.
Polyhedra	:	Capsid structures in baculoviruses, composed of the protein polyhedrin.
Polymer	:	A long sequence of monomers.
Polymerase	:	An enzyme that synthesises a copy of a nucleic acid.
Polymerase chain reaction (PCR)	:	A method for the selective amplification of DNA sequences. Several variants exist for different applications.

Polymorphism	:	Refers to the occurrence of many allelic variants of a particular gene or DNA sequence motif. Can be used to identify individuals by genetic mapping and DNA profiling techniques.
Polynucleotide	:	A polymer made up of nucleotide monomers.
Polynucleotide kinase (PNK)	:	An enzyme that catalyses the transfer of a phosphate group onto a 5′-hydroxyl group.
Polypeptide	:	A chain of amino acid residues.
Polystuffer	:	An expendable stuffer fragment in a vector that is composed of many repeated sequences.
Positional cloning	:	Cloning genes for which little information is available apart from their location on the chromosome.
Preformationism	:	Refers to the idea that all development is pre-coded in the zygote, and that development is simply the unfolding of this information. Now considered too simplistic.
Pribnow box	:	Sequence found in prokaryotic promoters that is required for transcription initiation. The consensus sequence is TATAAT.
Primary transcript	:	The initial, and often very large, product of transcription of a eukaryotic gene. Subjected to processing to produce the mature mRNA molecule.
Primer extension	:	Synthesis of a copy of a nucleic acid from a primer. Used in labelling DNA and in determining the start site of transcription.
Probe	:	A labelled molecule used in hybridisation procedures.
Proinsulin	:	Precursor of insulin that includes an extra polypeptide sequence that is cleaved to generate the active insulin molecule.
Prokaryotic	:	The property of lacking a membrane-bound nucleus, e.g. bacteria such as *E. coli*.
Promoter	:	DNA sequence(s) lying upstream from a gene, to which RNA polymerase binds.
Pronucleus	:	One of the nuclei in a fertilised egg prior to fusion of the gametes.
Prophage	:	A bacteriophage maintained in the lysogenic state in a cell.
Protease	:	Enzyme that hydrolyses polypeptides.
Protein	:	A condensation' (dehydration) heteropolymer composed of amino acid residues linked together by peptide bonds to give a polypeptide.
Proteome	:	Refers to the population of proteins produced by a cell.
Protoplast	:	A cell from which the cell wall has been removed.
Prototroph	:	A cell that can grow in an unsupplemented growth medium.
Purine	:	A double-ring nitrogenous base such as adenine and guanine.
Pyrimidine	:	A single-ring nitrogenous base such as cytosine, thymine and uracil.
Random amplified polymorphic DNA	:	PCR-based method of DNA profiling that involved amplification of sequences using random primers. Generates a type of genetic fingerprint that can be used to identify individuals.
Reading frame	:	The pattern of triplet codon sequences in a gene. There are three reading frames, depending on which nucleotide is the start .point. Insertion and deletion mutations can disrupt the reading frame and have serious consequences, as often the entire coding sequence becomes nonsense after the point of mutation.
Recessive	:	An allele where the expression is masked in the phenotype in heterozygous individuals.

Recombinant DNA	:	A DNA molecule made up of sequences that are not normally joined together.
Recombination frequency mapping	:	Method of genetic mapping that uses the number of crossover events that occur during meiosis to estimate the distance between genes.
Regulatory gene	:	A gene that exerts its effect by controlling the expression of another gene.
Renaturation kinetics	:	Method of analysing the complexity of genomes by studying the patterns obtained when DNA is denatured and allowed to renature.
Repetitive sequence	:	A sequence that is repeated a number of times in the genome.
Replacement vector	:	A bacteriophage vector in which the cloning sites are arranged in pairs, so that the section of the genorne between these sites can be replaced with insert DNA.
Replication	:	Copying the genetic material during the cell cycle. Also refers to the synthesis of new phage DNA during phage multiplication.
Replicon	:	A piece of DNA carrying an origin of replication.
Reporter gene	:	A gene used to disclose the function of potential regulatory DNA sequences upstream of the reporter gene
Restriction enzyme	:	An endonuclease that cuts DNA at sites defined by its recognition sequence.
Restriction fragment	:	A piece of DNA produced by digestion with a restriction enzyme.
Restriction fragment length polymorphism (RFLP)	:	A variation in the locations of restriction sites bounding a particular region of DNA, such that the fragment defined by the restriction sites may be of different lengths in different individuals.
Restriction mapping	:	Technique used to determine the location of restriction sites in a DNA molecule.
Retrovirus	:	A virus that has an RNA genome that is copied into DNA during the infection.
Reverse transcriptase	:	An RNA-dependent DNA polymerase found in retroviruses, used *in vitro* for the synthesis of cDNA.
Ribonuclease (RNase)	:	An enzyme that hydrolyses RNA.
Ribonucleic acid (RNA)	:	A condensation heteropolymer composed of ribonucleotides.
Ribosomal RNA (rRNA)	:	RNA that is part of the structure of ribosomes.
Ribosome	:	The 'jig' that is the site of protein synthesis. Composed of rRNA and proteins.
Ribosome-binding site	:	A region on an mRNA molecule that is involved in the binding of ribosomes during translation.
RNA processing	:	The formation of functional RNA from a primary transcript. In mRNA production this involves removal of introns, addition of a 5′ cap and polyadenylation.
S_1 *mapping*	:	Technique for determining the start point of transcription.
S_1 *nuclease*	:	An enzyme that hydrolyses (degrades) single-stranded DNA.
Saccharomyces cerevisiae	:	Unicellular yeast (baker's yeast) that is extensively used as a model microbial eukaryote in molecular studies. Also used in the biotechnology industry for a range of applications, as well as in brewing and bread-making.
Screening	:	Identification of a clone in a genomic or cDNA library (q.v.) by using a method that discriminates between different clones.
SCIDS	:	Severe combined immunodeficiency syndrome, a condition that results from a defective enzyme (adenosine deaminase).
Scintillation counter	:	A machine for determining the amount of radioactivity in a sample.
Selectable marker	:	Gene coding for resistance to an antibiotic or herbicide which can be used to select for transformed tissue or plants.

Selection	:	Exploitation of the genetics of a recombinant organism to enable desirable, recombinant genomes to be selected over non-recombinants during growth.
Sequence tagged site	:	Refers to a DNA sequence that is unique in the genome and which can be used in mapping studies. Usually identified by PCR amplification.
Sex chromosome	:	The non-autosomal X and Y chromosomes in humans that determine the sex of the individual. Males are XY, females XX.
Sex-linked	:	Refers to pattern of inheritance where the allele is located on a sex chromosome.
Silencing	:	The process whereby an organism shuts down the expression of a gene.
Single-locus probe	:	Probe used in DNA fingerprinting that identifies a single sequence in the genome. Diploid organisms therefore usually show two bands in a fingerprint, one allelic variant from each parent.
Single nucleotide polymorphism	:	Polymorphic pattern at a single base, essentially the smallest polymorphic unit that can be identified.
Somatic cell	:	Body cell, as opposed to germ-line cell.
Southern blotting	:	Method for transferring DNA fragments onto a membrane for detection of specific sequences by hybridisation.
Specific activity	:	The amount of radioactivity per unit material, e.g. a labelled probe might have a specific activity of 10^6 counts/minute per microgram. Also used to quantify the activity of an enzyme.
Sperm	:	The mature male gamete.
Structural gene	:	A gene that encodes a protein product.
Stuffer fragment	:	The section in a replacement vector that is removed and replaced with insert DNA.
Tandem repeat	:	A repeat composed of an array of sequences repeated contiguously in the same orientation.
Taq polymerase	:	Thermostable DNA polymerase from the thermophilic bacterium *Thermus aquaticus*. Used in the polymerase chain reaction.
TATA box	:	Sequence found in eukaryotic promoters. Also known as the Hogness box, it is similar to the Pribnow box found in prokaryotes, and has the consensus sequence TATAAAT.
T-DNA	:	Region of Ti plasmid of *Agrobacterium tumefaciens* that can be used to deliver recombinant DNA into the plant cell genome.
Terminal transferase	:	An enzyme that adds nucleotide residues to the 3′ terminus of an oligo- or polynucleotide.
Temperate	:	Refers to bacteriophages that can undergo lysogenic infection of the host cell.
Thermal cycler	:	Heating/cooling system for PCR applications. Enables denaturation, primer binding and extension cycles to be programmed and automated.
Thermus aquaticus	:	Thermophilic bacterium from which *Taq* polymerase is purified. Other bacteria from this genus include *Thermus flavus* and *Thermus thermophilus*.
Thymine (T)	:	Nitrogenous base found in DNA only.
Ti-plasmid	:	Plasmid of *Agrobacterium tumefaciens* that causes crown gall disease.
Tissue plasminogen activator (TPA)	:	A protease that occurs naturally, and functions in breaking down blood clots. Acts on an inactive precursor (plasminogen), which is converted to the active form (plasmin). This attacks the clot by breaking up fibrin, the protein involved in clot formation.

Totipotent	:	A cell that can give rise to all cell types in an organism. Totipotency has been demonstrated by cloning carrots from somatic cells, and by nuclear transfer experiments in animals.
Transacting element	:	A genetic element that can exert its effect without having to be on the same molecule as a target sequence. Usually such an element encodes a protein product (perhaps an enzyme or a regulatory protein) that can diffuse to the site of action.
Transcription (T_c)	:	The synthesis of RNA from a DNA template.
Transcriptional unit	:	The DNA sequence that encodes the RNA molecule, i.e. from the transcription start site to the stop site.
Transcriptome	:	The population of RNA molecules (usually mRNAs) that is expressed by a particular cell type.
Transfection	:	Introduction of purified phage or virus DNA into cells.
Transfer RNA (tRNA)	:	A small RNA (~75–85 bases) that carries the anticodon and the amino acid residue required for protein synthesis.
Transformant	:	A cell that has been transformed by exogenous DNA.
Transformation	:	The process of introducing DNA (usually plasmid DNA) into cells. Also used to describe the change in growth characteristics when a cell becomes cancerous.
Transgene	:	The target gene involved in the generation of a transgenic organism.
Transgenic	:	An organism that carries DNA sequences that it would not normally have in its genome.
Translation (T_l)	:	The synthesis of protein from an mRNA template.
Transposable element	:	A genetic element that carries the information that allows it to integrate at various sites in the genome. Transposable elements are sometimes called 'jumping genes'.
Trisomy	:	Aneuploid condition where an extra chromosome is present. Common example is the trisomy-21 condition that causes Down syndrome.
Uracil (U)	:	Nitrogenous base found in RNA only.
Variable number tandem repeat (VNTR)	:	Repetitive DNA composed of a number of copies of a short sequence, involved in the generation of polymorphic loci that are useful in genetic fingerprinting. Also known as hypervariable regions.
Vector	:	A DNA molecule that is capable of replication in a host organism, and can act as a carrier molecule for the construction of recombinant DNA.
Virulent	:	Refers to bacteriophage that cause lysis of the host cell.
Virus	:	An infectious agent that cannot replicate without a host cell.
Western blotting	:	Transfer of electrophoretically separated proteins onto a membrane for probing with antibody.
Xenotransplantation	:	The use of tissues or organs from a non-human source for transplantation.
X-gal	:	5-Bromo-4-chloro-3-indolyl-β-D-galactopyranoside: a chromogenic substrate, for β-galactosidase; on cleavage it yields a blue-coloured product.
X-linked	:	Pattern of inheritance where the allele is located on the X-chromosome. In humans, this can result in males expressing recessive characters that would normally be masked in an autosomal heterozygote.
YAC	:	Yeast artificial chromosome, a vector for cloning very large pieces of DNA in yeast.
Zygote	:	Single-celled product of the fusion of a male and a female gamete. Develops into an embryo by successive mitotic divisions.

References

Ahern, K.M., *Principles of Gene Manipulation*, Butterworths, London.

Benaim Pinto, C., *Microbiology and Microbial Biomass*, Prentice-Hall, London.

Bernard, R., *Industrial Microbiology*, Academic Publishers, UK.

Chang, J.C., *Handbook of Biochemical Engineering and Biotechnology*, John Wiley & Sons, New York.

Coolingwood, R.W., *Fermentation Technology and its Industrial Applications*, John Wiley & Sons, New York.

Desmond, S.T., *Genetic Engineering*, Cambridge University Press, New Delhi.

Downe, S.A., *Industrial Microbiology and Biotechnology*, John Wiley & Sons, New York.

Dugan, P., *Molecular Biology*, Plenum Publishing Corporation, London.

Goldman, M., *Biochemical Engineering*, Gordon and Breach, Science Publishers, New York.

Gould, G.W., *Textbook of Microbiology*, D. Van Nostrand, New York.

Harding, G., *Fundamentals of Biochemistry*, Prentice-Hall, London.

Hidy, M., *Biotechnology as an Intellectual Property*, Prentice-Hall, London.

Jackwerth, F., *Comprehensive Biotechnology*, Harcourt Brace Jovanovich, New York.

Jarvis, A., *Patents and Legal Protection for Biotechnology*, John Wiley & Sons, New York.

Jencks, W.P., *Expression of Foreign Proteins in Micro-organisms*, John Wiley & Sons, New York.

Kim, C.K., *Enzyme Biotechnology*, Marcel Dekker, New York.

Lewis, R., *Antibiotics-cloning of Biosynthetic Pathways*, Chilton Book Co., USA.

Mason, T., *Industrial Aspects of Biochemistry and Microbiology*, McGraw-Hill, New York.

McCaull, J. and Crossland, J., *Molecular Biology and Biotechnology*, Harcourt Brace Jovanovich, New York.

Mitchell, R., *Industrial Aspects of Biochemistry and Microbiology,* McGraw-Hill, New York.

Nuan, E., *Recent Advances in the Polymerase Chain Reactions*, Van Nostrand Reinhold, New York.

Odum, K., *Antibody Engineering and Perspective in Therapy*, W.B. Saunders and Co., New York.

Phillips, D.J.H., *Microbial Degradation of Halogenated Compounds*, Applied Science Publishers, London.

Reid, G.K., *Microbial Transformation of Pesticides*, Reinhold Publishing Corporation, New York.

Robert, H.T., *Handbook of Biochemistry*, Butterworths, London.

Sax, R.A., *Microbial Insecticides*, Pergamon Press, Oxford, London.

Vollenweider, R.A., *Industrial Biotechnology*, Blackwell Scientific Publications, New York.

Wyatt, G.M., *Fermentation and Enzyme Technology*, Reston Publishing Co., Reston, Virginia.

Index